User Centered Design for Medical Visualization

Feng Dong
Brunel University, UK

Gheorghita Ghinea
Brunel University, UK

Sherry Y. Chen
Brunel University, UK

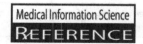

MEDICAL INFORMATION SCIENCE REFERENCE

Hershey · New York

Acquisitions Editor:	Kristin Klinger
Development Editor:	Kristin Roth
Editorial Assistants:	Ross Miller, Deborah Yahnke
Senior Managing Editor:	Jennifer Neidig
Managing Editor:	Jamie Snavely
Assistant Managing Editor:	Carole Coulson
Copy Editor:	Ashley Fails
Typesetter:	Michael Brehm
Cover Design:	Lisa Tosheff
Printed at:	Yurchak Printing Inc.

Published in the United States of America by
Information Science Reference (an imprint of IGI Global)
701 E. Chocolate Avenue, Suite 200
Hershey PA 17033
Tel: 717-533-8845
Fax: 717-533-8661
E-mail: cust@igi-global.com
Web site: http://www.igi-global.com

and in the United Kingdom by
Information Science Reference (an imprint of IGI Global)
3 Henrietta Street
Covent Garden
London WC2E 8LU
Tel: 44 20 7240 0856
Fax: 44 20 7379 0609
Web site: http://www.eurospanbookstore.com

Library of Congress Cataloging-in-Publication Data

User centered design for medical visualization / Feng Dong, Gheorghita Ghinea, and Sherry Chang, editors.
    p. ; cm.
  Includes bibliographical references and index.
  Summary: "This book features a comprehensive review of advances in medical visualization and human-computer interaction. It investigates the human roles during a visualization process, specifically motivation-based design, user-based design, and perception-and-cognitive-based design. It also provides real-world examples and insight into the analytical and architectural aspects of user centered design"--Provided by publisher.
  ISBN 978-1-59904-777-5 (h/c)
  1. Computer vision in medicine. 2. Diagnostic imaging--Data processing. 3. Imaging systems in medicine. 4. User-centered system design. 5. Human-computer interaction. I. Dong, Feng. II. Ghinea, Gheorghita. III. Chang, Sherry.
  [DNLM: 1. Diagnostic Imaging. 2. Computing Methodologies. 3. Equipment Design. 4. Human Engineering. 5. User-Computer Interface. WN 180 U84 2008]
  R859.7.C67U84 2008
  616.07'54--dc22
                    2007037649

British Cataloguing in Publication Data
A Cataloguing in Publication record for this book is available from the British Library.

Table of Contents

Selected Readings

Detailed Table of Contents

Chapter I

Madeleine Keehner, University of Dundee, UK

Peter Khooshabeh, University of California–Santa Barbara, USA

Mary Hegarty, University of California–Santa Barbara, USA

This chapter examines human factors relating to the use of 3D interactive medical visualization tools. The authors examine individual differences among users, discuss how these may impact the usefulness of medical visualizations, and suggest some implications for the design of these tools.

Chapter II

Yingjun Qiu, Beijing Sigma Center, China

Youbing Zhao, Siemens Ltd., China

Jiaoying Shi, Zhejiang University, China

This chapter introduces grid-based visualization and its applications to assist a wide range of applications including clinical practice. The authors have implemented a grid-based visualization system (Gvis), which utilizes large-scale computing resources to achieve large dataset visualization in real time and provides end users with reliable and interactive visualization services widely.

Chapter III

Raymond White, Sunderland University, UK

Robert Noble, The Robert Gordon University, UK

This chapter describes techniques and a software program that can be used to simplify interpretation of gait data. It can be viewed with an interactive display and a gait report can be produced more quickly with the key results highlighted. This allows referring clinicians to integrate the relevant gait measurements and observations and to formulate the patient treatment plan.

This chapter outlines and discusses how an increasingly popular approach of incorporating patient perspectives and experience in research can be used to inform the development of user-centered technology in healthcare, with particular emphasis on hand-held mobile devices.

This chapter presents a new visualization system which is cost effective and well-suited for interventional visualization. It allows users to view large time-resolved multidimensional datasets in real time with GPU Cluster Visualization. In addition, computational preprocessing can be hidden by rendering across distributed graphics cards, leading to improved frame-rates over a single graphics card solution.

This chapter introduces new visualization techniques which have been developed with the goal to improve diagnoses based on volumetric angiography datasets. The proposed passive visualization techniques comprise depth-based color coding techniques, different types of edge enhancement and the application of rendering techniques. The active visualization techniques support user interaction and include depth-based replacements of the mouse cursor and multiple views providing further insights.

This chapter studies how human computer interface influences the performance of specific scientific visualization tasks. Through an empirical study, the authors develop guidelines for selecting display environment for four commonly used volume visualization tasks, and compare the performance of three different stereo VR systems. In addition, the authors also carried out further investigation on performing 3D interaction tasks using tangible interfaces.

This chapter shows that image registration techniques can be effectively used to generate an overlay of visual and thermal images and provide a useful diagnostic visualization for the clinician.

Chapter IX

This chapter provides an overview for different software frameworks for real-time visualization. A number of well-known visualization algorithms are introduced. These algorithms are fully implemented in some open-source freely-available software frameworks, including Visualization Toolkit (VTK), MAF (Multimod Application Framework).

Chapter X

The chapter investigates visual and interactive aspects of navigation systems for orthopaedic surgery and suggests useful tools in order to enhance the surgeon usability of a navigation system. It provides detailed descriptions of the solutions proposed to overcome problems commonly found with navigation systems in orthopaedics.

Chapter XI

This chapter tackles the problem of multi-dimensional transfer function design. The new multi-dimensional transfer function design method introduced, which is region growing-based, significantly improves the effectiveness of multi-dimensional transfer function design, simplifies the task of user interaction, and helps users to save their time in the interactive design.

Chapter XII

X. Ye, Medicsight PLC, UK
F. Dong, Brunel University, UK

This chapter describes a method of applying medical visualization for human muscle modeling. It is an anatomically-based approach that attempts to provide models for human musculature based on the real morphological structures. Three major problems have been addressed: geometric modeling, deformation and texture.

Chapter XIII

Dongbin Chen, Brunel University, UK

This chapter provides a survey on image segment techniques, which are classified into a number of different approaches, including pixel-based, region-based, classification, deformable model, artificial neural network and texture-based. It provides valuable assistance for researchers and meets the ever-increasing demands in computing medical imaging systems.

Selected Readings

Medical Visualization has strong links to image processing. Especially, a user-centered design for medical visualization replies heavily on effective image analysis techniques. In this selected readings section, we include a number of presentations on latest techniques on image segmentation, retrieval, registration, formatting.

Chapter XIV

Chia-Hung Wei, University of Warwick, UK
Chang-Tsun Li, University of Warwick, UK
Roland Wilson, University of Warwick, UK

This chapter introduces a content-based approach to medical image retrieval. A case study, which describes the methodology of a CBIR system for retrieving digital mammogram database, is presented. It is intended to disseminate the knowledge of the CBIR approach to the applications of medical image management and to attract greater interest from various research communities to rapidly advance research

This chapter introduces 3D medical image segmentation by giving an overview of relevant methods with their advantages and limitations. Specifically, the authors discuss the issue of incorporating prior knowledge into the segmentation of anatomic structures and describe in detail the concept and issues of knowledge-based segmentation.

This chapter describes a vector-preserving framework to extend morphological operations to multi-channel images, and further propose a fully automatic multi-channel watershed segmentation algorithm that naturally combines spatial and spectral/temporal information. It also develops a parallel implementation strategy to speed up performance.

Chapter XVII

The chapter introduces biomedical image registration as a means of integrating and providing complementary and additional information from multiple medical images simultaneously for diagnostic decision making and treatment monitoring. Further, discussions on the future challenges and possible research trends of this field are presented.

This chapter introduces an object-oriented design and an open-source implementation for medical DICOM image reading. It produces an output data tree containing the information of the DICOM images and their related radiological studies, which can be browsed easily in a structured way through navigation interfaces coupled to it.

Preface

Medical visualization has attracted a lot of attention in the last two decades. It provides valuable assistance to the practice of medical professionals, including diagnosis, treatment planning, training and revision. Due to its strongly practical-oriented nature, a considerable number of examples have emerged which successfully apply medical visualization to support clinical practice, such as HipOp Project (Testi et al., 2004; Viceconti et al., 2004), Collaborators in Radiological Interventional Virtual Environments (Vidal et al. 2004), Blood Flow Visualization (Pivkin et al., 2005), and so forth. And the research interest in this area shows no sign of abating.

Medical visualization is an interdisciplinary area which involves a large number of diverse issues across computer and medical sciences. The primary goal of medical visualization is to provide high quality and fidelity display of human anatomy and structure through the rendering of medical data captured by modern equipments, such as CT, MRI, PET and Ultrasound, and so forth. Recently, great attention has been paid towards the visualization of complex 3D structures involved in human anatomy. This can be done either by extracting high quality surface models from 3D medical data, which is normally in volumetric form (Bertram, 2004; Livnat, 2004), or by carrying out direct rendering on the volumetric data (Mroz et al., 2000; Schulze & Rice, 2004).

Surface-based visualization requires high quality extraction of surface model from volumetric dataset. It is able to generate surface models that allow numerous manipulations with clinical meanings, such as shape measurement and analysis, model cutting for virtual surgery, and so forth. However, a critical challenge here is how to obtain surface model with sufficient medical accuracy. This issue also relates to image segmentation, which allows us to obtain region of interest from 2D and 3D images.

While the surface-based visualization is still a quite important approach in medical visualization, it is generally recognized that volumetric rendering allows us to see a great deal of fine details within medical data and also significantly improves the quality of 3D medical imaging (Dong et al., 2001). One of the most critical issues in volumetric rendering is to allow users to easily choose the most relevant information to visualize by constructing an adequate and interactive transfer function (Kniss et al., 2002).

However, just providing quality images is not the ultimate goal of using a computer to assist medical practice. To be clinically meaningful, useful information needs to be identified by carrying out analysis towards medical images. To this end, great efforts have been made in medical image analysis, which involves a large number of activities including lesion detection (Sluimer et al., 2006; Ye et al., 2007; Wei et al., 2007;), medical image registration (Hajnal et al., 2001; Napel et al., 2004; Krueger et al., 2007), segmentation (Manay & Yezzi, 2003; Aldasoro & Bhalerao, 2007; Noble & Boukerroui, 2007) and classification (Zhang, 2000; Petersen et al., 2002; Baese, 2003), organ shape measurement, analysis and motion tracking, in order to seek useful clinical information. Many of these practices require significant prior knowledge about human anatomy. Hence, the techniques and knowledge from human anatomy, image processing and analysis, jointly constitute vital input for medical visualization.

Currently, vast majority of existing medical visualization techniques polarize their efforts on data modeling and rendering. Their target is to generate high-quality images with a great deal of fine structure details, such as blood vessels, muscle fibers, and so forth. Such images convey significant visual information for clinicians. However, many of these works have put too much emphasis on producing decent images, while neglecting the human factors involved during a visualization process.

Previous experiences and examples have strongly suggested that simply using graphic techniques to display medical data may not provide adequate support for clinicians. As a new research trend, the interest in human factors within the medical visualization research community has been increasing over the last few years. Instead of simply generating high quality photo-realistic images, researchers have started to pay more attention to the human perspective. In fact, there is a growing body of evidence suggesting the strong need to study human factors as a basis for medical visualization design. Moreover, humans' perspective, thinking and interaction with images significantly affect their understanding of the information presented visually. As the ultimate goal of medical visualization is to accurately deliver clinical information for medical professionals, an effective visualization process should include users as an integral part of the course of action.

Therefore, this book attempts to reflect such a trend by collecting a number of different research works and surveys in medical visualization with particular emphasis on User-Centered Design (UCD). In general terms, UCD is an approach to provide rationale and justification to the design of a product from the perspective of people who will use it. There is an international standard for UCD methodologies (ISO13407, 1999), which outlines the general process of a development life cycle focusing on user-centered activities. This cycle includes: specifying the context of use, which identifies potential users of the product; specifying requirements, which defines and documents detailed user requirements; creating design solutions, which covers from initial concept to complete design for the product; and evaluating designs, which provides product assessment through usability testing.

A good practice of USD for medical visualization requires careful design from the perspective of users in order to meet their business objectives. Such a design has to be user-centered and task- oriented. Whether a medical visualization system or technique is intended for surgeons or for medical students should make a significant difference with respect to the design. As a medical visualization system clearly involves knowledge from both computer and medical science, which are two clearly distinguished disciplines, making user interface as consistent as possible can help users in their learning and minimize the time required for their training. Unavoidably, a medical visualization system may involve computing languages, instructions, and terminologies in its interface, therefore, for the purpose of facilitating users, it is important to keep the dialogue between the users and system in a natural sequence. No redundant information should be presented to the users, as irrelevant information adds unnecessary complexity. In particular, terminologies need to be defined clearly and their meaning should remain consistent. This helps to reduce unnecessary mental effort from the users and consequently allows them to concentrate on their tasks. Much human computer interaction research has shown that complicated interaction task can significantly frustrate users and distract them from their real task, which potentially lead to low efficiency and more errors. Also, providing adequate feedback to the user interaction is of great importance. Due to the limitation of computing facilities and increasing large scale of dataset, many user-wanted jobs, for example, rendering a large medical dataset, require considerable time to fulfill. In this case, to make the users confident on the actions that they have taken, proper feedback from the system, such as progress bar, need to be given to indicate the time remaining for the job. Such a feedback should be given at a proper level, as irrelevant diagnostic or status information can give rise to unnecessary confusion. Also, since a modern medical visualization system often involves a large number of functionality, providing adequate navigation mechanisms allows the users to familiarize themselves with the system. A proper navigation mechanism concerns many issues on computer interface, such as giving proper and consistent window titles and offering location indicators. Other mechanisms such as providing a navigation map should be considered. In between different view windows, such as the rendering window to present the 3D picture of a dataset, and the statistics window to illustrate the data distribution, clear and easy routes need to be defined to allow the users to switch between them for their specific tasks. In addition, providing sufficient flexibility and tolerance is of great user interests. Often users choose system functions by mistake, for example, start to render a wrongly-selected large dataset, which involves large computing resources. They should be given a clearly marked exit to leave the unwanted state, for example, immediate canceling of the dataset rendering.

Apart from the multidisciplinary issues already involved, a user-centered medical visualization further concerns a wide range of other issues in human-computer interaction and interface, design, usability, and so forth. This book endeavors to explore some of these issues by looking into the UCD in medical visualization from a number of selected perspectives:

- This book will look at the influence of human factors and individual differences to the design of visualization techniques and systems. This will also include the investigation on the effectiveness of different measures for human-computer interaction with respect to the implementation of a range of user tasks.
- An important usability issue from user perspective is the processing speed of visualization techniques. The book will cover different ways for accelerating the data analysis and rendering, including the use of grid-based and cluster-based systems to achieve real-time visualization.
- The usability of visualization techniques and systems heavily depends on the design of software systems. Apart from following the general code of practice in software engineering, medical visualization systems also features their own characteristics, that is, requires the integration of data analysis and high quality rendering. The book will provide some insight into this particular issue.
- Usability is strongly influenced by a number of underlying key techniques in medical visualization, such as image segmentation, registration and image retrieval, transfer function for volumetric rendering, and so forth. Despite many years of efforts, these fundamental image techniques have yet to become fully automatic, and therefore user involvement (interaction) is necessary in order to achieve quality results. This book will report some latest progress in these areas.
- As usability is also strongly practical-oriented, this book will provide a number of practical cases which are related to usability studies within different medical context, including clinical gait analysis, vascular visualization, navigation problem in orthopaedic surgery, and so forth.

ORGANIZATION OF THE BOOK

The book is organized into 18 chapters. A brief description of each of the chapters follows:

Chapter I. Individual Differences among Users of Medical Visualizations: Spatial Abilities and Patterns of Interactivity

This chapter examines human factors relating to the use of 3D interactive medical visualization tools. The authors examine individual differences among users, discuss how these may impact the usefulness of medical visualizations, and suggest some implications for the design of these tools.

Chapter II. Grid–Based Visualization and its Medical Applications

This chapter introduces grid-based visualization and its applications to assist a wide range of applications including clinical practice. To overcome the problem of the existing grid computing technology, which is mainly batch job-oriented without providing support for interactive visualization application, the authors have implemented a grid-based visualization system (GVIS), which utilizes large-scale computing resources to achieve large dataset visualization in real time and provides end users with reliable and interactive visualization services widely.

Chapter III. Reporting Clinical Gait Analysis Data

This chapter describes techniques and a software program that can be used to simplify interpretation of gait data. The software package described in this chapter can be viewed with an interactive display and a gait report can be produced more quickly with the key results highlighted. This allows referring clinicians to integrate the relevant gait measurements and observations and to formulate the patient treatment plan.

Chapter IV. Capturing Data in Healthcare Using Patient–Centered Mobile Technology

This chapter outlines and discusses how an increasingly popular approach of incorporating patient perspectives and experience in research can be used to inform the development of user-centered technology in healthcare, with particular emphasis on hand-held mobile devices.

Chapter V. Cluster–Based Multidimensional Visualization: Harnessing Computational Resources for Real–time Visualization

This chapter presents a new visualization system which is cost effective and well suited for interventional visualization. It allows users to view large time-resolved multidimensional datasets in real time with GPU cluster visualization. In addition, computational preprocessing can be hidden by rendering across distributed graphics cards, leading to improved frame-rates over a single graphics card solution. Finally, rendering on graphics cards offloads CPU cycles for generating the next timeframe in the visualization.

Chapter VI. Supporting Spatial Cognition in Vascular Visualization

This chapter introduces new visualization techniques which have been developed with the goal to improve diagnoses based on volumetric angiography datasets. The proposed passive visualization techniques comprise depth-based color coding techniques, different types of edge enhancement and the application of rendering techniques which have been inspired by illustrations in order to enhance depth perception of complex blood vessel systems. The active visualization techniques support user interaction and include depth-based replacements of the mouse cursor as well as multiple views providing further insights.

Chapter VII. 3D Interaction with Scientific Data through Virtual Reality and Tangible Interfacing

This chapter studies how human computer interface influences the performance of specific scientific visualization tasks. Through an empirical study, the authors develop guidelines for selecting display environment for four commonly used volume visualization tasks, and compare the performance of three different stereo VR systems. In addition, the authors also carried out further investigation on performing 3D interaction tasks using tangible interfaces.

Chapter VIII. Automated Overlay of Infrared and Visual Medical Images

This chapter shows that image registration techniques can be effectively used to generate an overlay of visual and thermal images and provide a useful diagnostic visualisation for the clinician. Medical infrared imaging captures the temperature distribution of the human skin and is employed in various medical applications. Often it is useful to cross-reference the resulting thermograms with visual images of the patient, either to see which part of the anatomy is affected by a certain disease or to judge the efficacy of the treatment.

Chapter IX. Software framework of Medical Visualization Algorithms

This chapter provides an overview for different software frameworks for real-time visualization. A number of well-known visualization algorithms are introduced. These algorithms are fully implemented in some open-source freely-available software frameworks, including Visualization Toolkit (VTK), MAF (Multimod Application Framework).

Chapter X. Navigation in Computer-Assisted Orthopaedic Surgery

The chapter investigates visual and interactive aspects of navigation systems for orthopaedic surgery and suggests useful tools in order to enhance the surgeon usability of a navigation system. The chapter provides detailed descriptions of the solutions proposed to overcome problems commonly found with navigation systems in orthopaedics, aiming at the fulfillment of critical user requirements in clinical practice by providing the user with a tightly guided procedure and an immediate graphical virtual environment.

Chapter XI. Multi-Dimensional Transfer Functions Design

This chapter tackles the problem of multi-dimensional transfer function design. The new multi-dimensional transfer function design method introduced in this chapter, which is region growing based, significantly improves the effectiveness of multi-dimensional transfer function design, simplifies the task of user interaction, and helps users to save their time in the interactive design.

Chapter XII. Graphical Modeling of Human Muscles

This chapter describes a method of applying medical visualization for human muscle modeling. It is an anatomically-based approach that attempts to provide models for human musculature based on the real morphological structures. Three major problems have been addressed: geometric modeling, deformation and texture.

Chapter XIII. Image Segmentation

This chapter provides a survey on image segment techniques, which are classified into a number of different approaches, including pixel-based, region-based, classification, deformable model, artificial neural network and texture-based. It provides valuable assistance for researchers to effectively select their appropriate segmentation methods in relation to their specific applications, and hence meets the ever-increasing demands in computing medical imaging systems.

Chapter XIV. A Content-Based Approach to Medical Image Database Retrieval

This chapter introduces a content-based approach to medical image retrieval. A case study, which describes the methodology of a CBIR system for retrieving digital mammogram database, is presented. It is intended to disseminate the knowledge of the CBIR approach to the applications of medical image management and to attract greater interest from various research communities to rapidly advance research in this field.

Chapter XV. Methods and Applications for Segmenting 3D Medical Image Data

This chapter introduces 3D medical image segmentation by giving an overview of relevant methods with their advantages and limitations. Specifically, the authors discuss the issue of incorporating prior knowledge into the segmentation of anatomic structures and describe in detail the concept and issues of knowledge-based segmentation.

Chapter XVI. Parallel Segmentation of Multi-Channel Images Using Multi-Dimensional Mathematical Morphology

This chapter describes a vector-preserving framework to extend morphological operations to multi-channel images, and further propose a fully automatic multi-channel watershed segmentation algorithm that naturally combines spatial and spectral/temporal information. It also develops a parallel implementation strategy to speed up performance.

Chapter XVII. Biomedical Image Registration for Diagnostic Decision Making and Treatment Monitoring

The chapter introduces biomedical image registration as a means of integrating and providing complementary and additional information from multiple medical images simultaneously for diagnostic decision making and treatment monitoring. Further, discussions on the future challenges and possible research trends of this field are presented.

Chapter XVIII. A Software Tool for Reading DICOM Directory Files

This chapter introduces an object-oriented design and an open-source implementation for medical DICOM image reading. It produces an output data tree containing the information of the DICOM images and their related radiological studies, which can be browsed easily in a structured way through navigation interfaces coupled to it.

REFERENCES

Aldasoro, R.; Bhalerao, A. (2007). Volumetric texture segmentation by discriminant feature selection and multi-resolution classification. *IEEE Trans. on Medical Imaging, 26*(1), 1-14.

Baese, A. (2003). *Pattern recognition in medical imaging.* Academic Press Inc.

Bertram, M. (2004). Volume refinement fairing isosurfaces. *Proceedings of IEEE Visualization,* (pp. 449-456).

Dong, F., Clapworthy, G., Krokos, M. (2001). Volume rendering of fine details within medical data. *Proceedings of IEEE Visualization,* (pp. 387-394).

Hajnal, J., Hill, D., Hawkes, D. (2001). *Medical image registration.* CRC Press.

ISO13407. (1999). *Human-centered design processes for interactive systems.* http://www.usabilitynet. org/tools/13407stds.htm.

Kniss, J., Kindlmann, G., & Hansen, G. (2002). Multi-dimensional transfer functions for interactive volume rendering. *IEEE Transactions on Visualization and Computer Graphics, 8*(4), 270-228.

Krueger, S., Wolff, S., Schmitgen, A., Timinger, H., Bublat, M., Schaeffter, T., Nabavi, A. (2007). Fast and accurate automatic registration for MR-guided procedures using active microcoils. *IEEE Trans. on Medical Imaging, 26*(3), 385-392.

Li, P., Napel, S., Acar, B., Paik, D., Jr., R., Beaulieu, C. (2004). Registration of central paths and colonic polyps between supine and prone scans in computed tomography colonography: Pilot study. *Med. Phys,31*(10).

Livnat, Y., & Tricoche, X. (2004). Interactive point-based isosurface extraction. *Proceedings of IEEE Visualization,* (pp. 457-464).

Manay, S., & Yezzi, A. (2003) Anti-geometric diffusion for adaptive thresholding and fast segmentation. *IEEE Trans. Image Processing, 12*(11), 1310-1322.

Mroz, L., Hauser H., & Gröller, E. (2000). Interactive high-quality maximum intensity projection. *Computer Graphics Forum,* 19(3), 341-350.

Noble, J., Boukerroui, D., Ultrasound image segmentation: A survey. *IEEE Trans. on Medical Imaging, 25*(8)987-1010.

Petersen, M., De Ridder, E., & Handels, H. (2002). Image processing using neural networks—a review. *Pattern Recognition, 35*(10).

Pivkin, I., Richardson, P., Laidlaw, D., Karniadakis, G. (2005). Combined effects of pulsatile flow and dynamic curvature on wall shear stress in a coronary artery bifurcation model. *Journal of Biomechanics, 38*(6),1283-1290.

Sluimer, I., Schilham, A., Prokop, M., Ginneken, B. (2006). Computer analysis of computed tomography scans of the lung: A survey. *IEEE Trans. Medical Imaging, 25,* 385-405.

Schulze, J., & Rice, A. (2004) Real-time volume rendering of four channel data sets. *Proceedings of IEEE Visualization, (pp. 598-599).*

Testi, D., Simeoni, M., Zannoni, C., Viceconti, M. (2004). Validation of two algorithms to evaluate the interface between bone and orthopaedic implants. *Comput Methods Programs Biomed, 74*(2), 143-150.

Viceconti, M., Chiarini, A., Testi, D., Taddei, F., Bordini, B., Traina, F., Toni, A. (2004). New aspects and approaches in pre-operative planning of hip reconstruction: A computer simulation. *Langenbecks Arch Surg, 389*(5), 400-404.

Vidal, F., Bello, F., Brodlie, K., John, N., Gould, D., Phillips, R., Avis, N. (2004). Principles and applications of medical virtual environments. *Proceedings of Eurographics 2004: State of the Art reports*, (pp. 1-35).

Wei, J., Sahiner, B., Chan, H., Hadjiiski, L., Roubidoux, M., Helvie, M., et al. (2007). Computer-aided detection of breast masses on prior mammograms. *Proceedings of SPIE, Medical Imaging*, (vol.6514).

Ye, X., Lin, X., Beddoe, G., & Dehmeshki, J. (2007). Efficient computer-aided detection of ground-glass opacity nodules in thoracic CT images. *Proceedings of the 29th IEEE Engineering in Medicine and Biology Society(EMBS). Lyon, France.*

Zhang, G. (2000). Neural networks for classification: A survey. *IEEE Transactions on Systems, Man and Cybernetics, Part C: Applications and Reviews, 30*(4).

Acknowledgment

The editors would like to acknowledge the help of all involved in the collation and review process of the book, without whose support the project could not have been satisfactorily completed.

Special thanks also go to all the staff at IGI Global, whose contributions throughout the whole process from inception of the initial idea to final publication have been invaluable. In particular, to Deborah Yahnke, who continuously prodded via e-mail for keeping the project on schedule. Her enthusiasm motivated me to initially accept her invitation for taking on this project.

In closing, I wish to thank all of the authors for their insights and excellent contributions to this book. I also want to thank all of the people who assisted me in the reviewing process. Finally, I want to thank my wife and child for the true support and encouragement during the months it took to give birth to this book.

Chapter I
Individual Differences Among Users:
Implications for the Design of 3D Medical Visualizations

Madeleine Keehner
University of Dundee, UK

Peter Khooshabeh
University of California–Santa Barbara, USA

Mary Hegarty
University of California–Santa Barbara, USA

ABSTRACT

This chapter examines human factors associated with using interactive three-dimensional (3D) visualizations. Virtual representations of anatomical structure and function, often with sophisticated user control capabilities, are growing in popularity in medicine for education, training, and simulation. This chapter reviews the cognitive science literature and introduces issues such as theoretical ideas related to using interactive visualizations, different types and levels of interactivity, effects of different kinds of control interfaces, and potential cognitive benefits of these tools. The authors raise the question of whether all individuals are equally capable of using 3D visualizations effectively, focusing particularly on two variables: (1) individual differences in spatial abilities, and (2) individual differences in interactive behavior. The chapter draws together findings from the authors' own studies and from the wider literature, exploring recent insights into how individual differences among users can impact the effectiveness of different types of external visualizations for different kinds of tasks. The chapter offers recommendations for design, such as providing transparent affordances to support users' meta-cognitive understanding, and employing personalization to complement the capabilities of different individuals. Finally, the authors suggest future directions and approaches for research, including the use of methodology such as needs analysis and contextual enquiry to better understand the cognitive processes and capacities of different kinds of users.

INTRODUCTION

The study of anatomy is a core component of medical training. With developments in computer graphics, interactive three-dimensional (3D) visualizations of anatomical structure and function are becoming increasingly prevalent in medicine for education, training, and simulation purposes. This chapter examines human factors relating to the use of these tools. We examine individual differences among users, discuss how these may impact the usefulness of medical visualizations, and suggest some implications for the design of these tools. We focus particularly on two variables that differ among individuals and that are especially relevant to using interactive 3D visualizations effectively. These are: 1) individual differences in spatial abilities, which affect a user's internal representation of the information presented; and 2) individual differences in interactive behavior, which affect how the user manipulates and interacts with the external visualization. We draw together findings on these issues from our own studies and from the wider literature, in order to make recommendations for design and suggest future directions and approaches for research on this topic.

BACKGROUND

The study of anatomical structure and function is a fundamental part of medical training. At some level, the goal of anatomy education is to provide students with high quality spatial mental models of human anatomy that they can use in medical practice. Resources such as diagrams, bench-top models, and cadaver dissection laboratories have long been used to provide students with an understanding of the 3D relationships among different anatomical structures. But compared with today's technologies, these traditional learning materials have a number of limitations. Printed diagrams are unavoidably restricted to two dimensions,

generally entail only cardinal views, and bear little resemblance to real anatomy. Bench-top models are often useable only once as they are of little value once they have been "dissected." Cadavers, although the most naturalistic of these materials, are rare commodities, whose use in medical schools is becoming increasingly restricted due to the expense of maintaining dissection laboratories. For teaching purposes, they also have the drawbacks of being opaque, restricting the learner's view of internal structures, and of being idiosyncratic, making standardization difficult.

With developments in medical informatics (Collen, 1995; De Dombal, 1996, van Bemmel & Musen, 1997), the medical establishment has begun to explore 3D visualizations as potential alternatives to traditional learning resources. Unlike physical teaching materials, computer visualizations are flexible, permitting designers and users to alter parameters such as anatomical variability, disease-state, or viewpoint perspective. They can also be easily reused with little cost and can be widely disseminated, allowing access outside the traditional constraints of the classroom. As a result, medical education has begun a dramatic shift towards introducing digital representations into its learning programs.

Medical educators are enthusiastically embracing the potential of these resources. The Association of American Medical Colleges (AAMC) foresees a future in which these tools play a central role in teaching, learning, evaluation, continuing education and certification within medicine and the allied health professions. They advocate the development of new core digital resources such as virtual patients, simulations, 2D and 3D images, and interactive cases, and recommend that these become an integral part of future medical education programs (Florance & Masys, 2002; Florance & Moller, 2002). Optimism about the educational potential of new technology is not limited to the medical domain. Researchers in the cognitive and learning sciences have seen visualizations as external aids that can "enhance" or "amplify" cognition (Norman, 1990; Card, MacKinlay & Schneiderman, 1999), with "remarkable potential to help students learn" (Gordin & Pea, 1995, p. 276).

However, despite much optimism about their educational potential, our understanding of how learners interact with 3D computer visualizations is relatively limited. Recently, researchers have begun to use cognitive research methods to examine the relationship between these external aids and internal thought processes, and to explore the full range of factors that affect learning from digital media (e.g., Zhang & Norman, 1994; Kirsh, 1997; Hutchins, & Kirsh, 2000; Gray & Fu, 2004; Hegarty, 2004; Hollan, Lowe, 2004;). A striking finding from these studies is that interactive visualizations are not equally effective for all users. Therefore, in this chapter we focus particularly on how individual differences among users affect both use of external visualizations and what is learned from these external aids.

The Relationship Between External Representations and Internal Cognition

In the cognitive science literature, a distinction has been made between "external visualizations" that exist outside the mind of an individual, such as diagrams, graphs, and computer visualizations, and "internal visualizations," such as visual mental images or mental models that are representations in a person's mind (Hegarty, 2004). External tools vary widely, ranging from simple pencil and paper to state-of-the-art interactive virtual simulations, but one key feature of such systems is that they allow the user to externalize some of the mental processing associated with a task. Virtual representations of 3D anatomical structures are a typical example of such external representations. In this section, we review some theoretical ideas about how *external* representations (such as 3D medical visualizations) are related to the internal representations of individual users.

One approach that is highly relevant is the theory of *distributed cognition* (Zhang & Norman, 1994). According to this theory, cognitive processes are distributed across both internal and external components. Cognition is not a process that occurs only in the mind of the individual; rather, cognition occurs both *internally* (in the mind) and *externally* (in the world). According to this approach, the "action space" within which a task is completed is distributed across the internal representations of the user and any external media that can be used to represent or explore ideas, concepts, or information. External representations are thus not merely peripheral aids to cognition. They *intersect with* the user's internal representation, making up a joint cognitive system (Hollnagel & Woods, 2005). Furthermore, the external representation is an obligatory component of the thinking space for a distributed problem. How the user manipulates or interacts with an external representation is as much a part of cognition as the unseen internal mental processes of reasoning or visualizing.

In distributed tasks, performance involves a tradeoff between the internal and external resources that are available to the individual. Internal cognitive processes include moment-to-moment attentional and representational resources such as working memory and long-term knowledge or expertise. External processes include the perceptual-motor processes that users engage to interact with an external display and observe the results. Importantly, the properties of external representations influence how we interact with them. They anchor and structure cognition and constrain the range of possible behaviors. As such, an external tool can change the very nature of a task. For example, different characteristics of external representations can mean that more or less of the task load is carried out internally (Zhang & Norman, 1994). An important question for visualization designers is what factors govern the moment-by-moment decisions by an individual of how to allocate a task to internal versus external resources.

Theories of *embodied cognition* assume that whenever possible, people minimize the reliance on internal memory and offload cognitive functions onto perceptual-motor processes (e.g., Kirsh & Maglio, 1994; Zhang & Norman, 1994; Ballard, Hayhoe, Pook, & Rao, 1997; Wilson, 2002). According to this approach, internal cognitive processes are relatively effortful and somewhat error-prone, so that the option of *manually* rotating an external visualization into a desired view is in general preferred over the option of *mentally* rotating a representation in one's head. A somewhat different view comes from *soft-constraints* models, which propose that external perceptual-motor processes are not necessarily preferred over internal cognitive processes. In this view, humans are simply biased towards finding the most efficient means of completing a task, so that we seek the most cost-effective tradeoff among the cognitive, perceptual, and motor resources available within a given task environment. Experimental studies using cognitive tasks that include interactive external tools have shown that the moment-to-moment allocation of resources is indeed flexible, and depends on the relative utility (operationalized as time) of using internal versus external resources (Gray & Fu, 2004; Gray, Sims, Fu, & Schoelles, 2006).

We can view the use of computer visualizations in medicine in the light of these theories. The idea is that having access to flexible and realistic renderings of anatomy should allow relatively effortful or inefficient internal cognitive processes to be offloaded onto less effortful or more efficient perceptual-motor processes, such as physically manipulating the external visualization and observing the results (Gordin & Pea, 1995; Kirsh, 1997; Card, MacKinlay, & Shneiderman, 1999). For example, rather than needing to imagine how an anatomical structure would look from a specific viewpoint or how a set of structures would appear if rotated into a different orientation, it is possible to perform the processes of rotation and perspective change

externally, by physically manipulating a virtual model. Similarly, virtual simulations can allow practice with understanding complex anatomical structures (e.g., the bile ducts of the liver), prior to performing surgical procedures that make heavy demands on spatial cognitive processes, such as laparoscopic cholecystectomy (a minimally invasive surgical procedure for removal of the gall bladder).

However, the kinds of reasoning and learning processes that are done with medical visualizations often involve more complex factors than the tasks studied to date in distributed cognition controlled experiments. In the real-world domain of medicine, using interactive visualizations effectively involves relatively complex reasoning to decide what is the most task-relevant information, as well as planning and executing the motor actions that reveal that information in ways that help the user achieve his or her goals. Thus, studies of how interactive visualizations are used in medicine can contribute to the development of theories of distributed cognition, as well as benefiting from this theoretical framework.

Types or Levels of Interactivity

One factor that is clearly important in determining how an interactive visualization is used is the type or level of interactivity that it allows. Medical visualizations can vary widely in the degree to which they permit interactive control by the user. While some are highly interactive and flexible, permitting free and unconstrained manipulations, others simply present information and do not permit the viewer to engage with them interactively.

Betrancourt (2005) distinguishes broadly between two main types of interactive capabilities: systems that allow relatively low-level control over pace and direction of the presentation (play, pause, rewind, etc.), and systems with more sophisticated capabilities such as altering the parameters in a simulation, or changing the viewpoint to allow exploration from different perspectives. Krygier, Reeves, Cupp, and Di Biase (1997) distinguish between resources that are *static* (e.g., images, maps, diagrams, graphs), *animated* (which express change or motion when activated), *sequential* (which present information in a predetermined linear sequence), *hierarchical* (which allow a non-linear exploration of embedded information or nested concepts), and *conditional* (which respond flexibly and directly to the user's manipulations). These different levels of interactivity may be more or less effective as properties of medical visualizations, depending on the characteristics of the task and the user.

Potential Benefits of Interactive Visualizations

There are several ways in which a 3D computerized visualization might help in cognitive tasks such as understanding anatomical relations, generating a mental model of anatomy, long-term learning about structure and function, or planning how to approach a specific medical or surgical task. Here we outline some of the reasons why 3D visualizations, particularly those that are inter-active, might be expected to augment cognition, that is, we describe the *potential* benefits of these external aids.

One potential benefit from dynamic visualizations is to provide additional depth cues in the display to better communicate the 3D structure of anatomy. Static 2D representations, such as photographs or diagrams, provide only *picto-rial* depth cues, such as shading and occlusion (nonetheless, well-rendered medical illustrations often use these cues very effectively). In contrast, rotating a dynamic visualization, even by a small amount, provides *motion-based* depth cues such as motion parallax, accretion, and deletion. These cues depend on a model's ability to move or turn, not on whether the movements are interactively controlled by the viewer, so this type of spatial information can be made available regardless of

whether a visualization's level of interactivity is *animated* (merely playable) or *conditional* (responding flexibly to user manipulations; Krygier et al., 1997). If designed and used effectively, this information should aid the viewer in constructing an accurate internal representation of 3D structure.

If the viewer is allowed to actively control the visualization, there may be further benefits from the correspondence between the motor commands made to control the visualization and the resulting movements observed. Research on perception and action indicates that monitoring the efferent commands used to control our muscles during active exploration may provide especially strong cues about spatial properties (e.g., Feldman & Acredolo, 1979; Christou & Bülthoff, 1999; Wang & Simons, 1999; Philbeck, Klatzky, Behrmann, Loomis, & Goodridge, 2001). Furthermore, congruent hand motions can facilitate imagined spatial rotations of 3D structures, while incongruent hand motions can impede these processes (Wexler, Kosslyn, & Berthoz, 1998; Wohlschlager & Wohlschlager, 1998).

These studies suggest that a naturalistic control interface allowing the manipulations made by users to be exactly mirrored in the movements of the visualization should be especially beneficial in helping learners to create an integrated spatial mental model of any structure they are viewing and exploring. Researchers in the field of human-computer interaction use the term 'direct manipulation' to refer to this kind of interface (Hutchins, Hollan, & Norman, 1985). They suggest that cognitive effort results when there is a gulf between the user's goals and the way to accomplish the task with the interface. Direct manipulation interfaces can bridge this gulf by providing proper feedback and control. In addition, direct manipulation systems provide a qualitative sense of direct engagement, which Hutchins et al. (1985) describe as "a feeling of first-personness, of direct engagement with the objects that concern us" (p. 318). Through direct engagement, the computer used as a tool becomes "invisible-in-use" and the focus changes to the higher-level task goals and intentions (Heer & Khooshabeh, 2004).

Shneiderman (1983) has identified key properties associated with direct manipulation systems, namely that they continuously represent the object of interest, use physical actions or labeled button presses rather than complex syntax, and allow rapid incremental reversible operations whose impact is immediately visible. According to Hutchins et al. (1985), "direct manipulation requires that the system provide representations of objects that *behave as if they are the objects themselves*" (p. 311, emphasis added). Control mechanisms for achieving this type of direct one-to-one mapping include hand-held control interfaces such as 3D mice, data gloves that track the user's hand motions, and sophisticated 3 or 6 degrees of freedom motion trackers, but these technologies can be too complex and costly for widespread use. Fortunately, the facilitating effects of hand movements are not critically dependent on a one-to-one mapping of the hand motion and the direction of the imagined rotation. Schwartz and Holton (2000) have shown that hand motions when using a tool can facilitate mental rotation even when the motions are not congruent with the rotations that result, provided the individual has an internal model of how the tool works. A more important feature of good design, therefore, is that the relationship between the control mechanism and the resulting changes on-screen is transparent and easily learnable.

Another potential benefit of interactivity arises when the visualization can be rotated in order to view the object or structure from different perspectives. In embodied cognition terms, if a user needs to imagine an object from a different orientation, rotating the external representation is an obvious way to intelligently offload an effortful internal cognitive process onto a less effortful external perceptual-motor process. In an interesting study about how people played the computer game *Tetris*, Kirsh and Maglio (1994) found that people often rotated the *Tetris* pieces on the computer screen rather than mentally rotating them. Strategically rotating or altering the viewpoint of a visualization in this way corresponds to what they call an *epistemic* action, that is, a physical action performed "to uncover information that is hidden or hard to compute mentally" (p. 513) and to what Kirsh (1997) refers to as a *complementary* action, which is performed in the world and relieves the individual of the need to perform an internal computation. Having interactive control over the perspective of an external visualization allows the user to select whether and when to implement this type of action, whereas a traditional, non-interactive resource does not.

In summary, our review of theories of distributed cognition, types of interactivity afforded by 3D visualizations, and the potential benefits of these visualizations for medical education make it clear why both the medical community and cognitive scientists are excited about the potential of these new external aids.

THE PARADOX: INTERACTIVE VISUALIZATIONS ARE NOT ALWAYS BENEFICIAL

Despite all the potential ways in which interactive visualizations might help to augment cognition, previous research has failed to show consistent benefits to users. The results of controlled studies that have compared interactive to non-interactive tools in visual-spatial tasks have been quite mixed.

Some studies have found clear advantages of interactive visualizations, especially for learning about 3D structure. Harman, Humphrey, and Goodale (1999) and James et al. (2002) showed that participants who were allowed to actively rotate 3D objects in an immersive virtual environment while learning their structure had faster recognition times in a subsequent test than participants who passively viewed the objects rotating, even though the rotations were identical in each case. They argued that providing learners with interactive control allowed them to focus on the views of the objects that were most important for later recognition (see also James, Humphrey, & Goodale, 2001). A similar advantage has been found for learners allowed to actively explore large-scale virtual environments (Peruch, Vercher, & Gauthier, 1995; Christou & Bulthoff, 1999). James et al. (2001) have suggested that an additional benefit from active exploration may result from the operation of motor processes during physical rotation, which enhance mental rotation abilities as discussed earlier (Wexler, Kosslyn, & Berthoz, 1998; Wohlschlager & Wohlschlager, 1998; Schwartz & Holton, 2000). Additionally, Kuhn and Ho (1980) have suggested that learners who are given interactive control are able to develop *anticipatory schemes*, which allow them to make use of the outcomes they observe.

By contrast, other studies have found that participants allowed to control an interactive visualization perform no better than participants who merely watch a visualization and are not allowed to interact with it or control it in any way. When participants had to infer structure from three-dimensional data presented on computer, Marchak and Marchak (1991) found that a group who used interactive controls to manipulate the representation performed no better than a group who simply watched the representation rotate automatically. Similarly, Zumbach, Reimann, and Koch (2001) showed that participants who actively navigated hypertext did not differ in knowledge acquisition from their partners who received the same information passively. In studies using virtual environments, active and passive explorations have been shown to produce equal levels of performance in both desktop and immersive environments (Wilson, Foreman, Gillett, & Stanton, 1997; Wilson, 1999; Melanson, Kelso, & Bowman, 2002; Foreman, Sandamas,

& Newson, 2004).

Finally, in some cases, individuals given access to interactive control have actually been found to perform worse than those who were not given this control. In a task that entailed searching for structure in 3D point clouds, Marchak and Zulager (1992) found that participants permitted to freely rotate the visualizations were more likely to erroneously report structure when there was none. Richardson, Wuillemin, and MacKintosh (1981) found that active participants made more errors and took more trials to learn a tactile maze than passive participants, and argued that it was the cognitive demands of regulating or making decisions that interfered with the active participants' learning processes. Huttenlocher (1962) found that adolescents who were simply presented with instances learned concepts faster than those who actively chose the instances to be presented, and she attributed the poorer performance of the active group to disruptions in memory processes arising from the demands of instance selection. These studies suggest that having interactive control can require additional cognitive effort that takes attention away from the main task.

There are several potential reasons for the inconsistent results concerning the benefits of interactivity.[1] One possible factor is how a user interacts with the representation. Provision of an interactive visualization does not guarantee that users will discover the *most effective* way to manipulate it in order to accomplish a task. Importantly, the quality of the information that users gain depends on how effectively they interact with the visualization. The way in which a user interacts with a visualization may be determined by external factors such as the type or level of interactive control available or the type of interface used to control it, or by internal factors such as expertise, prior knowledge, or an understanding of how the visualization can be used to achieve the task goals.

Secondly, the idea that 3D visualizations augment or improve cognition assumes that all users have the cognitive capabilities needed to make sense of the information represented, regardless of whether it is interactive or non-interactive. It is possible that individual differences in the general population determine how easily each user can mentally assimilate the information contained in a 3D visualization. This individual variability may be responsible for differences in task performance, because some individuals have trouble comprehending the external visualization that is supposed to help them complete the task.

So, are there individuals who do not have the ability to benefit from interactive visualizations, either because they do not know how to manipulate them effectively to gain helpful information, or because they cannot comprehend the spatial relations represented, or both? What are the characteristics of such individuals and what can this tell us about barriers to effective use? Can interactive visualizations be made more adaptive for these types of users? To date, little attention has been paid to individual differences among users, which is our focus in this chapter. In the next section, we discuss two user variables we have found to be important for interacting successfully with external visualizations. These are: 1) individual differences in *spatial abilities*, and 2) individual differences in *interactive behavior*.

User Variable I: Individual Differences in Spatial Abilities

The first important user variable, especially in the context of learning anatomy, is *spatial ability*. Spatial ability can be defined as the ability to mentally generate, maintain, and manipulate internal visual-spatial representations (Hegarty & Waller, 2005). Importantly, this ability varies significantly within the general population; some individuals have a facility for spatial thinking, while others find these processes very difficult (for reviews, see Eliot & Smith, 1983; Lohman, 1988; Carroll, 1993; Hegarty & Waller, 2005). In fact, there are several somewhat dissociable

spatial abilities that have been comprehensively documented through standardized testing. The most robust and well documented of these, *spatial visualization*, is involved in tasks that entail "apprehending, encoding, and mentally manipulating spatial forms" (Carroll, 1993, p. 309), suggesting that it measures a person's capability to generate and maintain internal visualizations.

Individual differences in spatial abilities are known to be important for learning and reasoning about anatomical relations. Consider this description of the human heart, which we adapted from several online descriptions:

The heart is a hollow, muscular organ that lies within the chest between the lungs, behind and slightly to the left of the breastbone. Two-thirds of its mass lie to the left of the body midline. It is slightly larger than a clenched fist and has the shape of a blunt inverted cone. The human heart has four chambers; the upper two, at the broad end of the heart, are called the atria, while the lower two, at the apex of the heart, are called the ventricles. There are valves between the atria and ventricles, which are like doors that open in one direction only. Oxygen-rich blood from the lungs flows into the left atrium, and from there it is pumped through the mitral valve, down into the left ventricle, the largest and strongest chamber in the heart. As the left ventricle contracts, the mitral valve is forced shut, and the blood is pushed out through the aortic valve into the aorta, which delivers the oxygen-rich blood to the body.

As this example illustrates, a detailed understanding of anatomy involves many spatial concepts, such as the shape of anatomical structures, where they are located relative to each other, how they are connected, and how different components operate as parts of a dynamic system. Given this kind of spatial content, it is perhaps not surprising that studies have shown that success in learning about anatomy is related to individual differences in spatial ability. Rochford (1985) found that medical students with lower spatial abilities achieved consistently lower marks than higher-spatial students in both practical anatomy examinations and multiple-choice anatomy questions classified as spatially three-dimensional. Although some low-spatial students were able to acquire a spatial understanding of anatomy with time, others never acquired this understanding. Findings such as these suggest that that there is a strong spatial component to the way anatomical knowledge is mentally represented. They also imply that individuals with lower spatial abilities will have a harder time acquiring, representing, and manipulating a spatial mental model of anatomy. Consistent with this prediction, spatial abilities have also been found to be important in performing medical procedures, such as in surgery and dentistry. In many of these procedures the internal structures of the body are not directly visible, so that medical professionals have to rely on their mental spatial representations of anatomical relations (for further discussion, see Hegarty, Keehner, Cohen, Montello, & Lippa, 2007).

While spatial abilities are known to predict anatomy learning through traditional methods, more recently they have also been shown to affect anatomy learning *from 3D computer visualizations* (Garg, Norman, Spero, & Maheshwari, 1999; Garg, Norman, & Sperotable, 2001;). In a study where multiple views of 3D anatomy were presented to medical students via an automatically rotating computer visualization, a subsequent test of anatomical knowledge showed a significant disadvantage to individuals with poor spatial abilities (Garg et al., 1999). For these students, learning was effective only if the display was restricted to a simple depiction entailing just two cardinal views. Such findings suggest that highly complex 3D computer visualizations might actually impair spatial understanding for low-spatial individuals.

In a study that involved learning about the structure of plant and animal cells, either with or without access to interactive 3D models, Huk

(2006) showed that higher-spatial individuals did better overall than lower-spatial learners, but importantly also found an interaction between spatial ability and learning with interactive 3D models. While higher-spatial learners did better with these 3D models than without them, the reverse was true for lower-spatial learners, whose performance was poorer when they had access to these models than when they did not. Moreover, the students' subjective reports of perceived cognitive effort were consistent with this interaction, that is, lower-spatial individuals experienced greater cognitive load when they learned with the 3D models, whereas the reverse was true for higher-spatial learners. Interestingly, the lower-spatial individuals spent more time interacting with the models, yet did worse on the learning test, consistent with their self-reports of higher cognitive load associated with the presence of these resources.

In the VIZMED (Visualizations for Medicine) research project at the University of California, Santa Barbara, we have been examining the relationship between spatial visualization ability and use of external representations in a task that involves inferring and interpreting cross sections of 3D anatomy-like structures. The ability to infer and interpret cross-sections is central to visual-spatial thinking in medicine, as well as science and engineering (Kali & Orion, 1996; Hsi et al., 1997; Orion & Chaim, 1997). For example, Russell-Gebbett (1985) identified two discrete skills involved in understanding 3D structures in biology: the abstraction of sectional shapes, and an appreciation of the spatial relationships of internal parts of a three-dimensional structure seen in different sectional planes. In medicine, the ability to infer and comprehend cross sections is involved in learning anatomy and interpreting medical images such as MRI or CT scans, which represent 2D cross-sections through 3D anatomy (Hegarty et al., 2007).

We developed a spatial reasoning task in which participants were asked to imagine and draw a cross-section of a 3D object. To control for prior knowledge, we initially created an unfamiliar anatomy-like 3D structure, designed to resemble an anatomical configuration, rendered as translucent so that the internal structure was visible (Cohen & Hegarty, in press; Keehner, Hegarty, Cohen, Khooshabeh, & Montello, in press)[2]. The unfamiliar structure was egg-shaped and included internal ducts that branched in different directions, similar to the biliary ducts of the liver (see Figure 1). The task was to imagine what a given vertical or horizontal cross section through the object would look like, if viewed from a specified viewpoint indicated by an arrow outside the structure, pointing towards the cross-section (see Figure 1). While they were performing this task, the participants had access to a 3D computer visualization of the structure that could rotate but which did not show the cutting plane. In different experiments, we varied the degree to which participants had interactive control of the visualization.

An informal task analysis indicates a number of separate cognitive components in this task. The first step is to encode the spatial characteristics of the stimulus object, such as the outer shape, the location and axis of the cutting line, and the spatial relationships among the ducts. A second step is to assume the perspective of the arrow. In Figure 1, this arrow points down at the stimulus object from above. To assume this perspective, we hypothesized that participants could either mentally rotate an internal representation of the object, or mentally change their perspective with respect to their internal representation of the object, or rotate the external visualization of the stimulus object to the viewing perspective indicated by the arrow. Participants also had to mentally imagine slicing the object and removing the section of the object between the viewer and the cross-sectional

Figure 1.

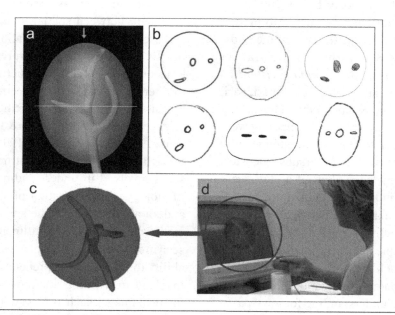

a) Printed stimulus of the 3D anatomy like object used in all of our studies, showing the cutting plane and viewing-direction arrow for one trial. b) The correct duct locations for this cross-section (upper left) and sample drawings by participants. c) The view of the object from the perspective of the arrow. d) An interactive participant manipulating the object using the unconstrained hand-held control device (Keehner et al., in press, Experiments 2 and 3). The highlighted area shows the screen view, and indicates that this participant rotated the object into the orientation that corresponds to the arrow perspective.

plane, and finally they had to infer and draw the configuration of ducts that would be visible in the resulting cross section.

Across all of our studies we have found that spatial ability predicts performance on our task, regardless of whether the individual has access to an interactive visualization, a non-interactive visualization, or no visualization, while they perform the task (Cohen & Hegarty, in press; Keehner et al., in press; Khooshabeh, 2006). Figure 2 shows this relationship (Keehner et al., 2007; Experiment 3), and indicates that spatial ability is important both when participants have interactive control over the visualization and when they watch a non-interactive visualization, which in this case showed the optimal views of the structure. This is consistent with previous findings demonstrating that spatial ability affects an individual's success in apprehending spatial structure from 3D visualizations (Garg et al., 1999; Huk, 2006).

In summary, it appears that spatial visualization ability is an important factor in comprehending and learning anatomical structure, both in general and from 3D computerized representations. Hegarty (2004) has suggested that there are at least three possible ways in which interactive visualizations could affect individuals of different abilities. First, such visualizations might "augment" performance equally for high-spatial and low-spatial individuals, so that students of all abilities are helped equally. Second, provision of an interactive visualization may be particularly effective for low-spatial individuals who have poor internal visualization abilities (acting as a cognitive "prosthetic" for these low-spatial learners). Third, spatial ability might be a necessary prerequisite for using external visualizations effectively, in which case access to these tools might actually increase the gap between individuals of different abilities by especially helping higher-spatial learners. This brief review indicates that high spatial

Figure 2.

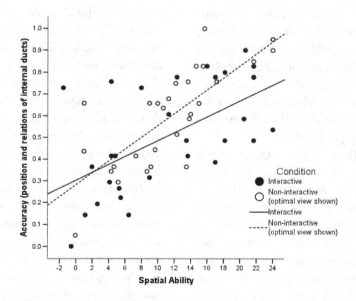

Relationship between spatial ability and task performance in Keehner et al., in press, Experiment 3 (performance was measured as accuracy of drawn duct locations within the cross-section and in relation to each other). The scatterplot indicates that these two variables were highly correlated in both the interactive condition (shown in Figure 1d) and the non-interactive condition, in which the participant had no direct control over the visualization but the on-screen object was pre-programmed to rotate into the arrow view for each trial, thus providing task-relevant information.

ability is important for benefiting from external visualizations (Cohen & Hegarty, in press; Garg et al., 1999; Huk, 2006; Keehner et al., in press), but to date we know of no situation in which an external visualization appears to compensate for low spatial ability. An important goal of future research will be to establish which aspects of 3D external visualizations produce difficulties for individuals with poorer internal visualization abilities, and how visualizations can be redesigned to compensate for these difficulties.

User Variable II: Individual Differences in Interactive Behavior

The second important characteristic of users that affects learning from interactive visualizations is individual differences in *interactive behavior*. As we discussed earlier, some theorists assume that individuals interact effectively with visualizations, either by adopting flexible tradeoffs between effort and outcome, as in the soft constraints model (Gray & Fu, 2004; Gray, Sims, Fu and Schoelles, 2006), or by always offloading effortful cognitive processes onto perceptual-motor processes, as in the embodied cognition approach (Kirsh & Maglio, 1994; Ballard, Hayhoe, Pook & Rao, 1997; Wilson, 2002; Zhang & Norman, 1994). But do all individuals use visualizations in the same way, and if there are individual differences in their use, are these predictable?

In some cases, all participants appear to use external visualizations in a consistent and adaptive way. For example, Garg et al. (2001) gave medical students interactive control over one of two 3D visualizations of the carpal bones of the wrist and hand. One model showed multiple views, varying by 10 degree intervals, while the other showed only key views, 180 degrees apart, i.e., the palmar (front) and dorsal (back) views of the hand. Students with the multiple views model did better than those with the key views model. Interestingly, an examination of the interactions showed that those with the multiple views model actually spent most time on the key views of 0

and 180 degrees and the views immediately adjacent to these, indicating that even though they had unrestricted access to multiple views of the structure, they actually restricted themselves primarily to the two key views. Consistent with this, responses to test questions indicated that the mental models of the structure these students acquired took the form of viewpoint-specific, 2-D projections of the key views.

This pattern is consistent with a study on 3D object recognition by James, Humphrey, and Goodale (2001). They used fictitious 3D objects presented in an immersive virtual environment, controlled by participants via an intuitive handheld interface. From analyzing the patterns of interactions, they identified that the critical information for learning the structure came from "plan" views, such as the front and side of the object, as these provide the most information about 3D structure with the smallest amount of movement. They also noted that while participants dwelled primarily on these "plan" views, they also moved the object back and forth around these views for extended periods of time. These intentional *wobbles* typically had a range of less than 45° around a central point (+/- 22.5°). The authors assumed that they provide more 3D spatial information than a static view alone because of the depth cues provided by motion. In both of these studies participants appeared to find the optimal way of using the interactive visualization and there were not large individual differences in how it was used.

In contrast, recent studies in other domains indicate that there can be large individual differences in how people use interactive visualizations, and people do not always use these visualizations optimally. For example, Lowe (2004, in press) has explored patterns of interactions among domain novices using animated weather maps, which are visually complex, dynamic, user-controllable visualizations. He found large individual differences both *spatially* (where in the visualization they focused their attention) and *temporally* (how much time they spent looking at different frames of the animation). Overall, the use of the interactivity was piecemeal, i.e., restricted both spatially and temporally. Lowe (2004) puts this down to a lack of domain knowledge and the complexity of the information presented in the visualization. He argues that merely making interactivity available is not sufficient for ensuring effective use, especially for users who are not expert in a particular domain, and suggests that designers of dynamic educational visualizations may need to be more proactive in helping learners extract relevant information (see also Betrancourt, 2005).

Our own research in the VIZMED project indicates that individual users differ in terms of what they do when given access to an interactive system (Cohen & Hegarty, in press; Keehner et al., in press). In some of our studies, participants were given access to an interactive visualization of a novel 3D object while they had to imagine and draw a cross-section of the object. As described earlier, in a typical trial a line indicated where the object had been sliced and they had to draw the cross section of the object from the perspective of an arrow, shown in the stimulus diagram (see Figure 1). In an early experiment, (Keehner, et al., in press, Experiment 1) we found that performance was better when participants viewed an interactive animation compared to when they viewed a non-interactive animation that merely showed the object rotating in space. However, in a second experiment (Keehner, et al., in press, Experiment 2) we used a yoked design in which we recorded the interactions of each "interactive" participant and played them back to a "passive" participant, who received exactly the same visual information as their "yoked" interactive partner but did not have any control over the visualization. In this situation, there was no effect of interactivity. That is, the interactive and passive-viewing groups had equivalent performance on the cross-section task.

Examination of the interactivity logs indicated that not all active users were able to manipulate the interactive visualization effectively, and differences in how they interacted with the representation strongly predicted performance on the cross section task. The most successful interactive participants adopted a strategy of rotating the visualization of the object to what we call the "arrow view", that is, the view of the object that one would see if one viewed it from the perspective of the arrow in the stimulus trial (see Figure 1). Less successful participants did not adopt this strategy. In a third experiment (Keehner et al, in press, Experiment 3) we introduced a non-interactive condition that mimicked the "ideal" movements of the visualization, based on the most successful patterns of interactivity that we had observed previously. Participants in this non-interactive condition, who had no control over the visualization but were exposed to task-relevant information on every trial, performed significantly better than interactive participants who had the means to control the visualization but who did not use it in a strategically useful way, and just as well as interactive participants who did use the visualization effectively. These findings suggest that accessing task-relevant information (in this case a particular view of the structure) is more important than interactivity per se. In the context of our task, merely having active control over the visualization did not guarantee success, whereas seeing the critical view(s) of the structure did. Most importantly, there were large individual differences in how effectively people used the visualization, which determined whether they saw the task-relevant information, and these differences in interactive behavior were correlated with task performance.

Taken together, these findings suggest that merely giving users control over a dynamic visualization does not guarantee that they will use it effectively. It is interesting to consider why there was low variability and high success in use of interactive controls in the studies of Garg et al. (2001) and James et al (2001) whereas there were large individual differences in use of interactivity in our own studies and those of Lowe (2004; in press). One important factor may be the expertise of the participants. For example, Lowe studied domain-naive participants, whereas Garg examined medical students studying anatomy, who had experience of learning other anatomical structures from 2-D diagrams and 3D resources such as physical models and dissected samples. Thus it is possible that these individuals had some insight into how to best manipulate the visualization to maximize their learning. A second difference is the nature of the stimulus. Lowe presented visually complex, dynamic 2-D maps, whereas Garg presented a 3D structure, which has inherent spatial properties that define its structure, such as cardinal axes, and moreover it is a familiar object (the hand) that we all have direct experience of manipulating in the real world. Similarly James et al. (2001) used a simple, albeit novel, object whereas the object used in the Keehner et al., experiments had a complex internal structure. Finally, the task in these experiments differed. In the Garg et al. and James et al. studies, the task was to learn the structure of an object, so that it could be recognized later from different views. In contrast the tasks in the Lowe and Keehner et al. studies involved complex inference and problem solving processes.

These findings have implications for the design of interactive visualizations, and suggest that both the properties of the intended users and the properties of the visualization may dictate whether and to what extent interactive control should be available, unconstrained, and unguided. In the next section we discuss some potential ways in which these insights might be implemented in visualization design.

SOLUTIONS AND RECOMMENDATIONS

The findings reviewed in this chapter can provide some potential avenues for visualization designers and implementers to enhance the effectiveness of interactive visualizations in medicine and related fields. First, it is clear from our own studies and

others that spatial ability has an important role in determining how well individuals can make use of the information contained in 3D medical visualizations. At present, virtual technologies are so new that little is known about how this variable impacts on their use. As we discussed earlier, further research is needed to establish which characteristics of visualizations might help or hinder individuals of differing spatial abilities, and whether there are issues that are unique to these forms of representation or whether general principles of spatial understanding apply.

Another variable we have discussed is individual differences in interactive behavior. What drives the variability, or similarities, among users in terms of how they interact with dynamic visualizations? One factor that has been identified in the wider literature as important for interactive behavior generally is the user's metacognitive understanding. Metacognition is often defined somewhat simplistically as "thinking about thinking". Metacogntive processes typically refer to higher order executive processes relating to one's own cognitive processes (Flavell, 1995). Metacognitive knowledge can include knowledge about our own cognitive preferences and styles, knowledge of the task at hand and its likely processing demands, and knowledge of cognitive and metacognitive strategies including when and where they may be helpful. Metacognitive regulation includes the implementation of strategies and processes to regulate and oversee learning, such as planning and monitoring cognitive activities and checking the outcomes of those activities. When an external visualization is interactive, the user is free to manipulate it in unpredictable ways. How a user interacts with an external visualization is therefore dependent on his or her metacognitive understanding of what the task entails and how the visualization can be used to help achieve the task goals.

However, previous research suggests that such metacognitive understanding is often lacking (Hegarty, 2004; Lowe, 1999, 2004; Rieber, Tzeng,

& Tribble, 2004). The ability of the user to grasp how to use an interactive visualization effectively probably depends on internal factors, such as previous experience and expertise, as suggested by some of the comparisons among studies that we have made. It is also likely to depend to some extent on properties of the visualization itself. We have alluded to some of the possible contributory factors, such as what is represented and how familiar it is to the user, the method of control, the range of interactive behaviors that are possible, the complexity of the visual information, and whether the representation is static or dynamic.

Kirsh (2004) views metacognition, like first-order cognition, as a situated or distributed process. While metacognition clearly involves internal processes, it also depends on skills that are oriented towards controlling external mechanisms or tools. In this distributed cognition view, metacognition is "a process that is partly in the world and partly in the head" (Kirsh, 2004, p. 6). If both internal and external factors are at work in shaping an individual's metacognitive understanding of a task, then both individual differences among users and differences among external tools might affect a user's metacognitive understanding of how to use an interactive visualization. Accordingly, in a review of the literature on interactive animations Betrancourt (2005) hypothesized that only certain types of learners (e.g., those with more experience) will benefit from certain types of interactivity. Designers of interactive tools should therefore consider how the features of their design might interact with the characteristics of the intended user. For example, if a tool is designed primarily for domain experts, different principles may apply compared to a visualization designed for domain novices.

Kirsh (2004) argues that good design helps users "discover" the affordances of an external representation in such a way that they can make effective use of them. Well designed "affordance landscapes", that incorporate effective cues and constraints, make metacognition easier. Zhang

and Norman (1994) propose that external visualizations anchor and structure cognition by constraining the range of possible behaviors, thereby constructing the "action space" for a task. This implies that designing visualizations to make task-relevant affordances more intuitively obvious might mitigate individual differences in performance.

In fact, our data from the VIZMED project indirectly support this view. We compared two experiments in which the task was again to imagine and draw a cross section of the novel object in Figure 1 (Keehner et al., in press). In these experiments, the external visualization of the novel object had different interfaces that allowed differing degrees of interactivity. In one, participants used two mouse-controlled slider bars, which allowed them to rotate the object around only the cardinal (horizontal and vertical) axes. In the other, they used a highly intuitive 3 degrees-of-freedom hand held motion-tracker to rotate the object around any axes, such that unrestricted rotations of the motion-tracker were exactly mirrored in unrestricted rotations of the visualization on the computer screen. The interactive participants in the more constrained condition did better than those in the less constrained condition. We suggest this difference may be due to (rather than in spite of) the more constrained interface, which effectively restricted possible rotations to the two axes containing views of the object that were important for completing the task. It is likely that this constraint changed the participant's internal representation of the task, allowing individuals to more easily "discover" the critical view. Consistent with this interpretation, in a related study of the cross section task in which participants used the more constrained interface (Cohen & Hegarty, in press), the majority of participants accessed the critical view on at least three quarters of the trials, a rate of access that was substantially higher than we observed with the more naturalistic, but also more unconstrained, interface. Thus our results are consistent with the somewhat counterintuitive theoretical claim (Betrancourt, 2005; Krygier, et al., 1997) that limited interactivity is more effective for novice users than full interactivity.

This approach helps to reconcile the apparently contradictory findings from the interactivity literature. The question of whether having active control over the visualization helps or hinders depends on factors such as the degree of transparency in how to best manipulate the representation in order to achieve the task goals. A very important aim of good design is to ensure that if interactivity is provided, how to use it is transparent. However, our studies also suggest that even with an intuitive interface, not all users may be able to discover how to use an interactive visualization effectively. For these users, it may be more effective to offer a non-interactive, but optimal, "play" mode that presents the most task-relevant information (but one in which the user can control the speed and direction of play; Lowe, in press; Schwan & Riempp, 2004), or to provide a tutorial in how to use the visualization effectively.

Given the large individual differences among users that we have observed, one recent trend that might be helpful in this domain is personalization. Personalized systems and interfaces are a part of a growing trend of technologies that lower the barrier of entry into computing (Jones, 2003). Our research suggests that because tasks in the medical domain rely on visuospatial and metacognitive abilities, two main factors that should be considered in personalized systems are spatial ability and metacognition.

A recent study suggests that domain knowledge might also be an important factor in personalized systems. Wang, Li, and Chang (2006) have developed a system to teach spatial geometric transformations, such as the cross-section task used in our research. Their Coordinate Tutor system takes into account spatial ability as well as cognitive style to personalize educational content. These two traits are explicitly measured by the tutor using psychometric tests of spatial ability

and a questionnaire to determine learning style. The results of an evaluation showed that adaptive tutoring is beneficial to spatial learning, but personalization based on domain specific knowledge, as well as spatial ability and learning style, is also necessary.

There may be other user characteristics that contribute to how effectively visualizations are utilized and whether they allow the user to achieve his or her goals. Discovering these user characteristics may depend on methodologies that are not typically applied in the development of medical visualizations. One methodological approach that may be helpful in this context is needs analysis. A crucial, but often neglected, step in the development of any technology is understanding the needs of potential users. The engineering community has traditionally used historical approaches, which look at legacy data of how previous developments were achieved and use those as lessons learned to improve future development (Zelkowitz, 1998). However, solely applying engineering methodology to developing medical visualizations is not appropriate because user needs are neglected in favor of improving the technology. We suggest that designers of medical visualizations could borrow research tools from cognitive psychology as discussed in this chapter.

A final approach that might be useful is contextual inquiry, a method pioneered by human-computer interaction designers based on ethnographic methods in anthropology. When using this method, designers of an interactive system act as apprentices and conduct in-situ interviewers with users, who in turn act as masters. The master-apprentice relationship is useful because the designers (apprentices) learn how the work is performed directly from the source (Beyer, 1997). Because different individuals explain things differently, in a contextual enquiry situation the designer can learn about individual differences in how users perform a given task. We believe that this method could be fruitful in studying the learning of anatomy for medicine, allowing researchers to gain important insights into the constraints of the training situation and the needs and capabilities of individual learners (e.g., Khooshabeh, 2004).

CONCLUSION

In this chapter, we have explored individual differences among users and discussed implications for the design of 3D medical visualizations. Our main conclusions are as follows:

- A useful theoretical framework for understanding individual differences among users of medical visualizations is the approach known as *distributed cognition*
- Distributed cognition theories claim that cognition occurs not only in the head but also in the world, via the use of external tools such as visualizations
- Embodied cognition theory predicts that users will intelligently off-load effortful internal cognitive processes onto external tools, while soft constraints models claim that we maximize cost-effectiveness by efficiently managing the tradeoff between internal and external resources available in a given task environment
- Given the characteristics of interactive 3D computer visualizations, they have much potential to augment or enhance cognition
- Paradoxically, however, research shows that interactive visualizations are not always beneficial
- Inconsistent findings on the benefits of interactive visualizations can result from *external* properties of the visualization or *internal* characteristics of individual users
- Two important *internal factors*, which differ among users, are spatial abilities and interactive behavior patterns
- Individual differences in *spatial abilities* affect the user's ability to comprehend the spatial relations within the visualization

- Individual differences in *interactive behavior* determine the user's ability to manipulate the visualization effectively to gain task-relevant information
- Interactive behaviors are strongly driven by the user's *metacognitive understanding* of the task and how the external visualization can be used to achieve the task goals
- According to distributed cognition theory, metacognition can be supported by good design. A well designed *affordance landscape* can help users discover the best way to interact with the visualization
- Given that users differ substantially from one another on important user variables, one approach that may be helpful for ameliorating the effects of individual differences in the future is *personalization*

Future Research Directions

The issues discussed in this chapter have raised a number of potential avenues for further research. Here we overview some empirical, applied, and theoretical questions that to date remain partially or totally unanswered, and provide potential topics for future research in this field.

One potential future direction is to systematically compare the effects of different types of control interfaces. Thus far, we have made this comparison only across experiments, using our cross-section task. Interfaces can differ in terms of the level of interactivity that they afford, the method of control, and task-relevant constraints (e.g., if rotation is only useful in one dimension, then constraining the interface to this dimension is task-relevant). Research on this question has implications for applied issues relating to real-world design, but also speaks to theoretical ideas about direct manipulation, the role of motor processes in spatial cognition, and the distributed nature of metacognition.

Another possibility is to vary the stimuli and examine effects on both task performance and interactive behavior. In order to fully understand the variables influencing interactivity and spatial comprehension, it is important to establish the potential contributions of the structure itself, to examine whether there are universal laws that apply to all external visualizations or whether these are moderated by the nature of the structure that is being represented. In our studies to date, we have used two different structures, the duct model shown in Figure 1 and a virtual 3D model of a human tooth, which is a more complex object. We have alluded to the fact that the structure represented in any visualization has intrinsic properties that may influence how easily its spatial relations are comprehended by different users and the subsequent development of a spatial mental model, as well as eliciting different patterns of interactive behavior. Important factors may include variables such as familiarity, regularity, intrinsic spatial markers (e.g., cardinal axes), and complexity. This research avenue speaks not only to applied issues relating to implementing visualizations in different real-world domains, but also to the theoretical relationship between the internal representation of the user and the external representation that is present in the world.

Finally, an important issue for future research is the influence of individual differences among users. In this chapter we have overviewed some findings on this question, but we still know relatively little about the range of user variables that may be important in this domain. There is much work to be done in answering this question, as individual differences are often neglected in experimental studies, which tend to average performance across all participants to reveal main effects. More research exploring individual factors would be an important contribution to basic science. Moreover, it would help us move towards applied goals such as personalization and adaptive tutoring, as tools for mitigating the differences among learners and helping to ensure that all individuals benefit from the powerful potential of computer visualizations in real-world cognitive tasks.

ACKNOWLEDGMENT

This research was supported by National Science Foundation grant 0313237. We thank Jerome Tietz for technical support, Cheryl Cohen for research contributions, and Meg Vallas for assistance with data coding.

REFERENCES

Ballard, D. H., Hayhoe, M. M., Pook, P. K., & Rao, R. P. N. (1997). Deictic codes for the embodiment of cognition. *Behavioral and Brain Sciences, 20,* 723-742.

Betrancourt, M. (2005). The animation and interactivity principles in multimedia learning. In R. E. Mayer (Ed.), *The Cambridge Handbook of Multimedia Learning* (pp. 287-296). New York, NY: Cambridge University Press.

Beyer, H., & Holtzblatt, K. (1997). *Contextual Design: A Customer-Centered Approach to Systems Designs*: Morgan Kaufman.

Card, S. K., MacKinlay, J. D., & Shneiderman, B. (1999). *Readings in information visualization: Using vision to think*. San Francisco: Morgan Kaufmann.

Carroll, J. (1993). *Human cognitive abilities: A survey of factor-analytic studies*. New York: Cambridge University Press.

Christou, C. G., & Bülthoff, H. H. (1999). View dependence in scene recognition after active learning. *Memory & Cognition, 27*, 996-1007.

Cohen, C. A, & Hegarty, M. (in press). Individual differences in use of an external visualization to perform an internal visualization task. *Applied Cognitive Psychology.*

Collen, M. F. (1995). *A history of medical informatics in the United States, 1950 to 1990.* Indianapolis, IN: American Medical Informatics Association.

De Dombal, F. T. (1996). *Medical informatics: The essentials.* Oxford, Boston: Butterworth-Heinemann.

Eliot, J., & Smith, I. M. (1983). *An international directory of spatial tests.* Windsor, Berks: Nfer-Nelson.

Feldman, A., & Acredolo, L. P. (1979). The effect of active versus passive exploration on memory for spatial location in children. *Child Development, 50,* 698-704.

Flavell, J. H., Green, F. L., Flavell, E. R., Harris, P. L., & Astington, J. W. (1995). Young children's knowledge about thinking. *Monographs of the Society for Research in Child Development, 60*(1), 1-113.

Florance, V. & Masys, D. (2002). *Next generation IAIMS: Binding knowledge to effective action.* Report Number N01-LM-9-3523.Washington, DC: Association of American Medical Colleges.

Florance, V. & Moller, M. T. (2002). *Better Health 2010: A report by the AAMC's better_health 2010 Advisory Board.* Washington, DC: Association of American Medical Colleges.

Foreman, N., Sandamas, G., and Newson, D. (2004). Distance underestimation in virtual space is sensitive to gender but not activity-passivity or mode of interaction. *CyberPsychology & Behavior, 7*(4), 451-457.

Garg, A. X., Norman, G., & Sperotable, L. (2001). How medical students learn spatial anatomy. *The Lancet, 357,* 363-364.

Garg, A. X., Norman, G. R., Spero, L., & Maheshwari, P. (1999). Do virtual computer models hinder anatomy learning? *Academic Medicine, 74*(10), S87-S89.

Gordin, D. N., & Pea, R. D. (1995). Prospects for scientific visualization as an educational technology. *The Journal of the Learning Sciences, 4,* 249-279.

Gray, W. D., & Fu, W.-T. (2004). Soft constraints in interactive behavior: The case of ignoring perfect knowledge in-the-world for imperfect knowledge in-the-head. *Cognitive Science, 28*(3), 359-382.

Gray, W. D., Sims, C. R., Fu, W.-T., & Schoelles, M. J. (2006). The soft constraints hypothesis: A rational analysis approach to resource allocation for interactive behavior. *Psychological Review, 113*(3) 461-482.

Harman, K. L., Humphrey, G. K., & Goodale, M. A. (1999). Active manual control of object views facilitates visual recognition. *Current Biology, 9,* 1315-1318.

Hegarty, M. (2004). Commentary: Dynamic visualizations and learning: Getting to the difficult questions. *Learning and Instruction, 14,* 343-351.

Hegarty, M., Keehner, M., Cohen, C., Montello, D. R. & Lippa, Y. (2007). The role of spatial cognition in medicine: Applications for selecting and training professionals. In G. Allen (Ed.) *Applied Spatial Cognition* (pp. 285-315). Mahwah, NJ: Lawrence Erlbaum.

Hegarty, M. & Waller, D. (2005). Individual differences in spatial abilities. In P. Shah & A. Miyake (Eds.). *The Cambridge Handbook of Visuospatial Thinking* (pp. 121 – 169). New York: Cambridge University Press.

Heer, J., & Khooshabeh, P. (2004, May 25-28). *Seeing the Invisible.* Paper presented at the Association for Computing Machinery Conference on Advanced Visual Interfaces Conference, Lecce, Italy.

Hollan, J., Hutchins, E., & Kirsh, D. (2000). Distributed cognition: Toward a new foundation for human-computer interaction research. *ACM Transactions on Computer-Human Interaction, 7*(2), 174-196.

Hollnagel, E., & Woods, D. (2005). *Joint Cognitive Systems: Foundations of Cognitive Systems*

Engineering. Boca Rotan: CRC Press - Taylor and Francis.

Hsi, S., Linn, M. C., & Bell, J. E. (1997). The role of spatial reasoning in engineering and the design of spatial instruction. *Journal of Engineering Education, April*, 151-158.

Huk, T. (2006). Who benefits from learning with 3D models? The case of spatial ability. *Journal of Computer Assisted Learning, 22,* 392-404.

Hutchins, E. L., Hollan, J. D., & Norman, D. A. (1985). Direct manipulation interfaces. *Human-Computer Interaction, 1*, 311-338.

Huttenlocher, J. (1962). Effects of manipulation of attributes on efficiency of concept formation. *Psychological Reports, 10*, 503-509.

James, K. H., Humphrey, G. K., & Goodale, M. A. (2001). Manipulating and recognizing virtual objects: Where the action is. *Canadian Journal of Experimental Psychology, 55*, 111-120.

James, K. H., Humphrey, G. K., Vilis, T., Corrie, B., Baddour, R., & Goodale, M. A. (2002). "Active" and "passive" learning of three-dimensional object structure within an immersive virtual reality environment. *Behavior Research Methods, Instruments, & Computers, 34*, 383-390.

Jones, A. (2003). *Grand Research Challenges in Information Systems Final Report*. Warrenton, Virginia: Computing Research Associates (CRA).

Kali, Y., & Orion, N. (1996). Spatial abilities of high school students in the perception of geologic structures. *Journal of Research in Science Teaching, 33*, 369-391.

Keehner, M., Hegarty, M., Cohen, C., Khooshabeh, P., and Montello, D. R. (in press). Spatial reasoning with interactive computer visualizations: The role of individual differences in distributed cognition. *Cognitive Science*.

Khooshabeh, P. (2004). *Learning Spatial Relationships: Ethnography and Experiment of an Echographic Training Simulation*. Unpublished Undergraduate Honors Thesis, Primary Reader: Professor Richard Ivry. Secondary Reader: Professor Frank Tendick, University of California, Berkeley.

Khooshabeh, P. (2006). *Quality of Information: Mental Representations and Small Scale Space*. Unpublished Masters Thesis, University of California, Santa Barbara.

Kirsh, D. (1997). Interactivity and multimedia interfaces. *Instructional Science, 25,* 79-96.

Kirsh, D. (2005). Metacognition, distributed cognition and visual design. In P. Gardinfors & P. Johansson (Eds). *Cognition, Education, and Communication Technology* (pp. 147-180). Mahwah, NJ: Lawrence Erlbaum.

Kirsh, D. & Maglio, P. (1994). On distinguishing epistemic from pragmatic action. *Cognitive Science, 18*(4), 513-549.

Krygier, J., Reeves, C., Cupp, J., & DiBiase, D. (1997). *Multimedia in geographic education: Design, implementation, and evaluation*. Retrieved March 16, 2006, http://horizon.unc.edu/projects/monograph/CD/Science_Mathematics/Krygier.asp

Kuhn, D., & Ho, V. (1980). Self-directed activity and cognitive development. *Journal of Applied Developmental Psychology, 1*, 119-133.

Lohman, D. F. (1988). Spatial abilities as traits, processes and knowledge. In R. J. Sternberg (Ed.), *Advances in the psychology of human intelligence* (Vol. 4, pp. 181-248). Hillsdale, NJ: Erlbaum.

Lowe, R. K. (1999). Extracting information from an animation during complex visual learning. *European Journal of Psychology of Education. 14*, 225-244.

Lowe, R. K. (2004). Interrogation of a dynamic visualization during learning. *Learning and Instruction, 14,* 257-274.

Lowe, R.K. (in press). Learning from animation: where to look, when to look. In R.K.Lowe and W. Schnotz (Eds.) *Learning from animation: Research and implications for design.* New York: Cambridge University Press.

Marchak, F. M., & Marchak, L. C. (1991). Interactive versus passive dynamics and the exploratory analysis of multivariate data. *Behavior Research Methods, Instruments, & Computers, 23,* 296-300.

Marchak, F. M., & Zulager, D. D. (1992). The effectiveness of dynamic graphics in revealing structure in multivariate data. *Behavior Research Methods, Instruments, & Computers, 24,* 253-257.

Melanson, B., Kelso, J., & Bowman, D. (2002). *Effects of active exploration and passive observation on spatial learning in a CAVE.* Retrieved October 2005, from http://eprints.cs.vt.edu/archive/00000602/

Norman, D. A. (1990). *Cognitive artifacts.* La Jolla, CA: Dept. of Cognitive Science, University of California, San Diego.

Orion, N., Ben-Chaim, D., & Kali, Y. (1997). Relationship between earth-science education and spatial visualization. *Journal of Geoscience Education, 45,* 129-132.

Peruch, P., Vercher, J.L., & Gauthier, G. M. (1995). Acquisition of spatial knowledge through visual exploration of simulated environments. *Ecological Psychology, 7*(1), 1-20.

Philbeck, J. W., Klatzky, R. L., Behrmann, M., Loomis, J. M., & Goodridge, J. (2001). Active control of locomotion facilitates nonvisual navigation. *Journal of Experimental Psychology: Human Perception and Performance, 27,* 141-153.

Richardson, B. L., Wuillemin, D. B., & MacKintosh, G. J. (1981). Can passive touch be better than active touch? A comparison of active and passive tactile maze learning. *British Journal of Psychology, 72,* 353-362.

Rieber, L. P., Tzeng, S-C., & Tribble, K. (2004). Discovery learning, representation, and explanation within a computer-based simulation: Finding the right mix. *Learning and Instruction, 14,* 307-323.

Rochford, K. (1985). Spatial learning disabilities and underachievement among university anatomy students. *Medical Education, 19,* 13-26.

Russell-Gebbett, J. (1985). Skills and strategies: Pupils' approaches to three-dimensional problems in biology. *Journal of Biological Education, 19,* 293-298.

Schwan, S. & Riempp, R. (2004). The cognitive benefits of interactive videos: learning to tie nautical knots. *Learning and Instruction, 14,* 293-305.

Schwartz, D. L. & Holton, D. L. (2000). Tool use and the effect of action on the imagination. *Journal of Experimental Psychology: Learning Memory and Cognition, 26,* 1655-1665.

Shneiderman, B. (1983). Direct manipulation: A step beyond programming languages. *Computer, 16*(8), 57-69.

van Bemmel, J. H., & Musen, M. A. (Eds.) (1997). *Handbook of medical informatics.* Heidelberg, Germany: Springer-Verlag.

Wang, H.-C., Li, T.-Y., & Chang, C.-Y. (2006). A web-based tutoring system with styles-matching strategy for spatial geometric transformation. *Interacting with Computers, 18*(3), 331-355.

Wang, R. X.-F., & Simons, D. J. (1999). Active and passive scene recognition across views. *Cognition, 70,* 191-210.

Wexler, M., Kosslyn, S. M. & Berthoz, A. (1998). Motor processes in mental rotation. *Cognition, 68,* 77-94.

Wilson, M. (2002). Six views of embodied cognition. *Psychonomic Bulletin and Review, 9,* 625-636.

Wilson, P. N. (1999). Active exploration of a virtual environment does not promote orientation or memory for objects. *Environment and Behavior, 31,* 752-763.

Wilson, P. N., Foreman, N., Gillett, R., & Stanton, D. (1997). Active versus passive processing of spatial information in a computer simulated environment. *Ecological Psychology, 9,* 207-222.

Wohlschlager, A., & Wohlschlager, A. (1998). Mental and manual rotation. *Journal of Experimental Psychology: Human Perception and Performance, 24,* 397-412.

Zelkowitz, M. V., Wallace, D.R. (1998). Experimental models for validating technology. *IEEE Computer, 31*(5), 23-31.

Zhang, J. & Norman, D.A. (1994). Representations in distributed cognitive tasks. *Cognitive Science, 18,* 87-122.

Zumbach, J., Reimann, P., & Koch, S. (2001). Influence of passive versus active information access to hypertextual information resources on cognitive and emotional parameters. *Journal of Educational Computing Research, 25*(3), 301-318.

Additional Reading

Cohen, C. A, & Hegarty, M. (in press). Individual differences in use of an external visualization to perform an internal visualization task. *Applied Cognitive Psychology.*

Garg, A. X., Norman, G. R., Spero, L., & Maheshwari, P. (1999). Do virtual computer models hinder anatomy learning? Academic Medicine, 74(10), S87-S89.

Garg, A. X., Norman, G. R., & Sperotable, L. (2001). How medical students learn spatial anatomy. The Lancet, 357, 363-364.

Gray, W. D., Sims, C. R., Fu, W.-T., & Schoelles, M. J. (2006). The soft constraints hypothesis: A rational analysis approach to resource allocation for interactive behavior. *Psychological Review, 113(3)* 461-482.

Gray, W. D., & Fu, W. (2004). Soft constraints in interactive behavior: The case of ignoring perfect knowledge in-the-world for imperfect knowledge in-the-head. Cognitive Science, 28(3), 359-382.

Gray, W. D. (2000). The nature and processing of errors in interactive behavior. Cognitive Science, 24(2), 205-248.

Harman, K. L., Humphrey, G. K., & Goodale, M. A. (1999). Active manual control of object views facilitates visual recognition. *Current Biology, 9,* 1315-1318.

Hegarty, M. (2004). Commentary: Dynamic visualizations and learning: Getting to the difficult questions. *Learning and Instruction, 14,* 343-351.

Hegarty, M., Keehner, M., Cohen, C., Montello, D. R. & Lippa, Y. (2007). The role of spatial cognition in medicine: Applications for selecting and training professionals. In G. Allen (Ed.) *Applied Spatial Cognition* (pp. 285-315). Mahwah, NJ: Lawrence Erlbaum.

Hegarty, M. & Waller, D. (2005). Individual differences in spatial abilities. In P. Shah & A. Miyake (Eds.). *The Cambridge Handbook of Visuospatial Thinking* (pp. 121 – 169). New York: Cambridge University Press.

Herzfeldt, B., & Rettig, M. (2003). Interaction Design Case: VasSol CANVAS. Paper presented at the Designing the User Experience (DUX), San Francisco, CA.

Hollan, J., Hutchins, E., & Kirsh, D. (2000). Distributed cognition: Toward a new foundation for human-computer interaction research. *ACM Transactions on Computer-Human Interaction, 7*(2), 174-196.

Hollnagel, E., & Woods, D. (2005). *Joint Cognitive Systems: Foundations of Cognitive Systems Engineering.* Boca Rotan: CRC Press - Taylor and Francis.

Huk, T. (2006). Who benefits from learning with 3D models? The case of spatial ability. *Journal of Computer Assisted Learning, 22,* 392-404.

Hutchins, E. L., Hollan, J. D., & Norman, D. A. (1985). Direct manipulation interfaces. *Human-Computer Interaction, 1,* 311-338.

James, K. H., Humphrey, G. K., & Goodale, M. A. (2001). Manipulating and recognizing virtual objects: Where the action is. *Canadian Journal of Experimental Psychology, 55,* 111-120.

Jones, A. (2003). *Grand Research Challenges in Information Systems Final Report.* Warrenton, Virginia: Computing Research Associates (CRA).

Keehner, M., Hegarty, M., Cohen, C., Khooshabeh, P., and Montello, D. R. (in press). Spatial reasoning with interactive computer visualizations: The role of individual differences in distributed cognition. *Cognitive Science.*

Kirsh, D. (1997). Interactivity and multimedia interfaces. *Instructional Science, 25,* 79-96.

Kirsh, D. (2005). Metacognition, distributed cognition and visual design. In P. Gardinfors & P. Johansson (Eds). *Cognition, Education, and Communication Technology* (pp. 147-180). Mahwah, NJ: Lawrence Erlbaum.

Norman, D. A. (1990). *Cognitive artifacts.* La Jolla, CA: Dept. of Cognitive Science, University of California, San Diego.

Rieber, L. P., Tzeng, S-C., & Tribble, K. (2004). Discovery learning, representation, and explanation within a computer-based simulation: Find-

ing the right mix. *Learning and Instruction, 14,* 307-323.

Shneiderman, B. (1983). Direct manipulation: A step beyond programming languages. *Computer, 16*(8), 57-69.

Wang, H.-C., Li, T.-Y., & Chang, C.-Y. (2006). A web-based tutoring system with styles-matching strategy for spatial geometric transformation. *Interacting with Computers, 18*(3), 331-355.

Wexler, M., Kosslyn, Stephen., Berthoz, Alain. (1998). Motor processes in mental rotation. *Cognition, 68,* 77-94.

Wilson, M. (2002). Six views of embodied cognition. *Psychonomic Bulletin and Review, 9,* 625-636.

Zelkowitz, M. V., Wallace, D.R. (1998). Experimental models for validating technology. *IEEE Computer, 31*(5), 23-31.

Zhang, J. & Norman, D.A. (1994). Representations in distributed cognitive tasks. *Cognitive Science, 18,* 87-122.

ENDNOTES

[1] One methodological factor that might account for some of the mixed results on the effects of interactivity is whether the provision of interactive control is confounded with the specific visual information that a user receives. Manipulating a visualization changes what appears on the screen, and therefore interactive and non-interactive users may not receive the same visual information, and even different interactive users may not see the same thing. It is possible that differences in the visual information available, rather than interactivity per se, account for some differences in task performance. Some researchers have taken care to

overcome this confound by using a "yoked" design in which the interactions of each active participant are recorded and played back to a yoked participant who therefore receives the same visual information but has no control over the visualization.

[2] In more recent studies we have generalized our findings to imagining cross sections of a real anatomical object (Khooshabeh, 2006).

Chapter II
Grid–Based Visualization and its Medical Applications

Yingjun Qiu
Beijing Sigma Center, China

Youbing Zhao
Siemens Ltd., China

Jiaoying Shi
Zhejiang University, China.

ABSTRACT

Traditional visualization approaches cannot handle new challenges in the visualization field such as visualizing huge data sets, communicating between existing visualization systems and providing interactive visualization services, widely. In this chapter, the authors introduce an emerging research direction in the visualization field, grid-based visualization, which aims to resolves the above problems by utilizing grid computing technology. However, current grid computing technology is almost batch job-oriented and does not support interactive visualization applications natively. In this chapter, the authors implement a grid-based visualization system (GVis) which utilizes large-scale computing resources to achieve large dataset visualization in real time and provides end users with reliable interactive visualization services, widely. In GVis system, current grid computing technology is extended to support interactive visualization applications.

INTRODUCTION

Brief Introduction of Visualization

Visualization is the process of transforming scientific data or sampled data into graphical image by utilizing computer graphics and image processing technologies (Drebin, 1988; Kaufman, 1991; Kaufman, 1997). By transforming raw data into understandable graphical image, visualization allows scientists and researchers to gain understanding and insight into the data and the subjects that are studied. Due to this capability, visualization has been widely used in a variety of science and commercial areas since its arising, such as medicine, biology, biological chemistry, atmospheric physics, earth physics, computational fluid dynamics, finite element analysis, meteorology, oil and gas exploration and production, and so

forth (Funchs, 1989; Shi, 1995; Lum, 2002; Bethel, 2003). Figures 1, 2 and 3 present some examples of medical and scientific visualization.

User interactivity is an important feature of user-centered visualization applications, which allows doctors, researchers and scientists to explore the data more directly and effectively. For example, when viewing medical imagery with moderate to high levels of transparency, doctors can perform operations such as moving, rotation, selection and zooming of the visual representation to gain enhancement and efficiency in the visual perception of the image (Russell, 1987). Interactive visualization can also make computational steering enabled as scientists or doctors can change the parameters of simulation dynamically and see the effect of this change immediately.

According to the conceptual model proposed by Harber and McNabb (1990), the overall visu-

Figure 1. Visualization of a tooth with different three dimensional transfer functions (From Chuck Hansen, University of Utah)

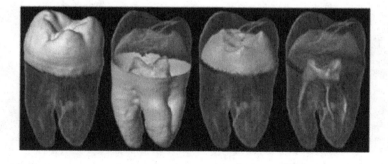

Figure 2. Illustrating ganglion cells (Lum, 2002)

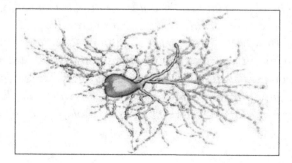

alization process is divided into three smaller procedures: data preprocessing such as enrichment/enhancement/reduction, data transformation to geometry, and geometry rendering. Figure 4 presents a pipeline to describe the actual series of procedures in visualization process.

In this pipeline, the original data either comes from data repositories or is generated online from active scientific simulation. During the initial preprocessing, data required for visualization is derived from the original raw data, for example, by extraction, approximation, and interpolation. Afterwards, the preprocessed data is transformed into geometry elements with color, lighting and texturing attributes. Finally, geometry elements is rendered to produce the final 2D image by computer graphics and image processing methods, for example, modeling transformation, clipping, back face culling, screen space transformation, Z-buffer, shading and anti-aliasing. Geometry

rendering is the most important and complex procedure in visualization process, which often involves complicated computation and is memory demanding.

Visualization Techniques

Classification of Visualization Techniques

Volume data visualization (Drebin, 1988; Kaufman, 1991; Nielson, 1999) is one important branch of visualization, which is used in many application domains especially in medical area. Compared to surface data which solely determines the outer shell of an object, volume data is able to describe the internal structure of a solid object. A volume is a regular 3D array of data values, voxels. Therefore, visual representation of volume data

Figure 3. Images of black hole simulations (Bethel, 2003)

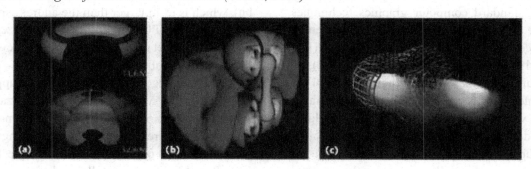

Figure 4. Conceptual model of visualization pipeline

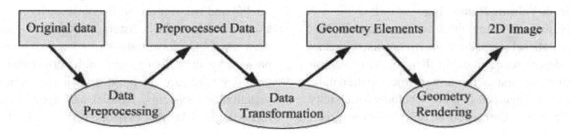

often provides much more interior information of an object then surface data (See Figure 1).

In terms of the underlying rendering techniques, visualization from volume data can be divided into surface rendering and direct volume rendering (Udupa, 1989). Surface rendering is an indirect geometry-based technique which is used to visualize structures in 3D scalar or vector fields by converting these structures into immediate geometrical representation first, and then using conventional computer graphics techniques to render these surfaces. Direct volume rendering is a technique for the visualization of 3D scalar data sets without using immediate geometrical representation.

Surface Rendering

Surface rendering is an indirect method to obtaining an image from volume data set. This is due to its requirement of constructing surfaces in the data. Intermediate surfaces are constructed by mapping data values onto a set of geometric primitives in a process known as iso-surfacing. The surfaces can then be rendered into a displayable image using standard computer graphics techniques. There are a number of techniques to implement surface rendering, for example, cuberilles (Herman, 1979), marching cubes (Lorenson, 1987), and iso-surfaces (Pekar, 2001; Tenginakai, 2001).

Due to the process of constructing surfaces, each volume element of the data should be considered whether it is inside or outside of the iso-surface. This process may result in a loss of accuracy especially when visualizing small or fuzzy details. Information on the interior of surfaces can also get lost in this process.

Direct Volume Rendering

Volume rendering does not use intermediate geometrical representation, in contrast to surface rendering techniques. In the process of volume rendering, first each volume element in the dataset has to be mapped to a color value with opacity. Afterwards, the composed RGBA (for red, green,

blue and alpha) result is projected onto the 2D viewing plane from the desired viewpoint to obtain the final image. A big advantage of direct volume rendering is that the interior information of the volume data can be displayed, which enables users to view the 3D data as a whole. Disadvantages are the difficult interpretation of the interiors and the much longer time to perform volume rendering than surface rendering.

Ray casting (Levoy, 1988), splatting (Westover, 1990) and shear-warp (Lacroute, 1994) are some typical direct volume rendering approaches. Today, with the rapid advance of graphics hardware, 2D and 3D hardware texture mapping (Cullip, 1993; Cabral, 1994) has become a widespread volume rendering method.

Parallel Visualization Techniques

Visualization applications are often computation and memory intensive, especially in medical applications where huge data sets are commonly used. For instance, the well-known visible human data set consists of 6.5GB (2048x1216x1877 voxels, 12 bit), which is even larger than the address space of conventional PC. The ability to visualize the enormous dataset in interactive rate is far beyond the capabilities of commodity PCs.

To handle huge volume data set and support real-time interactivity, an interactive visualization system has to employ special high-performance graphics hardware based on multiprocessing and parallel memory organization, for example, SGI Onyx2 and FUZION. Parallel techniques must also be applied in these visualization systems to implement parallel visualization algorithms.

With the rapid advances of graphics hardware for PC and the significant decrease of its price since the 1990s, PC clusters or loose coupled networked PCs, has gradually become an alternative way, instead of special high performance graphics hardware, to build high performance visualization systems. Parallel and distributed technologies like MPI (MPI), PVM (PVM) and

DCE (DCE) are widely used in these systems to develop parallel and distributed visualization applications.

The main idea of parallel visualization is to divide a large visualization task into several smaller subtasks which can be executed in parallel by different visualization units so that large dataset can be handled properly. In general, parallel visualization algorithms can be classified into two categories: sort first and sort last (Molnar, 1994). Sort first method decomposes the final image in screen space, and each visualization unit renders a 2D tile of the final image. In this method, each visualization unit must keep the whole dataset. Sort last method on the other hand decomposes the whole dataset into several parts, each of which is rendered by one visualization unit. Then the partial rendered frames are combined into the final image. This method does not enforce each visualization unit to keep the entire dataset. Compared to sort first method, sort last method scales better but increases the latency of rendering.

Challenges in Visualization Field

While tremendous advancement has been made in the field of visualization in recent years, conventional visualization techniques and visualization systems are facing severe challenges.

First, enormous datasets are being generated for visualization in medical or scientific domains nowadays. For instance, in the medical area, the size of the dataset for building a colorful digital human brain is about 4.5 PetaBytes (1PetaBytes $= 10^{15}$Bytes) (Foster, 1999). The ability for effectively handling these enormous datasets, particularly in interactive rate, is far beyond the capabilities of both the visualization systems based on special high performance graphics hardware and those based on PC clusters.

Second, conventional visualization systems are usually employing special graphics hardware and tailored for specific software platforms, and are often involving a static collection of computation

and rendering resources so that these systems do not scale well to allocate and utilize geographically distributed and heterogeneous resources in large scale environment.

Third, visualization software and tools which have been developed in the past two decades are usually incompatible with each other. The visualization software packages cannot be used together to solve larger and complete problems. It is also difficult for existing visualization systems to communicate with each other and integrate as a larger system to support collaboration.

Fourth, a new requirement in the visualization field is to integrate visualization systems seamlessly with scientific computing process so that simulation data can be visualized online rather than being downloaded to local storage and being visualized later. Visualization has always been driven by scientific applications which generate a huge amount of data to be visualized. Traditionally, these generated data are downloaded and stored locally before visualization is performed. However, it takes much more effort to keep this increasing data. Furthermore, it causes a high delay for scientists to obtain visual representation of the data, which is unacceptable in many research studies.

Finally, visualization systems must enhance their capabilities to provide services in on a much larger scale even over Internet to numerous users and to provide an integrated environment for users to perform remote and collaborative visualization at distributed locations. As the size of the generated dataset is increasing rapidly, visualization tends to be carried out in consolidated visualization centers that can provide extreme computing and storage capabilities. This produces urgent needs for remote visualization capabilities of visualization systems, through which remotely located users can perform visualization on their desktops or mobile devices while the actual data and computation is carried out remotely. This is extremely important for medical applications, where remote visualization of large medical datasets and collaborative visualization among doctors in geographically distributed sites are increasingly needed. However, collaboration in visualization systems is always a complicated issue due to difficulties of coordinating the activities of multiple simultaneous users, handling the balance of bandwidth and latency, dealing with synchronization, and considering the different work habits of each involved user (Coleman, 1996).

Some of these problems have existed for many years, such as large dataset support. Others are new requirements for visualization, such as large scale collaborative visualization and seamless integration with science computing. The emerging grid infrastructure and technologies bring new ideas for developing visualization applications and building visualization systems to deal with these critical problems in visualization field.

The Grid

Grid Introduction

Grid computing (Foster, 1999, 2001, 2002, 2003, Berman, 2002) technology has emerged and had quickly grown as an important new field in the last decade, which changes the way we perceive and use computing resources. "Grid computing distinguishes from conventional distributed computing by its focus on large-scale resources sharing, innovative applications, and, in some case, high-performance orientation" (Foster, 2001). The grid effectively integrates all kinds of resources over Internet such as networking, communication, computation and information to form a single virtual platform to provide consistent, secure and pervasive services to end users. The core of the grid is coordinated resource sharing and problem solving in dynamic, multi-institutional virtual organizations (VOs) (Foster, 2001). Due to this extremely immense capability, the gird has been applied in many application domains and is transforming science, business, health and society.

The development of grid computing is firstly driven by large scale science applications, for example, computational biology, genomics, high-energy physics, which usually demand for tremendous computation and storage resource, which cannot be fulfilled by localized computing platforms and infrastructures (Foster, 1999; Berman, 2002). To satisfy the tremendous resource demand for these applications, widely distributed resources must be utilized effectively and efficiently through sophisticated software infrastructure. This has been the first generation of grid computing systems. In this generation, the grid focuses on integrating geographically-distributed high performance computation resources through network software infrastructure as a single powerful platform to fulfill the execution of a range of science applications. Several grid projects emerged in this generation and had been very successful, for example, FARNERT (FARNERT), I-WAY (Foster, 1997).

The rapid advancement of commodity computer (Moore's Law) and the speedy advancement of network bandwidth (Gilder, 2002) result in more and faster capable hardware and network components around the Internet. For example, today a commodity computer is even ten times faster than a Cray supercomputer in 1980s (Foster, 2003). The second generation of grid systems focuses on providing core technologies such as middleware, libraries and tools to support large-scale data and computation applications by utilizing distributed commodity computers. Globus (Globus), Legion (Legion) and Cactus (Cactus) are some typical grid middleware and systems that have been developed in this generation. We will talk about these grid middleware in detail in a later section. This generation has also seen a growing number of large-scale grid development projects, such as DoE's Science Grid (DoE Science Grid), NSF's TeraGrid (TeraGrid) and the UK e-Science Grid (e-Science).

To the current third generation of grid systems, the emphasis has been shifted to global collaboration through common computation and data infrastructure which is built with open and standard service-oriented approaches, such as OGSA (Foster, 2002; OGSA) and WSRF (WSRF). The grid has been redefined as "the computing and data management infrastructure that will provide the electronic underpinning for a global society in business, government, research, science and entertainment" (Foster, 2003). The ultimate goal of the grid is to effectively integrate geographically-distributed and heterogeneous resources like computation, networking, communication, information and knowledge, which belong to different individuals, institutions and organizations, to act as a whole virtual platform to provide exuberant services to end users.

Grid Architecture

To make the grid infrastructure a reality, open standards and new technologies should be defined and developed to achieve flexible, secure and coordinated resource sharing and collaboration among dynamic virtual organizations. Grid architecture has been proposed to identify fundamental system components for the construction of grids, specify the purpose and function of each component and

indicate the interaction between these components (Foster, 2001). The following will introduce two open and extensible grid architectures with focus on well-defined protocols and services.

The Layered Grid Architecture

The layered grid architecture was firstly proposed in Foster (2001), which consists of five layers, as shown in Figure 5.

The grid fabric layer provides the resource entities for sharing in the grid, for instance, computation resources, storage resources and rendering resources. Fabric components implement the operations that occur on specific resources and provide APIs for higher levels to perform sharing operations. The connectivity layer enables the resources in the fabric layer to be connected and exchange data with each other. Core communication and authentication protocols that are required for network transactions are defined in this layer. Building on the connectivity layer, the resource layer defines the protocols for the operation of managing and sharing individual resources. It implements these protocols by calling the functions in the fabric layer to access and control local resources. While the resources layer focuses on operation on individual resources, the collective

Figure 5. The layered grid architecture and its relationship to the Internet protocol architecture. Because the Internet protocol architecture extends from network to application, there is a mapping from grid layers into Internet layers (Foster, 2001).

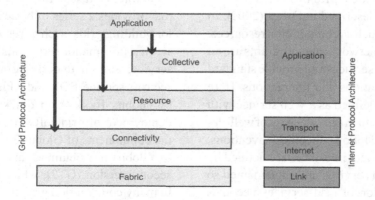

layer is focused on integration of collections of resources and interactions among them. The final layer, application layer, calls the functions in the lower layers to operate and organize resources in different virtual organizations. Through the five layers' architecture, resources can be shared and utilized across distributed virtual organizations effectively and securely.

Protocols are the core of this grid architecture, which are defined between layers for interaction and communication. Each layer component implements an APIs for calling its functions. The SDK implemented in this grid architecture helps users to construct a grid system quickly.

Open Grid Service Architecture (OGSA)

The Open Grid Service Architecture (OGSA) framework is a new grid architecture proposed by Globus community and IBM at Global Grid Forum (GGF) 4 (GGF). It is built on the convergence of grid computing and Web services (Web Services) which has rapidly advanced in industry in recent years. Web services establish a collection of standards of new technologies for distributed computing by the effort of industry-leaders, for example, IBM, Microsoft and HP, and the World Wide Web Consortium (W3C). These standards include, for instance, SOAP (SOAP), WSDL (WSDL), UDDI (UDDI), and WSFL (WSFL). With these new technologies, Web services support a service-oriented approach to facilitate service discovery, service description and service interaction to implement grid mechanisms.

OGSA is fully described in Foster (2002). In OGSA, resources such as computation resources, storage resources, networks and programs are all represented as grid services and provide standard interfaces for operations and interactions. Here the grid service is defined as a Web service with special capability, which provides a set of well-defined interfaces and follows specific conventions. A core set of consistent interfaces are defined by OGSA that all grid services are implemented so that the construction of grid services becomes

quite easy. OGSA provides a series of essential grid services to support automatic service discovery, dynamic service creation, lifetime management, notification and manageability of grid services. It also defines and provides a bundle of higher level services such as security protocol mapping, distributed data management and workflow to support the diverse requirements of different applications in the grid environment.

Grid Middleware

In the evolution of grid systems, there are a growing number of grid middleware, libraries and tools that have been developed for building software infrastructure and key services to support resource sharing and collaboration across large scale environments. Some of the middleware and tools are complying with the architecture models we introduced in the last section, while others are not, since they are concentrated on specific domains to support different requirement and address different problems. The following introduces some of the middleware which are the most significant to date.

Globus

The Globus (Globus) project is a U.S. multi-institutional research effort that seeks to develop the core technologies for the construction of computation grids. It has been based on the successful experience of I-WAY project. Globus project developed a software infrastructure—Globus Toolkit (GT) that provides a series of basic services and tools for building grids, such as resource management service, information service and data management service, and an underlying authentication and security service. SDK and APIs are also provided by Globus Toolkits for quick development and deployment of grid software. Figure 6 presents the components of Globus Toolkit 3.0 (GT3).

Globus has obtained much success from its second version (GT2), which has been utilized in many computation grid projects. The Layered

Grid Architecture model is proposed and implemented in GT2. After that, it evolved to version 3 (GT3) with the introduction of the Open Grid Service Architecture (OGSA) framework. GT3 contains a reference implementation of OGSI (OGSI) to provide essential services defined in OGSA model, such as grid service definition, service creation and notification, and so forth. Based on these essential services, higher level services are implemented to provide resource management, information management and data management in large scale grid. Globus is continuing its evolution with the trends of more combination and cooperation between the grid and Web service communities. WSRF (WSRF) was proposed in January 2004 in place of OGSI, which addresses the combination of grid and Web service architecture to facilities large scale collaboration across virtual organizations. GT4 takes this new trend and is developed according to WSRF model.

Legion

Legion (Grimshaw, 1997; Legion) is an object-based grid computing system which was firstly developed at the University of Virginia. It provides a software infrastructure to integrate geographically-distributed high performance computers and enable seamless interaction among them. Through this software infrastructure, Legion presents as a single virtual computer for users to develop programs and applications, at their workstations, regardless of scale, physical location and underlying operating system of this virtual computer.

Different from Globus, Legion utilizes object-oriented approach to implement a grid infrastructure so that it gains the advantages of data abstraction, encapsulation, inheritance and polymorphism. All the components are encapsulated as objects in Legion. Legion defines a set of core objects, including host objects, vault objects, implementation objects and caches, binding agents, context objects and context spaces, to provide basic services required by the grid system. Legion is responsible for the management of these objects and the interaction between these objects. User objects are also supported in Legion to extend the capabilities of system-level objects.

Condor

Condor (Condor) is a software package developed by Wisconsin-Madison for executing batch jobs on

Figure 6. Components of Globus Toolkit 3.0. GT3 contains an OGSI reference implementation which provides the basic mechanisms for grid service definition, grid service creation, lifetime management, notification and manageability. System-level services are also provided in GT3 for resource management (e.g, GRAM), information management (e.g., MDS) and data management (e.g., GridFTP).

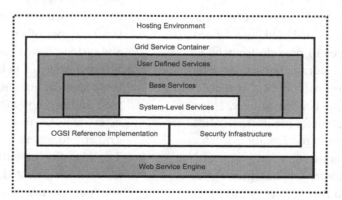

a variety of UNIX computers, particularly those that would be idle. Condor presents features such as automatic resource location and job allocation, check pointing, and the migration of processes. These features are implemented without modification of the underlying UNIX kernel. However, users need to link the Condor libraries with their programs to enable these features.

Condor manages a dynamic resource pool and allocates computing resources from this pool to execute the batch jobs submitted by users. The activities on all the participating computing resources are monitored by Condor for determining which machine is available so that it can be placed into the resource pool. When a machine gets busy, it leaves the resource pool.

Condor was developed in 1986 and has been utilized in many universities and research institutions. It is also widely used in commercial areas. While condor is designed for executing batch jobs, it does not support interactive applications such as visualization.

Grid-Based Visualization and its Medical Applications

The emerging grid infrastructure and technologies give people brand new conception on how to build visualization systems and create visualization applications to take these challenges, which may give new opportunities to medical visualization applications:

1. Since the grid technologies can effectively integrate widely distributed and heterogeneous resources to provide tremendous computation and storage power, large dataset visualization will not be a bottleneck in the visualization field any longer. This is extremely important for medical visualization in which huge, high-resolution data sets are commonly required.

2. Open and standard technologies developed by the grid community facilitate the integration of diverse systems on the grid. Therefore, medical visualization systems built with these open technologies will be easier to integrate and interoperate.

3. The grid infrastructure is also provided with the capabilities for effective resource sharing and collaboration in large scale environment, which can give a strong support to achieve remote and collaboration visualization among distributed organizations. This will foster remote and collaborative diagnosis and operations among multiple distributed hospitals.

Grids will effectively link visualization data source, distributed computational and storage resources, visualization devices, and users across a widely-distributed virtual organizations. With such a background, grid-based visualization becomes a hot research subject in both visualization and the grid field.

In the last several years, much work has been done in this field, including grid-enabled visualization applications, grid-based visualization middleware and integrated visualization systems based on the grid. We will give a brief survey on this subject in another section. Although grid-based visualization owns a bright vision, it actually faces many challenges nowadays. Here we give a list of difficulties for grid-based visualization.

•   Transplanting existing visualization applications and systems onto grid platform is really hard work. In the past ten years, a large number of visualization applications and systems have been built to fulfill activities in a range of fields. However, most of these applications and systems do not scale well and are not capable of dealing with heterogeneous resources in a large scale grid environment.

•   The majority of current grid technology is batch job-oriented, which does not give much support for interactive applications, such as visualization. To enable visualization applications to fit into grid environment, existing grid technology should be extended to support interactivity of the grid.

- The grid is still on its way to becoming mature. Much more work needs to be done in the future, including building high speed network infrastructure around the world, deploying tremendous computation nodes and connecting them with the underlying network infrastructure, and developing open and standard software infrastructure to support flexible, secure and coordinate resource sharing. Grid-based visualization depends on the maturity of the grid infrastructure.

In the remainder of this chapter, we will first introduce the evolution of grid-based visualization research. Then we will illustrate the important issues to be considered while building a grid-based visualization system. After that, we give solutions to the important issues by presenting a grid-based visualization system of our own—GVis. The results of our solution with medical datasets included will also be presented as reference. Lastly, we will give our own opinions of the future trends on grid-based visualization and conclude this chapter.

SURVEY ON GRID-BASED VISUALIZATION

With the increasing development of the grid and scientific visualization, grid-based visualization has emerged as an important research field. Much work has been done to explore this new direction. *Computer Graphics & its Applications* had a special issue on grid-based visualization in March 2003. In this section, a survey of research work on grid-based visualization is presented to give the reader an understanding of the general research background. From these research works,

we believe that grid-based visualization will have a large influence on the future visualization research and applications. In the following, we will categorize research on grid-based visualization into several subsections.

Utilize General Grid Middleware to Extend Existing Visualization Systems

Early research simply used distributed computing capabilities of the grid to accelerate the visualization process. As we know, many existing visualization applications are not grid-enabled. It is not easy for these applications to utilize large-scale computation and storage resources, and provide service widely. By utilizing existing grid middleware, such as Globus or Cactus, these legacy applications can be extended to catch capabilities to deal with a much larger dataset and provide visualization service to end users more widely and collaboratively. Examples of this kind of research include Aeschlimann (1999), Knops (2002), gViz (gViz), DVR (DVR, 2002), and so forth.

In 1999, Aeschlimann proposed a grid-based distributed visualization framework DV (1999). It was a framework for distributed non-interactive visualization. With the framework, a visualization task can be divided into "active frames" and then distributed dynamically to idle computing nodes. However, it is more computing- oriented and cannot support user interactive visualization.

Knosp et al. also proposed a volume rendering framework (Knosp, 2002) which was based on the resource management, information services and data transferring tools provided by Globus Toolkit. Like Aeschlimann (1999], it can support dynamic task division and resource allocation. However, the main disadvantage is that their framework which can only support sort-first parallel rendering method is not general enough. Besides that, it does not have a separate grid-supporting layer to build visualization applications on heterogynous platforms.

gViz is a UK eScience project carried out by the Leeds University and NAG. (http://www.nag.co.uk). The aim of the project is to make the IRIS Explorer from NAG grid-enabled so that grid-based visualization, combination of visualization and simulation, computational steering, and multi-user collaboration can be achieved.

Another example is the DVR (DVR) system developed by the Virtual Observatory (www.aus-vo.org) and AstroGrid (www.astrogrid.org) in Australia. It can provide remote visualization of astronomical data on the Internet. DVR is based on Globus Toolkit 3 and the rendering is performed in a cluster using ShearWarp volume rendering; the rendering result is transmitted to the client side Java applet. With server side written in C++, it cannot utilize heterogeneous computing resources and the user interactivity is also constrained by the client side Java applet.

These works of grid-based visualization is somehow intuitive. Another category of grid-based visualization research focuses to bridge grid system and visualizations; in this category, special grid middlewares are developed for visualization applications to seamlessly integrate with the grid.

Develop Special Grid Middleware to Integrate Visualization and the Grid

Most visualization applications are designed without consideration of grid capability so that it is not easy for them to be integrated with grid systems and benefit from that. Developing special grid middleware is an effective approach to make visualization applications grid-enabled. With the capability of special grid middleware, visualization applications are able to be executed on grids and visualization systems are able to seamlessly integrate with other computing grid systems. VLAM-G (Belloum, 2003), GVK (Kranzlmüller, 2003), GriKSL (GridKSL) are examples of this kind of special grid middleware.

VLAM-G is a virtual laboratory middleware developed by the University of Amsterdam. It provides middleware and toolboxes for grid-based scientific computing and visualization which include user interface, session manager, collaboration support, flow manager, runtime system, and so forth. VLAM-G is based on Globus 2 to utilize its resource management and information management. Though VLAM-G is a powerful platform for virtual laboratory operation, the emphasis of it is on the integration of scientific computing and visualization. Consequently, it is natural that VLAM-G cannot support interactive visualization well.

Grid Visualization Kernel GVK from the CrossGrid project is another example of grid visualization middleware based on Globus. The concept of GVK can be divided into two main parts, the interface between the simulation and the visualization, and the implementation of the visualization pipeline. The advantage of GVK is that it enables the user to define arbitrary visualization pipeline configurations using the well-known data-flow approach. With GVK, the visualization pipeline can be split at any point, and the processing modules can be distributed across the grid as desired. GVK tried to provide universal modules for visualization applications; the published materials lack enough implementation details on this.

The GriKSL project is developed by the Albert Einstein Institute and Konrad Zuse Center for Information Technology in Germany. The GriKSL project is aimed to develop new tools and techniques to move compute-intensive applications to the Cactus environment. It concentrates on three main areas: application-oriented techniques and tools to allow scientists and developers to utilize distributed resources of the Cactus; tools and techniques which allow describing and handling really huge data sets; tools for remote and distributed data visualization which allow users to analyze and visualize simulation results in Cactus environments. The main disadvantage of GriKSL is that it focuses on integrating the scientific back-end of Cactus and the front visualization end seamlessly, thus it is tightly coupled with Cactus and can only support non-interactive visualization process.

Large-scale grids are intrinsically distributed, heterogeneous and dynamic, which engenders big challenges for building grid-based visualization systems. These characteristics of grids are not quite considered when existing visualization applications are designed and developed. On the other hand, many grid systems are designed for batch applications so that they are unable to be used for visualization applications directly. Building new grid-based visualization system gives us an opportunity to consider all these situations more deeply and comprehensively.

Build New Grid-Based Visualization System

Building new grid-based visualization system involves constructing a grid platform to integrate large scale distributed resources to support visualization, and developing new visualization applications on the grid platform with consideration of the intrinsic characteristics of grids.

Researchers at the Computational Visualization Center of University of Texas at Austin proposed a grid-enabled visualization system (CCV, 2003). Grid middleware Globus is used for resource management and data management and a grid portal is provided for access to a set of dedicated visualization servers. For real-time interactivity, CORBA connection is used between clients and visualization servers.

Bethel et al. in the Lawrence Berkeley National Laboratory (LBNL) have also done much in the field of grid-based visualization. They developed an object order visualization back-end VisaPult (Bethel, 2003) for visualization of T-bytes-sized scientific data. They made the system grid-enabled by connecting it to grid middleware Cactus. A noticeable contribution of their work is a high through-output data transfer scheme using connectionless UDP protocols. In addition, a Web-based VisPortal is developed to enable access to a rich set of visualization tools.

Grimstead et al. developed a distributed, collaborative Resource-Aware Visualization Environment (RAVE) that supports automated resource discovery across heterogeneous machines (Grimstead, 2003). RAVE runs as a background process using grid/Web services, enabling a user to share resources with other users and supports a wide range of machines. The local display device may render all, some, or none of the data set remotely, depending on its available resources. This enables scientists and engineers to collaborate on their works.

CAD & CG state key lab in Zhejiang University in China has also built a grid-based visualization system GVis (Shi, 2004; Zhao, 2004; Qiu, 2005), which aims at utilizing heterogeneous computation resources in large scale to support large dataset visualization in interactive rate and provide widespread visualization services to end users. It consists of a complete grid runtime environment (GVRE) which enables interactive visualization application to execute reliably in a grid environment, an extensible visualization framework (GVVF) with various parallel rendering methods and volume rendering algorithms implemented, and an integrated user interface (GVisPortal) for users to access GVis system remotely. GVis is fully implemented in Java™, which makes it a cross-platform system.

Compared with the other two categories of grid-based visualization systems, this category focuses more on the integrated system architecture and the construction of a grid-supporting environment for general purpose resource, task and data management.

The remainder of this chapter will focus on the research work of the last category. Building new grid-based visualization systems is the biggest challenge, while on the other hand, new grid-based visualization systems will be more powerful, efficient and practical than those that are just extended from existing visualization systems. In the next section, we will introduce the important issues and problems involved in building grid-based visualization systems.

GRID-BASED VISUALIZATION SYSTEM: GVis

Building new grid-based visualization systems is one of the most important research subjects on grid-based visualization, which is also the most challenging subject. In this section, we will introduce the important issues that must be fully considered when building a grid-based visualization system. With these issues in mind, we design and build GVis system. The architecture and detailed implementation of GVis system will be illustrated in this section.

Important Issues and Problems

Grid-based visualization systems utilize computer resources in a large-scale grid environment, where resources are always distributed, dynamic and heterogeneous. These characteristics of grid resources quite hinder researchers and developers from building efficient, reliable and stable visualization systems for scientific or medical use. However, on the other hand, scientists and doctors request high efficiency, reliability and stability of visualization systems to be able to provide effective and efficient visualization services with high interactivity. In summary, to build a grid-based visualization system, the following four important issues must be given full consideration and be resolved properly.

1. Distributed and Heterogeneous Resource Management

Grid-based visualization systems mostly distinguish themselves from traditional visualization systems by utilizing large-scale resources which are distributed and heterogeneous. The resources are often different from each other on their categories and performance. For example, some are personal computers with low performance, and some are special high-performance servers. The resources are often incompatible with each other too, holding different hardware architectures, running on different kinds of operating systems, providing different technologies and interfaces to communicate with them. Visualization task must be able to be executed on any resources if only with appropriate performance and functionality, regardless of their locations, hardware architectures and platforms. Therefore, strong resource management must be implemented to hide these underlying differences and provide open and standard interface to describe the performance and functionalities of resources.

2. Dynamic Resource Scheduling and Execution

In traditional distributed visualization systems, visualization tasks are often distributed and executed on a static group of computers. However, resources in a grid-based visualization system are intrinsically dynamic. New resources may join the visualization system to provide service at any time, while existing resources may stop working or even crash at any time. In addition, performance of resources may fluctuate more or less all the time. If some resources are no longer available or the performance of these resources becomes too low, visualization tasks executed on these resources should be migrated onto other resources dynamically. Therefore, it is not feasible and practical to partition and distribute visualization task statically. Dynamic resources mapping and scheduling mechanisms must be implemented to achieve dynamic execution of visualization task. As a practical visualization system, multi-task and multi-user support is also a necessity. The systems must enable multiple visualization tasks, which can be submitted by the same user or different users, to be executed concurrently and efficiently. Therefore, resources must be scheduled effectively to make sure the efficiency and stability of each visualization task. This is critical for a grid-enabled system to support multiple visualization tasks which may be submitted by multiple users.

3. Distributed Execution of Visualization Pipeline

A really big challenge of building a grid-based visualization system is how to apply visualization pipeline to a distributed grid environment. As described in a previous section, visualization pipeline contains three critical procedures including data preprocessing, data transformation and geometry rendering. On a single machine, it is executed as a whole and continuous data flow. But in a grid-based visualization system, usually the visualization pipeline must be partitioned and distributed onto different computers to be executed. How do you perform the partitioning of visualization pipeline? There can be two different approaches: static partitioning and dynamic partitioning. The pipeline is partitioned into several fixed stages by static approach, each of which is executed as a different component on distributed computers. While in the dynamic approach, the pipeline can be partitioned into different numbers of stages dynamically, and each of the stages can be executed on distributed computers. The dynamic approach can be more flexible and practical than the static approach, especially in grid environment. Dynamic partitioning should be performed with consideration of many important factors, such as the dataset, the performance of computation resources and user interactivity. For instance, if the data set is too large and transferring data between different resources is costly in a visualization system, it is recommended that data transformation and geometry rendering should be executed on the same resource to reduce the latency. However, dynamic approach also involves much more complexity; we should keep a good balance between flexibility and complexity. In addition, parallel computing technology is often employed within distributed visualization pipeline to improve the efficiency of each stage of the pipeline. To achieve the partitioning and execution of the visualization pipeline, efficient, flexible and robust distributed and parallel visualization algorithms must be implemented.

4. Visualization Services and Usability

The eventual goal of building a grid-based visualization system is to widely provide comprehensive visualization services to end users. Users should be able to access the visualization systems and consume the visualization services remotely and easily at distributed locations. Remote accessing is probably one of the most important capabilities of grid-based medical visualization systems. That is because in such systems, users and computation resources for visualization are usually widely distributed at different locations. The ability of visualization must be delivered to remote users and doctors as services. In addition, an intuitive user interface must be provided for users to access the services and perform visualization interactively. And the user interface should also remain consistent whenever the users access the visualization systems from Windows desktops, Linux desktops or even mobile platforms.

How to Build a Grid-Based Visualization System

With all the above considerations in mind, here we give some recommendation of building a grid-based visualization system.

First, utilize existing grid middleware such as Globus Toolkit to integrate distributed, heterogeneous and dynamic resources in a large-scale environment. With the functions provided by grid middleware, high-level user-defined services can be implemented to provide task management including task submission, task distribution, task migration, and so forth. However, most of the existing grid middleware are batch-oriented, which are designed for high latency computation-intensive applications rather than interactive applications like visualization. Therefore, grid middleware should be carefully chosen according to the requirements of visualization applications; extension of grid middleware may also need to be made to support visualization on the grid.

Second, visualization pipeline partitioning is implemented within distributed and parallel visualization architecture. An appropriate parallel rendering approach should be chosen according to the involving dataset and computation resources in a grid-based visualization system. Sometimes, a mixture of different parallel rendering approaches can benefit the system much more. The visualization architecture should be flexible and scalable enough to utilize large scale resources dynamically. At last, efficient rendering algorithms should be developed to perform underlying rendering.

Third, visualization ability can be encapsulated as standard grid services (extended Web services) and widely delivered to remote users through a grid portal (GridPort). Through the grid portal, users can easily access the visualization services remotely from their desktops at distributed locations. A grid portal can provide a consistent user interface Web sites so that the users can utilize Web browsers to communicate with the systems and perform remote visualization. However, sometimes Web applications are not provided with satisfied user interactivity which is extremely important for medical applications; in that case desktop applications can be developed in Java™ or other cross-platform languages to enable users to access the visualization systems from different platforms.

GVis Architecture

GVis is an interactive grid-based visualization system which integrates large-scale resources to achieve large dataset visualization in real time and provide end users with efficient interactive visualization services, widely. It has been fully implemented with Java™. The system is scalable, extensible, multi-task-enabled, cross-platform and easy to use.

As shown in Figure 7, GVis system consists of three components, which are GVis Runtime Environment (GVRE), GVis Visualization Framework (GVVF) and GVis user interface Portal (GVisPortal). GVRE is the underlying software infrastructure of GVis system, which is based on Globus Toolkit 3.0.; GVRE consists of four function modules to provide large-scale information management, dynamic and heterogeneous resource management, visualization task management, and centric data management. To enable visualization applications to be executed in grid environment, GVRE provides several critical mechanisms such as resource mapping, dynamic resource scheduling, visualization task distribution, task monitoring, and task migration. GVVF is a visualization framework fully implemented with Java™, which takes charge of the partitioning and execution of visualization pipeline in grid environment. It involves a distributed parallel visualization architecture in which various parallel rendering approaches and volume rendering algorithms have been implemented. GVVF is an extensible framework where new parallel rendering methods and rendering algorithms can be implemented and added into this framework. The third component, GVisPortal, is the portal of GVis system, which provides user interface for end users to consume visualization services effectively and remotely. Through GVisPortal, users can customize and submit visualization tasks, view the running status of visualization tasks, and, the most important, interact with visualization application and view the rendered data set. GVisPortal has no dependency on the detailed implementation of GVRE and GVVF. GVisPortal is also fully Java™-based, which makes it possible to run on a variety of software

Figure 7. GVis Architecture

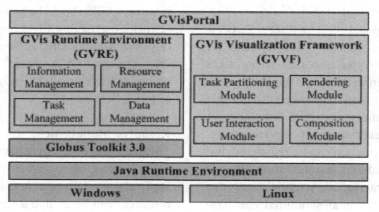

platforms and hardware architectures with a consistent UI. The three-tier architecture makes GVis a scalable and extensible visualization system, while fully Java™-based implementation makes it cross-platform and easy to deploy.

GVRE

Through extending Globus Toolkit 3.0 (GT3), GVRE is built to provide functions including information management, resource management, visualization task management and data management. GVRE provides a transparent grid environment in which interactive visualization applications can be executed efficiently and reliably. GVRE also provides mechanisms to enable user interactivity in grid applications, which is a contribution to the current batch-oriented grids.

As we mentioned in a previous section, GT3 is a general grid middleware used for construction of grid systems. GT3 provides basic mechanisms for creating and managing user-defined grid services. It also provides system-level grid services to accomplish dynamic resource management, large scale information management, and secure and reliable data management in grid environment. However, GT3 itself does not provide support for users to interact with applications in grid;

neither does it implement resource scheduling or any fault tolerant mechanism for applications to execute reliably on grid. Therefore, based on the basic services and tools provided by GT3, we create our own resource management service and task management service as an extension of GT3, which support heterogeneous resource management, dynamic resource scheduling, and reliable execution of visualization task. Through task management service, GVRE enable user interactivity of visualization application in grid environment.

Figure 8 describes the overview of GVRE. There are four different kinds of services deployed in GVRE architecture to accomplish information management, resource management, task management and data management.

Information Management

As mentioned in previous sections, a grid-based visualization system involves large scale distributed resources which are usually dynamic and heterogeneous. Resources can be different in their hardware architectures, software platforms, functionalities and performance. Resources are also dynamic so that new resources can join in and existing resources can exit at any time. How do you make a visualization system aware of this information so that it can perform adjustments according to the change?

In GVRE, a global directory service, GVis Information Index Service (GIIS) is built for resource discovery and resources query. GIIS keeps the information of all live resources, such as CPU architecture and frequency, OS name and version, main memory size, hard disk capacity, video memory size and acceleration performance. The resource information can be registered, un-registered, updated and searched through a set of well-defined interfaces. Actually, GIIS also keeps the information of all submitted visualization tasks such as the resources being involved in executing the task, the status of the task, and so forth, which can be used to measure the load of the system and to help achieve efficient task management (refer to Task Management).

As GVis system may utilize a huge number of resources, GIIS should be provided with capabilities of high reliability, high concurrency and quick response. Additionally, GIIS must be scalable with the scale-up of GVis system. By reason of this, we build GIIS using LDAP (OpenLDAP) instead of Index Service in GT3.

Resource Management

The main goal of resource management is to hide heterogeneity of resources from visualization applications. Through resource management, resources can be used in a standard way, so that resources can be shared among different organizations effectively and easily (Czajkowski, 1999). In GVis system, resources exist as grid services, which is consistent with the OGSA architecture model. Resources can be used by invoking in-

Figure 8. Overview of GVRE architecture

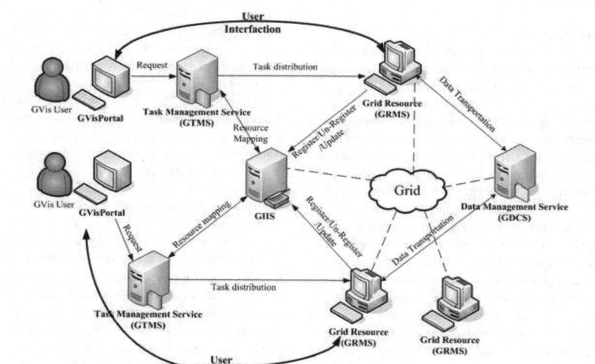

terfaces of grid services. In GVRE, we develop GVis Resource Management Service (GRMS) and deploy GRMS on each resource to manage this resource in a grid environment. GRMS is responsible for collecting resource information, registering, unregistering and updating resource information to GIIS. GRMS dealing with requests for resource utilization from visualization applications then validates and schedules these requests. After a request has been accepted and scheduled, the corresponding visualization application will be launched on the resource and managed by GRMS.

Task Management

Task management is the core component of GVRE. It provides several key functions and mechanisms. First, it provides a mechanism to describe a visualization task. With this mechanism, visualization task is strictly described with a Task Request Specification (TRS) file which is in XML format. A TRS file usually has a content of resources requirement, and execution arguments of a visualization task, such as parallel rendering approach, rendering algorithm, and so forth. Second, after a visualization task is submitted, task management will parse the TRS file and perform automatic resource mapping according to the resource requirement in TRS file. Third, visualization task will be partitioned and distributed to selected resources by this module. After the task has been accepted and distributed successfully, a task session will be created to save information such as the resource requirement and execution arguments of this task. The resources involved in the execution of this task and the status of this task are also saved in the task session. Actually, task session information is updated and synchronized to GIIS every a few minutes. Fourth, an interactive connection between user client and visualization task is established for the user to interact and view the result. Last but not least, task management takes charge of task monitoring of the current task and performs task migration if the resources

involved in the execution of this task encounter special problems, such as low performance or system crash. Task migration is a very important feature of a GVis system, which makes the system much more fault-tolerant and much more reliable. Based on these aforementioned functions, task management enables multiple task support in a GVis system.

Task management is performed by GVis Task Management Service (GTMS) which is deployed on special servers in a GVis system. There may be multiple GTMS in a GVis system to make the system capable of dealing with a number of requests and enable multi-task support.

Data Management

The data management component is always an integrant part of large-scale distributed system. In a GVis system, data management is provided to store large visualization datasets and transport data between distributed resources dynamically. GVRE contains a centralized data center, GVis Data Center Service (GDCS), which performs the functions of data management. After a visualization task starts to be executed, a visualization application will send requests for data transporting from the data center to the computation resource to be rendered.

Centralized data management makes functions including data storing, data updating and data synchronizing much easier to implement, which also makes execution of a visualization task easy to distribute.

GVVF

GVRE provides underlying functions for visualization applications to execute on dynamic and heterogeneous resources efficiently and reliably, but not visualization applications themselves. Visualization applications are developed in GVVF.

As we mentioned in foregoing sections, a big challenge for building a grid-based visualization system is how to apply visualization pipeline into a grid environment. We achieve this target by GVVF. GVVF is a visualization framework which implements different kinds of parallel rendering approaches and different kinds of volume rendering algorithms to perform partitioning and execution of visualization pipeline. In GVVF, traditional pipeline is expanded and partitioned into four parts and then distributed onto different resource nodes to execute, as illustrated in Figure 8. Four function modules are involved in the execution of visualization pipeline in GVVF, each of which is executed on a different kind of resource node and all together to finish a visualization task.

Partitioning Module

A partitioning module is running on a task partitioning resource node, which performs task partitioning according to the execution arguments of visualization task including parallel rendering approaches and rendering algorithms. It acts as a coordinator in the whole execution process of a task, which makes the decision of choosing rendering nodes and composition nodes from a list

of resource candidates. It will also decide how to partition the visualization task according to the performance of each rendering nodes dynamically. Currently, two kinds of partition methods are supported by the partitioning module: screen space partitioning and object space partitioning, which are corresponding to sort-first and sort-last parallel rendering approaches, correspondingly.

Rendering Module

The rendering module is running on rendering resource nodes. Usually, a number of rendering nodes are involved in a task to perform parallel rendering to achieve high efficiency and low latency. The rendering module will get its partial work of the whole task from the partitioning module and then perform rendering to get a partial image. When the task is partitioned by screen space method, each rendering module will render part of the ultimate image. On the other hand, if the task is partitioned by object space method, each rendering module will render part of the object dataset. The rendering algorithm to be used is chosen by the partitioning module according to execution arguments of the visualization task.

Figure 8. Distributed visualization pipeline in GVVF

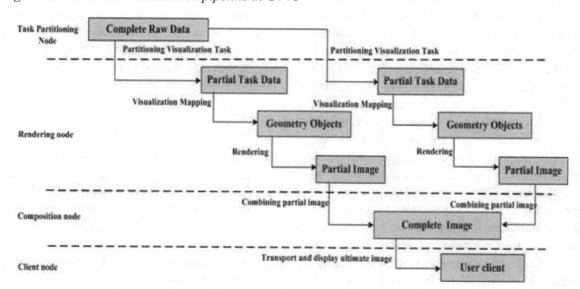

Currently, only two different volume rendering algorithms are supported, 2D and 3D hardware texture-based direct volume rendering methods. However, additional volume rendering and surfacing rendering algorithms can be implemented and integrated into GVVF easily.

Composition Module

In the third step of the pipeline, partial image from rendering nodes will be combined into ultimate image. Usually only one composition node is involved in visualization task due to the cost and latency caused by composition. The same as that of rendering module, to use which composition algorithm also depends on which parallel rendering approach is used. If screen space method is adopted at the task partitioning step, then composition is just a simple step to join partial images from different rendering modules into a whole complete image. On the other hand, if object space method is adopted when a task is partitioned, composition involves recombining the rendered frames from different rendering modules to generate the complete image.

User Interaction Module

The user interaction module is running on the client node where users access the GVis system and perform remote visualization. Through this module, users can view the final image of visualization and interact with visualization task. The user's input are received by this module and transferred to the composition module to rendering modules to perform interactive visualization. At the same time, a complete visualization image generated by composition module is transported to this module and displayed to users. The connection between user interaction module and composition module is established after the visualization task begins to execute. Actually, the connection is part of the task session of current task which is created by GTMS (see Task management). This architecture is ready to support shared visualization of a data set among multiple users.

GVisPortal

GVisPortal provides a portal for users to access the GVis system and perform visualization remotely and collaboratively on their desktops. It implements a unified user interface for end users to perform two different kinds of interaction. First, through the user interface, users can customize and submit a visualization task, view session information of a visualization task, and terminate a visualization task. Second, through the user interface, users can interact with a visualization task. When the task is executing, users can modify execution arguments of current visualization task, and view visualization results such as moving, zooming and rotating image. Figure 10 is a snapshot of GVisPortal user interface.

Besides the unified user interface, an API is also developed in GVisPortal for external applications to access visualization service in GVis system, which facilitates the integration of GVis system with other systems.

Instead of a Web-based grid portal, GVisPortal is implemented as a Java application running on client nodes, which provides strong supports for users to access a GVis system and perform interactive visualization which is extremely important for medical applications. Full implementation with Java™ makes GVisPortal a cross-platform portal, which can be easily deployed and executed on many important platforms, such as Windows and Linux.

Workflow of a GVis System

In this section, we introduced the architecture of a GVis system, which consists of three main components: GVRE, GVVF and GVisPortal. The following figure describes the overview of a GVis system and illustrates how these components work together.

First, GVRE is the underlying runtime environment which provides the management of resources, information, task, and data in

Figure 10. User interface of GVisPortal

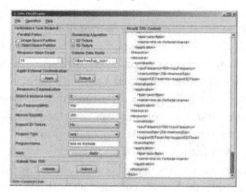
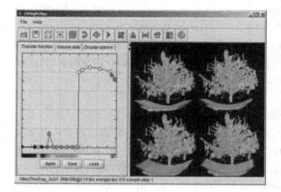

Figure 11. Overview of GVis system workflow

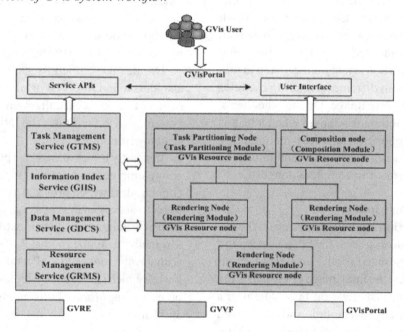

GVis system. Visualization services are also implemented and managed by GVRE. Second, GVisPortal provides an end user interface for users to access the GVis system and to submit visualization tasks. After a visualization task is submitted, the task description file will be parsed for resource mapping, and then visualization programs implemented in GVVF will be launched on the selected resources to execute the task. Users are able to communicate and interact with the visualization program and view the final image through GVisPortal.

GVis Implementation

In a previous section, we mentioned that several important issues should be considered when building a grid-based visualization system. In this section, we will illustrate the detailed implementation of the GVis system and see how the important issues are handled within the implementation.

Heterogeneous and Dynamic Resource Management

In GVRE, we develop a standard grid service, GRMS, to manage resource in a GVis system. With this grid service deployed on each resource, heterogeneity of resources is hidden from visualization applications. Instead, standard interfaces of a grid service are exposed and can be invoked by resource users. For example, resource information such as architecture, functionality and performance can be obtained by invoking the grid service interface exported by GRMS. Request for resource utilizing can also be performed by standard interface invoking. In this way, resource can be used in a standard way regardless of its architecture, platform, and its location.

GRMS also collects information and current state of resource and saves them in GIIS. With information and the state of all live resources in GIIS, the GVis system is able to map and use the resource effectively although the resource is dynamic.

Dynamic Resource Mapping

It is difficult to select resources to execute a visualization application statically in a large scale environment. Resources are dynamic and may change their status quickly in a grid system. Through the task management service (GTMS) in GVRE, dynamic resource mapping is performed to match and select resources automatically for a visualization task. Users just need to specify the number of resource and performance requirements of each resource in a TRS file when submitting a visualization task. GTMS contains a TRS parser to parse the file to obtain the resource requirement. After that, GTMS performs resource mapping according to the resource requirement for the task with resource information in GIIS, then partitions the visualization task into different parts and launches the visualization application on selected resources to execute the visualization

task. Dynamic resource mapping makes it possible to distribute and execute visualization applications in the GVis system dynamically.

Task Migration

Resources involved in the execution of a visualization task may stop working due to low performance, network failure or system crash. In that case, visualization task should be migrated to other resources. GTMS provides corresponding mechanisms to achieve this feature. First, after a visualization task is accepted and distributed to resources to execute, a task session will be created to hold and manage information of this task, such as resource requirement, execution arguments and current resources involved in this task. The task session information will also be synchronized into GIIS. Second, GTMS will monitor the performance and status of each resource involved in this task. A situation such as low performance or no response of resources will be detected by GTMS. On detecting these exceptions, GTMS will select other resources according to the resource requirement of this task and finish the migration.

Task migration is a very important feature of GVis system, which makes the system much more fault tolerant and reliable. Together with dynamic resource mapping, task migration mechanism effectively handles the second issue of building grid-based visualization system—dynamic resource scheduling and execution.

Distributed Visualization Pipeline

GVVF implements a distributed visualization pipeline to visualize a large dataset with multiple resources in GVis system. The pipeline is partitioned and distributed to different resources to execute in parallel. Several optimizations have been applied in the implementation of distributed a visualization pipeline for high efficiency and low latency.

A visualization pipeline is not partitioned between data to geometry transformation and geometry rendering because geometry data is usually very large. It is costly to transfer this data on a network between different resources, which will result in a high latency for interactive visualization.

The entire visualization task is partitioned into several units, appropriately, according to the performance of each rendering unit, no matter what parallel rendering approach is applied. In screen space method, the ultimate screen space is divided into different parts according to the rendering capability of each rendering unit. On the other hand, in object space method, the object database is divided into different parts. Load balance among rendering units can be achieved with this method to improve the efficiency.

High performance rendering algorithms including 2D and 3D hardware texture-based direct volume rendering are developed with JOGL (JOGL) in GVVF to perform underlying rendering. As we know, in a visualization system, most of the computation time is spent on rendering. Therefore, performance of the underlying rendering algorithms will highly affect the efficiency of the visualization pipeline.

Data transferring between different modules in GVVF is implemented with Java NIO Socket Channel (J2SDK) directly to reduce the latency.

Access Visualization Services with GVisPortal

Visualization services are built within GVis system through GVRE and GVVF and provided to end users through GVisPortal. A service APIs and an ultimate user interface are implemented in GVisPortal. Users can either develop applications to access the visualization services with the service APIs or access the services with the end user interface directly. GVisPortal is running on client desktops for end users to access the GVis system remotely. In addition, GVisPortal enables users to submit multiple visualization tasks, manage these tasks and interact with them respectively.

GVisPortal is fully developed with Java, which makes it easy for users to access the GVis system on different platforms, such as Windows and Linux.

GVis Testbed and Result

To test the effectiveness of our solutions of building a grid-based visualization system, we built a testbed for the GVis system and carried out several experiments on the GVis system. The results show that GVis can be well used for distributed and collaborative visualization including medical applications.

The testbed contains three types of computer nodes which are connected with each other by campus network in Zhejiang University in China, as illustrated in Figure 12. The first part contains eight PC nodes and one server node in CAD & CG lab of Zhejiang University. Each of these computer nodes is connected into campus network by a 100Mibts/s network interface. The second part is a high-performance PC cluster with 32 nodes. Computer nodes in the PC cluster are connected with each other by a gigabits network, where the peak bandwidth between every two computer nodes can reach 3GBits/s. The PC cluster is connected into the campus network by a 100Mibts/s network interface. The last part is a remote client PC connected to campus network with 10Mibts/s network interface. The GVis system is deployed on these computer nodes.

Different kinds of operating systems are installed on the computer nodes in our testbed, including Windows XP, Windows 2003 Server, Debian/GNU Linux and Redhat Linux. J2SDK (J2SDK) 1.4.2_08 is installed on each of these computer nodes for Java™ applications to execute.

Table 1 contains the detailed information of our testbed.

Within the testbed, several experiments are carried out on the GVis system with different

Figure 12. Testbed for GVis system

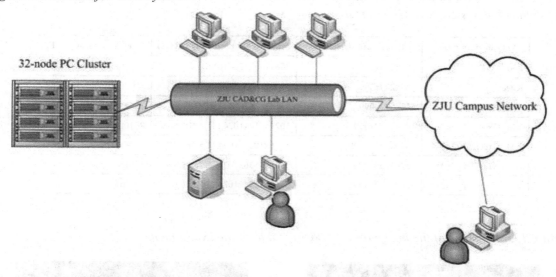

Table 1 Resource nodes in the testbed for the GVis system

Parameters	Lab PC nodes	Lab Server Node	PC Cluster Nodes	Remote Client PC Node
CPU	Intel P4 2.4G	Dual Intel P4 2.4G	Dual Intel P4 2.4G	Celeron 1.2G
Main Memory	512MB	1GB	1GB	245MB
Video Card	Nvidia 5700LE	Nvidia 5950	Nvidia 5950	S3 ProSavage
Video Memory	128MB	256MB	256MB	16MB (Share)
Network Interface	100Mbps	1000Mbps	1000Mbps x3	10Mbps
OS	Windows / Linux	Redhat Linux	Windows 2003 Server	Windows XP
Java Version	J2SDK1.4.2_08	J2SDK1.4.2_08	J2SDK1.4.2_08	J2SDK1.4.2_08

sizes of visualization datasets. In the experiments, users access the GVis system from one of the lab PC nodes and the remote client PC. The following table contains the detailed information of the experiment's results. We use foot and knee data set to show how the GVis system can support medial applications. Additionally, to acquire huge datasets, we use arrays of the christmas tree data sets, as shown in Table 2.

As a grid-based distributed platform, GVis can also support multi-task visualization and collaborative visualization. As shown in Figure 14, multiple medical visualization tasks can be

submitted and run with GVis. In the same manner, shared view and control of the same dataset from different sites can be easily supported by GVis, which means collaborative visualization of large volume datasets can be achieved with the GVis system.

From the results, we can see that the GVis system enables large datasets to be visualized in real time and provide the capability for users to interact with the visualization remotely and collaboratively, even from a computer with very low performance to perform local visualization, such as the remote client PC node in our testbed.

Table 2. Result of the experiments (The interactive FPS data is collected on the client nodes where users access the GVis system with GVisPortal)

Volume data name	Volume data size (Bytes)	Memory for rendering (Bytes)	Average interactive FPS
Foot	256x256x256	256x256x256 (16MB)	15~20fps
Knee	379x229x305	512x256x512 (64MB)	15~20fps
XMasTree	512x512x999	512x512x1024 (256MB)	10~15fps
XMasTreeDup_2x1x1	1024x512x999	1024x512x1024 (512MB)	8~10fps
XMasTreeDup_3x2x1	1536x1024x999	1536x1024x1024 (1.5GB)	3~5fps
XMasTreeDup_3x3x1	1536x1536x999	1536x1536x1024 (2.25GB)	3~5fps
XMasTreeDup_5x3x1	2660x1536x999	2660x1536x1024 (3.75GB)	2~3fps

Figure 13. Snapshots of the image on the GVisPortal from the experiments

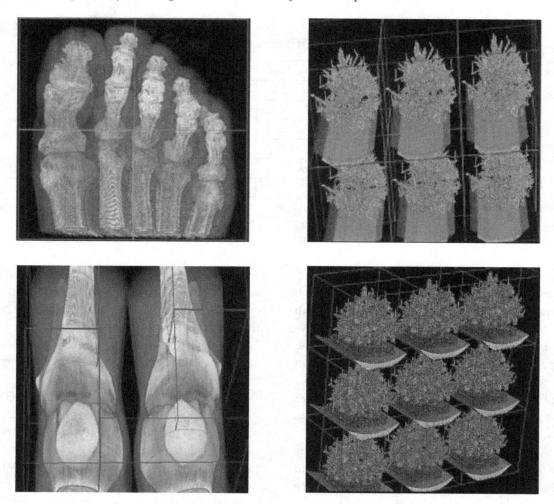

Figure 14. Screen snapshot to show that multiple medical visualization tasks can be launched and run from the GVis system

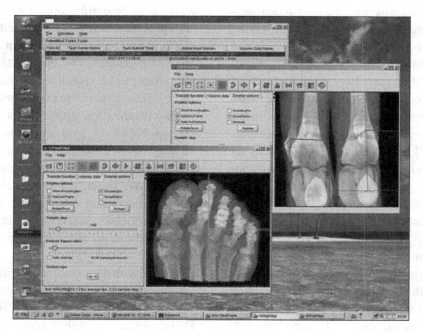

CONCLUSION

In this chapter, we first introduced the basic concept and techniques in visualization field, and then we presented big challenges faced by visualization. The emerging grid infrastructure and technologies show its high potential to deal with these challenges, which favors a new research direction in both grid and visualization fields. We also introduced the research work that has been done in this new field in recent years, among which the most important category is building new grid-based visualization systems. Several important issues should be considered when building a grid-based visualization system, such as heterogeneous resource management in large scale, dynamic resource scheduling, distributed execution of visualization pipeline and comprehensive visualization services. However,

interactive visualization on the grid requires some extensions to existing grid middleware and technologies. We present a grid-based visualization system, GVis, which was built in ZJU CAD lab, to look through the solutions to deal with these issues and problems.

GVis is a scalable and extensible grid-based visualization system which integrates distributed resources in large scale to achieve large dataset visualization in interactive rate and provide reliable interactive visualization services to end users, widely. It is a fully Java™-based system with a cross-platform feature. In GVis, we built our own task management services as an extension to GT3 to support interactivity and fault tolerance on the grid so that interactive visualization can be performed reliably in GVis.

A testbed was built in ZJU CAD lab to experiment the effectiveness of the GVis system. The results of our experiments show that grid-based visualization is capable of dealing with large dataset visualization by utilizing distributed computation resources in large scale and providing real time interactivity for end users, which can be effectively applied to medical fields. Grid-based visualization can also extend the scale of providing visualization services. Future work in the GVis system field includes scaling up the range of utilizing resource and providing service, enabling more kinds of rendering algorithms for visualization, and providing more usability for end users.

Future Research Directions

The rapid advancement in medical and scientific areas brings big challenges into the visualization field, such as large dataset visualization particularly in interactive rate, and large scale collaborative visualization. The emergence of grid infrastructure and related technologies encourage people to explore new approaches to take the challenges, which results in a new research direction—grid-based visualization. With much successful experience having been gained in the past, we expect that future research work in this field will focus on the following issues.

First, grid-based visualization will rely on data grid infrastructure to accomplish data integration. Today, huge data for visualization is being generated in a large range of applications around the world, and the same is in the future. These distributed data around the world tend to be used in a more cooperative way to solve hard problems across different domains. For instance, medical imagery from different organizations can be utilized together for more efficient and accurate medical diagnosis. Therefore, data grid infrastructure will be involved in grid-based visualization to accomplish reliable data storing, efficient and secure data transportation in a large-scale environment.

Second, there is an increasing trend that visualization will integrate with scientific computing on the grid. Scientific computing and simulation activities are being transplanted onto a grid platform and benefiting from that. However, the huge data generated by these activities are usually unable to be visualized immediately online for scientists to perform computational steering. With visualization applications being moved onto grid platform, grid-based visualization will be able to provide seamless integration between scientific computing and visualization directly on the gird. We should notice that this integration does not mean that visualization itself will able to be performed in real time. To achieve that, new visualization algorithms and techniques must be developed on the grid.

Third, with data, computational resources and visualization devices being gathered by the grid, the ways of people performing visualization will also change accordingly. Users will be more likely to perform remote visualization since enormous data are beyond the capabilities of local resource and must be performed on remote resources in the grid. Users will have many more chances to work together on visualization since data, computational resources and visualization devices can be shared across different organizations on the grid. Grid-based visualization systems must be capable of providing such an integration platform for users to do remote and collaborative visualization work, and to exchange their ideas, information and knowledge in visualization.

Fourth, future visualization tends to be user-centric, which is especially true for medical visualization. Therefore, more attention must be paid to usability in grid-based visualization. As the grid promises to provide consistent and pervasive services to end users, grid-based visualization systems must enable users to access persistent visualization services at any time, from any distributed locations, and with any devices. Consistent user experience should be enabled in these systems whenever users consume the visualization services from their desktops or even mobile devices. Intuitive user interfaces should be provided in these systems for more effective understanding and exploration of data. The systems will also need to enable stable services so that users can stop and then continue their visualization work at a later time, from a different location or with different collaborators.

Although grid-based visualization is still in its early stage, we believe, with the increasing maturity of grid infrastructure and technologies, that grid-based visualization will be the right way to bring people into the future of visualization.

ACKNOWLEDGMENT

We would like to thank Dr. Wei Chen for his kind help on the project, Ms. Yaping Zhang for some experimental results in this chapter, and Mr. Ke Yang for the English proofreading.

The work in this chapter is supported by the National Grand Fundamental Research 973 Program of China (No. 2002CB312105, No. 2003CB716104) and the National Natural Science Foundation Key Project of "Digital Olympic Museum" of China (No. 60533080).

REFERENCES

Aeschlimann, M., Dinda, P., Kallivokas, L., López, J., Lowekamp, B., & O'Hallaron, D. (1999). Preliminary report on the design of a framework for distributed isualization. *Proceedings of the International Conference on Parallel and Distributed Processing Techniques and Applications* (PDPTA'99). Las Vegas, NV.

Belloum, A., Groep, D., Hendrikse, Z., Hertzberger, B., Korkhov, V., et al. (2003). VLAM-G: A grid-based virtual laboratory. *Future Generation Computer Systems, 19*(2), 209-217.

Berman, F., Fox, G., & Hey, T. (2002). Grid computing—making the global infrastructure a reality. John Wiley & Sons, Ltd.

Bethel, E., & Shalf, J. (2003). Cactus and visapult: An ultra-high performance grid-distributed visualization architecture using connectionless protocols. *IEEE Computer Graphics and Applications, 23*(2), 51-59.

Cabral, B., Cam, N., & Foran, J. (1994). Accelerated volume rendering and tomographic reconstruction using texture mapping hardware. *Proceedings of the 1994 Symposium on Volume Visualization,* (pp. 91-98). New York, NY: ACM Press.

Cactus. http://www.cactuscode.org.

Center for Computational Visualization of University of Texas at Austin. (2003). Grid- enabled visualization. Poster of NPACI All-hands Meeting. San Diego, CA.

Coleman, J., Goettsch, A., Savchenko, A., Kollmann, H., Wang, K., Klement, E., & Bono, P. (1996). TeleInViVoTM: Towards collaborative volume visualization environments. *Computers & Graphics, 20*(6), 801-811.

Condor. http://www.cs.wisc.edu/condor/.

Cullip, T., & Neumann, U. (1993). *Accelerating volume reconstruction with 3D texture mapping hardware.* Chapel Hill, NC: University of North Carolina.

Czajkowski, K., Foster, I., & Kesselman, C. (1999). Resource co-allocation in computational grids. *Proceedings of the 8th IEEE International Symposium on High Performance Distributed Computing* (HPDC-8), (pp. 219-228).

DCE. http://www.opengroup.org/dce/.

DoE Department of Energy Science Grid. http://www.doesciencegird.org.

Drebin, R., Carpenter, L., & Hanrahan, P. (1988). Volume rendering. *Computer Graphics, 22*(4), 65-73.

DVR. http://www.aus-vo.org/soft_dvr.html.

e-Science. http://www.e-science.clrc.ac.uk and http://www.escience-grid.org.uk/.

FAFNER. http://www.npac.syr.edu/factoring.html.

Foster, I., Geisler, J., Nickless, W., Smith, W., & Tuecke, S. (1997). Software infrastructure for the I-WAY high performance distributed computing experiment. *Proceedings of the 5th IEEE Symposium on High Performance Distributed Computing,* (pp. 562-571).

Foster, I., & Kesselman, C. (1999). *The grid: Blueprint for a new computing infrastructure.* San Francisco, CA: Morgan Kaufmann.

Foster, I., Kesselman, C., & Tuecke, S. (2001). The anatomy of the grid: Enabling scalable virtual organizations. *International J. Supercomputer Applications, 15*(3).

Foster, I., Kesselman, C., Nick, J., & Tuecke, S. (2002). The physiology of the grid: An open grid services architecture for distributed systems integration. *Open Grid Service Infrastructure WG, Global Grid Forum.*

Foster, I., & Kesselman, C. (2003). *The grid 2: Blueprint for a new computing infrastructure.* San Francisco, CA: Morgan Kaufmann Publishers.

Fuchs, H., Levoy, M., & Pizer, S. (1989). Interactive visualization of 3D medical data. *IEEE Computer,* 46-50.

Global Grid Forum. http://www.ggf.org.

Gilder, G. (2002). *Gilder's law on network performance. Telecosm: The world after bandwidth abundance.* Touchstone Books.

The Globus Projects. http://www.globus.org.

GriKSL. http://www.aei.mpg.de/~tradke/GriKSL/.

Gridport. http://gridport.net/main.

Grimshaw, A., Wulf, W., et al. (1997). The legion visio of a worldwide virtual computer. *Communications of the ACM, 40*(1).

Grimstead, I., Avis, N., & Walker D. (2003). Automatic distribution of rendering workloads in a grid-enabled collaborative visualization environment. *Proceedings of the 2004 ACM/IEEE conference on Supercomputing.*

gViz. http://www.visualization.leeds.ac.uk/gViz/.

Haber, R., & McNabb, D. (1990). Visualization idioms: A conceptual model for scientific visualization systems. In: G. Nielson, B. Shriver, & L. Rosenblum (Eds.), *Visualization in scientific computing,* (pp.74-93). Los Alamitos, NM: IEEE Computer Society Press.

Hadwiger, M., Berger, C., & Hauser, H. (2003). High-quality two-level volume rendering of segment data sets on consumer graphics hardware. *Proceedings of the IEEE Visualization 2003 Conference,* (pp. 301-308).

Herman, G., & Liu, H. (1979). Three-dimensional display of human organs from computer tomograms. *Computer Graphics and Image Processing, 9*(1), 1-21.

JavaTM 2 SDK. Standard edition documentation version 1.4.2 http://java.sun.com/j2se/1.4.2/docs.

JOGL. Java-openGL binding. https://jogl.dev.java.net/.

Kaufman, A. (1991). *Volume visualization.* IEEE Computer Society Press.

Kaufman, A. (1997). Volume visualization: Principles and advances. *Proceedings of SIGGRAPH.* Los Angeles, CA.

Knosp, B., Wang, S., & Ni, J. (2002). Grid-based volume rendering. *Proceedings of the International Conference of Supercomputing*. Baltimore, MD.

Kranzlmüller, D., Heinzlreiter, P., & Volkert, J. (2003). Grid-enabled visualization with GVK. *Proceedings of 1st European Across Grids Conference 2003*. Santiago, Spain.

Lacroute, P., & Levoy, M. (1994). Fast volume rendering using a shear-warp factorization of the viewing transformation. *Proceedings of ACM SIGGRAPH'94* (pp. 451-458). New York, NY: ACM Press.

Legion. http://www.cs.virginia.edu/~legion/.

Levoy, M. (1988). Display of surfaces from volume data. *IEEE Computer Graphics and Applications, 8*(3), 29-37.

Lorenson, W., & Cline, H. (1987). Marching cubes: A high resolution 3D surface construction algorithm. *Computer Graphics (Proceedings of SIGGRAPH`87), 21*(4), 163-169.

Lum, E., & Ma, K. (2002). Hardware-accelerated parallel non-photorealistic volume rendering. *Proceeding of NPAR 2002 Symposium on Non-Photorealistic Animation and Rendering,* (pp. 67-75).

Molnar, S., Cox, M., Ellsworth, D., & Fuchs, H. (1994). A sorting classification of parallel rendering. *IEEE Computer Graphics and Applications, 14*(4), 23-32.

Moore's Law as Explained by Intel. http://www.intel.com/research/silicon/mooreslaw.htm.

Message Passing Interface. http://www.mpi-forum.org/.

Nielson, G., & Hamann, B. (1999). Techniques for the interactive visualization of volumetric data. *Proceeding of IEEE Visualization 1999 Conference,* (pp. 45-50).

The Open Grid Services Architecture. http://www.globus.org/ogsa/.

Open Grid Services Infrastructure (OGSI) Version 1.0. S. Tuecke, Czajkowski K., Foster, I., Frey, J., Graham, S., Kesselman, C., Maguire, T., Sandholm, T., Vanderbilt, P., Snelling, D.; Global Grid Forum Draft Recommendation, 6/27/2003.

OpenLDAP. http://www.openldap.org.

Pekar, V., Wiemker, R., & Hempel, D. (2001). Fast detection of meaningful isosurfaces for volume data visualization. In: T. Ertl, K. Joy, & A. Varshney (Eds.), *Proceedings of IEEE Visualization 2001,* (pp. 223-230).

Qiu, Y., Shi, J., Zhao, Y., & Chen, W. (2005). GVis: An architecture for grid-enabled interactive parallel visualization. *Proceedings of the 5th Conference on Virtual Reality and Visualization 2005* (CCVRV'05). Bejing, China (in Chinese). *Journal of Computer Research and Development, 42,* Supplement A, 612-617.

Russell, G., & Miles, R. (1987). Display and perception of 3D space filling data. *Applied Optics, 26*(6), 973-982.

Shi, J., & Cai, W. (1995). *Algorithms and systems of scientific visualization*. Science Press (in Chinese).

Shi, J., Zhao, Y., Qiu, Y., & Chen, W. (2004). A case study on grid-enabled visualization. *Journal of Computer Research and Development, 41*(2), 2231-2236 (in Chinese).

Simple Object Access Protocol (SOAP). http://www.w3.org/TR/soap/.

Tenginakai, S., Lee, J., & Machiraju, R. (2001). Salient iso-surface detection with model-independent statistical signatures. In: T. Ertl, K. Joy, & A. Varshney (Eds.), *Proceedings of IEEE Visualization 2001,* (pp. 231-238).

UDDI.org. http://www.uddi.org/.

Udupa, J., & Herman G. (1989). Volume rendering vs. surface rendering. *Communication of ACM, 32,* 1344-1366.

Web Service. http://www.w3.org/2002/ws/.

Westover, L. (1990). Footprint evaluation for volume rendering. *Proceedings of SIGGRAPH'90. ACM SIGGRAPH Computer Graphics, 24*(4), 367-376.

Web Services Description Language. http://www.w3.org/TR/wsdl/.

Web Services Flow Language (WSFL 1.0). (2001). Frank Leymann, IBM Software Group. http://www-306.ibm.com/software/solutions/webservices/pdf/WSFL.pdf.

Web Service Resource Framework. http://www.globus.org/wsrf/.

Zhao, Y., Chen, W., Qiu, Y., & Shi, J. (2004). GVis: A Java-based architecture for grid- enabled interactive visualization. *Proceedings of the 3rd international conference on grid and cooperative computing- GCC. Lecture Notes in Computer Science, 3252,* 704-711. Wuhan, China: Springer-Verlag.

Additional Reading

The following additional readings are highly recommended for understanding the background and technology described in this chapter.

Belloum, A., Groep, D., Hendrikse, Z., Hertzberger, B., Korkhov, V., et al. (2003). VLAM-G: A grid-based virtual laboratory. *Future Generation Computer Systems, 19*(2) 209-217.

Berman, F., Fox, G., & Hey, T. (2002). Grid computing—Making the global infrastructure a reality. John Wiley & Sons, Ltd.

Bethel, E., & Shalf, J. (2003). Cactus and visapult: An ultra-high performance grid-distributed visualization architecture using connectionless protocols. *IEEE Computer Graphics and Applications, 23*(2), 51-59.

Brodlie, K., Duce, D., Gallop, J., Walton, J., & Wood, J. (2004). Distributed and collaborative visualization. *Computer Graphics Forum, 23*(2), 223-251.

Buyya, R. (2001). The virtual laboratory project: Molecular modeling for drug design on grid. *IEEE Distributed System Online, 2(*5).

Center for Computational Visualization of University of Texas at Austin. (2003). Grid- enabled visualization. *Poster of NPACI All-hands Meeting.* San Diego, CA.

Charters, S., Holliman, N., & Munro, M. (2003). Visualization in e-demand: A grid service architecture for stereoscopic visualization. *Proceedings of UK e-Science Second All Hands Meeting.*

Chervenak, A., Foster, I., Kesselman, C., Salisbury, C., & Tuecke, S. (2001). The data grid: Towards an architecture for the distributed management and analysis of large scientific datasets. *Journal of Network and Computer Applications, 23,* 187-200.

E-Science. http://www.e-science.clrc.ac.uk and http://www.escience-grid.org.uk/.

EuroGrid project. http://www.eurogrid.org.

Foster, I. (2005). Service-oriented science. *Science, 308*(May).

Foster, I., Kesselman, C. (1999). *The grid: Blueprint for a new computing infrastructure.* San Francisio, CA: Morgan Kaufmann.

Foster, I., & Kesselman, C. (2003). *The grid 2: Blueprint for a new computing infrastructure.* San Francisco, CA: Morgan Kaufmann Publishers.

Foster, I., Kesselman, C., Nick, J., & Tuecke, S. (2002). The physiology of the grid: An open grid services architecture for distributed systems integration. *Proceedings of the Open Grid Service Infrastructure WG, Global Grid Forum.*

Foster, I., Kesselman, C., & Tuecke, S. (2001). The anatomy of the grid: Enabling scalable virtual organizations. *International J. Supercomputer Applications, 15*(3).

Grimstead, I., Avis, N., Walker, D. (2004). Automatic distribution of rendering workloads in a grid-enabled collaborative visualization environment. *Proceedings of the 2004 ACM/IEEE conference on Supercomputing.*

Java-OpenGL Binding. https://jogl.dev.java.net/.

Knosp, B., Wang. S., & Ni, J. (2002). Grid-based volume rendering. *Proceedings of the International Conference of Supercomputing.* Baltimore, MD.

Kranzlmüller, D., & Heinzlreiter, P. (2003). Visualization services on the grid—the grid visualization kernel. *Parallel Processing Letters, 13*(2), 125-148.

Kranzlmüller, D., Heinzlreiter, P., & Volkert, J. (2003). Grid-enabled visualization with GVK. *Proceedings of 1ˢᵗ European Across Grids Conference.* Santiago, Spain.

Kranzlmüller, D., Rosmanith, H., Heinzlreiter, P., & Polk, M. (2004). Interactive virtual reality on the grid. *Proceeding of the 8ᵗʰ IEEE International Symposium on Distributed Simulation and Real-Time Applications* (DS-RT'04). IEEE.

Shalf, J., & Wes Bethel, E. (2003). The grid and future visualization system architectures. *Proceeding of IEEE Computer Graphics and Applications.*

The Global Grid Forum. http://www.gridforum.org.

The Globus project. http://www.globus.org.

Zhao, Y., Chen, W., Qiu, Y., & Shi J. (2004). GVis: A Java-based architecture for grid- enabled interactive visualization. *Proceedings of the 3ʳᵈ international conference on grid and cooperative computing - GCC. Lecture Notes in Computer Science, 3252,* 704-711. Wuhan, China: Springer-Verlag.

Chapter III
Reporting Clinical Gait Analysis Data

Raymond White
Sunderland University, UK

Robert Noble
The Robert Gordon University, UK

ABSTRACT

Gait analysis is a special investigation that can assist clinical staff in the decision making process regarding treatment options for patients with walking difficulties. Interpretation of gait analysis data recorded from 3D motion capture systems is a time consuming and complex process. This chapter describes techniques and a software program that can be used to simplify interpretation of gait data. It can be viewed with an interactive display and a gait report can be produced more quickly with the key results highlighted. This will allow referring clinicians to integrate the relevant gait measurements and observations and to formulate the patient treatment plan. Although an abbreviated analysis may be useful for clinicians, a full explanation with the key features highlighted is helpful for movement scientists. Visualization software has been developed that directs the clinician and scientist to the relevant parts of the data simplifying the analysis and increasing insight.

INTRODUCTION

Gait analysis is the systematic measurement, description and assessment of those quantities thought to characterize human bipedal locomotion (Davis et al., 1991). Kinematic, kinetic, electro-myographic (EMG) and temporo-spatial data of the subject is acquired and analyzed during the gait analysis process. Human gait is a cyclical event and by convention the gait cycle begins and ends at initial foot contact of the same leg. That is, it represents two steps.

The purpose of clinical gait analysis is to communicate reliable, objective data on which to base clinical decisions. It can also be used to quantify outcomes and may ultimately predict the effects of various interventions for a patient with ambulatory difficulties. This requires a multi-disciplinary team to synthesize, analyze and evaluate the large number of variables used to describe a person's gait and to provide a clear course of surgical, orthotic, prosthetic, pharmaceutical or therapeutic intervention.

Clinical gait analysis techniques using 3D motion capture systems have several inherent sources of errors due to limitations of the modeling software used, skin movement artifacts and marker placement errors (Kadaba et al., 1989). The current cost of gait analysis for a patient is high and is estimated to be equivalent in cost to six MRI scans. This is an important limitation of these techniques. Also, the current method of presentation of clinical gait analysis data is not readily understood by many clinicians and this also inhibits the widespread use of these techniques.

At present there are no universally accepted techniques for interpretation of clinical gait analysis data, but a consensus has developed in some areas, notably in cerebral palsy gait. Clinical gait analysis begins to provide a scientific basis to determine how neuromuscular impairments correspond to abnormal movements. Traditionally, clinicians report changes in joint angles following surgery as an outcome measure of the effectiveness of the surgical procedure, for example, increased knee flexion following hamstring lengthening. This does not give any indication of functional improvements to the patient's gait and therefore gait analysis data can be an important adjunct to the clinical examination. For gait data to be useful in the management of the patient, both the clinical examination data (a static, passive assessment) and the gait data (a dynamic or functional assessment) should correspond.

In most gait laboratories clinicians normally require only summary information from the gait recording provided by the gait analysis team (movement scientists). The movement scientists carry out is an comprehensive investigation of the data and therefore needs detailed information to support the quality of their reporting to the clinical team. However, both the clinician and the movement scientist would benefit from the data processing being automated and the

reporting to be simplified and presented in an easily comprehensible, standardized format. This will lower the cost of a gait assessment and may improve the consistency of the reporting. This chapter describes the development of a software package that shows how clinical gait analysis data can be presented in alternative ways and can offer simplifications that may aid understanding and reduce costs.

Three-dimensional motion capture systems such as Vicon (Oxford Metrics, Oxford, UK) offer accurate, high-resolution recordings of human locomotion. These systems acquire, and display three-dimensional motion data on patients while walking and are able to integrate analogue data to enable simultaneous acquisition of force plate, EMG and video data.

The Vicon system has a specifically designed software package, Polygon (Oxford Metrics, Oxford, UK) to generate interactive multimedia reports from the captured 3D data. This software produces the graphical data used in clinical reports.

BACKGROUND

Bipedal gait represents each person's unique solution of how to get from one place to another. There is a natural variability to a person's gait as motor tasks cannot be repeated identically from walking trial to walking trial. Therefore, intra- and inter-subject variability are natural elements of movement patterns associated with functional tasks (Manal et al., 2004). This natural variation is an important consideration when analyzing the gait of patients' with walking disabilities.

Diagnosis and rehabilitation of patients with locomotor disorders is increasingly supported by gait analysis data (Barton et al., 1995). Cerebral palsy is a locomotor disorder that can prevent or inhibit walking and cause a lack of muscle coordination and spasms due to an injury to the brain prior to or shortly after birth. Children with cerebral palsy are the most commonly assessed patient group using gait analysis techniques. This is due to the unpredictable nature of surgical outcomes and other forms of intervention intended to improve their gait (Gage, 1991).

Gait analysis data is usually reported as a time history of kinematic and kinetic variables expressed as a percentage of the gait cycle in the form of line graphs (see Figures 1- 4).

Normal movement implies that the time history of the pattern lies within a range of values that are distributed about a time varying mean. That is, a normative range is established for comparison with a patient's gait. A clinical gait report may contain over 50 graphs when kinematic and kinetic data of the pelvis, hip knee and ankle are presented in the three orthogonal planes. The clinical team visually assess deviations and interprets the patient's gait by comparison with the normative data range (Manal et al., 2004). The data from the gait analysis is also compared with the data from the clinical examination.

Many studies have recognized the challenging nature of analyzing gait data and the need for simplification of the graphical output of the 3D motion capture systems (Chau, 1991a; Manal et al., 2004). A variety of approaches have been tried to aid the analysis of gait data including fuzzy logic, neural networks, artificial intelligence and multi-variate statistical techniques that have been described (Chau, 1991a; 1991b). Manal et al. (2004) developed a type of thermometer scale for color coding the magnitude and direction system of movement pattern deviations relative to normative kinetic and kinematic values.

However, our approach differs from that previously described in gait studies as we have employed visualization techniques. Spence (2001) states that the use of iconic displays can be an aid to the understanding of complex data. Card (1999) describes the techniques of visualization as using vision to think. The software developed in this study therefore uses these principles to represent gait data.

METHOD

Interrogation of the kinetic (forces, moments and powers) and kinematic (joint rotation angles) output graphs from a multi-media authoring tool such as Polygon (Oxford Metrics, Oxford, UK) can be automated using simple analytical techniques. This can save time in the analysis process if only the graphs showing out-of-range data are displayed and salient features highlighted. Graphs of kinematics and kinetics are assessed in terms of three properties: their pattern, range and timing (PRT). The pattern refers to the general shape of the graph and the number and height of specific peaks and troughs. The range refers to the total spread in the angle from minimum to maximum. The timing refers to where particular peaks, troughs or crossing points occur in the cycle. Therefore, software was developed as an aid to automating the analysis of the graphical output of the gait data. Visualization techniques were used to aid the interpretation of this data.

Individual cerebral palsy patient graphs (see Figures 1, 2 and 3) were compared to normative curves to detect whether any of the following occurred:

1. Out-of-range data at initial foot contact
2. Out-of-range data greater than the mean ± 2SD
3. Out-of-range peak and trough values
4. Out-of-phase peak and trough values
6. Incorrect slope of the graph at a selected point in the cycle

Each curve is stored as a dataset of 51 points, representing one gait cycle. The point in the gait cycle at which a given stance phase event occurs is read in from the system (i.e., initial contact IC, opposite foot off OFO, opposite foot contact OFC, toe-off, TO). Finding a value from the graph at one of these events is simply a matter of reading from the corresponding curve.

At each point, the mean value and standard deviation (SD) of the normative curve is known. An out-of-range value, at a given point in the cycle, is then taken to be one which is more than two standard deviations from the normative value. The ± 2 SD value was arbitrarily selected since there are currently no guidelines. An alternative choice could have been to select the mean ± 1SD.

The patient data may show variations from the normal range (± 2 SD) such that the peak amplitude may be high or low or its phase may be early or late. The following paragraphs describe how amplitude and phase deviations are calculated. If the peak value is missing in the subject's data, the method still gives an answer, although its meaning is uncertain.

To find the phase difference of the peak value, the subject's curve is moved horizontally until it gives the best match to the normal curve. For example, in Figure 1, sliding the subject's right knee curve to the left by about 5% lines up with the peak value in the normal curve. The program therefore calculates the root mean square (RMS) value of these differences in the patient data compared to the normative range.

It is important to limit the part of the curve which is being compared to the peak of the normal curve. If too little of the curve is compared, the result may be affected by noise. It is therefore not sufficient to simply look for the maximum value of the curve. If too much of the curve is used, the result may be inaccurate. In principle the normal curves should be inspected for each joint and a suitable value chosen per curve and per peak. In practice two positions have been used on the normal curve, for example, the toe-off frame to initial contact frame.

It is also important to limit the shift being applied to the subject's curve. As a match could probably be found (erroneously) by shifting the curve half a cycle. The horizontal shift is therefore limited to a specified amount. This is read in from a data file and is currently 12 steps in either direction, although this is self-selected.

The peak value is found by taking the selected part of the subject's curve and shifting it one time increment from the maximum shift to the left to the maximum shift to the right. At each step a difference from the normal curve is computed and the position with the least difference is taken to be the best match. The shift at the best match is the required phase shift of the peak.

The difference at each step is computed as follows. The selected part of the subject's curve has a number of points (N) and a time shift of a given number of time steps (Tshift). Suppose the part of the normal curve selected as having the peak runs from time step Tstart to Tend, where:

$$Tend + 1 - Tstart = N$$

Calling the subject curve at time step T, Subject [T] and the normal curve Normal [T], we are comparing Subject [T + Tshift] with Normal [T] from T = Tstart to T = Tend. The comparison at each point seeks to find the difference and these differences add up to give a total difference. The difference is therefore calculated at point T as:

$$difference [T] = (Normal [T] - Subject [T + Tshift])^2$$

Subtracting gives the difference and squaring makes the difference positive, so all the errors add up. The total difference for the curve is given by summing up the N points of the curve (Box 1).

This is then calculated for each value of Tshift and the minimum resulting total difference is

Box 1.

$$\text{Total difference} \left(\text{Tshift}\right) = \sum_{Tstart}^{Tend} \text{difference} \left[\text{T}\right], \qquad \text{Tshift} = -12, .., 12$$

chosen as the position of best fit. The value of Tshift then gives the amount by which the peak is early or late:

Time difference = Tshift for minimum total difference

Having found the required time shift, the peak can then be moved vertically to line up with the normal curve. A similar method is used to find the minimum difference between the shifted subject curve and the normal curve as the subject curve is shifted vertically.

Having identified peak and trough values, the range is simply the difference. This is compared to the value obtained for the mean curve. The slope of a graph was estimated by using the range from the adjacent trough to peak values.

The four main components to the software are:

a.   **Reduction of graphs and simplified display:** This involves interrogation of the graphs for out-of-range data and eliminating data within pre-set limits. Methods of highlighting out-of-range data are described below.

b.   **Clinically relevant data from gait analysis:** The kinetic and kinematics graphs are assessed for their pattern, range and timing. A rule-based method is described for assessing the graphs.

c.   **Clinical verification of gait data:** Use of hypothesis buttons to observe the dynamic effects of the clinical examination data

d.   **Icon Interface:** Presentation of the graphical results is made using an icon interface. These components are combined into the integrated display screen showing the outputs of the software. They can be displayed collectively or individually for greater visualization.

Figure 1. Sagittal plane motion of the knee

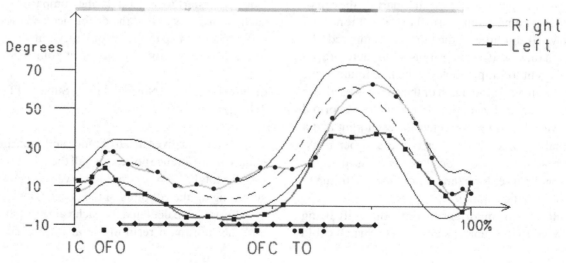

The angle vs. time graph shows the sagittal plane motion of the knee for a normal range within the black lines and the mean value shown dotted. Cerebral palsy gait is shown as "■" (left leg) and "●" (right leg). The graph shows two areas were the left knee is out of range and highlighted by the horizontal lines marked with "◆". Also shown is the thermometer scale after Manal and Stanhope (2004).

Reduction of Graphs and Simplified Display

There may be in excess of 50 graphs to analyze if kinematic (joint rotation angles) and kinetic (forces, moments and powers) and EMG data are interrogated and only limited parts of certain graphs may be clinically important.

The software was developed to eliminate graphs that are within the normal range (mean ± 2 SD) so that the user can concentrate on the more important out-of-range graphs. The out-of- range features of the displayed graphs are highlighted using different techniques to assist the user. Figure 1 shows sagittal plane motion of the knee. The black lines are the mean value for normal knee motion ± 2 standard deviations (SD). The left leg data for the patient is shown by the red line and the right leg is shown by the green line. The patient data shows increased knee flexion in early stance, hyperextension in terminal stance

and delayed flexion in swing. The out of range difference is shown by a purple horizontal line and is only flagged if the joint is out of range for more than three consecutive frames, so minor excursions are ignored.

Along the top of Figure 1 there is a thermometer scale that shows an alternative method of encoding out of range values (Manal et al., 2004). This uses a scale from red (below) to blue (above) the normal range. The further the value is below (or above) the range, the brighter the red (or blue). The graphical output is supported by text (not shown in Figure 1) explaining what has been found. For example, the average deviation from the mean of left knee flexion = - 10° and the range is 15 ° less than expected.

The normal curve can be divided into the ranges of interest and similar analysis can be carried out on these ranges. If swing phase knee flexion (2nd peak) is of interest, its peak value and whether it occurs early or late can be highlighted

Figure 2. Delayed knee flexion

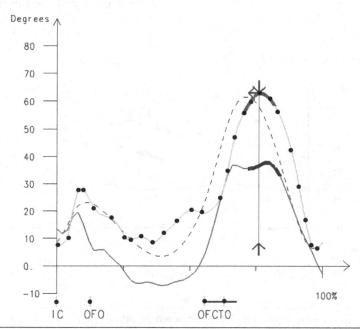

The angle vs. time graph shows the peak knee flexion of the right leg as indicated by the thickened line. The arrows indicate a delay and loss of range.

as shown in Figure 2. The horizontal position of the curve is offset by 8% (4 frames) to the right indicating a delay in knee flexion.

Clinically Relevant Data from Gait Analysis

For gait data to be useful in the management of the patient, both the clinical examination data and the gait data should correlate well. Clinicians report changes in joint angles or limb segment position following surgery as an outcome measure of the effectiveness of the procedure. This does not, however, give any indication of functional improvements to the patient's gait.

In the previous section, parts of graphs outside the normal range (mean ± 2SD) were highlighted. To facilitate analysis of pathological data, a rule-based method was developed using 20 clinical features reported by Gibbs (2000). Three of these have been used to illustrate the software. Many more rules exist and can also be included in the software.

Rules Applied

Rule 1 states that a patient with spasticity of the hip flexors may have increased pelvic tilt prior to toe-off. It would be useful to highlight the pelvic tilt graph prior to toe-off to see if this has increased and by how much. The rules can also be used to confirm the static examination findings and quantify the dynamic effects on the patient's gait. This is called the "hypothesis" mode in the software. Several rules, however, may have the same gait deviation.

Rule 2 states that delayed maximum knee flexion in swing and a reduced rate of flexion prior to and after toe off may be associated with spasticity of rectus femoris.

Rule 3 states that knee extension at toe-off is associated with spasticity of rectus femoris.

An illustration of the design of the software is shown in the following 2 examples.

Example of Rule 1: Increased anterior tilt of the pelvis prior to toe-off of the right leg may be due to spasticity of the hip flexors. Comparing

Figure 3. Pelvic tilt example of Rule 1

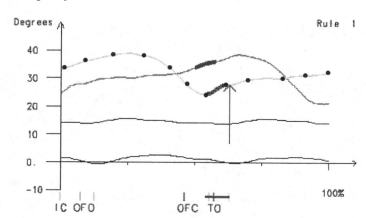

The angle vs. time graph shows an example of Rule 1 where increased anterior tilt of the pelvis (lumbar lordosis) prior to toe-off (TO) of the right leg may be due to spasticity of the hip flexors.

the patient values with the normal data (mean + 2 SD), increased pelvic tilt has occurred (lordosis) if the average difference over the four frames is more than 2 SD (see Figure 3).

The following features can be seen on the graph:

1. The horizontal brown line at the bottom shows the range over which the rule applies
2. The brown arrow runs from the mean value of a normal curve to the right leg curve of the patient
3. Thickened areas of the right and left curves show the four frames prior to toe-off for each curve
4. Text also appears stating the conclusions of the rule

Example of Rule 2: Delayed maximum knee flexion in swing and a reduced rate of flexion prior to and after toe-off may be associated with spasticity of rectus femoris. The normal graph of sagittal plane knee flexion is shown by the black dotted line in Figure 2 with a peak in mid-swing. A best fit can be found for the peak and hence the delay in the peak obtained. This reduced rate of flexion prior to and after toe-off, corresponding to a slope on the graph at the appropriate point is interpreted as a reduced range of flexion. The figure shows the display that appears if this rule is activated. Various indicators on the graph show why it has been triggered:

1. The curves are highlighted at the peaks and an arrow pointing left shows the peak is delayed.
2. The range is indicated at the peak value and the frames around toe-off (at which the slope is considered reduced) is indicated.
3. A text message lists the possible problems connected with the rule. Optionally, text could be added to explain why the rule fired.

A graph, similar to Figure 2 or 3, is displayed automatically for each rule that is initiated, when data is presented to the program. The annotations highlight the reason why the graph has been presented. The text explains the possible associated problems. In this way, the user is quickly directed to important parts of the data.

Clinical Verification of Gait Data

If the clinical examination of the patient reveals that they have spasticity of the hip flexors, then the gait analysis graphs would be expected to show an increase at the anterior tilt prior to toe-off (Rule 1). If several rules have the same suggested problem as one of their outputs, there will be several parts of different graphs to be considered.

A series of hypothesis buttons are available so that when the clinical examination reveals a musculo-skeletal problem, all the rules that have the associated problem as outputs are run. Those that are triggered produce graphs as shown in Figures 2 and 3. Those that are not triggered also produce graphs, but without the blue arrows. This allows the user to see all the rule-related data associated with this problem, with significant out-of-range data highlighted. Figure 4 shows a typical example. The hypothesis button for rectus femoris spasticity generates graphs for Rules 1, 2 and 3.

Rule 3 states that knee extension at toe-off is associated with spasticity of rectus femoris.

Rule 3 is activated and has the blue indicators on it. Rules 1 and 2 do not and only have the thickened line showing the point of the graph the rule is looking at and the event markers.

Icon Interface

The volume of data produced from motion capture systems make the analysis process very time consuming. Furthermore, clinicians are not always familiar with analyzing this type of graphical data. For these reasons, an icon interface has been

Figure 4. Knee flexion only Rule 3 is activated

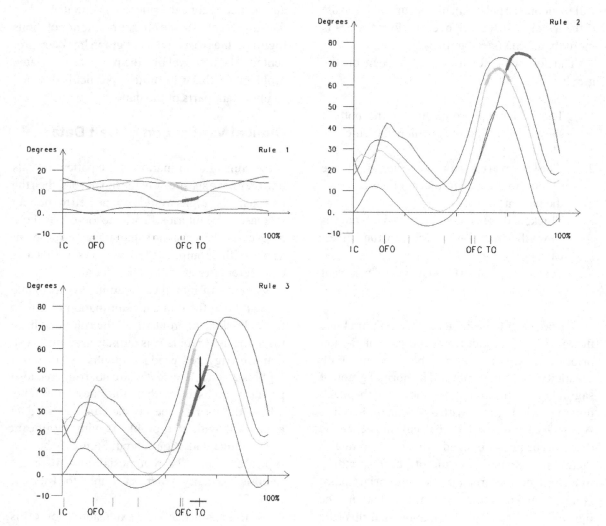

Clinical examination has found rectus femoris spasticity. This generates graphs for Rules 1, 2 and 3. Rule 3 is activated and so has the arrow indicators on it. Rules 1 and 2 do not; so they only have the thickened line showing the point of the graph the rule is looking at and the event markers.

developed that presents the useful information to the user extracted from the graphs.

There are two features of the graphical outputs that characterize the gait cycle, the foot-to-ground events (IC and TO) and the pattern, range and timing (PRT) of the graphs. Rule 1 was typical of the former, where the critical issue was the pelvic tilt prior to toe-off. Rule 2 is typical of the

latter, referring to a delayed peak and a reduced range (Figure 2).

A previous section discussed general properties of individual graphs related to PRT. Using the normal curve, the peaks, ranges and troughs of each graph can be identified. Values can be calculated for the delay or excess height of a peak or trough and whether a range is too large

Figure 5. The icon interface

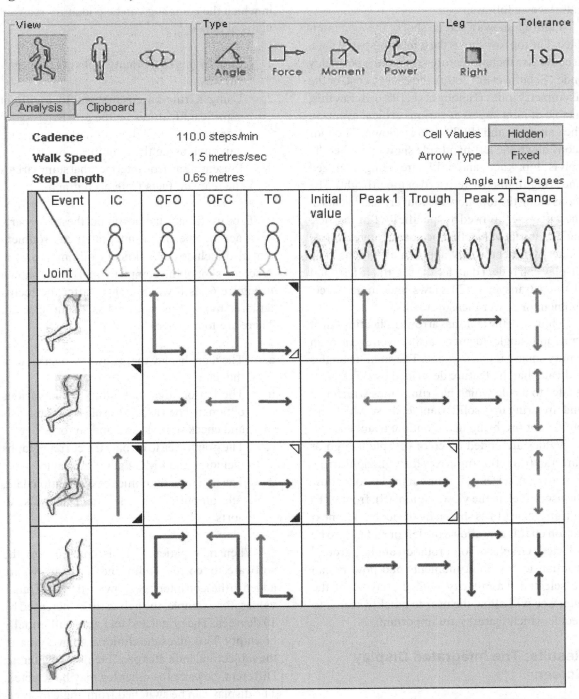

Shows a basic diagrammatic form of the icon interface. The icons on the top row show: a) the three orthogonal views, and b) the joint angle, force, moment and power data that can be selected. The display area shows the joint selected on the left side of the screen and top row shows the position in the gait cycle.

or small. This analysis can be input to an icon interface as follows.

Figure 5 shows a screen shot of the icon interface. The top row shows the temporo-spatial data. It could also include features such as the normalcy index Schutte et al. (2000), the energy cost, or the asymmetry index (Herzog et al., 1989). Below this, a table of joint angles at various critical events in the gait cycle and (PRT) data is shown. The four icons down the left-hand side shows whether the pelvis, hip, knee, and ankle are being analyzed and is highlighted in red (left) or green (right). The icons along the top show the four critical events in the gait cycle followed by specific PRT properties, such as initial value, first peak and range. Not all values will necessarily apply to all graphs. The display can reflect data for the sagittal (S), frontal (F) and transverse (T) views and angle, force, moment or power measurements.

The rest of the table has arrows indicating out of range joint angles (degrees) at the given event, or an empty square if it is in range. The small triangles indicate that the feature described by this square relates to a rule which has run. Rules which run and fire bring up a solid triangle; those which run but do not fire bring up an outline triangle.

Values are coded by color (purple is high or early) and direction (up arrow for high, right arrow for early). A series of buttons at the bottom allow the user to select the view, sagittal (S), frontal (F) or transverse (T) as shown by the icons. The next button on this row allows the left or right leg to be selected. Graphs of joint rotation angles, ground reaction forces, joint moments and powers can be selected. Familiarity with the layout of the interface will allow the user to quickly scan it to decide which features are important.

Results: The Integrated Display Screen

Successful interpretation of motion capture data depends upon finding the pertinent information from a large amount of data and making a correct deduction. This chapter has discussed four ways in which the computer can help identify relevant items of data by:

1. Simplifying individual graphs in a meaningful way
2. Using a rule-based analysis to highlight significant features on the graphs
3. Comparing clinical examination data with gait data, using the hypothesis mode
4. Presenting an icon interface that summarizes the relevant facts from each graph

To be useful as a diagnostic aid, these four parts must act together in an integrated environment that also includes the clinical examination data. A screen shot of the complete interface is shown in Figure 6, as it would appear after the rectus femoris hypothesis button has been selected. There are four areas:

a. The icon display that allows an overview of the data
b. The button area that contains the various options needed to run the rule-based analysis and check hypotheses, and so forth
c. The graph area to display the current graphs including the EMG data if available
d. The text area for clinical examination data, rule output and single graph analysis reports

When new patient data is entered into the software, the corresponding indicative arrows are added to the icon interface showing the out of range values; for example, the pelvic tilt is increased by 10 degrees. The graph and text area will initially be empty. This gives the clinician an overview of the subject and indicates possible areas of interest. Different views or the other leg may be selected. The display can be switched from angle to force, moment or power as required. Selecting a square containing one of the joint icons adds the corresponding graph for that joint to the graph area.

Figure 6. The integrated display screen

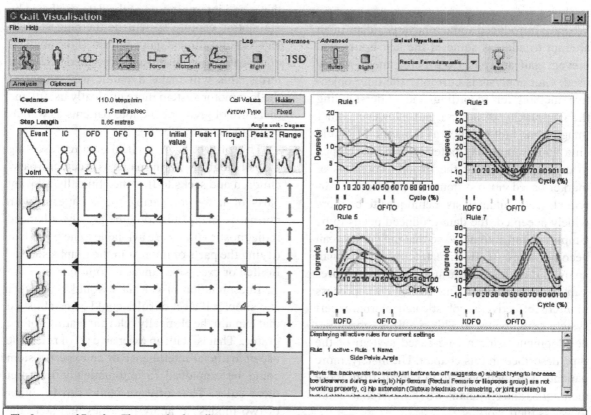

The Integrated Display. The icon display allows an overview of the data. The button area contains the various options needed to run the rule-based analysis, check hypotheses, and so forth. The graph area displays the currently requested graphs, including the EMG data if available. The text area displays clinical examination data, rule output and single graph analysis.

This also displays the corresponding analysis for the graph in the text area. All computed values for peaks, troughs, ranges and out-of-range sequences are listed. This allows a clinician to identify any parts of the graph which are out of range and their variation from normal.

Selecting the rules button resets the display to its initial state, runs the rules and brings up graphs (as for example in Figure 6) for any rule (s) that is triggered. Messages derived from the output of any rule that is triggered are also listed, pointing towards possible areas of investigation. Selecting a hypothesis button resets the display and brings up all graphs related to that hypothesis.

Visualization techniques have been used in the integrated display in two ways: in the icon interface and in the interrogation of the graphical display. The integrated display therefore is designed to follow the users thought patterns and to assist in their analysis (Noble et al., 2005).

The next stage in development of reporting gait analysis data is to achieve agreement amongst the gait analysis community regarding the establishment of a set of rules that can be programmed into an expert system. That is, features on the graphical display along with clinical examination (and imaging data) can be used to identify the cause and severity of the gait disability. This work therefore represents a starting point for much further development in the interpretation of gait data.

CONCLUSION

We have introduced some innovative ideas in an attempt to address some of the key issues that prevent gait analysis from being more widely used. Gait analysis is currently the only objective method for recording and understanding the complexity of human gait. However, other imaging modalities, such as dynamic MRI and cine fluoroscopy may potentially be developed to overcome some of the major limitations of marker-based video systems. In order for the current clinical gait analysis techniques to be more widely accepted, the data produced needs to be simplified and automated so that the process can become more cost effective. Interpretation of gait analysis data for clinical use currently requires a multi-disciplinary team. To make the process more cost effective, a sophisticated internal expert system could be used. This requires substantial development using a rule-based system of the type described in this chapter. Ultimately, more patients will then be able to benefit from these techniques and clinicians will have a reliable tool to assess their work.

Gait data is of necessity and complex, but simpler methods of display need to be developed. The use of icons as described in this chapter is a potential solution to this problem. In the future, the gait analysis process should provide a treatment program for the patient and ultimately, it is hoped that the gait analysis process will be able to likely predict the outcome of various interventions.

Future Research Directions

The present camera-based systems using reflective markers for 3D motion capture will be superseded by marker-less tracking systems. Hence some of the technical issues regarding the errors due to marker placement and movement artifacts will not be pertinent. Developments in computer modeling techniques will allow prediction of the effects of wearing an orthotic device, or how changes in muscle tone may affect gait. However, the synthesis and interpretation of the data produced by 3D motion capture systems is the biggest challenge facing clinical gait analysis. If the analysis of the data is automated and described in clinical terms, this will make dynamic assessment of the locomotor system more clinically useful and therefore of greater benefit to patients as well as being more cost effective.

This project takes cyclical data representing the pathological walking patterns of cerebral palsy children and seeks to find the clinically relevant parts of it by comparing these patterns with normative data. This could be greatly enhanced if diagnostic rules were available to help in identifying the parts of interest in the graphs such as limited or excessive ranges of joint motion.

Interpretation of gait data would be quicker and simpler if a set of rules could be established that explain the clinically relevant features of the graphs. That is, with an extensive set of rules, the use of artificial intelligence or an expert system could be employed to automatically interpret those rules. The software could run in either of two modes: to apply the rules and state the clinical interpretation, for example increased plantarflexion of the ankle occurs in the swing phase of gait if there is weakness in tibialis anterior, or the user could ask questions which the expert system would answer in the light of the rules and the data.

The software package currently looks at cyclical walking data and could in principle be extended to any cyclical function of the body, from heart rate data to the evaluation of a golf swing. The system needs both normal data and a set of rules for interpretation.

For new applications, normal data could be collected and stored. Eventually it might be built into a shared database where all users contribute. Rules could be built up from experience in the community. A more exciting research direction would be to include diagnostics with the data (once an expert had studied the subject) and to apply machine learning (e.g., neural networks, case-based reasoning) to the data to build up rules automatically.

An extension of the system might be used in other medical applications. For example, following anesthesia, a patient might do simple repetitive tests until the system verified they were fit to drive.

Analysis of cyclical data is not limited to the medical field. Other areas include condition monitoring of rotating machinery. Rules relating to the machine's condition could be written, or derived by the system and relevant performance highlighted by the system to alert the user as to a pending wear condition.

ACKNOWLEDGMENT

The authors wish to acknowledge the contribution to this work made by Richard Longair, during his honors year computing project.

REFERENCES

Barton, G., & Lees, A. (1997). An application of neural networks for distinguishing gait patterns on the basis of hip-knee joint angle diagrams. *Gait and Posture, 5,* 28-35. Gage, J. (1991). *Gait analysis in cerebral palsy.* London: Mac Keith Press.

Card, S., Mackinlay, J., & Shneiderman, B. (Eds.). (1999). *Readings in information visualization: Using vision to think.* San Francisco, CA: Morgan Kaufmann.

Chau, T. (2001a). A review of analytical techniques for gait data. Part 1, Fuzzy, statistical and fractal methods. *Gait and Posture, 13,* 49-66.

Chau, T. (2001b). A review of analytical techniques for gait data. Part 2, Neural networks and wavelet methods. *Gait and Posture, 13,* 102-120.

Davis, R., Ounpuu, S., Tyburski, D., & Gage, J. (1991). A gait analysis data collection and reduction technique. *Human Movement Science, 10,* 575-587.

Gibbs, S. (2000). *Guide to the interpretation of gait deviations.* Scotland: The Dundee Royal Infirmary.

Herzog, W., Nigg, B., Read, L., & Olsson, E. (1989). Asymmetries in ground reaction force patterns in normal human gait. *Medicine and Science in Sports and Exercise, 21,*110-114.

Kadaba, M., Ramakrishnan, H., Wootten, M., Gainey, J., Gorton, G., & Cochran, G. (1989). Repeatability of kinematic, kinetic, and electromyographic data in normal adult gait. *Journal of Orthopaedic Research, 7,* 849-860.

Manal, K., & Stanhope, S. (2004). A novel method for displaying gait and clinical movement analysis data. *Gait and Posture, 20,* 222-226.

Noble, R., & White, R. (2005). Visualisation of gait analysis data. *Paper presented at the International Conference on Information Visualisation.* London.

Spence, R. (2001). *Information visualization.* Essex: ACM Press.

Schutte, L., Narayanan, U., Stout, J., Selber, P., & Gage, J. (2000). An index for quantifying deviations from normal gait. *Gait and Posture, 11,* 25-31.

Additional Reading

Awad, E. (1996). *Building expert systems: Principles, procedures and applications.* St. Paul, MN: West Publishing Company.

Darlington, K. (2000). *The essence of expert systems.* Essex, England: Prentice Hall.

Gurney, K. (1997). *An introduction to neural networks.* London: UCL Press.

Goodwill, C., Chamberlaine M., & Evans, C. (1997). *Rehabilitation of the physically disabled adult.* London: Stanley Thornes.

Haupt, R. (1998). *Practical genetic algorithms.* New York, NY: John Wiley & Sons.

Inman, V., Ralston, H., & Todd, F. (1981). *Human walking.* Baltimore, MD: Williams & Wilkins.

Inselberg, A. (1997). *Multidimensional detective.* Phoenix, AZ: IEEE Symposium on Information Visualization, (InfoVis '97).

Kirtley, C. (2005.) *Clinical gait analysis: Theory & practice.* Oxford: Churchill Livingstone.

Michalewicz, Z., Schmidt, M., Michalewicz, M., & Chiriac, C. (2006). *Adaptive business intelligence.* New York, NY: Springer Verlag.

Negnevitsky, M. (2002). Artificial intelligence: A guide to intelligent systems. New York, NY: Addison Wesley.

Nigg, B., & Herzog, W. (1999). *Biomechanics of the musculo-skeletal system.* Chichester: John Wiley & Sons.

Perry, J. (1992). *Gait analysis. Normal and pathological function.* Slack Inc.

Petrovski, A., & McCall, J. (2005). Smart problem solving environments for medical decision support. In: H-G. Bayer et al. (Eds.), *Proceedings of the Genetic and evolutionary computation conference* (GECCO). Washington, D.C.: ACM Press.

Pirolli, P., & Rao, R. (1996). Table lens as a tool for making sense of data. In: T. Catarci, M. Costabilem, S. Levidaldi, & G. Santucci (Eds.), *Workshop on advanced visual interfaces.* Washington, D.C.: ACM Press.

Russell, S., & Norvig, P. (2002). *Artificial intelligence: A modern approach.* Essex, England: Prentice Hall.

Robertson, D. (1997). *Introduction to biomechanics for human motion analysis.* Waterloo: Waterloo Biomechanics.

Robertson, D., Caldwell, G., Hamill, J., Kamen, G., & Whittlesey, S. (2004). Research methods for biomechanics. *Human Kinetics,*

Rose, J., & Gamble, J. (1994). *Human walking.* Baltimore, MD: Williams & Wilkins.

Smidt, G. (1990). *Gait in rehabilitation.* New York, NY: Churchill Livingstone.

Soderberg, G. (1986). *Kinesiology–application to pathological motion.* Baltimore, MD: Williams & Wilkins.

Winter, D. (1990). *The biomechanics and motor control of human gaits.* Waterloo: University of Waterloo Press.

White, R., Agouris, I., Selbie, R., & Kirkpatrick, M. (1999). The variability of force platform data in normal and cerebral palsy gait. *Clinical Biomechanics, 14*(3), 185-192.

Whittle, M. (1996). *Gait analysis: An introduction.* Oxford: Butterworth-Heinemann.

Williams, M., & Lissner, H. (1977). *Biomechanics of human motion.* Philadelphia, PA: Saunders.

Zatsiorsky, V. (1998). Kinematics of human motion. *Human Kinetics,*

Zajac, F., & Neptune, R., & Kautz, S. (2002). Biomechanics and muscle coordination of human walking Part I: Introduction to concepts, power transfer, dynamics and simulations. *Gait and Posture, 16,* 215-232.

Chapter IV
Capturing Data in Healthcare Using Patient–Centered Mobile Technology

Sarah Pajak
Brunel University, UK

Lorraine H. De Souza
Brunel University, UK

Justin Gore
Northwick Park Hospital, UK

Christopher G. Williams
General Dynamics, UK

ABSTRACT

This chapter outlines and discusses how an increasingly popular approach of incorporating patient perspectives and experience in research can be used to inform the development of user-centered technology in healthcare, with particular emphasis on hand-held mobile devices. The chapter draws on a program of research and technological developments between an acute hospital trust and the Schools of Health Sciences and Social Care (SHSSC) and Information Systems, Computing and Mathematics (SISCM) at Brunel University in West London. The authors critically review existing literature and discuss the development of a new prototype mobile device for use by healthcare professionals in capturing patient information at the front end of hospital care.

INTRODUCTION

A three-year research project funded through the Knowledge Transfer Partnership (KTP), due for completion by the end of 2007, has focused on evaluating patient and staff experiences in rela-
tion to the radical redesign of an acute district general hospital. A key aim of the research is to benefit these groups in an accident and emergency (A&E) environment, through the identification and development of technological tools designed to improve the patient journey which can be uti-

lized by clinicians. Patients and staff have been observed in real-time field settings to establish positive outcomes, as well as areas that could be improved through the introduction of these evidence-based tools. The acute trust's re-development program, recognized at national level, is a consequence of a forward-thinking approach to developing and evaluating hospital services and is underpinned by current National Health Service (NHS) policy and reform.

Motivation for the research project is fueled by the potential in disseminating the lessons learned and benefits afforded by the tools across the NHS on a national basis. One key output has been the development of a prototype mobile device (in the form of a personal digital assistant (PDA)) for recording and sharing patient information in an emergency care environment. The impetus for this development arose out of the initial findings of the research that highlighted two key issues of concern to patients and staff: communication and waiting times. It was evident that the ways in which patient information and data were recorded during emergency consultations, and then relayed to staff that needed to use the information for clinical decision making could be problematic, thereby impacting on the patient journey. Hence, we have recommended a possible technological solution.

Rather than focusing on the detailed findings of the main research, this chapter is centered upon describing how the research is being used to feed into the technological development. The chapter begins with the political context surrounding the advent of patient-centered care and associated NHS reform. This leads into an account of the re-development program at the hospital trust involved. The methodology employed in studying staff and patient perspectives at the hospital is presented, followed by a brief account of the key findings around collection and communication of patient information. The application of technology to address the identified issues is then proposed which includes a review of exist-

ing systems. The advantages of the utilization of hand-held mobile technology with its flexibility of application, portability and potential for linking with other systems, steers direction for the subsequent proposal of the patient-centered PDA "proof of concept." The chapter concludes with a look towards future trends in the field.

NHS POLICY AND REFORM

As healthcare has a strong political component, it is important to place the advent of patient-centered care and healthcare re-development into a political context. The election of a new Labor Government in 1997 brought a pledge to alter perceived 'failures' in the NHS, and to build upon and learn from areas of success where they occurred (nhs.uk Web site). The Labor party had been particularly critical of the market approach of the previous Conservative administration. They aimed to remove competition but maintain the purchaser-provider spilt (Levitt et al., 1999). The approach by the new government to commit to bringing an end to internal markets was viewed as "eclectic and pragmatic" (Ham, 2004, p.54).

The 1997 white paper, *The New NHS: Modern, Dependable,* set out the new political approach which was focused on partnership and integrated working, and was driven by performance (although these concepts and new ways of working were being established across certain organizations in health and social care before this time). This created the basis for further NHS reforms outlined in the NHS Plan (Department of Health, 2000) and Delivering the NHS Plan (Department of Health, 2001). It appeared that efforts were being made to give greater authority and decision making power to patients and frontline staff. Ham (2004) outlined how the policies to deliver the NHS Plan, while offering important differences, were to some extent "similar in a number of respects to those that lay behind the internal market (p.67), and this is particularly the case with offering greater patient choice" (Ham, 2004).

However, establishing the patient position at the center of the NHS goes beyond simply offering greater choice in a healthcare environment. Not only the desire for patient involvement, but the general expectation of this participation has perceptibly intensified in the development and design of NHS services. This is both a political and social shift which is reflected not only by governmental approaches to policy and reform, but change program developed by certain public agencies and awareness- raising by various user groups. The heart of the NHS Plan being presented as a vision of "a patient-centred service" (Department of Health, 2000, p.8) is a testament to this.

The evolution of thinking away from clinicians primarily holding the power and control over patient care is in part a consequence of a number of well publicized NHS scandals. Kennedy (2001) in the Bristol Royal Infirmary Inquiry, a seminal report on certain failings surrounding children's heart surgery at the hospital, showed how NHS culture may directly impact on the patient experience, for better or worse. This report highlighted how cultures of nursing, medicine and management, for example, can be seen as traditionally distinct and internally closely-knit.

Kennedy (2001) surmises that his report is:

An account of a hospital where there was a 'club culture:' an imbalance of power, with too much control in the hands of a few individuals. It is an account in which vulnerable children were not a priority, either in Bristol or throughout the NHS. (p.2)

This statement is important as it clearly indicates that the issues identified were not unique to Bristol but may apply to the NHS as a whole. This does not necessarily mean that the majority of clinicians were not delivering good quality care to their patients, but the consequence of such a view is that patients are now being offered greater responsibility over their care.

The NHS Improvement Plan (Department of Health, 2004), along with the plans presented in 2000-2003 outlined previously, proposed new targets centered upon increases in workforce and new structures within both the NHS and the Department of Health. This formed part of a ten-year reform process. The NHS Plan set out how increased funding and reform aimed to redress geographical inequalities, improve service standards and extend patient choice. It outlined a new delivery system for the NHS, as well as changes for social services and a range of professional groups.

The Healthcare Commission's statutory duty to assess the performance of healthcare providers and include the use of patient surveys further mirrors the importance placed upon patient involvement in national standards. The Healthcare Commission asserts that Patient Focus (a domain in its own right) should have the following specific outcome: "Healthcare is provided in partnership with patients, their carers and relatives, respecting their diverse needs, preferences and choices" (Healthcare Commission website, 2004).

Attempts have been made in the NHS to translate the principles around user-centered services and integrated working into frontline care. Change management models such as those under the umbrella of process redesign have become particularly popular (Iles & Sutherland, 2001; McNulty & Ferlie, 2002). Old professional cultural barriers are to be knocked down in favor of modernized services built around the patient. We focus here on one organization that has attempted to put the rhetoric into practice.

THE ACUTE HOSPITAL TRUST

While it is becoming more common-place to find evidence within hospital trusts of involvement and consultation with patients in the design of services, it is less so the case that efforts are explicitly made from the outset to achieve an outcome which goes beyond the realms of the service provision itself. In this respect, the re-development program presented in this chapter, and associated research project focusing on patient experience, may be unique in their end-point ambition. The project involves a trust that has gained a reputation for its clinically-led innovation (recognized in the NHS Plan) and has attempted to develop a transformational change model designed to be an 'exemplar' for modernizing local hospitals (Figure 1). With various external NHS pressures and changes in strategy aside, the trust is keen on using the research findings for further service innovation and the collaboration with the university is aimed at producing technological development that may be used more widely to improve staff working practices, care processes and patient care across the NHS.

The re-development program has focused upon integration of hospital and community services, rapid throughput and expert teams. Ensuring more appropriate and timely referrals to the hospital from more highly trained general practitioners (GPs) and community services, is a key aim of the hospital model (which incorporates a smaller hospital bed base). This approach has been developed, at least in part, in conjunction with expert clinicians and public and patient groups via public feedback sessions and involvement of committees that include user representatives. These consultations have suggested that the desire expressed for patients to be cared for and treated

Figure 1. Key hospital model objectives

A major drive for improved patient care and better health for the local population by providing services that deliver care to patients at the right time in the right place

Developing a 'whole systems' approach where effective health services can be provided locally by harmonizing primary care, local hospital and more specialist services (e.g., chronic disease management) to prevent inefficiencies, gaps in provision, delays and duplication of effort

Staff, patients and the local community to be involved in the development, implementation and communication of the project

in their own homes (where appropriate), would be medically more beneficial. Staff satisfaction levels and views towards the working environment are also expected to improve as a result of the changes taking place at the hospital. Our evaluation of the model will assess to what extent these aims are being fulfilled.

On a departmental level, the A&E model has introduced systems which revolve around specialist teams incorporating multi-skilled staff (e.g., nurse practitioners), with the aim to reduce unnecessary delays and improve the overall emergency service for patients. In addition, multi-disciplinary working is a central philosophy of the program and we focus here on a key theme related to this: sharing of information between professionals.

RESEARCH METHODOLOGY

Nationally, research identifying patient and staff views relating to hospital services is mainly conducted through regular patient and staff surveys, the results of which are collated and published with free availability for all (e.g., Healthcare Commission surveys). The distinguishing feature which sets the current research aside from this bulk collection of data is the in-depth qualitative exploration of experiences and pathways within the hospital setting, from the patients' and staffs' perspectives. Appropriate NHS ethical approval has been granted for this ongoing project.

The various phases of data collection involved many hours of observations and tracing of patient pathways within the 'majors' A&E department. Researchers, in teams and individually, gradually built up a picture of the key elements of the patient pathway. Combining this with interviews with patients, who gave informed consent to participate, and staff views, it was possible to establish areas of concern which lent themselves to potential technological development.

Patients were traced while on the 'majors' section of the A&E department from the point of admission to either discharge home or onto a ward, where appropriate. Patient notes were also studied to establish aspects of patient care which may have been missed in patient interviews, or to confirm observations. The periods of observation began in 2003 and have been carried out during a number of updates leading to the present day. Current findings are based upon 73 patient maps conducted so far in the A&E department.

Where possible, all elements of patient care were observed. This commonly included interactions between patients and a range of health professionals. In particular, we focused on the assessments made by staff of the patient's condition (known as 'clerking'); from nurses who carried out initial assessments to doctors taking histories and requesting further assessment. Patients were observed having cannulas fitted, drips topped up, blood samples taken, being referred to the x-ray room, waiting for test results, and exchanging information with doctors, nurses, healthcare assistants and porters. Doctors also were observed writing up patient notes and accessing previous assessment results.

CAPTURING PATIENT INFORMATION: THE PATIENT/STAFF PERSPECTIVE

Through collation of observations and interviews to the point of 'saturation' (where we felt no new findings would emerge), key themes evolved regarding the A&E patient pathway. As mentioned previously, we are focusing here only on a limited number of initial findings that have been used by the research team to develop a technological prototype. The evaluation project is an ongoing process and further data collection is due to take place.

An understanding of the structure of staffing has been achieved as a result of the research. The A&E team consists of a nurse manager, nurse practitioners who may specialize in emergency care or surgery, and generic nursing staff. The A&E doctors are headed by a consultant (who is available for consultation) and also includes higher level doctors such as registrars and staff grade doctors and junior doctors (Senior House Officers and House Officers). The junior doctors such as Senior House Officers (SHOs) working on the unit are typically on six-month placements, rotating across specialties, while the senior doctors are more permanently based in A&E. The porters and administrators are the remaining staff component and critical to the smooth running of the service. The hospital model itself relies upon integration between this team of staff which makes up A&E and doctors from other specialties, such as medicine or surgery, who are referred to when necessary.

When doctors carry out the initial clerking of a patient, this involves taking a full history and carrying out an examination, ordering tests and so forth (this procedure may last approximately 10 to 25 minutes depending on the individual patient). If a different specialty is required following a visit from the A&E doctor, the patient may be expected to repeat elements of the procedure which has already taken place. For example, the notes recorded by a junior doctor in A&E from an initial clerking procedure may be repeated by a doctor from the surgical team who requires the same information, perhaps with additional facts included.

All patients who enter A&E are issued a hospital identification number. These numbers, along with basic information including a patient's name, address and date of birth, are printed onto a sheet of stickers which is placed within the patient file. The stickers are to be attached to patient notes and samples such as blood or urine which have been taken from the patient, as required. A trolley positioned in the center of the majors department holds all patient notes and is located adjacent to the white board which tracks which bay a patient is in, their time of arrival and doctor/nurse responsible for their care. This is particularly relevant in the context of the

4-hour governmental target for A&E outlined in the NHS Plan (2000) and implemented in 2004, as a means to manage waiting times.

As highlighted, a key philosophy of the hospital model is to integrate working, modernize the environment and enhance the patient journey. There is much evidence that these attempts are improving both staff and patient experiences (to be reported elsewhere). One area for improvement is that some patients have voiced some concerns with the clerking phase of their journey, and sharing of information between professionals. During this interaction between patient and clinician, observations were made by the researchers, and patients openly commented, that there was some repetition of questions asked and information requested from various professionals. This issue is known to be a general problem across the NHS and other health and social care systems. Being asked to repeat information resulted in patients experiencing frustration and some concern over the quality of their care, along with causing potentially unnecessary delay to the patient journey.

Following observations and discussions between the researchers and clinicians, the reasons suggested for such repetition became clear. Clinicians commented that some repetition was necessary in order to confirm certain clinical suspicions, but that due to poor note taking skills and/or a lack of communication between some of their colleagues, elements of clerking had, at times, to be unnecessarily repeated and notes re-written. In addition, the problem of lost notes was also raised, leading to delay and potential repetition for patients and staff.

TECHNOLOGICAL POSSIBILITIES

These findings led us to consider one of a number of possible technological outputs from our KTP project. In collaboration with colleagues from Brunel University and the trust, discussions took place to formulate a solution to the problems around recording and sharing clerking information as reported by patients and staff. Establishing a proof of concept to lead, ideally, to a handheld mobile prototype will be explored in the following sections.

Handheld Computer Systems in Healthcare

Problems and attempted solutions around capturing patient information have been addressed by others and are not unique to our project. The research described above, however, has uncovered a need to harness or develop a system that is more efficient at managing relevant information within a busy emergency scenario (i.e., during clerking). In this context, clinicians need quick and easy access to a system that can record and produce detailed data on an ongoing basis at the point of care. We have postulated that this could be achieved with the use of a Personal Digital Assistant (PDA). PDAs are often used in implementations within hospitals due to their user-friendly size, cost and ability to communicate via fixed and wireless networks. It is important to provide some context of previous work in this area to see how our developmental idea fits into the evidence base.

Using PDAs to Record Data

A typical example of such an application could be seen in the work of Oyama et al. (2002) in their implementation of a piece of software that enabled clinicians to enter historical and laboratory patient data at the point of care. Once entered into the PDA's database, patient records would then be merged with a centralized patient record database located on a server, and could be printed to provide reports for inclusion in clinical notes (Oyama et al., 2002).

A slightly different approach was taken by Bird and Lane (2006), as their system was used with 12 first-year medical students in more controlled settings and with the aim of assessing whether or not the use of PDAs would result in benefits in emergency care, via improved access to procedural and patient documentation (Bird & Lane, 2006). PDAs were provided to all 12 of the students and criteria set for the recording of patient information. The trial was conducted over a three-year period and compared to a previous, totally paper-based trial that also lasted for three years. It was concluded that utilizing PDAs did not alter emergency medicine procedures or patient resuscitation documentation, when compared to the equivalent paper-based trial.

Another system for documenting patient procedures and resuscitation information was developed by Rosenthal and Wolford (2000). They cited the limitations of many existing systems as being cumbersome or prone to data loss, and developed a piece of software for use with PDAs that allowed clinicians to enter basic demographic information (although evidence supporting an explanation of this claim was not wholly apparent). Clinicians typically entered their details onto the PDA in around one minute where the information was transferred to a desktop computer and onto a pre-existing database. The researchers concluded that the system presented a cost-efficient method of improved data capture, a reduction of burden upon secretaries and increased tracking capabilities (Rosenthal & Wolford, 2000).

Lapinsky et al. (2001) designed and implemented a system using PDAs for an Intensive Care Unit (ICU) team at Mount Sinai Hospital, Canada. It included hospital and medical reference materials and enabled patient details to be captured using the PDA's specialist application through the use of a customized template. The use of templates proved cumbersome as they merely provided an outline for the information to be entered and did not assist the user with data entry. Lapinsky et al. (2001) found that the lack of a network interface restricted the benefits of the system, as the information contained on the PDAs was isolated. Access to external data sources

could have benefited both the patient records and reference applications.

The work of Serif et al. (2005) is also relevant to this discussion. This study involved the development of a system that enabled back pain data to be captured and visualized in mobile form through the use of a PDA. The system encapsulated pain drawings that allowed patients to locate the source of pain and also an appropriate scoring system for evaluating the degree of pain. The detailed documentation of the design, implementation and evaluation of the system showed that tried and tested methods of documenting patient conditions could be successfully digitized. The use of a wireless LAN also aided the usefulness of this system.

While some limitations have been identified, the above studies, in particular those by Oyama et al. (2002), Rosenthal and Wolford (2000) and Serif et al. (2005) indicate the possibility that PDAs could be an effective way to enhance the capture of patient information in certain healthcare environments. However, despite being the closest set of examples to our development (particularly as they facilitated the entry of patient information at the point of care), the above devices mainly originated from outside the UK. Further, more development is required focusing on the clerking phase of the patient journey.

Using PDAs for Monitoring or Reference

The above examples illustrate how PDAs can be developed to assist the recording of patient data. However, it appears that these are rare and most developments center around the use of PDAs mainly for monitoring and reference purposes.

Newlan et al. (2002) developed software for commercially available PDAs which displayed real-time physiological outputs from a patient monitor. The software had the ability to display several waveforms at once and operated over a

Wireless Local Area Network (WLAN) within a hospital or outside a hospital via the General Packet Radio Service (GPRS), thus allowing caregivers to monitor patients remotely. The software also had the ability to store the information being conveyed onto the PDA's removable memory. The implications of this with regard to patient confidentiality meant that security had to form a core part of the software. The authors described the use of hybrid public key cryptography for the encryption of data, of individual user logins in authenticating members of staff, and of firewalls to regulate access through the wireless network. This included handshake protocols and encryption algorithms to protect the transmission of usernames or passwords and to prevent data corruption or modification (Newlan et al., 2002).

The PDA-based reference system for clinicians developed at the Western General Hospital in Edinburgh used a WLAN that was constructed with particular attention paid to the implications such a network would have on sensitive medical equipment within the hospital. These PDAs were used to provide functions such as access to the hospital's patient database, x-ray and endoscopic images, medical reference materials and guidelines, papers and journals. Other features included note taking at the point of care, and the experimentation of digital note taking for speech recognition or transcription by secretaries, however, the system did not enable details to be captured, only accessed (Turner et al., 2005). The use of off-the-shelf packages did not compromise the final system, as was initially expected by the authors. Usability problems were averted through the use of 'pick lists' to speed up data entry and standard interface widgets to aid familiarization. Interference with hospital equipment was not an issue, nor was security with the use of Virtual Private Network (VPN) technology in establishing secure communication links.

The previous example is highly relevant given the nature of the research presented in this chapter, and the hospital context within which the devel-

opments would be employed. However, despite the authors' detailed account of the design and implementation of the system, their description of the evaluation of both the project and system lacked sufficient detail. Furthermore, the availability of detailed electronic medical information for use by any computer system is quite unique within a UK hospital. This was in part due to the sporadic development and procurement of hospital information systems within the UK NHS since its inception in the late 1940s.

The Mobile Medical Data (MOMEDA) system (Pattichis et al., 2002) provided both clinicians and patients with mobile access to information. Patients were able to access information regarding medical conditions and expected treatments both before and after hospital attendance (Pattichis et al., 2002). Clinicians were able to obtain medical records and images using a mobile phone, which meant that those who regularly travelled between different hospitals could still access patient details offsite using the mobile phone network. This is particularly relevant within the context of the hospital model we are focusing on where integration with community services and flexible, multi-disciplinary working is fundamental.

The importance of the MOMEDA system is its ability to operate outside hospital premises using the commercial mobile phone network. Despite this being a highly attractive feature, particularly for mobile clinicians, the associated cost of transmitting detailed images across the mobile network would more than likely attract a high cost due to the volume of data that would need to be transmitted. Systems such as the PDA-based medical records system outlined by Turner et al. (2005) had a distinct advantage over systems such as MOMEDA, in that communication costs did not escalate as system usage increased, as the WLAN was a privately operated network.

Part of the work carried out by Sommers et al. (2001) at Virginia Commonwealth University (VCU) was in providing 15 medical students with PDAs for use as a reference tool. The results of the study indicated that students felt the PDAs had many benefits including accessing medical reference and documentation, treatment guidelines and patient monitoring (Sommers et al., 2001). This system was developed with the specific needs of a university hospital medical school in mind. The PDA software was heavily customized for use by students and designed and constructed in an entirely different way to the PDA-based system developed by Turner et al. (2005) at Edinburgh's Western General Hospital. Despite the evaluation highlighting the perceived usefulness of the system at VCU, caution should be exercised, as students are much more likely to be familiar with the use of mobile devices, removing the usability barrier typically encountered by researchers in such applications where user acceptance may be a more prominent obstacle.

The work carried out by Aziz et al. (2005) at St. Mary's Hospital, London looked at the possible use of PDAs to replace the current system of pagers used by a hospital surgical team. The study looked at efficiencies that could be gained in communication between team members, and assessed this through the length of time members took to respond to calls using PDAs compared to pagers. The PDAs used also functioned as mobile phones and provided access to the Internet and reference materials pre-loaded onto each of the PDAs. Results of the trial showed that the bi-directional PDA-mobile phones enabled faster communication between the team when compared to pagers. It was also found that initially there was some aversion from members of the team to embracing new technology and change (Aziz et al., 2005). This, in contrast with the results of the trial at VCU (Sommers et al., 2001) highlights the impact end-users can have on the system under development.

In summary, this section presents a comparative discussion of current PDA systems used to manage patient information in a healthcare context. Some studies have shown the potential for the use of handheld mobile devices in recording

patient data. However, from studying the relevant literature, it appears these are rare developments. Most other applications of handheld technology within healthcare in the UK or abroad seem to facilitate monitoring procedures (e.g., patients' vital signs) or the provision of reference materials for clinicians often in terms of conveying specific clinical information. These studies, nonetheless, also provide an insight into the possibility of using PDAs in conjunction with wider data systems. This previous work has led us to begin developing a technology that may be applied to solve the problems around capturing patient information at the front end of care, and information that needs continuous updating. How can clinicians record clear and valid patient information during clerking procedures that can be used in a busy and ever-changing emergency setting?

A TECHNOLOGICAL SOLUTION

As highlighted above, published findings suggest the use of PDAs in electronically capturing patient details is an emerging field, both within the UK and abroad, and is one which is conducive to further development. Most developments are related to non-UK contexts and capture only a small subset of patient information. Further, the systems may not be customizable to other areas of medicine, where often only patient resuscitation details are recorded (see for example, Bird & Lane, 2006; Rosenthal & Wolford, 2000). Many systems involve more primitive components and may not be accepted as industry standard, or particularly robust given the nature of each application.

This evidence has reinforced the aim of our research project to develop a piece of software to record patient information on attendance to the A&E department of an acute hospital, particularly during clerking phases. The software is intended to form part of a proof-of-concept that can be extended to other areas of healthcare by being customizable, robust in design, and above all, applicable to an NHS hospital where procedures and IT infrastructures often differ.

The need for this type of mobile technology is elicited directly from the experiences of the patients and staff in our study. The findings suggest that repetition of assessments may occur because previous assessments have not been recorded in the notes properly or communicated effectively. Further, doctors and nurses continually move around the hospital system, as do patients. For example, an attendance to A&E may result in patients being referred to an assessment area, then referred for investigations such as x-ray (where results need to be relayed to doctors quickly), and possibly being admitted to a ward. Further referrals may then follow (e.g., outpatient referrals, or discharged back to community care settings).

The PDA mobile device may not only have the capability of keeping up with changeable physical locations, but also benefit clinicians through immediate provision of and sharing of information between and within various services throughout the hospital (potentially throughout the UK, given the existence of the national electronic records program). Note-taking problems, as observed in some instances during our research such as illegibility and loss of documentation, would also be overcome. Additionally, and most importantly in terms of clinical governance issues, having the ability to track which clinician has been responsible for clerking or treating a patient through a user sign-in feature when utilizing the PDA, would be of significant benefit over the relatively fallible system currently in operation.

The proposed PDA solution is based upon the digitization of the 'clerking form' (called the 'Adult Inpatient Assessment Protocol') currently used in the A&E department at the hospital. Clinicians complete the protocol following completion of a full history and examination of the patient. The protocol may not be completed in its entirety, as the latter part requires the recording of various test results and patient observations. During completion, the protocol is kept with the patient's notes in the A&E department. It is currently only available in paper form, and following patient discharge is stored in the hospital's archive together with other patient notes.

During development of the proof of concept, specific requirements were obtained from a combination of primary documentation used at the hospital and interviews undertaken with staff. The current IT developments within the trust were established with a meeting with the relevant Director of Information Management and Technology.

This technology addresses a number of key requirements:

- Mobility of device
- Ability to record patient information gathered during the clerking phase incorporating extended text-based notes and diagrams
- The ability to produce the equivalent paper-based records for inclusion in patient notes
- Consideration of appropriate security measures
- Adaptability in the device to allow for revisions to protocol and software

The PDA idea was developed using a simulation model on a computer where certain sections of the paper-based 'clerking protocol' were mapped onto the model to mirror the key stages of the clerking phase of the patient journey. When transformed to the PDA, it was envisaged that this process would guide the clinician through required fields and clarify the current stage of the patient journey while allowing the clinician to clearly record detailed relevant information. This illustrates the patient-centered nature of this proposed device. Figures 2 and 3 outline the process through which the PDA would operate in a hospital setting. An administrator would have access to the XML (Extensible Mark-up Language) document defining the appearance of the protocol (thus allowing alterations to be made). The hospital intranet would be used to link the system together.

Figure 2. Overall system architecture design

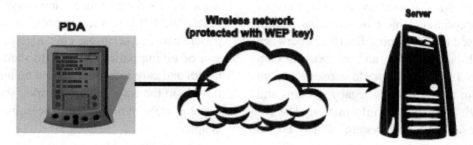

Figure 3. PDA use in context of hospital intranet

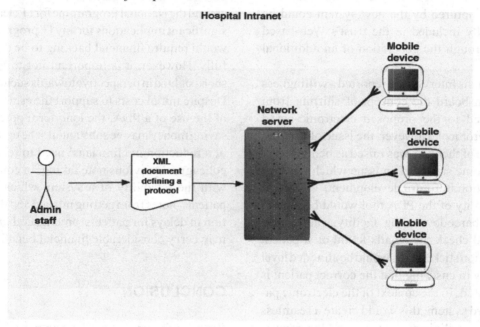

PDA EVALUATION

With an outline system specification formulated from the original initial research findings (indicating patients have concerns with repetition, while clinicians are concerned with poor notes), further clarification was sought on these issues with the system's prospective end users through direct observation at the hospital and interviews with relevant staff (n=7). This qualification was

sought with full consideration being given to the pressures typically encountered each day by clinical staff. Outlining the PDA concept to staff also proved useful in determining the general opinion amongst clinicians in the application of technology to this area.

IT managers at the trust indicated that the development of modular, Web-based systems would be the best option in future IT developments. It has been ascertained that the majority of patient data held by the trust is contained in information 'silos' on legacy systems, most of which were command line-based systems. Recent work focused on developing interfaces between a new Web-based system and the existing data structures. The system would retrieve patient details from the underlying legacy systems and generate views of patient information. The extensible design of a new system, shortly due to go live at the time of writing, would be able to accommodate the inclusion of patient data from other sources. This therefore, would mean that any data captured by the new system could be successfully included in the trust's Web-based system through the generation of an additional Web page.

Clinicians interviewed reported a willingness to take on board the concept of shifting from paper-based to the proposed electronic-based clerking protocol. However, the issue of training for the use of the PDA was raised as being necessary for some staff and an issue which requires consideration in future development.

The utility of the PDA tool would be greater still if a barcode reading facility was able to record and check the details found on a patient identification sticker. This would be an added level of security in ensuring that the correct patient is being treated. In the context of the electronic patient record system, this would create a seamless link between clinician clerking and the generic patient record. Data protection issues also would need to be fully addressed, as in any new data collection system.

FUTURE TRENDS

The PDA developments discussed in this chapter may contribute to UK-wide efforts to collect patient information and transfer patient records to an electronic format, although more research and testing is required. The National Programme for

IT (Connecting for Health Web site, 2007) aims to modernize the current computer systems used within the NHS, thereby improving the flow of patient care and services. This, together with the aim of giving patients access to their personal health and care information, and an ambition to transform the way the NHS works, shows there is some clear synergy with the subject of this chapter.

The highly publicized financial constraints currently facing many parts of the NHS and current issues that have been cited in the media around the National Programme for IT clearly have significant implications for any IT program which would require financial backing to be developed fully. However, it is important not to be overly short-sighted in perspective towards such a project. Despite initial costs to support the establishment of the use of a PDA, the long-term potential for saving money may be substantial. The opportunity of a reduction in clinicians' need to repeat their colleagues' previous note taking, in conjunction with the reliability of a system which protects patients' notes from getting mislaid and the reduction in delays for patients, amongst other factors, may carry considerable financial benefits.

CONCLUSION

We have shown that patient experience research can uncover 'critical areas' in the patient journey where improvements are required (e.g., clerking phase in A&E), thereby providing scope and detail to develop patient-centered technology for use at the front end of care. The PDA software prototype described here for capturing patient data has the potential to reform the way hospital clinicians currently record and share patient clerking details. This may be a further step towards revolutionizing healthcare systems within the field of hand-held mobile technology. More evaluation of the use of such a development and how it may link in with current and new hospital IT systems across the NHS is required, but the implications for staff working and patient experience have the potential to be far reaching. In the context of the national IT program for electronic patient records and the political emphasis on patient-centered care, these observations are particularly salient.

Future Research Directions

There are many varied opportunities related to the work presented by the authors in this chapter for consideration as future research directions. As the NHS continually evolves and hospital and healthcare services are further developed, opportunities for developing advanced technologies will continually present themselves.

Another focus of the authors' research is the organizational culture of hospital services, and in particular how cultures may vary between specialist and non-specialist areas within a hospital. Related to this is the role of the patient and the perceived control they have over their care and treatment. Traditional clinical boundaries are being challenged in this era of patient-centered modernization and there is a need for providing healthcare professionals with tools for addressing the cultural shift. This is especially relevant in respect to hospital re-developments, particularly as they often seek to build services around the patient journey. These insights, both from within our evaluation and across other studies, may enable the development of further technologies in a comparable way to the work described here. For example, computer-based interactive training tools focusing on optimum care pathways and multi-disciplinary working may be developed, where professionals can learn how to implement the best approaches and assess how various clinical scenarios may lead to different outcomes (such as in the case of 'simulation modelling').

In addition, with particular emphasis on the topic of this chapter, future research opportunities may relate to the potential for investigation of

working towards an entirely paper-free environment within an accident and emergency department context. Support for the smooth integration of such a system may include elements such as bar code readers on PDAs which link together patient information in a more seamless manner. The addition of barcode scanners or other peripheral devices (depending on the intended application) may assist in data capture and help minimize clerical errors. The longer-term implication might be for the majority of services across this and other UK hospitals to utilize electronic protocols, provided they were properly evaluated and proved successful. This could contribute to an evidence base that indicates the possibility of a hospital-wide paper-free environment.

Other important work may include the way in which data entered should be validated or verified. The challenge in this area is that although it should improve the accuracy of the data entered, it should do so without compromising the dynamic and user-friendly way in which protocols are designed, deployed and displayed. Furthermore, future developments could include a simple tool for the quick and concise creation of new protocols for use with this system. Work could also focus on system integration issues, such as software metrics and security measures as both would assist the integration of such a system into existing information systems at other hospitals and health trusts.

The scope for the application of technology within healthcare is near limitless and changes occurring in the NHS today are cutting edge. In addition to the clear patient and staff benefits resulting from such applications, the potential financial considerations and commitments would also be substantial. As a consequence of this, research which either evaluates the potential efficacy of proposed devices or provides an increased evidence base for the success of existing tools is fundamental to the ongoing 'modernisation' of the NHS.

ACKNOWLEDGMENT

The authors would like to express their thanks to the following people who contributed to and supported this work: Professor Zahir Irani, Professor Ewan Ferlie, Professor Les Mayhew, Lynne Greenstreet, Paul Parkin, David Powell, Sir Graham Morgan, Mr. Michael Burke, Dr. John Riordan, Yvonne Slater, Dr. Vincent Mak, Dr. Alan Warnes, Dr. Nicki Panoskaltsis, Dr. David King, Doug Irish, Manil Chouhan, Pooja Goel, Harnaik Johal, Sajita Sachchithanantham, Rick Juniper and all the staff and patients who kindly took part in the research. We would also like to extend our appreciation to the Department of Health for funding the project through the Knowledge Transfer Partnership (KTP) scheme and NHS R&D Support Funding.

REFERENCES

Aziz, O., Panesar, S., Netuveli, G., Paraskeva, P., Sheikh, A., & Darzi, A. (2005). Handheld computers and the 21st century team: A pilot study. *BMS Medical Informatics and Decision Making, 5*(28).

Bird, S., & Lane, D. (2006). House officer procedure documentation using a personal digital assistant: A longitudinal study. *BMC Medical Informatics and Decision Making, 6*(5).

Connecting for Health. Retrieved April 1, 2007, from http://www.connectingforhealth.nhs.uk/.

Department of Health. (2000). *The NHS plan: A plan for investment, a plan for reform.* London: HMSO.

Department of Health. *The creation of the National Health Service.* Retrieved April 13, 2006, from http://www.dh.gov.uk/AboutUs/HowDH-Works/HistoryOfDH/HistoryOfDHArticle/fs/en?CONTENT_ID=4106108&chk=ujPIOa.

Ham, C. (2004). *Health policy in Britain: The politics and organisation of the National Health Service* (5th ed.). Hampshire: Palgrave Macmillan.

Healthcare Commission. (2004). Retrieved April 13, 2006, from http://ratings2004.healthcarecommission.org.uk/.

Iles, V., & Sutherland, K. (2001). *Organisational change.* NCC SDO.

Kennedy, I. (2001). *Learning from Bristol: Public inquiry into children's heart surgery at the Bristol Royal Infirmary 1984-1995.* London: The Stationery Office.

Lapinsky, S., Weshler, J., Mehta, S., Varkul, M., Hallett, D., & Stewart, T. (2001). Handheld computers in critical care. *Critical Care, 5*(4), 227-231.

Levitt, R., Wall, A., & Appleby, J. (1999). *The reorganized National Health Service* (6th ed.). United Kingdom: Stanley Thornes Ltd.

McNulty, T., & Ferlie, E. (2002*). Re-engineering healthcare: The complexities of organisational transformation.* Oxford: Oxford University Press.

Newlan, S., van Dam, T., Klootwijk, P., & Meij, S. (2002). Ubiquitous mobile access to real-time patient monitoring data. *Computers in Cardiology, 22-25,* 557-560.

NHS Modernisation Agency. (2005). *Improvement leaders' guide: Process mapping, analysis and redesign.* London: HMSO.

NHS.UK. (2006). *About the NHS.* Retrieved April 12, 2006, from http://www.nhs.uk/england/aboutTheNHS/history/default.cmsx.

Oyama, L., Tannas, H., & Moulton, S. (2002). Desktop and mobile software development for surgical practice. *Journal of Pediatric Surgery, 37*(3), 477-481.

Pattichis, C., Kyriacou, E., Voskarides, S., Pattichis, M., Istepanian, R., & Schizas, C. (2002). Wireless telemedicine systems: An overview. *IEEE Antenna's and Propogation Magazine, 44*(2), 143-153.

Rosenthal, M., & Wolford, R. (2000). Resident procedure and resuscitation tracking using a palm computer. *Academic Emergency Medicine, 7*(10), 1171.

Serif, T., Ghinea, G., & Frank, A. (2005). A ubiquitous approach for visualizing back pain data. *Proceedings of the International Conference on Computational Science and its Applications* (ICCSA 2005), (pp. 1018-1027).

Sommers, K., Hesler, J., & Bostick, J. (2001). Little guys make a big splash: PDA projects at Virginia Commonwealth University. *Proceedings of the 29th annual ACM SIGUCCS conference on User services,* (pp. 190-193).

Turner, P., Milne, G., Kubitscheck, M., Penman, I., & Turner, S. (2005). Implementing a wireless network of PDAs in a hospital setting. *Personal and Ubiquitous Computing, 9*(4), 209-217.

Additional Reading

Ancona, M., Dodero, G., Minuto, F., Guida, M., Gianuzzi, V. (2000). Mobile computing in a hospital: The WARD-IN-HAND project. Symposium on Applied Computing. *Proceedings of the 2000 ACM symposium on Applied Computing* (SAC '00), (pp. 554-556).

Andrade, R., Wangenheim, A., Bortoluzzi, M., & De Biasi, H. (2003). A strategy for a wireless patient record and image data. *International Congress Series, 1256* (June), 869-872.

Beach, M., Miller, P., & Goodall, I. (2001). Evaluating telemedicine in an accident and emergency setting. *Computer Methods and Programs in Biomedicine, 64,* 215-223.

Berglund, M., Nilsson, C., Révay, P., Petersson, G., & Nilsson, G. (2007). Nurses' and nurse students' demands of functions and usability in a PDA. *International Journal of Medical Informatics, 76*(7), 530-537.

Campbell, C., Clark, L., Loy, D., Keenan, J., Matthews, K., Winograd, T., et al. (2007). The bodily incorporation of mechanical devices: Ethical and religious issues (part 1). *Cambridge Quarterly of Healthcare Ethics, 16*(2), 229-239.

Editorial. (2005). *Journal of Visual Communication in Medicine, 28*(3), 101.

Honeybourne, C., Sutton, S., & Ward, L. (2006). Knowledge in the palm of your hands: PDAs in the clinical setting. *Health Information and Libraries Journal, 23*(1), 51-59.

Kho, A., Henderson, L., Dressler, D., & Kripalani, S. (2006). Use of handheld computers in medical education. A systematic review. *Journal of General Internal Medicine, 21*(5), 531-537.

Kuziemsky, C., Laul, F., & Leung, R. (2005). A review on diffusion of personal digital assistants in healthcare. *Journal of Medical Systems, 29*(4), 335-342.

Lee, T. (2007). Patients' perceptions of nurses' bedside use of PDAs. *CIN: Computers, Informatics, Nursing, 25*(2), 106-111.

Luo, J. (2006). Mobile medical sources: Medical information anytime and anywhere. *Primary Psychiatry, 13*(10), 19.

Luo, J. (2007). The medical evolution of personal digital assistants. *Primary Psychiatry, 14*(1), 20-22.

May, C., Finch, T., Mair, F., & Mort, M. (2005). Towards a wireless patient: Chronic illness, scarce care and technological innovation in the United Kingdom. *Social Science & Medicine, 61*(2005), 1485-1494.

Patel, N. (2002). Health informatics governance: Researching deferred IS/IT mechanisms. *Proceedings of the 36th Hawaii International Conference on Systems Sciences* (HICSS'03).

Reynolds, P., Harper, J., Dunne, S., Cox, M., & Myint, Y. (2007). Portable digital assistants (PDAs) in dentistry: Part I. *British Dental Journal, 202*(7), 409-413.

Smordal, O., & Gregory, J. (2003). Personal digital assistants in medical education and practice. *Journal of Computer Assisted Learning, 19*(3), 320-329.

Sugden, B., &Wilson, R. (2004). Integrated care and electronic transmission of prescriptions: Experience off the evaluation of ETP pilots. *Health Informatics Journal, 10*(4), 277-290.

Swarts, J. (2005). PDAs in medical settings: The importance of organization in PDA text design. *IEEE Transactions on Professional Communication, 48*(2), 161-176.

Van Sinderen, M., van Halteren, A., Wegdam, M., Meeuwissen, H., & Eertink, E. (2006). Supporting context-aware mobile applications: An infrastructure approach. *IEEE Communications Magazine, 44*(9), 96-104.

Ward, M. (2007). The doctor's PDA and smartphone handbook: A guide to handheld healthcare. *Journal of Telemedicine & Telecare, 13*(3), 162-162.

Wilcox, R., & Whitham, E. (2003). Reduction of medical error at the point-of-care using electronic clinical information delivery. *Internal Medicine Journal, 33*(11), 537-540.

Willmot, M., & Sullivan, F. (2000). NHSNet in Scottish primary care: Lessons for the future. *British Medical Journal, 321,* 878-881.

Yi, M., Jackson, J., Park, J., & Probst, J. (2006). Understanding information technology acceptance by individual professionals: Toward an integrative view. *Information & Management, 43*(3), 350-363.

Chapter V
Cluster–Based Multi–Dimensional Visualization:
Harnessing Computational Resources for Real–Time Visualization

Douglas R. Janes
University of Wisconsin–Madison, USA

Michael J. Schulte
University of Wisconsin–Madison, USA

Ethan K. Brodsky
University of Wisconsin–Madison, USA

Walter F. Block
University of Wisconsin–Madison, USA

ABSTRACT

There is a growing need for high-frame-rate low-latency visualization solutions as medical practice moves toward interventional procedures. We present a cost-effective visualization system well suited for off-line visualization and interventional procedures. Users can view large time-resolved multi-dimensional datasets in real time with GPU cluster visualization. In addition, computational pre-processing can be hidden by rendering across distributed graphics cards, leading to improved frame-rates over a single graphics card solution. Finally, rendering on graphics cards offloads CPU cycles for generating the next time frame in the visualization. We have developed a network arbitration protocol for GPU cluster visualization called "token scheduling." Our protocol reduces communication latency, which in turn lowers visualization latency and improves system stability and scalability. In addition, we evaluate GPU cluster behavior and performance through a timing analysis. This analysis leads to a better understanding of cluster size needed to achieve the desired frame rate of a given problem.

INTRODUCTION

In the current medical clinical imaging paradigm, referring physicians usually order a diagnostic procedure to answer a clinical question. Technologists perform a set of prescribed scans that are specified and designed in advance to answer the specific question. Images are reconstructed and stored before being reviewed later by a radiologist at a Picture Archiving and Communication System (PACS). A PACS can post-process images from many modalities and enhance images when viewing off-line. Although these off-line still images are successfully used to diagnose many ailments, there is a growing need to interactively render multiple dimension image volumes, often containing time-varying information. These capabilities are necessary as imaging expands beyond anatomical diagnostic imaging to address functional clinical questions and interventional procedures, where processing must be performed in real time.

In addition to interventional procedures, interactive visualization of high-resolution images can convey additional information through motion. High resolution and motion are a large part of human perception and can naturally enhance insight provided by visualization; enabling the user to observe behavior not easily seen in still images. For example, viewing 3D medical images in real time can enable or enhance many interventional medical procedures. In contrast-enhanced MR angiography of the chest and abdomen, real-time imaging enables technologist to coach the patient to initiate a breath-hold as intravenous contrast arrives in the chest. Later, interactive visualization of the flow patterns in the MR exam can inform the radiologist about complex pathology such as dissections and abnormal vascular networks.

Currently, only top medical centers have access to real-time visualization of 3D medical image volumes. Very little interventional MRI is being performed outside research centers for several reasons, with visualization being one of the chief reasons. The remaining facilities view low-resolution time-resolved visualization (Figure 1) on PACS systems off-line, often with poorly responsive interaction when the number of dimensions of data grows. If the tools are not responsive or are not easy to use, the radiologists will not utilize them. Thus, new visualization solutions are needed to help overcome these problems.

One such visualization solution, called graphics processing unit (GPU) Cluster Multi-dimen-

Figure 1. Current clinical solutions have reduced resolution and cinematic rate (right), the full resolution image as seen on a PACS system (left)

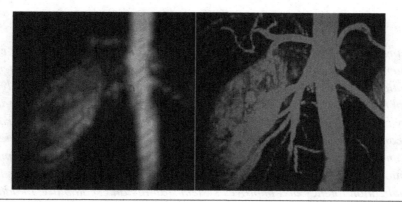

When playing back time-resolved image volumes on a commercial PACS system, resolution is reduced. Cines using images similar to the left image can deliver a vague indication of contrast flow in the body, but lacks detail for precise control in an interventional system.

sional Real-time Visualization, uses the combined resources of a computer cluster to generate an animated interactive visualization of large, complex data sets. GPU Cluster Multi-dimensional Visualization enables users to visualize complex models and image sets in real time. Multi-dimensional visualization refers to the visualization of 3D volumes with additional overlaid data. For example, in medical imaging it is useful to overlay 3D spatial data with additional information, such as flow vectors. GPU Cluster Visualization is a distributed computing solution where computation and rendering are performed in parallel on a computer cluster. This method can extend currently developed complex n-dimensional single time-frame visualization models to time-rendered models that are interactive at the full cine frame rate in real time.

This approach offers significant advantages over recorded visualization cines, since it allows users to visualize, manipulate, and interact with multi-dimensional datasets in real time. A key component of this approach is the ability to dynamically select a sub-volume of interest to analyze. For example, the user can visualize the body at various scales. GPU Cluster Visualization is beneficial since it provides the ability to visualize large complex time-varying 3D image volumes and datasets, without the prohibitive cost of supercomputers. It is also beneficial for datasets that are too large to be stored on a single graphics card, require significant pre-processing before it is rendered, or cannot be visualized in real time by a single computer due to memory constraints.

Acquiring MRI image data fast enough to produce time-varying 3D image volumes at reasonable frame rate and resolutions is challenging. The spatial encoding mechanisms in MR only allow a relatively small number of detectors to acquire data simultaneously; unlike ultrasound and CT where thousands of sensors can sample data

Figure 2. The 4D Cluster Visualization (4DCV) user interface

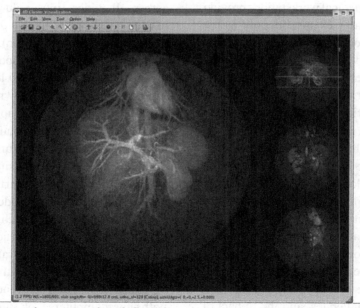

The 4DCV interface runs on the master node and allows the user to interactively manipulate the displayed image. The main image (at left) is a time-resolved 3D MIP which can be seen from arbitrary viewpoints and with arbitrary cut planes. The three smaller images (at right) show axial, coronal, and sagittal slices which can be used as an aid for image manipulation.

at once. Consequently, our group has conducted significant research to enable faster acquisition times. One method, time-resolved Contrast-Enhanced MR Angiography (CE-MRA), provides time-varying three-dimensional data for cinematic interactive visualization. Such methods are essential for delivering the full promise of MRI in diagnostic angiography and guiding intravascular procedures. We have previously shown that the high image contrast between vessels and background in CE-MRA allows accelerated imaging using an under-sampled 3D projection (3D PR) trajectory (Barger, Block, Toropov, Grist, & Mistretta, 2002; J. Liu et al., 2006), known as Vastly under-sampled Isotropic PRojection (VIPR) imaging. Angiography exams are visualized using a Multi-Planar Volume Reformat (MPVR) tool that allows the user to interactively view a Maximum Intensity Projection (MIP) image of the data from various viewing perspectives. When working with 4D MRA exams (three dimensions plus time), the added time dimension and large anatomical coverage can increase the memory requirements for visualization tools by a factor of 20 or more over conventional techniques. Current medical workstations provide some capability for large exams, but only with a substantial loss of resolution at very modest frame rates during interactive operations. We present a method for interactively visualizing 4D and multi-dimensional volumetric data, as shown in Figure 2, with no loss in resolution using powerful graphics cards and distributed processing.

In this chapter, multi-dimensional visualization and its user interface implications are presented through an in-depth look at GPU Cluster Visualization and its behaviors. An implementation of 4D Cluster Visualization (4DCV) is discussed as we review our approach of providing interactive real-time visualization applications. We present background literature, the challenges facing real-time GPU Cluster Visualization applications, our approach to these challenges, and the impact of this technology on multi-dimensional GPU cluster visualization.

BACKGROUND

Over time, low latency rendering for visualization has moved from primarily supercomputers to primarily graphics cards. Supercomputers are capable of fast rendering, due to high parallelism present in graphics rendering, at a premium cost. In recent years, graphics processors have increased in parallel processing capability and clock speed. This combined with direct rendering on GPU hardware, using Graphics languages like OpenGL (Shreiner, Woo, Neider, & Davis, 2005), enable low-latency, low-cost rendering for visualization. In addition, OpenGL and visualization packages built on top of OpenGL, like Open Inventor (Wernecke, 1994), provide high-level languages for rapid development of rendering algorithms. Finally, distributed GPUs are being used to reduce rendering latencies even further.

A scientific visualization study of parallel pipelined rendering on a supercomputer studied using inter-volume and intra-volume parallelization for pipeline rendering of time-varying volume data (Chiueh & Ma, 1997); from one time frame across all nodes (intra-volume parallelization) to each node working on its own separate frame (inter-volume parallelization). They found that a hybrid between the two methods worked well since it was the best at hiding I/O latency and time to first frame viewed, also known as startup latency. They targeted an efficient approach to hide the I/O latency involved with loading and processing large 128^3 time-varying volumetric datasets of a time-dependent turbulence simulation. The super computer processors were partitioned into groups, called virtual rendering nodes, to exploit inter-volume parallelization in hiding I/O latencies. In addition, the processors in each group were used to exploit intra-volume parallelism. This work was before modern GPUs with multiple rendering pipelines existed and thus rendering images even with supercomputers took significant amounts of time. They found that the ideal number of virtual groups were in the range of 4 to 8 nodes for 16 to 64 cluster node solutions. Current midrange commodity GPUs now have 12+ parallel rendering pipelines, which exceeds the group size of all the efficient solutions in this study; so inter-volume parallelism is accounted for to some degree on graphics cards. One requirement in this system is that the rendering time of sub-volumes needs to be large enough to cover the cost of synchronization and compositing all the intermediate results into the final image.

Research has also focused on using clusters for visualization. One technique uses software library interfaces that interpret OpenGL commands and then in turn re-distribute the rendering across several nodes in a cluster. Chromium is one such framework (Humphreys et al., 2002). Chromium processes streams of graphics API commands, re-distributing them according to a configuration file and the capabilities of nodes in the cluster. It is a flexible framework that allows many cluster topologies without requiring re-development of OpenGL programs by providing a library that processes OpenGL commands to match configurations specified by the user.

Cluster rendering algorithms tend to utilize OpenGL primitives or vertex-based rendering. Medical visualization, on the other hand, typically deals with volume element- (voxel-) based rendering, frequently called "volumetric rendering." In this case, data is stored in voxels, where each voxel can store one or many data values associated with a location in the volume. One major difference between rendering from volumetric data as opposed to primitives is volumetric data will often be significantly larger. In volumetric data visualization, where the volume data is also generated by the cluster, network and CPU resources of the cluster are needed for data generation where possible. GPU Cluster Visualization frees up resources needed to manage data transfers by scheduling data transfers ahead of time; thus allowing more CPU cluster cycles and more network bandwidth for generating real-time volumetric data, such as data for MRI image reconstruction.

Another cluster-based visualization solution (Tomov et al., 2004) combined Chromium, Open Inventor (Wernecke, 1994), and VTK (Schroeder, Martin, & Lorensen, 2002) to visualize large 3D volume on a commodity-based cluster. They experimented with both volumetric rendering and objects built with several OpenGL primitives. Their system used a master/slave configuration, where the master node captured user input and broadcasted the information to the slave nodes, where each slave ran an application to visualize a separate part of a global scene. They found that the communication of data was a large bottleneck in their system. This bottleneck could be alleviated by using display lists in the OpenGL primitive rendering case. However, their 1Gbit network was fully utilized causing a bottleneck when rendering volumetric data at even a volume size of 16MB. For reference, a 256^3-voxel volume with one 2-byte datum per voxel is 32MB. Thus a specialized solution that also provides capabilities for generating and pre-processing data is needed when volumetric data is visualized in real time.

Noting the need for more computational power for real-time and interventional MRI, Redmond et al. (2004) introduced the technique of 4D Cluster Visualization. This technique focuses on producing real-time interactive cines of volumetric time-resolved data by rendering MIP images, reading back the 2D rendered result, and sending the 2D result to a central cine console, for viewing. In 3D graphics, 3D objects must be transformed or projected from 3D space to 2D space for display on a screen. A frequent projection algorithm used in medical imaging is MIP. In this method, each voxel or volume element is projected onto the 2D screen space, where only the maximum value along each projection line is kept for each pixel in the final image. Modern graphics cards are capable performing these MIP computations at a rapid rate, making pre-loading of data the dominant bottleneck.

Several issues led to the introduction of GPU Cluster Visualization. First, the memory capacity of one graphics card is not enough to hold large numbers of volumetric datasets. The time needed to load, pre-process, and render large datasets leads to unacceptable frame rates and response times, when using a single node for visualization. Second, GPU clusters allow the volumetric dataset to be generated and rendered in real time by reconstructing MRA image data on the same cluster. Essentially, there is more than rendering that goes into visualizing data. Third, parallel processing can hide latency, thus increasing the performance of the overall system.

MULTI-DIMENSIONAL VISUALIZATION CHALLENGES

Multi-dimensional visualization allows information to be conveyed from large multi-variate datasets and enables processing multi-variate data mapped to 3D space, where each voxel has multiple data points of associated information,

for example, multiple images can be rendered simultaneously to convey additional information (Figure 3). When considering a human computer interface that allows good human control, system response time must be considered. In a study of remote manipulator control from video feedback (Liu, Tharp, French, Lai, & Stark, 1993), operators were able to achieve interactive manipulation without degradation in their performance with 500ms response times for experts and 100ms response times for novices. In addition, experts were able to interactively manipulate the system down to 1-second response time, with only a small increase in manipulation error. Lower response times were shown to have little impact on user performance. From our preliminary studies, we have noted that response times above 400ms have noticeable lag in response and the object appears to have a noticeable amount of update lag, where the visualization viewing perspective moves past the mark when the mouse stops. Response times between 400ms and 200ms appear more fluid

Figure 3. Multi-dimensional images have multiple data values per voxel

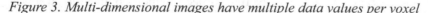

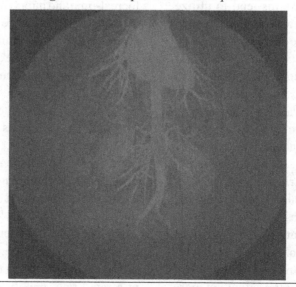

In this image two 3D volumes are being rendered at the same time. This can be done by having two data points for each voxel. The first point consists of an early image that shows arteries, shown in red. The second point is taken from a later image where the veins, shown in blue, are displayed by taking the difference between the artery volume and the current volume. This is just one way that multi-dimensional images can be used to enhance visualization.

with less lag. In updates above 100ms, manipulation no longer appears to have any lag. Response times below 100ms only make manipulation appear sharper. For interventional systems, a more thorough study needs to be made since the flow rate or movement rate of objects in the image dictates the response time needed for accurate manipulation and control.

To convey the information present in a real-time multi-dimensional interactive visualization, systems are challenged with producing high image resolution visualization cine while achieving high frame rate at a fast response time. One way to minimize response time and maximize frame rate is to use a supercomputer. Although this is a valid solution, it is cost prohibitive in many situations.

A cost effective alternative is the use of GPU Cluster Visualization. A GPU cluster can meet both frame rate and response time requirements of many visualization workloads. The frame rate needs to be variable to convey information such as motion. The maximum frame rate achievable by a given cluster can be increased by adding more nodes until the maximum frame rate achievable due to serial operations is reached. This can be performed dynamically at runtime. The response time needs to be fast for adequate manipulation. If the response time is too slow, user interaction becomes sluggish or weighty. Motion continues to occur after the user stops manipulating the volume being visualized, such as by manipulating the mouse. At the other extreme, once an acceptable response time is met, using faster response times unnecessarily puts pressure on the system network, which is a precious resource for generating future data to be visualized.

Large multi-variable volumetric visualization datasets can stifle real-time performance due to long data transfer latencies. In addition, the data grows at the rapid pace of $O(n^3)$, where n is one dimension of a regular cube of volumetric data. This necessitates consideration of where and when data is processed in the visualization application, requiring precise control of rendering along with a delicate balance of inter-volume and intra-volume rendering to achieve a responsive design.

Finally, the user interface, scalability, extensibility, image serialization, and timing jitter present challenges to overcome when creating a GPU Visualization Cluster. User interface design, for MRI systems, is a complex issue of balancing functionality and complexity. Ease in growing the system and porting to other applications are critical to system adoption. The more applications a hardware system can efficiently support, the better the solution. Image serialization entails viewing medical images in chronological order. Timing jitters occur when frames are not displayed at a regular rate. All of these challenges should be addressed from an end-users perspective.

GPU CLUSTER VISUALIZATION

GPU Cluster Visualization utilizes clustered graphics cards to remotely visualize multi-dimensional data in the form of an interactive 3D cine. In our application, 4D Cluster Visualization (4DCV) is being developed for standalone GPU Cluster Visualization, as well as an essential part of an interventional MRI system. In addition, the cluster has been intentionally designed for low utilization of GPUs and CPUs and to meet specific response time and frame rate targets; allowing the interventional system to perform medical image reconstruction and data generation concurrently on the same cluster in real time. GPU Cluster Visualization supports latency hiding for loading images across the network, in addition to hiding the latency of pre-processing MRI images. Network bandwidth is one of the critical resources of MRI image reconstruction, due to the high communication bandwidth needed to reconstruct MRI images. Rendering on a slave node reduces network traffic as the data will already be present on the slave nodes; thus, data transfer time is spared by sending a much smaller 2D image across the network, compared to the 3D volumetric data needed to render the 2D image.

User Interface

For generations, people have used high-speed cameras to gain insight into fast processes, such as, running and impact, and used slow cameras, such as in time-lapse photography, to gain insight into slow processes. Motion in medical imaging allows the observance of flow rates (Figure 4) and motion in the body—not easily interpreted using still images. One example is the hemodynamic significance of stenosis. By watching the time-resolved flow of an injected contrast agent near a stenosis, the extent of the blockage and flow from collateral vessels to distal tissue can be appreciated. Fast frame rates are needed to observe rapid motion, such as flow in a moving heart; while slower frame rates are sufficient for viewing flow rates in a vascular system or larger view. The GPU Cluster Visualization framework accommodates both situations by offering a variable frame rate solution.

4DCV is a remote visualization solution that allows users to view images off-line at a location that is convenient to them. To bring about this flexibility, the system has been designed to operate with a standard office, 100Mb Ethernet link to the master node. Faster network connections enable faster frame rates and faster response times, but are not necessary for vascular flow visualization. Since 10 frames per second(fps) is seen as a sufficient frame rate for this application (Redmond et al., 2004), faster networks like 1Gb Ethernet, Myrinet, and Infiniband will be an essential element for interventional systems to reduce the latency from image capture to image viewing in real time.

The flexibility to automatically operate on slow or fast networks without user intervention is

Figure 4. In angiography the ability to observe and quantify flow rates is important

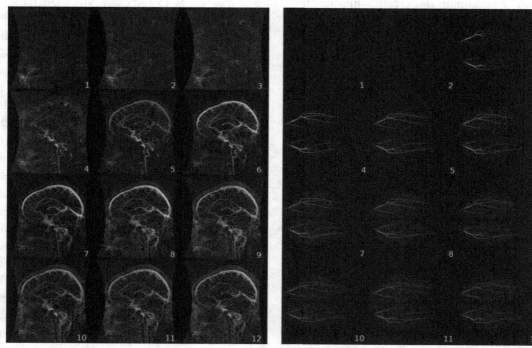

While looking at static images gives some sense of flow rate, it is easier for human perception to visualize the above sequences as an animated series. An animated series shows how flow rates change over time. In brain CE-MRA (left) the rate of enhancement can be easily seen in initial images, where differences in later frames are increasingly more difficult to see. In leg CE-MRA, image enhancement is more subtle across the entire series.

done by limiting the amount of data transferred to the master node from the slave nodes. The image size versus resolution tradeoff comes down to the resulting number of pixels that need to be transferred to generate a human interpretable image on the master node. Each pixel must be explicitly communicated in compressed or uncompressed form across the network. Also, image size, as viewed on the master can be increased once the image arrives at the master node. Thus, frame rate and response time are dependent on the total pixel count in the image, not in the eventual display.

The GUI interface as seen by the user is largely determined by the 3D visualization application being run on the cluster. Because GPU Cluster Visualization is a wrapper application that aids in combining the resources of several 3D visualization applications, each slave node runs its own copy of the 3D visualization application. GPU Cluster

Visualization naturally extends a 3D visualization application to an interactive cine with the full manipulation and feature set present on the original 3D visualization system. Adding motion combined with real-time interactive manipulation can increase understanding of behavior, giving further insight than the 3D visualization of a single time-frame snapshot.

A simple few-featured interface versus an intricate full-featured interface has long been an MRI user debate. GPU Cluster Visualization simplifies the issue by allowing higher resolution images to be viewed in real time, resulting in a higher standard baseline; eliminating the need for lower resolution options. GPU Cluster Visualization is part of a solution to reduce the compute time to real-time levels and part of a solution to enable the real-time use of MRI scan techniques.

Figure 5. Sampled images from an MRI angiography study visualization cine

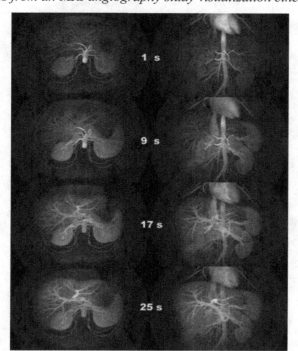

The select frames are shown from two perspectives side by side, axial view (right) and coronal view (left). Contrast flow is seen by the increased illumination of blood vessels and organs as the contrast agent spreads through the body.

The 4DCV user interface shown in Figure 2 demonstrates the information presented to the user in the 4DCV application; where the large center pane contains the interactive cine viewed by the user and the smaller panes on the right contain key views for axial, sagittal, and coronal references. Figure 5 shows an example of a 4-frame MRI time-resolved angiogram, viewed from the axial and coronal views. One can see the flow of contrast through the patient as time progresses from 1s to 25s.

Real-Time GPU Cluster Visualization

In 4DCV a distributed GPU cluster is used along with token scheduling to provide real-time visu-

alization by hiding latency and managing large datasets. This produces a visualization application capable of interactive and responsive visualization of time-varying volumetric medical datasets.

Distributed GPU Visualization Cluster Model

A distributed GPU visualization cluster enables real-time rendering of 3D model cines that tax the resources of a single node system. In the single rendering node model, volumetric data is sent to a single node and then rendered and viewed on the same node. Our multi-dimensional GPU Cluster Visualization model is a master-slave model (Figure 6), where slave nodes are equipped with graphics

Figure 6. 4DCV Block Diagram

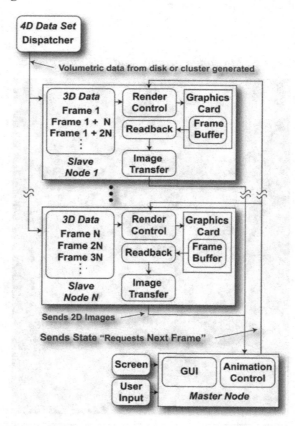

The master node controls the cine by requesting images and receiving images on scheduled boundaries. In standalone mode, images are read from disk. In interventional mode, data is generated on the cluster.

cards for rendering images from multi-dimensional data. In 4DCV, render processing is distributed by rendering each image on a separate slave node where the rendered images are sent to the master node for viewing. This model works for 4DCV since the dominating time is transferring the volumetric data to the rendering node, not the rendering time on the GPU. In addition, rendering on one node reduces network traffic significantly, since distributed rendering operations like volumetric data distribution and compositing of images are not needed. However, 4DCV does not handle the case where data distribution times are small and render times are high. When using longer, more complex latency rendering schemes of volumetric data, GPU Cluster Visualization needs to be modified to utilize parallel rendering or intra-volume parallelization. Hence, each node would render its volumetric data and send a 2D image to a slave node for compositing the image and then send the image to the remote master node. Either way, sending volumetric data across the network needs to be strictly planned to free necessary bandwidth for generating volumetric data for rendering later images in the sequence.

To reduce response time and frame-to-frame jitter, network bandwidth to the master node must be arbitrated. Consider the case with four slave nodes shown in Figure 7. This example shows that the latency for four transmissions will take around *4t* time units. In the arbitrated case, the latency of each packet is *t* from the start to the end of the transmission. Arbitration ensures only one frame is transferred at a time, thus producing faster response times and serializing the data transfers. Data on the master also needs to be processed sequentially, thus the arbitrated network has the added benefit of enabling a straightforward method of processing images sequentially in cine fashion. Sequential communication on the master link decreases latency without significant impact on throughput, allowing the frame rate to approach the full rate supported by the network.

Reduced data communication, offloaded CPU cycles, larger memory sizes, and larger GPU bandwidth are realized by having GPUs on each slave node. Rendering large volumetric datasets on slave nodes before transferring the data to the master node is a form of compression, because in 4DCV the resulting rendered image is smaller than the 3D volumetric dataset used to create the image. Real-time compression can further reduce data transmission times. Having a GPU on each slave node permits offloading CPU cycles that can then be used for real-time generation of more voxel, multi-variate data, or supporting scientific calculations needed for visualization. Finally, clustered GPUs increase the effective memory size and bandwidth of the collective rendering engine. They also increase the data transfer rate of the system from CPU to GPU since each card has a connection to the cluster. This combined

Figure 7. Image transmission latency

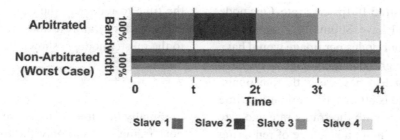

Due to large image sizes, arbitrating network bandwidth to the master node produces faster response times. In the top arbitrated bar, 100% of bandwidth is used for each individual image resulting in low transfer latency.

with the added GPU computational power yields higher frame rates with faster response times not available with a singe GPU solution.

Timing analysis

A timing analysis is useful in determining the size and performance of the cluster necessary to reach a desired latency and frame rate specification. Regardless of the GPU cluster configuration, the master node has a fixed amount of time to process each image in the cine:

$$\tau_m = \frac{1}{f} \qquad (1)$$

Where τ_m is the time available for each image in the cine on the master and f is the frame rate. When a cluster is used, the amount of compute time available for each frame increases with the addition of each slave node.

$$\tau_s = \frac{1}{f} N \qquad (2)$$

In 4DCV, the compute time available to pre-process image data and render the image on slave nodes, τ_s, is described by equation 2, where N is the number of slave nodes in the cluster. equation 2 holds true no matter how image computation is distributed among cluster nodes. If each image is computed on a single node, then all of the image computation time is available on one node. If image computation is spread across multiple nodes then all of these nodes equally divide the image computation time. Consider an 8-node cluster with a desired 10 fps cine rate. One node per image would have 800ms of computation time available, four nodes per image would have 200ms each and eight nodes per image would have 100ms each. In each of these cases, the total image computation time is 800ms; the computing time per image changes with the frame rate and size of the cluster. The main advantage of rendering on one node is less overhead from distributed computing. The main advantage of rendering on

multiple nodes is a potentially shorter rendering latency, where image rendering latency must be long enough on one node to justify the distributed rendering overhead.

When generating image frames for a time-varying visualization; computation can be divided into two categories: t_r the time to render the image and t_u the time to update state and prepare for the next image. In order for visualization to be performed on one system equation 3 must hold true.

$$\tau_m \leq t_r + t_u \qquad (3)$$

When equation 3 is false, the application will benefit from GPU Cluster Visualization.´ As the desire for more realistic visualization and faster frame rates continues to increase, GPU Cluster Visualization can take up the slack between current technology and computational demands of highly detailed visualizations with large datasets, volume visualization, and/or time-varying data.

In order for the frame rate to be met on a cluster, the time for image generation, t_i, assigned to a node plus the time to update to the next image must be less than the total time allotted to process a frame on each node (equation 4).

$$\tau_s \geq t_i + t_u \qquad (4)$$

In 4DCV, images are rendered on slave nodes; where image generation is made up of the components needed to generate images in a distributed fashion and display them locally, which includes: the time to render t_r, the time to read back the frame buffer t_{rb}, and the time to transfer the image to the master node, t_t, shown in equation 5.

$$t_i = t_r + t_{rb} + t_t \qquad (5)$$

Finally the time on the slave to update to the next frame, τ_u, is simply the time allocated on the slave per frame minus the time to generate an image; shown in equation 6, where N_i is the number of slave nodes working in parallel to generate a single image time-frame. This leads to the observation that growing the size of the cluster directly impacts the complexity of visualization possible on the cluster. In other words, adding more nodes translates into more time for image update and data generation on the cluster while still achieving the same or higher frame rates. It is a basic, but important concept for understanding the workloads that can benefit from GPU Cluster Visualization.

$$\tau_u = \frac{\tau_s}{N_i} - t_i \qquad (6)$$

Using the timing analysis above, the number of nodes required to meet an applications frame rate can be calculated using equations 7-9. For a given frame rate f, equation 7 can be used to calculate the number of nodes needed to render images on a cluster, N_r. equation 8 can be used to calculate the number of nodes needed to meet frame update computational demands, N_u. Finally, the total number of nodes needed in the system for a given problem, $N_{cluster}$, can be calculated with

equation 9. For more accurate results, data distribution needs to be decided before calculating the cluster size needed. This is because update and rendering times may not scale depending on the 3D visualization application being used.

$$N_r = t_i f \qquad (7)$$

$$N_u = t_u f \qquad (8)$$

$$N_{cluster} = \lceil N_r + N_u \rceil \qquad (9)$$

The response time of the system is based on the serial latencies of the system once the graphics card has been prepared for rendering. equation 10 is basically a sum of all the latencies depicted in Figure 8 with the addition $1/f$ to account for the potential delay between user input and the timed request for the next frame.

$$response\text{-}time = t_{ss} + t_i + t_{is} + t_{su} + \frac{1}{f} \qquad (10)$$

Where t_{ss} is the time to send state to the slave node, t_{is} is the time to perform image setup, and

Figure 8. Timing block diagram

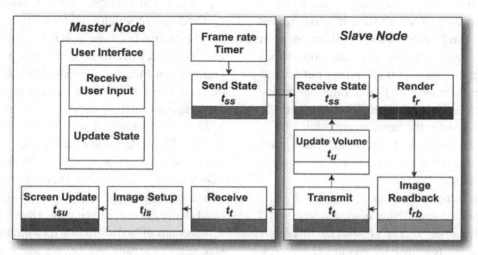

Several latencies contribute to the overall system response time. As each image is rendered, the path from sending state to screen update is taken. When each slave node is responsible for rendering multiple image volumes, the update volume path is taken between rendering passes.

Table 1. Cluster analysis using equations 1-10

Example	Frame-rate (f) fps	Image Generation (t_i) sec	Image Update (t_u) sec	Render Nodes (N_r)	Update Nodes (N_u)	Cluster Node Count ($N_{cluster}$)	Time Per Slave (τ_s) sec	Response- time (sec)
1	11	0.05	0.5	0.55	5.5	7	0.63	0.166
2	30	0.1	0.1	3	3	6	0.2	0.158
3	20	0.2	2	4	40	44	2.2	0.275
4	20	0.07	0.1	1.4	2	4	0.2	0.145
5	5	0.4	4	2	20	22	4.4	0.625

Several scenarios are shown where frame rate, image generation and image update times are varied to show several cluster behaviors. For these examples assume tss = 2ms, tis = 3 ms, tsu = 20 ms

t_{su} is the time to update the screen on the master node.

Table 1 gives examples of the size of cluster necessary to meet the needs of various 4DCV scenarios, where each time-frame is rendered by only one node ($N_i = 1$).

Higher frame rates can be achieved by adding more nodes to the system. In Table 1 the frame rate in Example 2 is faster than the frame rate in Example 4. This is a product of having more cluster nodes in Example 2. Adding cluster nodes can also overcomes longer image generation times. Comparing Example 1 and 2, it can be seen that the response time of Example 2 is shorter due to its faster frame rate, even though it has a longer image generation time. In Example 5, five frames per second can be achieved with this setup, even though the image update and generation times would lead to a time of 0.23 frames per second on a single node system. Frame rates can be increased until serial processing limitations are the bottleneck, chiefly the items in equation 10. For example, the frame rate can be increased until the image transfer latency to the master becomes the bottleneck.

Response time is largely decided by the performance of the string of dependent serial operations, namely t_{ss}, t_i, t_{is}, t_{su} and $1/f$. In Table 1 Example 1, the response time is larger than Example 2 even though the image generation time is almost double. This is because the frame period in equation 10 accounts for the delay between frames. The master node accumulates user input and then sends a render request to a slave node at timed intervals determined by the frame rate. The difference between response times in equation 1 and 2 is due to the more frequent render requests made in Example 2. This shows that response time can be reduced by having a higher frame rate. In this case, the frame rate represents the maximum rendering rate capable on the system. Interactive frame rate is logically independent from the cine frame rate in theory. If slower animation rates with faster response times are desired, simply choose an animation rate that is a factor of the frame rate. For example, the time frame can be updated on every other render update.

The main advantage of 4DCV is that preprocessing latency can be hidden. Modest size GPU clusters can hide a fair amount of latency and perform at various frame rates with relatively low response times. Example 5 in Table 1 shows a 22-node cluster that can hide 4 seconds of latency. Example 1 shows a 7-node cluster hiding 0.5 seconds of latency. One disadvantage of 4DCV latency-hiding is that the cluster node count increases quite rapidly when additional latency needs to be hidden, limiting its effectiveness to a few seconds of latency hiding for a modest cluster size and frame rate. But given enough resources there does not appear to be a theoretical limit on the amount of latency that can be hidden; one could in theory hide days of latency if enough nodes were available.

Data Management

Volumetric data size grows as $O(n^3)$, such that the total amount of data grows rapidly with volume size. For example, assuming one 16-bit short value is saved for each element: 64 x 64 x 64 requires 0.5 MB, 256 x 256 x 256 requires 32 MB, and 512 x 512 x 512 requires 256 MB. Larger volumes will continue to be advantageous for some time in the future, as volume size determines the field of view and resolution of the final medical image. One objective of GPU Cluster Visualization is to allow increasingly larger volumes to be processed in real time. To accomplish this, data management and communication must be considered when rendering from large time-varying volumetric datasets.

In medical voxel-based rendering, one method of processing volumetric data is to project data onto a 2D surface using a Maximum Intensity Projection (MIP). The image is a projection of the information in each voxel producing a 2D image that is smaller than the input data used to generate the image. Considering maximum theoretical Ethernet transfer rates, without accounting for communication overhead and network traffic, a 32MB data transfer of volumetric data taking a minimum of 250ms or a maximum of 4 fps is achievable. Comparing this to an ideal 100Mbit Ethernet connection which can theoretically transfer a 1024 x 1024 image with 1 byte per pixel at approximately 12 fps or a 512 x 512 image with 24-bit color at approximately 16 fps; it becomes apparent that data transfers need to be carefully planned to keep them from stifling performance and overwhelming the network.

4DCV manages its data by keeping all of the data for a given volume on one slave node in the cluster. This method works because the rendering time for one volume is sufficient to sustain 10+ fps with the use of low-end graphics cards (Janes,

Brodsky, Schulte, & Block, 2006). Thus major network data transfers in standalone mode are reduced to two types: loading volumetric data on cluster nodes at startup and the transfer of rendered images to the master node at runtime. Images are loaded at startup into slave node main memory allowing visualization of time-varying data too large to fit in the memory of one commodity graphics card or too large to sustain high-frame rates with limited bandwidth to the memory on one graphics card.

For multi-dimensional visualization where rendering times can easily exceed the allowable response time limit, one alternative is to turn to parallel rendering where each node or a subset of nodes has a portion of the volumetric data for each frame. Using this alternative, rendering time can be reduced; but the overhead of synchronization and compositing images needs to be amortized in order for the solution to be fruitful. Again, the main objective of GPU Cluster Visualization is to increase frame rates and decrease response time where possible using commodity-based systems

Token Scheduling

4DCV is built on a master-slave model where the master node provides a user interface and implicitly controls the slave nodes. The slave nodes render images according to requests from the master node and arbitrate the use of network bandwidth to the master node. Arbitration allows efficient use of the master network resources and reduces latency in the system, specifically targeting response time. This arbitration is performed by an internally developed Token Scheduling arbitration protocol inspired by Token Ring Networks.

Token Scheduling removes all arbitration computation and communication off of the network connection to the master node. This is accomplished by passing a token between the slave nodes in a circular fashion to provide arbitration of the master network bandwidth with low overhead. As shown in Figure 9, when a slave node receives a token, it is allowed to transmit an image across the network to the master node. When the last byte of the image transmission leaves the slave node, it passes the token to the next slave node.

Arbitrating the master node network bandwidth leads to better response times. The response time is reduced by causing the slave nodes to take turns using the network, as illustrated in Figure 7. In addition, Token Scheduling automatically serializes the image transmission, eliminates frame-to-frame jitter and significantly reduces frame-timing jitter. It also enables a straightforward method to adjust the frame rate and response time, based on the requirements of the end user.

Latency

Image generation from 3D volumetric datasets is performed in two steps: pre-processing and rendering from volumetric data. Pre-processing includes generation, distribution, pre-render conditioning, and loading of volumetric data in preparation for rendering. Rendering includes the projection of 3D volumetric data onto a 2D plane for viewing. All of these operations incur some latency, where operations independent of viewing perspective can potentially be hidden. However, operations dependent on viewing perspective, either directly or indirectly, cannot be hidden. 4DCV by default loops on the medical visualization cine. If all of the images fit into the memory of the graphics cards collectively, pre-processing only has to be performed once, which significantly reduces the size of the cluster ($t_u = 0$ -> $N_u = 0$). But, if at least one volumetric dataset time frame does not fit in the slave nodes graphics card memories, t_u will be non zero. Therefore, pre-processing will need to be performed in real time creating a need for latency-hiding.

In 4DCV, computational and communication latency cannot be completely eliminated. By use of

Figure 9. Token scheduling functional diagram

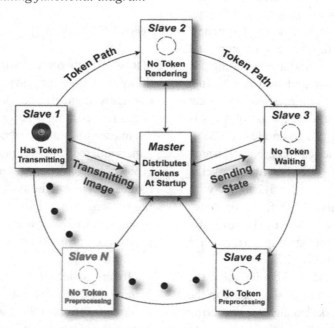

Master node network bandwidth is arbitrated by passing a token among slave nodes. Only the slave node with the token is allowed to transmit images to the master.

parallel resources, 4DCV hides several latencies, making them transparent to the user. Using cluster resources along with scheduling provided by Token Scheduling, pre-processing can be hidden by using a two-phase algorithm, depicted in Figure 9. In the first phase, each slave pre-processes the volumetric data needed to render the next frame it has been assigned. In the second phase, each slave renders the next image to be viewed and transmits it to the master node. Phase changes are driven by events. Phase one is entered when either the image is first assigned or at the end of phase two. Phase two begins when a render request has been received. All of this works due to a carefully planned allocation of cluster resources based on equations 1-9.

In GPU Cluster Visualization, the latency effects of several operations cannot be hidden. These latency effects show up in the response time, and because each operation is dependent on the previous operation, their effects add together as demonstrated by equation 10. These operations include: rendering on slave nodes, image transfer from master to slave, and master operations, such as image conditioning and screen update. Response time is measured from the time the user provides input to the time the screen updates. Because of this, rendering cannot be started until user input is provided. Thus, rendering latency along with all of the operations that are dependent on the output of the rendering operation cannot be hidden from the operator.

In addition to latency hiding, latency reduction can also be performed with distributed computing. 4DCV uses inter-volume rendering, where separate images are constructed simultaneously. This is a straightforward method to increase frame rates, but it suffers from lower response times since user input is needed well in advance. Intra-volume rendering, where a single image is rendered on multiple machines, suffers from distributed rendering overhead that can outweigh the increased read-back and rendering bandwidth. Chiueh and Ma (1997) used distributed computing

to perform inter-volume rendering. They enumerate several significant memory management and I/O latencies that need to be overcome. Typical inter-volume rendering challenges (Chiueh & Ma, 1997; Tomov et al., 2004) include distributing data to nodes, collecting results from nodes, compositing, and synchronization. All of these memory management latencies complicate the design of distributed systems, especially when considering inter-volumetric rendering of large datasets. Therefore, achieving fast response times and high frame rates are difficult when high-resolution images and multi-variate input datasets are used.

Scalability

Adding more nodes to 4DCV linearly increases data generation, pre-rendering, and rendering time available for each time frame; allowing more complex frames and multi-dimensional volumetric data to be generated and visualized. When running 4DCV without real-time data generation, performance scales well with adding slave nodes until the volumetric data fits collectively in the graphics card memories, where pre-processing of data no longer needs to be performed in real time. This also boosts performance since cluster nodes will not be needed to hide pre-processing. Once this occurs, adding more nodes no longer increases the performance of the system. When real-time data generation is also performed, the cluster also scales based on the application generating real-time data. One consideration that needs to be made for large clusters is GPU utilization. If GPUs are only used for rendering frames, having a graphics card on each slave node leads to low GPU utilization and limited benefit. In this case, it makes sense to have groups of cluster nodes that supply volumetric data to nodes with graphics cards. Decoupling the cluster in this fashion allows the benefit of GPU Cluster Visualization with less hardware.

GPU Cluster Visualization provides straight-forward management of serial operations to achieve high-frame rates for limited resources. This allows one solution to work with a wide range of master-to-cluster link bandwidths; from a slow wireless connection to a high-speed connection. The master can manage the master-slave connections simply by varying the image size transferred and the rate at which images are requested. For a properly balanced cluster, images are provided at the requested rate. When image transfer time is less than local rendering time, 4DCV can provide images faster than the frame rate possible by rendering on the master node itself.

Computation performed on each slave node is highly independent requiring little communication with other slave nodes. Communication consists of three types of messages during normal operation. The first message is from the master to a single slave node. The master sends the state needed to render the next time frame, implicitly notifying the slave to render a new image. The next message type is the slave node replying back to the master by sending back the newly rendered image. The third message type is a handshake between two slave nodes when the token is passed from one slave to another. Thus, all of the connections are point-to-point and precisely timed, eliminating contention or bottlenecks in the communication, no matter how many nodes are present. This achieves low network utilization, which is required for image reconstruction and volumetric data generation.

Any number of nodes can be supported by 4DCV. To capitalize on the scalable computational time provided by GPU Cluster Visualization, 4DCV can be run as a standalone single node system, a master with one slave node, or a master with many slave nodes. All of these configurations run from one executable where slave nodes and master node are specified by one command line switch. This is possible due to the scalable nature of Token Scheduling, which can be extended to support runtime cluster size scaling. In the one slave version, the slave is its own neighbor allowing it to send images one after another.

Extensibility

Visualization applications can be ported to work within the 4DCV framework with relatively few software changes. The main change consists of adding a small interface to the existing visualization application to enable communication between the 4D Cluster Visualization framework and the visualization application. The essential API consists of a few runtime functions: get rendering state, set rendering state, frame buffer read back, and frame buffer update, in addition to setup functions that specify images size and image file names. More advanced functionality in 4DCV is enabled by having the master node visualization program accumulate user input, where the state is passed to the slave node when a new image is to be rendered. The state basically consists of pre-processed mouse and keyboard commands, which are encapsulated into one state packet to give an absolute reference for rendering images.

Extending GPU Cluster Visualization is not limited to medical visualization. Scientific visualization and potentially non-visualization programs can be run on a GPU Cluster Visualization system. Sending the frame buffer contents to the master node does not have to be limited to just images. Arrays of any type, including floating point numbers, can also be sent. Transferring arrays of data to the master node allows use in other areas that can benefit from clustered GPUs like General Purpose GPU (GPGPU) scientific computing.

In an effort to make 4DCV more accessible, it has been designed to work well using commodity hardware. Having interactive 3D cinematic visualization more accessible to all users can accelerate the movement from diagnostic to interventional medical imaging in research and clinical settings. GPU Cluster Visualization can boost current technology to enable cinematic visualization of higher complexities.

Future growth is planned for 4DCV, as part of a real-time MRI image reconstruction and visualization system (Brodsky, Isaacs, Grist, & Block, 2006). In order to enable this growth, utilization of cluster resources used to perform real-time visualization are kept to a minimum. This is done by keeping data local where possible and rendering is largely performed on the graphics cards in the cluster, enabling the use of the cluster CPUs for real-time image reconstruction.

Implementation

The MR research group at the University of Wisconsin-Madison is working to translate the current diagnostic capabilities of MR angiography (4D MRA) into a real-time imaging system to guide and monitor interventional procedures. In this pursuit, 4DCV (Redmond et al., 2004; Janes et al., 2006) is being developed as a visualization platform for this purpose and as a standalone visualization application, where rendering of 3D images is performed on slave nodes by a modified version of a MPVR tool (Brodsky & Block, 2003).

A standalone version of 4DCV is currently implemented on a Linux cluster using commodity graphics cards, OpenGL, sockets, Qt, and an internally developed Token Scheduling protocol (Janes et al., 2006). Our current cluster hardware consists of seven HP zx2000 machines, each with an Itanium II processor, an HP NVIDIA Quadro4 980 XGL graphics card with 128MB of memory, and 4 GB of main memory, connected through a 100Mbit Ethernet LAN.

The implementation of 4DCV, illustrated in Figure 6, shows promising results. With lower-end graphics cards and commodity PCs, the system

Figure 10. Cluster timing example

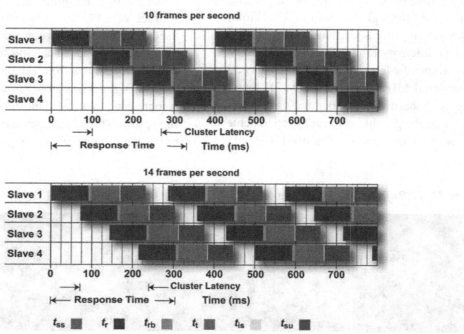

In a four node cluster using the numbers from our preliminary GPU cluster both 10 fps and 14 fps cine frame rates are presented. At the end of the 4th bar, when image transmission is complete, the slave is ready to update to the next image. In fact, the image can be updated during image transmission as long as it does not lengthen transmission latency.

can manipulate a large 256^3 voxel volume at 10 frame/s cine with roughly a 331 ms response time (Figure 10; Janes et al., 2006). These numbers do not include the time to pre-process images, since each node renders only one image. 4DCV rendering is performed on graphics cards, freeing CPU resources to perform MRI image reconstruction on the same cluster. The interactivity and ease of use of the 4DCV system and user interface is enhanced through feedback from radiologists who use the system to view time-varying images for interventional radiology.

The 4DCV application behaves identically to the 3D MPVR application (Brodsky & Block, 2003), with the addition of a cine created from the time-varying data. The thickness, orientation, and viewing angle of a targeted volume can be interactively specified to isolate the relevant structures of interest for the interventionalist (Redmond et al., 2004) at the full frame rate and response time. The target MIP volume is specified by two cut planes, where the user can specify the placement of each plane through the master GUI. Windowing-leveling is processed in hardware for isolation of image intensity ranges, adding the ability to focus on specific features in addition to targeting the rendered MIP volume. Finally, 3D textures along with hardware-accelerated interpolation support on the graphic cards are used to achieve fast low-artifact rendering (Figure 11).

FUTURE TRENDS

Real-time GPU Cluster Visualization stands to benefit from the current trends in commodity hardware improvements. GPU hardware performance continues to increase as memory size and speed increases, more graphics pipelines are added on chip, and graphics cards provide multiple GPU solutions, like SLI and Crossfire. The recent addition of programmable rendering pipelines show promise in delivering higher rendering algorithmic freedom and higher performance levels, opening new areas of hardware acceleration. GPUs and their use are rapidly changing. Current developments can be viewed on the developer pages for NVIDIA and ATI as well as the Web page for General Purpose GPU (gpgpu.org). CPUs are also increasing in performance by developing multiple core solutions and more efficient cores. Finally, networks continue to increase in bandwidth and decrease in latency.

In medical imaging, the computational resources of GPU Cluster Visualization can be used to enhance the human computer interface, by extracting and displaying in real time additional information from the data, adding to the user's insight. The number of coils used in MRI is increasing in order to improve SNR and imaging speed, which increases the need for parallel processing to render the images from each coil.

Figure 11. MIPs from oblique angles

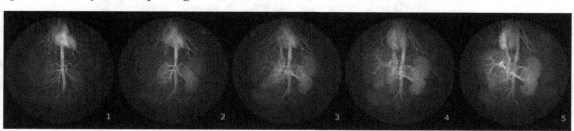

Our current GPU Cluster Visualization application uses 3D textures to reduce MIP artifacts when viewing a 3D voxel volume from oblique angles. The CE-MRA exam MIP time-series above shows a 3D time series where time progresses from left to right.

In addition, large volumetric datasets, large matrix visualization with overlays, segmentation, increased resolution and frame rates, 4D-CT and CE-MRI for interventional procedures, MRI with Diffusion Tensor overlays, PET with CT overlays, and virtual endoscopy with body motion can all benefit from GPU Cluster Visualization. To enable these benefits sooner using commodity hardware, it is important to offload CPU cycles and free network bandwidth for image reconstruction.

Several non-medical applications also show promise of benefiting from GPU Cluster Visualization. These visualization applications generally consist of 3D volume/surface models with overlays of scalar, vector, tensor field or gradient data, with ether slow data generation or rendering. Weather research is an important visualization field. 3D terrain surfaces including air and/or water volumes have good potential to be enhanced when visualizing ocean currents, tectonic plate shifting, volcanic activity, and geoscience modeling. Other areas include molecular modeling, finite element analysis, computational fluid dynamics, atmospheric flow models, high-energy physics, electron density maps, and severe weather modeling.

CONCLUSION

GPU Cluster Visualization enhances the human computer interface by enabling interactive medical cinematic visualization of large time-varying 3D volumetric datasets to better convey information. Specifically, motion is added, by processing datasets in real time to produce an interactive cine. The system can maintain fast response times with relatively high image resolution and user selectable frame rate for the cine application while frame rates can be varied to match the clinical application. This is all done in a highly runtime-scalable solution, where the user can specify the number of frames to be visualized. The visualization cluster can be configured to meet user require-

ments; ranging from one visualization machine to a large cluster. All of this is a step closer to reducing the complexity of an MRI interface. When coupled with an interventional system, the higher base image resolution enables viewing of higher-resolution images by the technologist.

Several challenges were addressed for designing a balanced system that is capable of high-frame rates and a low response time. This was done by managing serial latency with Token Scheduling to reduce response time by arbitrating the critical master link. In addition, communication was reduced by transferring 2D images from the cluster slave nodes to the remote master node, rather than transferring the 3D volumetric datasets. This approach enables extensions to lower bandwidth network links to the master including busy office networks and wireless connections, as well as faster frame rates on faster cluster networks. Parallelizable latencies are reduced by parallel processing before user perspective input is needed, thus effectively hiding them from the user where possible. When the cluster is large enough to pre-process and load the next time frame for the next render request, pre-processing of data is transparent to the user. In this case, pre-processing and loading latency are fully hidden; where pre-processing can include disk accesses when viewing off-line, or image reconstruction when using for interventional procedures. In general, applications will need both latency reduction and latency hiding to be responsive.

GPU Cluster Visualization increases the CPU and GPU memory and computational time available to process each time frame. We described the behavior of adding more nodes to one implementation, 4DCV, in equations 1-9, as well as a method to calculate the size of a cluster needed to meet the needs of a given workload. A significant amount of scheduling and data management stems from the large amount of volumetric data needed to process high-resolution MRI images, since these images grow at a very fast rate compared to the resulting image resolution. 4DCV exploits inter-volume parallelism to manage data; each time frame is processed on only one node to reduce dominant memory transfers, making room for real-time image reconstruction.

A high degree of scalability and extensibility is achieved by the use of a distributed CPU/GPU cluster. A computationally-scalable solution is achieved that can render complex datasets in real time because of several key elements including Token Scheduling, distributed computation, distributed rendering, viewing image size being smaller than multi-dimensional volumetric size, and low cluster overhead. Token scheduling handles network control, image sequencing, render requests, and image transfer control with low overhead. Additionally, increased computational resources coupled in real time allows applications to better meet the needs of the user by offering higher frame rates and image resolution. 4DCV is extendable to other visualization areas, in general and also from existing 3D visualization applications in a straight-forward manner. Any visualization application that includes volumetric rendering, volumetric data sizes larger than the visualized image size, and long rendering times could benefit from GPU Cluster Visualization.

FUTURE RESEARCH DIRECTIONS

In this work, a real-time GPU visualization cluster has been developed in preparation to combine with real-time image reconstruction or simulation data generation. The main strand of future GPU cluster research would be combining the real-time visualization engine along with real-time data generation, image reconstruction or scientific simulations on the same GPU cluster using GPU or CPU resources.

An additional research direction is evaluating the minimum frame rate and maximum response times needed for such tools when used in various interventional procedures. This would aid in the clinical acceptance of all such work. In addition,

the interplay with the myriad of settings available to MRI could be evaluated for 4D medical applications to improve clinical practice of interventional procedures. Additional clinical applications like applicability to 4D CT visualization when used for interventional operations could be evaluated.

Research in the GPGPU arena for medical imaging is still in its infancy. There is a great need to develop algorithms and methods to benefit the greater medical image community. Graphics hardware is continually getting improvements, leading to faster solutions. The latest improvement is highly general purpose languages for GPGPU processing like NVIDIA's CUDA and ATI's CTM. In these new platforms, programming graphics cards uses the C/C++ programming language to program the highly parallel hardware, instead of programmable shaders though a graphics library, for example, OpenGL. The visualization and some or all of the data generation could be moved to this highly flexible, highly promising programming interface for GPGPU solutions. SLI, Crossfire and Quadro Plex are also examples of increasingly high performance graphics cards with higher throughput. In addition to graphics cards, there are also other hardware acceleration methods like SIMD, the Cell processor, DSP and FPGA. All of these hardware platforms have the potential for providing significant speedups for visualization applications, with varying effort to achieve performance enhancements.

Using GPU clusters for visualization can significantly reduce communication overhead when visualizing large or high-resolution images. Due to reduced communication overhead, appropriate resolution images could be rendered and sent to portable devices without significant decrease in performance. The performance could be sufficient for review of medical records wirelessly. Research on how portable user interfaces could be useful in clinical practice or in scientific research would be applicable for such applications. While GPU clusters increase usability by providing a fast and responsive interface, there is still a need to develop better interfaces for 3D visualization that provide increased intuition about the present location within the anatomy of the patent. In present clinical practice, most interventionalists use 2D fluoroscopy or use two orthogonal planes. To bridge the gap when shifting from two orthogonal planes to 3D, new and innovative user interface solutions will be needed.

Using GPU clusters for extremely large simulations could also be researched. Where rendering times are long, individual frames in a time-resolved series must be rendered in a distributed fashion to achieve sufficiently reduced rendering times needed for fast response times. Investigating how to use and time cluster resources to achieve higher throughput and shorter response times in the overall system would be fruitful.

ACKNOWLEDGMENT

We thank the support of our funding through NIH NCI 1R01CA116380-01A1.We also thank Yijing Wu and Yan Wu for their assistance with image generation.

REFERENCES

Barger, A., Block, W., Toropov, Y., Grist, T., & Mistretta, C. (2002). Time-resolved contrast-enhanced imaging with isotropic resolution and broad coverage using an undersampled 3D projection trajectory. *Magnetic Resonance in Medicine, 48*(2), 297-305.

Brodsky, E., & Block, W. (2003). Interactive visualization of time-resolved contrast-enhanced magnetic resonance angiography (CE-MRA). *Proceedings of the 14th IEEE Visualization 2003,* (pp. 108). Seattle, WA: IEEE Computer Society.

Brodsky, E., Isaacs, D., Grist, T., & Block, W. (2006). 3D fluoroscopy with real-time 3D non-cartesian phased-array contrast-enhanced MRA. *Magnetic Resonance in Medicine, 56*(2), 247-254.

Chiueh, T., & Ma, K. (1997). A parallel pipelined renderer for time-varying volume data. *International Symposium on Parallel Architectures, Algorithms and Networks 1997 (I-SPAN '97),* (pp. 9-15). Taipei, Taiwan: IEEE.

Humphreys, G., Houston, M., Ng, R., Frank, R., Ahern, S., Kirchner, P., & Klosowki, J. (2002). Chromium: A stream-processing framework for interactive rendering on clusters. *SIGGRAPH 2002, Proceedings of the 29th annual conference on computer graphics and interactive techniques, 21*(3), 693-702. San Antonio, TX: ACM Press.

Janes, D., Schulte, M., Brodsky, E., & Block, W. (2006). Rapid vascular rendering using 4D cluster visualization. *ISMRM workshop on real-time MRI, (p. 6).* Santa Monica, CA.

Liu, A., Tharp, G., French, L., Lai, S., & Stark, L. (1993). Some of what one needs to know about using head-mounted displays to improve teleoperator performance. *Robotics and Automation, IEEE Transactions on, 9*(5), 638-648.

Liu, J., Redmond, M., Brodsky, E., Alexander, A., Lu, A., Thornton, F., et al. (2006). Generation and visualization of four-dimensional MR angiography data using an undersampled 3-D projection trajectory. *IEEE Transactions on Medical Imaging, 25*(2), 148-157.

Redmond, M., Brodsky, E., Hu, Y., Grist, T., Schulte, M., & Block, W. (2004). The 4D cluster visualization project. *Proceedings of the SPIE medical imaging 2004: Visualization, image-guided procedures, and display, 5367,* 28-38. San Diego, CA: SPIE.

Schroeder, W., Martin, K., & Lorensen, B. (Ed.). (2002). *The visualization toolkit an object-oriented approach to 3D graphics* (3rd ed.). Kitware.

Shreiner, D., Woo, M., Neider, J., & Davis, T. (Ed.). (2005). *OpenGL programming guide: The official guide to learning OpenGL, version 2.* Addison-Wesley.

Tomov, S., Bennett, R., McGuigan, M., Peskin, A., Smith, G., & Spiletic, J. (2004). Application of interactive parallel visualization for commodity-based clusters using visualization APIs. *Computers & Graphics, 28*(2), 273-278.

Wernecke, J. (1994). *The inventor mentor: Programming object-oriented 3D graphics with open inventor, release 2.* Addison-Wesley.

Additional Reading

Aeschlimann, M., Dinda, P., Kallivokas, L., Lopez, J., Lowekamp, B., & O'Hallaron, D. (1999). Preliminary report on the design of a framework for distributed visualization. *Proceedings of the international conference on parallel and distributed processing techniques and applications (PDPTA'99)*, (pp. 1833-1839). Las Vegas, NV: CSREA Press.

Ahrens, J., Law, C., Schroeder, W., Martin, K., & Papka, M. (2000). *A parallel approach for efficiently visualizing extremely large, time-varying datasets* (Technical Report No. #LAUR-00-1620) Los Alamos National Laboratory.

Anupam, V., Bajaj, C., Schikore, D., & Schikore, M. (1994). Distributed and collaborative visualization. *Computer, 27*(7), 37-43.

Blackwell, M., Nikou, C., DiGioia, A., & Kanade, T. (2000). An image overlay system for medical data visualization. *Medical Image Analysis, 4*(1), 67-72.

Brown, C. (1994). *UNIX distributed programming.* New York, NY: Prentice Hall.

Crockett, T. (1997). An introduction to parallel rendering. *Parallel Computing, 23*(7), 819-843.

Fernando, R. (2004). *GPU gems: Programming techniques, tips, and tricks for real-time graphics.* Addison-Wesley.

Foley, J., Van Dam, A., Feiner, S., & Hughes, J. (Ed.). (1995). *Computer graphics: Principles and practice in C.* Addison-Wesley.

Heng, Y., & Gu, L. (2005). GPU-based volume rendering for medical image visualization. *Proceedings of the 27th annual international conference of the engineering in medicine and biology society (IEEE-EMBS), (pp.* 5145-5148). Shanghai, China: IEEE.

Luebke, D., Harris, M., Krüger, J., Purcell, T., Govindaraju, N., Buck, I., et al. (2004). GPGPU: General purpose computation on graphics hardware. *SIGGRAPH '04: ACM SIGGRAPH 2004 course notes,* (p. 33). Los Angeles, CA: ACM Press.

Owens, J., Luebke, D., Govindaraju, N., Harris, M., Kruger, J., Lefohn, A., & Purcell, T. (2005). A survey of general-purpose computation on graphics hardware. *Eurographics 2005, State of the Art Reports,* 21-51.

Pharr, M., & Fernando, R. (2005). *GPU gems 2: Programming techniques for high-performance graphics and general-purpose computation.* Addison-Wesley.

Prince, J., & J. M., L. (2006). *Medical imaging signals and systems.* Pearson Prentice Hall.

Tomandl, B., Hastreiter, P., Rezk-Salama, C., Engel, K., Ertl, T., Huk, W. J., et al. (2001). Local and remote visualization techniques for interactive direct volume rendering in neuroradiology. *Radiographics: A Review Publication of the Radiological Society of North America, Inc, 21*(6), 1561-1572.

Wittenbrink, C. (1998). *Survey of parallel volume rendering algorithms* (Technical Report No. HPL-98-49 (R.1)) Hewlett-Packard Laboratories.

Additional Web References

ATI developer. http://ati.amd.com/developer/index.html.

General-purpose computation using graphics hardware: Courses page. http://www.gpgpu.org/cgi-bin/blosxom.cgi/Miscellaneous/Courses/index.html.

NeHe productions OpenGL tutorials. http://nehe.gamedev.net/.

NVIDIA developer zone. http://developer.nvidia.com/page/home.html.

Chapter VI
Supporting Spatial Cognition in Vascular Visualization

Timo Ropinski
University of Münster, Germany

Jennis Meyer-Spradow
University of Münster, Germany

Frank Steinicke
University of Münster, Germany

Klaus Hinrichs
University of Münster, Germany

ABSTRACT

In this chapter, we introduce visualization techniques which have been developed with the goal to improve diagnosis based on volumetric angiography datasets. In particular, we propose passive as well as active techniques to make analysis of 3D angiography datasets more efficient and effective. The passive visualization techniques emphasize the depth structure of a dataset and require no user interaction. The proposed passive visualization techniques comprise depth-based color coding techniques, different types of edge enhancement and the application of rendering techniques which have been inspired by illustrations in order to enhance depth perception of complex blood vessel systems. The active visualization techniques presented within this chapter support user interaction and include depth-based replacements of the mouse cursor as well as multiple views providing further insights. We will also present the results of a user study we have conducted in order to evaluate the techniques.

INTRODUCTION

Due to the decreasing costs necessary for medical scans and the increasing availability of appropriate scanners, the amount of volumetric datasets acquired during medical diagnosis is rising. Although medical image data is traditionally viewed sequentially 2D slice by 2D slice, this method is insufficient for large scale datasets consisting of hundreds of slices. This inherent complexity demands the development of interactive visualization techniques supporting an efficient and effective analysis. Since the medical datasets acquired using different imaging technologies differ in the way they are explored, specialized techniques have to be developed. In this chapter, we will introduce interactive visualization techniques which support the exploration of angiography datasets. We will show how the depth perception and thus the spatial cognition of these datasets can be improved and thus results in a more efficient as well as effective diagnosis. After discussing the major drawbacks of current non-invasive diagnostic methods based on angiography datasets, we will describe our

visualization and interaction techniques which eliminate most of the presented shortcomings. Finally, we will introduce the results of a user study we have conducted in order to evaluate the proposed techniques.

BACKGROUND

Cerebral angiography is commonly used to detect significant stenosis as well as aneurisms. While stenosis are constrictions, aneurisms are expansions of a vessel arising from a too thin vessel membrane. Both stenosis as well as aneurisms cause an increased risk of stroke and must therefore be identified and treated early. There are several ways to treat detected abnormalities. The most common cerebral interventional procedure to treat aneurisms is the endovascular embolisation, where the aneurism needs to be packed with coils. This process, as well as other treatments, require a good spatial comprehension of the vessel structures. While in other areas of medical imaging, 2D visualizations of the in-most

Figure 1. Side-by-side view of two angiography images. A conventional 2D angiography (a) and a volumetric dataset obtained by a 3D rotational angiography (b).

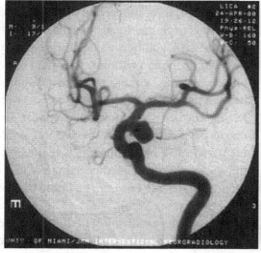 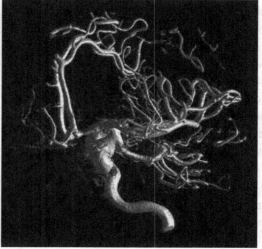

a.   b.

cases, inherently 3D datasets, may be sufficient to communicate the desired information; this is not the case in angiography, since for an angiogram diagnosis, complex spatial relationships need to be analyzed. An example of such a complex structure within a cerebral vessel structure with an aneurism is shown in Figure 1. While Figure 1 (a) shows a 2D representation of a classical 2D angiogram, Figure 1 (b) shows a 3D rendering of a volumetric angiography dataset. These images show that the vessel structures segmented from angiography datasets are of a complex nature in terms of furcations and the number of vessels overlapping in depth. The perception of these structures is hampered by the absence of perspective distortion. Since physicians need to conduct measurements within an angiography image, for example, measuring the length or thickness of a vessel, distances need to be preserved in the image. Thus an orthographic projection has to be used in the visualization process leading to the loss of perspective distortion.

To improve depth perception, physicians often view angiograms under motion by rotating them interactively. Because of the rigidity of the structures, the rotation of a vessel complex may give clues about its structure. However, since an orthographic projection is used, no motion parallax is present. Thus the dynamic change of occlusion is the only depth cue arising when rotating the dataset.

The most common technique used for visualizing vessel structures is the maximum intensity projection (MIP). In contrast to this direct rendering technique, model-based approaches generate and visualize a model of the vessel system to support generation of high- quality images. The initial work on this topic has been done by Gerig et al. (1993). Hahn et al. describe an image processing pipeline to extract models of vascular structures in order to generate high-quality visualizations (Hahn, 2001). In 2002, Kanitsar et al. have proposed a model-based visualization

technique based on curved planar reformation (Kanitsar, 2002). Oeltze and Preim (2005) have introduced the usage of convolution surfaces to further enhance visualization quality especially at vessel furcations. While all other techniques focus on visualizing the vessel structures without contextual information, the *VesselGlyph* provides also context information given by surrounding tissue (Stratka, 2004).

In this chapter, we introduce monoscopic visualization techniques to enhance depth perception. Lipton (1997) presents a classification of monoscopic depth cues. He states that lighting and shading provide a basic depth cue, whereas shadows give cues about the relative position of objects while the shading of an object gives information regarding its shape. Similar to the shading of plain surfaces, the texture of rough surfaces gives an important cue about an objects' shape. Furthermore, Lipton mentions the influence of brightness and color. He describes that bright objects appear to be closer to the viewer than dark ones. This effect is related to the diminution in visibility of distant objects caused by intervening haze. Additionally, a bluish haze of distant objects is described, which results from the scattering of red light in the atmosphere. Besides shadows, occlusions give hints about the interposition of objects. This effect has also been described by Ware (2004) as an important monoscopic depth cue and is exploited by physicians during visual diagnosis. In addition to occlusion, physicians also exploit motion parallax, the effect of nearby objects moving by more rapid than distant ones. Motion parallax as well as relative size, that is, letting further away objects to appear smaller due to perspective distortion, are both related to the perspective projection of the real world onto the viewers retina. Further explanations about monoscopic depth cues can be found in the work done by Pfautz (2000).

A detailed comparison of the influence of depth cues on depth perception has been described by Wanger (1992). Different models have been proposed for evaluating the interplay of depth cues. These models consider combinations of different depth cues and postulate how these depth cues contribute to the overall depth perception. The models incorporate, for instance, the weighted linear sum (Bruno, 1988), a geometric sum (Dosher, 1986), or the reliability of depth cues in the context of other cues and additional information (Young, 1993).

Besides simulating depth cues based on natural phenomena, the computer graphics and visualization communities have explored, to what extent illustrative techniques may support spatial cognition. Luft et al. (2006) describe a technique to enhance the perceptual quality of images containing depth information. The authors use the difference between the original depth buffer and a low-pass filtered copy to determine spatially important areas in a scene. Based on this information they introduce additional depth cues by locally enhancing the contrast, color and other parameters of the image and thus improve the perception of complex scenes.

Tarini et al. (2006) combine different techniques to enhance a viewer's perception of the three-dimensional structure of complex molecules. Among the techniques used are a method for efficient computation and storage of ambient occlusion terms and new edge-cueing techniques.

Winnemöller et al. (2006) present a method that abstracts video imagery by modifying the contrast of visually important features. The method reduces contrast in low-contrast regions using an approximation to anisotropic diffusion, and artificially increases contrast in higher contrast regions with difference-of-Gaussian edges. The authors evaluate the effectiveness of their abstraction framework in a user study.

Rusinkiewicz et al. (2006) use a non-photorealistic shading model to exaggerate shading in order to communicate surface geometry to users. The shading model is based on dynamically adjusting the effective light position for different areas of

the surface and thus reveals detail regardless of surface orientation.

VISUALLY SUPPORTING DEPTH PERCEPTION

Based on discussions with physicians and people from the visualization community, we have further improved our techniques for enhancing depth perception in angiography (Ropinski, 2006). Based on these discussions we have further improved our techniques. Especially, physicians have expressed their desire for interactive visualization techniques. Therefore, this section is split into two subsections: The first describes passive visualization techniques which do not require any user interaction, and the second introduces so-called active visualization techniques, which enable the user to explore vascular datasets interactively. Although the passive techniques allow interactive frame rates, they can be applied also when presenting still images in presentations or on print media, while the active visualization techniques can be exploited only when performing a diagnosis using a computer.

Passive Depth Enhancement

When developing the passive visualization techniques presented within this section, we had the goal in mind to keep the representation *compact*. Thus we decided to avoid additional complexity in terms of geometry or color variation that is required when applying some of the conventional depth cues used in computer graphics. For example, shadows which are commonly known to support depth perception of computer-generated images (Wanger, 1992) introduce additional shadow borders. Since these borders cause a high contrast, they are very likely to draw the user's attention and thus may lead to longer viewing times. Therefore, we have decided not to exploit shadow casting and other well-known depth cues.

Color Coding Depth Information

When using color coding, the image colors are used to code the depth information. Thus the selection of colors is limited and if the color of an object is changed, its observed distance will also be changed. However, when visualizing vessel systems, except for the shading information, the color channel usually contains no relevant information. Therefore, we are able to apply the depth-based color coding techniques which will be described below.

Figure 2 gives an overview of the techniques. Figure 2 (a) shows a standard rendering of an angiography dataset, the other images show the same dataset with color mapping applied. For color coding depth information, we normalize the depth values present in an image and apply an appropriate color mapping function. During the normalization we search for the smallest and the largest depth values present in the image and linearly scale the interval between them to lie in [0,1]. Thus we get for each pixel a normalized depth value between 0 and 1 specifying the distance from the viewer. Based on this normalized depth value, we can perform a color look up in a 1D color mapping texture, to get the depth-based color coding. Different color mappings for encoding depth information are shown in Figure 3. Thus the color coding techniques primarily diverge in the type of color mapping function they use. Since usually only one angiogram is viewed at a time and the resulting colors in the image serve only the spatial comprehension within this particular view, the colors do not have to be comparable across different views or datasets and the normalization is not constraining. To combine the color determined by using the color mapping

Figure 2.¹ Color coding depth information. Standard rendering without color coding depth (a), chromadepth (b) and pseudo chromadepth encoding (c).0 normalized depth value 1.

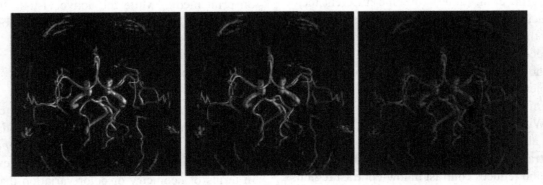

Figure 3.¹ Generated color mapping schemes used to produce color coded depth images the mappings are shown for a normalized depth value increasing from left to right. Chromadepth (a), pseudo chromadepth (b), reduced chromadepth (c), wrong chromadepth (d) and inverse gray-value mapping (e).

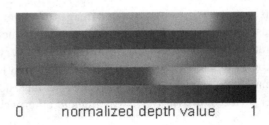

0   normalized depth value   1

function with the final image, several approaches are possible. In order to still provide shape cues provided by phong shading, we use a weighted blending between the current color and the color provided by the color mapping function. In the figures shown within this chapter we have used a blending factor of 0.5.

Figure 2 (b) shows the application of a chromadepth rendering. Chromadepth is a well-known technique for encoding depth information in the color channel (Steenblik, 1987; Bailey, 1998). Although chromadepth should be supported by wearing diffraction grating glasses to achieve optimal results, one can perceive depth in chromadepth pictures also without these glasses. The color coding as shown in the mapping function in Figure 3 (a) is exploiting the fact that light with different wavelengths is refracted differently by the lens of the eye. In addition to the chromadepth technique, Figure 2 (c) shows our proposed pseudo chromadepth technique (Ropinski, 2006), whereas the color mapping function shown in Figure 3 (b) is used. It uses the colors red (780nm) and blue (450nm) for a normalized depth value of 0 resp. 1. These colors have a maximized difference in wavelength and thus differ in the way they are refracted by the lens of the eye. Thus a maximum *depth contrast* can be given for near and distant objects. We have decided to choose blue instead of purple which would have had a smaller wavelength, possibly leading to an enhanced depth contrast. This selection is based on the findings presented by Berlin and Kay (1969) who have conducted a study analyzing the occurrence and the evolution of color names as they are used in different languages around the world. They found, that the usage of terms for primary colors is surprisingly consistent in different cultures. Besides the conclusion that the distinction of the primary colors seems to be determined neurologically, their results may lead to the conclusion, that we are more sensitive to perceive these colors. This would also match with the physiology of the eye incorporating s-, m- and l-type cones for sensing, blue, green and red light.

To allow a continuous color transition, we have linearly interpolated red and blue in the RGB color space leading to a purple color tone. With this color interpolation we no longer support the refraction characteristics of the eye, since purple light has a smaller wavelength then blue light and purple objects should thus appear further away than blue objects. However, in our evaluation we had very good perception results for pseudo chromadepth (Ropinski, 2006). This result leads to the question whether the refraction characteristics or the mental model has major influence on the perception process. To investigate this issue, we have generated two additional color mappings. Figure 3 (c) shows a so-called reduced chromadepth color mapping. It is the equivalent to our pseudo chromadepth mapping, but instead of interpolation within the RGB color space we use green for the medium values and interpolate between red and green, respectively, blue and green. Furthermore we have generated a chromadepth color mapping, without any correlation between refraction characteristics and the associated depth value (see Figure 3 (d)). We have evaluated all of these color mappings together with an inverse gray-scale depth mapping as shown in Figure 3 (e). This gray-scale mapping is inverse to the usual depth buffer color coding, that is, farther away objects are rendered darker, while closer objects are rendered lighter. This is due to the fact that the time to respond to a signal varies according to the color used; dark colors lead to a relative high response time whereas light colors ensure quick response times. Thus light objects are perceived slightly closer to the viewer.

Edge-Based Depth Enhancement

Ware (2004) states that occlusion "is probably the strongest depth cue" (p. 265). This is due to the binary nature of occlusions which leaves not much space for misinterpretation. In the WIMP (=window-icon-mouse-pointing) paradigm we get a sense of depth, although the windows do not expand in depth, have the same distance to the viewer and no depth information is given except the occlusion. This is also reflected in the vocabulary used when talking of the *topmost* window. Thus as Ware has stated, occlusion is the strongest (depth cue), since when an object overlaps another, we receive it as *in front of* the other object, despite that there are other depth cues present, stating the opposite.

Occlusion is already present when using regular volume rendering techniques. However, we further emphasize occlusion by introducing contour edges, because occlusion is harder to perceive when the overlapping objects have a similar surface shading resulting in a low contrast. Although no surface shading is applied, the contour rendering of an angiography dataset in Figure 4 (a) shows clearly the occlusion relationship. To achieve this effect, we apply an image-based edge enhancement technique (Saito, 1990) to angiography images. The edge enhancement is done by applying a three by three pixel-wide filter kernel. Since we are interested in silhouettes as well as contours, we had to take into account also the depth value at a pixels position in order to determine if it belongs to a contour edge. In our implementation, this is done in real time by exploiting fragment shader programmability, resulting in an image mask where all edge pixels

are flagged. Based on this mask we manipulate the final image color in order to get an edge overlay effect.

When applying edge enhancement techniques, it is important that the thickness of a vessel as displayed on the screen is not affected by the thickness of its edges. Otherwise, it would not be possible to measure and compare the dimensions of vessels having a different distance to the viewer. Therefore, we ensure that the edge is visualized only on top of those pixels belonging to the vessel by using edge coloring only at those pixel positions, where the current color is different from the background color. We introduce different techniques of edge coloring, which are similar to the depth color coding as described above. Thus our edge overlay technique initially accesses the edge mask. In cases where an edge is present, we access the current pixels' color and determine whether it is a background pixel. In cases where no background pixel is present, we fetch the normalized depth value at the current position and apply one of the color mapping functions shown in Figure 3, before blending the resulting color with the current pixel color. All this is done interactively within a fragment shader.

Figure 4 (b) shows a pseudo chromadepth rendering with enhanced edges, where the edges have a uniform color, that is, no depth color cod-

Figure 4.[1] *Contour of an angiogram (a), contour overlaid over standard rendering (b) and pseudo chromadepth applied to contour overlaid over an inverse gray-scale color mapping (c).*

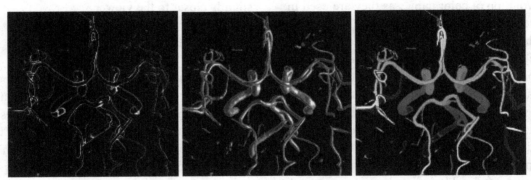

ing is used for the edges. Figure 4 (c) shows an inverse gray-scale color mapping overlaid with pseudo chromadepth colored edges.

Illustration-Inspired Depth Enhancement

In addition to the passive visualization techniques introduced above, we have also integrated concepts published by other authors into our volume visualization framework in order to evaluate whether they can improve depth perception in vascular visualization. We apply a color quantization described by Winnemöller et al. (2006) to the original image before we apply the depth-based color coding. Thus we can apply our technique in the same way it is described above, by only performing a pre-processing on the input image which provides us with the color quantization. Figure 5 (d) shows an example combined with pseudo chromadepth and for comparison Figure 5 (c) shows the original pseudo chromadepth image.

Figure 5.[1] Phong shading (a), depth darkening (b), pseudo chromadepth (c) and toon-based pseudo chromadepth (d).

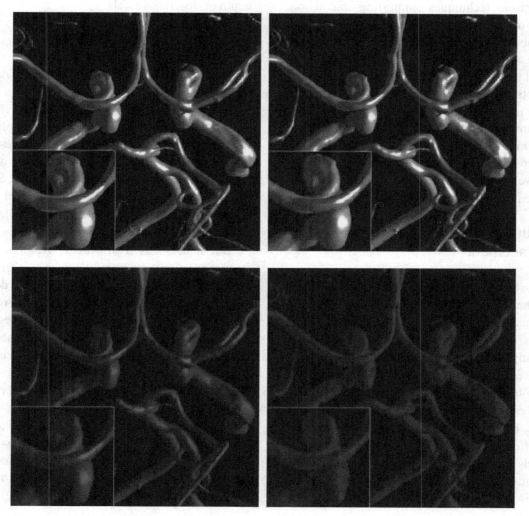

Furthermore, we have implemented and evaluated the depth darkening technique (Luft, 2006). Depth darkening performs a blurring of the depth buffer before performing the depth test. Thus it is possible to emphasize the depth relation between neighboring objects. An example of a 3D angiogram rendered using depth darkening is shown in Figure 5 (b); again to show a comparison, the phong-shaded vessel structure is shown in Figure 5 (a).

Active Depth Enhancement

To meet the desire of physicians for interactive exploration, we have also developed active visualization techniques supporting interaction, since often angiography images are examined interactively using a computer. As described above, the most obvious technique is rotating the vessel structure. Due to the changing occlusion of parts of the vessel structure, the user obtains a depth impression very easily. We will introduce additional active techniques to support the user in recognizing the depth structure of vessels while s/he concentrates on regions s/he is interested in, and we try to minimize the visualization of unwanted information that may distract the user.

Depth-Based Mouse Cursor Replacement

In most desktop applications, a computer mouse together with its screen representation is used for interaction. Normally the screen representation is an arrow-shaped cursor that is used to point at certain points of interest or to interact with objects. We alter this representation and provide additional depth information with the mouse cursor.

The user is not only interested in one depth value, but would like to compare depth values on different positions, for example, which of two vessels is nearest and which is further away. For this purpose we change the shape of the cursor and use a so-called cross-hair cursor instead of the standard cursor. A cross-hair cursor consists of two perpendicular lines, elongating along the x- and y-axis. Their intersection point is centered at the original mouse cursor position and can be moved by using the mouse.

To show different depth values simultaneously, we use a depth-dependent color coding for every point of the cross-hair cursor. The color of every point is chosen according to the depth value at the current position. The cross-hair is colored in real time while the user moves with the mouse over the angiography image. The remaining image stays untouched. As the cross-hair is moved by the mouse, the user can control the two perpendicular lines easily and exploit their color to compare the depth of different vessels.

Coding Schemes

A possible color scheme maps the range of depth values in a one-to-one manner to different colors, for example, a red to black gradient. Then vessels being close to the viewer will be colored in bright red shades, when the user moves the cross-hair over them, and vessels further away will be colored using a darker red or black. Such a mapping scheme has the advantage that it is always comparable, that is, the same color always represents the same depth value.

But it also has a drawback: Angiography images may contain many depth values from a relatively large depth range. Mapping the depth values in a one-to-one manner to colors may result in very small and hard-to-detect color nuances (see Figure 6 (a)). This problem can be addressed by choosing not only a red to black gradient, but using the whole color spectrum, for exampel, as when using the chromadepth technique as described above. But it can be further improved.

Preliminary tests have indicated that users prefer to compare vessels lying on the cross- hair lines without moving the cursor. Hence it is possible to show the user not only small *absolute* differences, but also larger *relative* differences (see

Figure 6 (b)). To do this, we count the number of different depth values covered by both lines of the current cross-hair cursor and divide the available color interval in the same number of subintervals before mapping every depth value to a color. As an example, consider that the cross-hair cursor crosses three vessels with the (normalized) depth values 0.7, 0.9, and 0.8, and these values should be visualized with a red to black gradient. In this case the gradient will be divided into three intervals—bright red, dark red, and black—and the cross-hair will be colored with these different colors at the appropriate locations. If an absolute mapping had been applied, all three values would be mapped to slightly different shades of dark red.

Of course in some situations with a large amount of different depth values, the proposed mapping yields only a small advantage, but in most cases it enhances the visualization. Especially, when applied to the very sparse angiography datasets it is easy to find an appropriate mapping.

However, the user has to take into account that the color coding is only valid within one position of the cross-hair cursor, because the relative depth situation may change when the cursor is moved. The use of a gradient with more than two colors may further improve the visualization as seen in Figure 7.

SplitView Visualization

Another very intuitive way to perceive depth information is changing the viewing position in order to look from the left or from the right. But when switching the view, the user may loose orientation within the vessel structure. Showing both views simultaneously solves this problem (see Figure 8). Usually the user is not interested in the whole vessel structure from a side view but concentrates on some details in the image.

Therefore, we divide the vessel structure in two parts, and in the side view we visualize only the part being in focus. Looking from the front view,

Figure 6.[1] The cross-hair cursor visualized depth information. Here a mapping inspired by the chromadepth gradient is used.

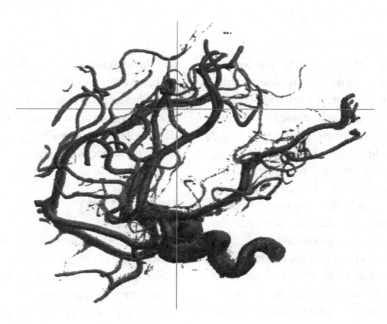

Figure 7.[1] *Color coding of the depth structure. The detail images show the differences when using an absolute mapping (a) and a relative mapping (b).*

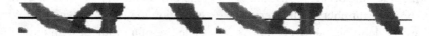

Figure 8.[1] *The left image shows a front view of the angiography data; the right image shows a clipped side view. The current plane is marked red.*

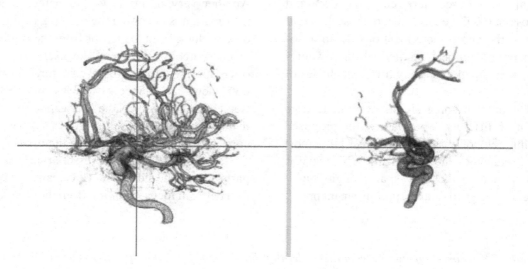

we cut along a plane that is determined by two vectors: the first vector points from the eye of the viewer to the mouse cursor, the second is the up vector. This results in a vertical plane that divides the vessel structure in a left and a right part. In the side view only the left part is visualized, that is, the parts of the vessel structure being behind the cutting plane as seen in Figure 8. The cutting plane and the side view are calculated and visualized in real time, so the user can alter the view with the mouse and see the result immediately.

To illustrate vessels that cross the cutting plane, the intersections are marked with red color. To clarify the relation between both views, we use a cross-hair cursor whose horizontal line is contin-

ued through the side view. Furthermore, this line makes it easier for the user to orientate her or herself. This technique needs a short familiarization, but has two big advantages: the user can perceive depth relations immediately and also very small depth differences are clearly visible.

USER STUDY

To evaluate the techniques and strategies described in this chapter, we have performed two laboratory studies temporally separated by approximately three months. In the first study, preliminary versions of the proposed concepts have been examined. Based on the results of this study we were able to identify implications for the development of other techniques to be evaluated in the second study.

The goal of both studies was to measure the effectiveness and efficiency of the depth perception when viewing static as well as interactive 3D angiogram datasets. Since the influence of depth cues is task dependent (Ware, 2004; Knill, 2005), we have chosen tasks similar to the diagnosis and analysis performed by physicians. However, there is no standardized viewing procedure, so we have decided to keep the task simple and hence minimize the influence on the perception of depth cues.

Experimental Design

When evaluating the proposed techniques we used objective as well as subjective evaluation techniques. During the subjective evaluation, we have exploited *think aloud techniques*, where subjects are requested to verbalize their exact thoughts while performing an activity and questionnaires both performed by an evaluator during and after the test series. In order to be able to get an empirical evaluation of the proposed techniques, we have implemented a user test application including *protocol analysis* via a logging mechanism. Thus all relevant data that has been evaluated has been automatically recorded during the test. The test application shows different series of angiogram images sequentially. Each of the 10 (for the initial study) and 9 (for the second study) series contains 5 angiogram images consisting of different vessel structures rendered with one of the techniques described above. As an independent variable for the empirical evaluation, we have chosen these different techniques used to render the vessels.

In each image, two flashing square-shaped outlines of equal size have highlighted two pre-defined vessels. Before each image has been shown, we have presented a message requesting the user to select either the front-most or the back-most of

two highlighted vessels. In order to not distract the user, the outlines displayed only the first *800 ms* when each image appears. In case the user wants to review these regions later on, she could make them pop up by pressing the spacebar. The corresponding selection could be simply performed by clicking with the mouse cursor inside or close to the area of the corresponding outline (see Figure 10). We have measured the time needed as well as the accuracy for the selection for each image. Although each user was aware of the fact that we measure the time, we asked them to primarily focus on performing a correct selection than on being fast.

In order to get also a subjective evaluation of the proposed techniques, the user had to answer a short questionnaire consisting of six questions displayed on the screen after each image series. The questions covered depth impression, confidence to have performed a correct selection, approximation of selection time, reliability of the images, whether the images are considered usable for daily work and how appealing the images appear. Each question had to be answered on a six-point Likert scale, were 1 is considered as a positive answer and 6 is considered as a negative one.

In contrast to the initial laboratory study, in the second laboratory test we have performed a formal user questionnaire immediately afterwards in order to get subjective comments of the participants after they performed the test. In addition to the empirical evaluation, these comments have given valuable hints about further implications for the design process. Detailed information about the first user study can be found in our previous work (Ropinski, 2006). In this section only the most important results from which we have implicated new directions are briefly described.

Initial Laboratory Study

For the first preliminary laboratory study, 14 participating users had to compare the depths of two vessels contained in an angiogram. The

Figure 9.[1] *The SplitView seen from bird's eye view. The right view shows the vessel structure in a side view. The current slice is marked red. The region before is clipped.*

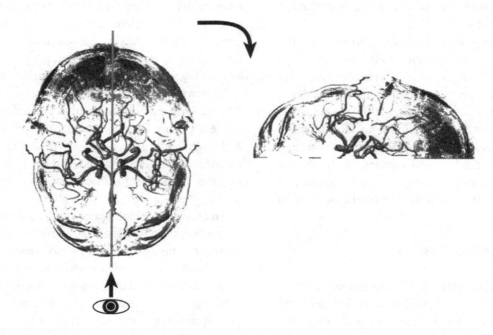

Figure 10. Participant in the laboratory environment using a LCD and an autostereoscopic display

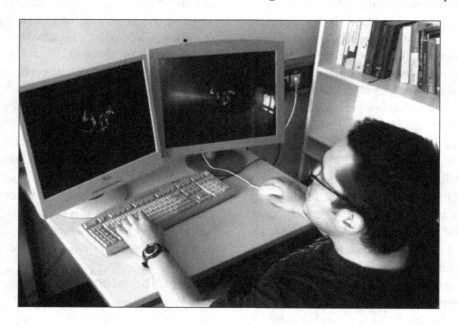

participants partly were familiar with medical imaging techniques because they were involved in medical visualization projects. Since we wanted to eliminate the influence of structure from motion, we made the task static, that is, the users were required to estimate the depths based on a single image without exploiting depth through motion phenomena.

We compared the proposed passive visualization techniques to a standard 3D visualization as shown in Figure 1 (b) as well as a stereoscopic visualization displayed using an autostereoscopic display. Hence the participants did not have to be equipped with inconvenient stereo glasses. During the tests we showed each user ten series, each consisting of five different images rendered using the same visualization technique. Since the perceptual interpretation of a single depth cue shown in isolation is affected by a prior presentation of a different depth cue in the same setting (Domini, 2003), we had to ensure that all of the images a user was confronted with either showed a different dataset or showed the same dataset from a different perspective. The series include:

standard rendering (see Figure 1 (b)), stereoscopic rendering, chromadepth (see Figure 2 (b)), pseudo chromadepth (see Figure 2 (c)), overlaid edges (see Figure 4 (b)), blended edges, perspective edges, edge shading, depth of field (10%), and depth of field (10%) combined with pseudo chromadepth. For a detailed explanation of these visualization techniques we refer to Ropinski (2006). Because of their diverse functionality, we decided not to evaluate a combination of depth of field with any of the edge-based techniques.

Results and Implications

The average percentage of incorrect selections, the mean time used to perform a selection as well as the average results of the questionnaire, are presented in the diagrams shown in Figures 11.

In an informal interview conducted immediately after the user study, the users were asked to denote their preferred visualization technique. Only two users said that they prefer to work with the autostereoscopic display, four preferred the chromadepth, four the pseudo chromadepth, one

Figure 11.[1] Results of the initial user study

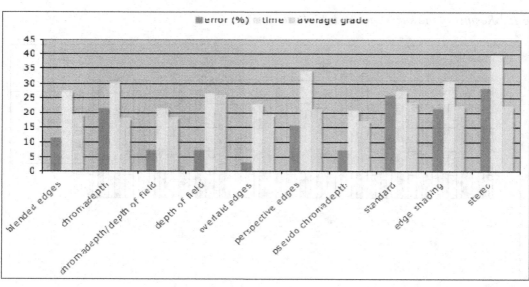

user the depth of field, two users the edge shading and one user the standard rendering technique. As shown in Figure 11, the standard rendering technique as well as the stereoscopic one did not lead to good results. While with the standard technique, this is obvious since the depth information is not available, we expected better results for stereoscopically rendered images. We believe the reason for the bad results is that only four of the participating users had prior experience using autostereoscopic displays. Although we asked each participant to test the display before the study and we ensured that there was time available for finding the sweet-spot before viewing the stereoscopic series, the users seemed to have problems perceiving the stereoscopic images.

Chromadepth uses more hues than pseudo chromadepth and should therefore allow to better measure differences in depth. However, Figure 11 indicates that when using pseudo chromadepth the users have achieved on average more correct and faster selections. It reduces the error rates by about 18% in comparison to the average error rate given by the standard technique. We have performed a statistical analysis that has revealed, that the hypothesis,

H1: Pseudo chromadepth reduces the error rate when performing depth estimations based on static angiography images,

can be assumed as true with a level of significance of at least 95%. Furthermore, pseudo chromadepth received a slightly better average grade in the questionnaire. This may be due to the fact which came up in the following interview, that six users were overwhelmed by the amount of hues present in a chromadepth image. However, we did not explain the color coding in advance; so maybe chromadepth would be more effective and efficient in case we would have explained the techniques before performing the study as done in the second study.

Depth of field also gave quite good results in terms of correctness. However, the response time has been increased, which we ascribe to the fact, that some users may have had the impression that the picture is out of focus and hence did need some time to try to get it in focus. This is also reflected in the bad average grade shown in Figure 12. Therefore, and because of some follow-up comments of physicians, we decided not to work with depth-of-field techniques anymore.

Figure 12.[1] Results of the survey to the initial user study

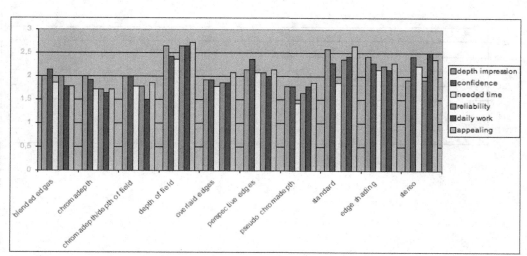

Although the overlaid edge technique did lead to very few wrong selections, the edge techniques in general seem neither to be very effective nor efficient. Especially, the perspective edge technique might be distracting and lead to over 15% of selection errors and quite long selection times. In contrast to these findings, physicians subjectively appreciated the overlaid contour edges to analyze local depth relations.

Second Laboratory Study

For the second laboratory study, analogously to the procedure in the initial study 11 participating users had to reveal the depth of two vessels contained in an angiogram image. Again, the participants partly were familiar with medical imaging techniques.

Besides the techniques we have evaluated in the initial study that was constrained to static images, we have included the passive visualization concepts described above as well as the interactive approaches introduced above. In contrast to the first study we have explained the basic concepts of the color coding techniques, in particular, chromadepth as well as pseudo chromadepth, in order to provide the participants an insight to the functionality. Thus, obscurities could be diminished before they influence the test results; for example, one participant had a red/green dysfunction, which disturbs the depth perception when viewing color coded angiogram images. Based on follow-up discussions of our previous work, we wanted to explore whether the mental model or the refraction characteristics of the color mapping have major influence on the depth perception.

Again, after each image series, the participants had to answer the questionnaires described above. After finishing the static image series, the interactive techniques were shown to the participants in a volume visualization application. The user had to accomplish informal simple tasks formulated by the evaluator using standard desktop devices, that is, mouse and keyboard. In contrast to the evaluation of depth when viewing static images, the users were able to change occlusion relations through motion, that is, the users were able to rotate the dataset.

Figure 13.[1] *Results of the second user study*

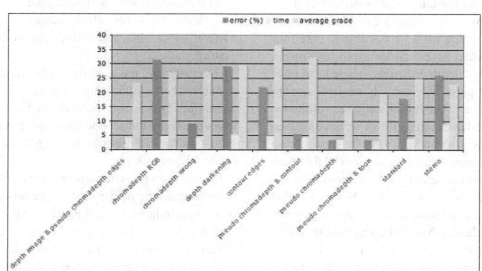

The interactive tasks to be performed have not been logged, but think aloud comments during accomplishing the tasks as well as the results from a questionnaire have been evaluated. Furthermore, *post-task walkthroughs* have been performed afterwards. The post-task walkthroughs have been used in order to give valuable hints about why the participants have done which action in order to achieve which goal by reviewing their procedures.

Results and Discussion

The average percentage of incorrect selections, the mean time used to perform a selection as well as the average results of the questionnaire are presented in the diagram shown in Figure 13.

It can be clearly seen from Figure 13 that each technique in which pseudo chromadepth color coding is involved returns quite good results in terms of the number of errors. Hence, as pointed out in hypothesis H1, it indicates again that when using this technique the error rate is reduced.

The combination of the pseudo chromadepth images with other visualization techniques did not improve the depth perception. The usage of toon shading in combination with pseudo chromadepth returns the same results in terms of the error rate, whereas the additional contours slightly degrade the results by approximately 2%. Unfortunately with this degrade we were not able to take into account whether it is primarily due to performing local or global depth decisions, where local ones incorporate parts of vessels lying in the same vicinity. Since in the initial study the results for chromadepth have been quite bad, we have focused in this study also on verifying the assumption that using chromadepth is not beneficial for depth perception when viewing angiogram images. As described above, we have used the color coded images, where we have used a color coding not correlating the depth with the wavelength. Using this technique, we have applied the same colors, but with wrong assignments with respect to the corresponding depth. That means the wavelength of the individual color does not correlate to the corresponding depth, but it has been assigned randomly.

However, an interesting observation comes up from the fact that using this wrong chromadepth color coding results in fewer errors than using correct chromadepth color coding. The same is true for the usage of pseudo chromadepth color coding which also improves depth perception in comparison to chromadepth, although the wavelength used in the pseudo chromadepth does not correlate with the human visual sense for depth perception, that is, purple has a smaller wavelength than blue. This leads to the assumption that a variety of hues does not support the users when depth perception is intended. Therefore, we formulate the hypothesis:

H2: When viewing angiogram images the applied color gradient with two hues, that is., pseudo chromadepth, not correlating with wavelength refraction characteristics, is preferable to the usage of more hues exploiting wavelength refraction characteristics, that is, chromadepth.

Again, we have revealed this hypothesis in a statistical analysis, which shows that it can be assumed as true with a significance level of at least 95%. However, chromadepth might be more efficient when combining with diffraction grating glasses.

Furthermore, the average grades of all questions show best results for the pseudo chromadepth technique. This is also indicated by the fact that users preferred the pseudo chromadepth encoding as shown in Figure 14 in comparison to the chromadepth techniques.

Again, using an autostereoscopic display has not increased the performance. The think aloud comments indicated that this was due to the fact that the square-shaped highlights have been rendered in a monoscopic way, such that it was difficult for the user to evaluate to which vessel the boxes referred to.

Figure 14.[1] Results of the survey to the second study

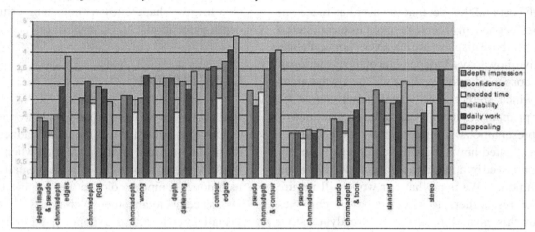

Although in both studies we told the participants that the time is not essential when accomplishing the tasks, we have measured the required time. There are no significant differences in terms of the required time. However, as it can be seen in Figure 11 and Figure 13, in both studies using the autostereoscopic display in general requires more time in order to evaluate depth.

The results of the survey evaluating the usage of the interactive techniques described above as well as further talks with physicians indicate that users prefer to view interactive visualizations over viewing static. Especially, the opportunity to change the view via rotating the dataset has been evaluated as very helpful by each participant. On a five-point Likert-scale, where 1 corresponds to not helpful, and 5 corresponds to very helpful, participants evaluated the feature of being able to rotate the vessel structures with 4.73 as the average. Evaluation of the color-coded chromadepth cursor as well as the red-color depth cursor was diverse. While medical visualization experts evaluate the cross-hairs as very helpful (chromadepth: 4.5, red-color: 4.0), in particular, non-experts revealed these techniques as not beneficial (chromadepth: 2.5, red-color: 2.0). However, many participants especially used the horizontal line of the cross-hair in order

to evaluate depth using a scan line analogue.

Independent of the experience with medical visualization, nearly all participating users have evaluated the SplitView as very helpful (in average 4.5). In particular, the reddish cutting slice in the right view (see Figure 8) has been evaluated as very helpful (in average 4.73). Although we assumed that the usage as well as interpretation of the result of this technique requires some effort to get used to it, the users remarked that after a short period of practice, the handling is intuitive instead of complex.

FUTURE TRENDS

We believe that efficient as well as effective depth perception is essential in order to provide a good spatial comprehension during the analysis of angiography datasets. Although some medical-oriented institutions already exploit stereoscopic visualization techniques to allow better spatial comprehension, these techniques are far away from being ubiquitous. The reason for this is that the user has to be either instrumented, that is, by wearing stereo glasses, or s/he has to use an autostereoscopic display. Due to the relatively high cost and the fact that the user has to stay in the sweet-spot in order to perceive a correct stereo image, these displays are not a very popular alternative, nowadays. Independent of the evolution of stereoscopic hardware there will be always areas in which stereoscopic visualization cannot be the primary choice, for example, on printouts or in presentations. Therefore, it should be further investigated how far spatial comprehension can be improved by applying appropriate visualization techniques. We hope that our work will inspire other researchers to develop new techniques with this goal. Furthermore, already existing visualization techniques may be evaluated to determine how far they can be used to support depth perception; and it may also be of interest to apply different lighting models or to apply ambient occlusion techniques.

To get further directions, we have conducted informal interviews with physicians who work with angiography datasets. These interviews have revealed that in addition to the required interactive rotation of a dataset in order to better perceive its depth relation, the possibility to switch between combinations of the different visualization techniques is much welcomed. Especially, to turn on and off the contour highlighting has been appreciated, since the color coding was considered as valuable to achieve a global spatial comprehension, while the contour highlighting was used to get local insights. Thus to exploit this effect on static media, it would be necessary to develop an automatic combination mode allowing to mix these visualization techniques with different weights depending whether local or global information is important for a certain image area. Another open issue is the development of an appropriate lighting model, optimally supporting spatial comprehension in angiography. While in general the phong lighting model was preferred to the toon-based color coding, the highlights were perceived as distracting in some image areas. Therefore, it would be necessary to

evaluate in how far existing lighting models are able to give shape cues without tampering the depth perception.

CONCLUSION

In this chapter we have proposed passive as well as active visualization techniques developed with the goal to improve depth perception when viewing 3D angiograms. The passive visualization techniques comprise color coding depth values as well as edge enhancement techniques. As active visualization techniques supporting user interaction, we have introduced a multiple view system called the SplitView, which allows showing different perspectives of the same dataset in order to support spatial comprehension. Furthermore, we have introduced a depth-based replacement of the mouse cursor. All these techniques can be applied in monoscopic environments and do not require any additional hardware. The passive techniques can even be applied when reproducing the angiograms on print media or in presentations.

To compare the introduced approaches with each other as well as to existing ones, we have conducted a user study. The evaluation has indicated that angiography seems to benefit from color coding depth information. Especially, our pseudo chromadepth technique is promising to improve spatial comprehension. With our study we were able to show that the mental model on which the color coding of the depth information is based is more important than different refraction characteristics of the eye when confronted with different wavelengths. Furthermore, we have received positive feedback by physicians, who deal with MR as well as CT angiography on a daily basis. They have considered especially the color coding as very helpful to better perceive the global depth relations within an angiogram, while they preferred to use the contour enhancement for dissolving local relationships, where the used colors would be quite similar.

Although the passive techniques presented within this chapter have been developed for static images, they can be applied in real time and are therefore also usable in interactive visualization applications.

FUTURE RESEARCH DIRECTIONS

We believe that there are mainly two areas where future research would be necessary regarding the concepts proposed in this chapter. One research area would be to investigate how to improve the described techniques and how to develop new techniques inspired by our concepts. The other area would be to evaluate how the proposed techniques could be used in other application domains. In the following paragraphs we will briefly describe both possible directions.

In the future it would be necessary to evaluate how subtle the color changes in the pseudo chromadepth technique can be, while still improving the depth perception. It would be nice to come up with images, where the color gradient is not that omnipresent but can still be exploited in the comprehension process. Additionally, the influence of different edge detection techniques should be explored more deeply in order to come up with *optimal* depth perception. While the edge detection techniques can be already considered as a non-photorealistic rendering technique, the usage of other non-photorealistic rendering techniques could be investigated. For instance, a combined visualization with the surface curvature could be helpful.

Furthermore, it would be interesting to explore how to exploit perception-based visualization techniques, as the ones proposed in this chapter, in the surgical domain. For instance in neurosurgery the surgeon operates by looking through a surgery microscope. By providing two oculars it is ensured that the surgeon can perceive a stereoscopic image. However, it is very exhausting to look through the microscope permanently, and in fact each surgical microscopy system has an additional display where the focus object is shown. The drawback of this display is the fact that it is monoscopic. Thus these surgical microscopy environments could possibly benefit from visualization techniques similar to those presented in this chapter in order to make the additional display more valuable. Additionally, it could be helpful to have a look at different datasets from other medical domains in order to find out in how far these domains may benefit from the proposed techniques.

REFERENCES

Bailey, M., & Clark, D. (1998). Using chromadepth to obtain inexpensive single-image stereovision for scientific visualization. *Journal of Graphics Tools, 3*(3), 1-9.

Bruno, N., & Cutting, J. (1988). Minimodality and the perception of layout. *Journal of Experimental Psychology, 117,* 161-170.

Domini, F., Caudek, C., & Skirko, P. (2003). Temporal integration of motion and stereo cues to depth. *Perception & Psychophysics, 65,* 48-57.

Dosher, B., Sperling, G., & Wurst, S. (1986). Tradeoffs between stereopsis and proximity luminance covariance as determinants of perceived 3D structure. *Journal of Vision Research, 26*(6), 973-990.

Gerig, G., Koller, T., Szekely, G., Brechbühler, C., & Kübler, O. (1993). Symbolic description of 3-D structures applied to cerebral vessel tree obtained from MR angiography volume data. IPMI '93: *Proceedings of the 13th International Conference on Information Processing in Medical Imaging* (pp. 94-111). Springer-Verlag.

Hahn, H., Preim, B., Selle, D., & Peitgen, H. (2001). Visualization and interaction techniques for the exploration of vascular structures. *VIS '01:*

Proceedings of the conference on Visualization (pp. 395-402). IEEE Computer Society.

Kanitsar, A., Fleischmann, D., Wegenkittl, R., Felkel, P., & Gröller, E. (2002). Cpr: Curved planar reformation. *VIS '02: Proceedings of the conference on Visualization* (pp. 37-44). IEEE Computer Society.

Knill, D. (2005). Reaching for visual cues to depth: The brain combines depth cues differently for motor control and perception. *Journal of Vision, 5*(2), 103-115.

Lipton, L. (1997). *Stereographics developers handbook*. StereoGraphics Corporation.

Luft, T., Colditz, C., & Deussen, O. (2006). Image enhancement by Unsharp masking the depth buffer. *SIGGRAPH '06: Proceedings of the 33rd annual conference on Computer graphics and interactive techniques* (pp. 1206-1213). ACM Press.

Oeltze, S., & Preim, B. (2005). Visualization of vascular structures: method, validation and rvaluation. *IEEE Transactions on Medical Imaging, 24*(4), 540-548.

Pfautz, J. (2000). *Depth perception in computer graphics*. Doctoral dissertation, University of Cambridge, UK.

Ropinski, T., Steinicke, F., Hinrichs, K. (2006). Visually supporting depth perception in angiography imaging. *Proceedings of the 6th International Symposium on Smart Graphics* (pp. 93-104). Springer.

Rusinkiewicz S., Burns, M., & DeCarlo, D. (2006). Exaggerated shading for depicting shape and detail. *SIGGRAPH '06: Proceedings of the 33rd annual conference on Computer graphics and interactive techniques* (pp. 1199-1205). ACM Press.

Saito, T., & Takahashi, T. (1990). Comprehensible rendering of 3-D shapes. *SIGGRAPH '90:*

Proceedings of the 17th annual conference on Computer graphics and interactive techniques (pp. 197-206). ACM Press.

Steenblik, R. (1987). The chromostereoscopic process: A novel single image stereoscopic process. *Proceedings of SPIE - True 3D Imaging Techniques and Display Technologies.*

Straka, M., Cervenansky, M., Cruz, A., Kochl, A., Sramek, M., Gröller, E., & Fleischmann, D. (2004). The vesselglyph: Focus & context visualization in ct-angiography. *VIS '04: Proceedings of the conference on Visualization* (pp. 385-392). IEEE Computer Society.

Winnemöller, H., Olsen, S., & Gooch B. (2006). Real-time video abstraction. *SIGGRAPH '06: Proceedings of the 33rd annual conference on Computer graphics and interactive techniques* (pp. 1221-1226). ACM Press.

Tarini, M., Cignoni, P., & Montani, C. (2006). Ambient occlusion and edge cueing to enhance real-time molecular visualization. *IEEE Transactions on Visualization and Computer Graphics, 12*(6).

Wanger, L., Ferwerda, J., & Greenberg, D. (1992). Perceiving spatial relationships in computer-generated images. *IEEE Computer Graphics and Applications, 12*(3), 44-51, 54-58.

Ware, C. (2004). *Information visualization*. San Francisco, CA: Morgan Kaufmann.

Winnemöller, H., Olsen, S., & Gooch B. (2006). Real-time video abstraction. *SIGGRAPH '06: Proceedings of the 33rd annual conference on Computer graphics and interactive techniques* (pp. 1221-1226). ACM Press.

Young, M., Landy, M., & Maloney, L. (1993). A perturbation analysis of depth perception from combinations of texture and motion cues. *Journal of Vision Research, 33*(18), 2685-2696.

ADDITIONAL READING

Braunstein, M. (1976). *Depth perception through motion.* Academic Press.

Braunstein, M., & Andersen, G. (1984). Shape and depth perception from parallel projections of three-dimensional motion. *Journal of Experimental Psychology and Human Perception, 10*(6),749-760.

Brubaker, L., Bullitt, E., Yin, C., Van Dyke, T., & Lin, W. (2005). Magnetic resonance angiography visualization of abnormal tumor vasculature in genetically engineered mice. *Cancer Research, 65*(18), 8218-8223.

Glushko, R., & Cooper, L. (1978). Spatial comprehension and comparison processes in verification tasks. *Journal of Cognitive Psychology, 10*(4), 391-342.

Julesz, B. (1964). Binocular depth perception without familiarity cues. *Science, 145*(3630), 356-362.

Mayhew, J., & Longuet-Higgins, H. (1982). A computational model of binocular depth perception. *Nature, 297,* 376-378.

Orkisz, M., Bresson, C., Magnin, I., & Champin, O. (1997). Improved vessel visualization in MR angiography by nonlinear anisotropic filtering. *Journal of Magnetic Resonance in Medicine, 37*(6), 914-919.

Parker, D. Goodrich, K., Alexander, A., & Buswell, H. (1998). Optimized visualization of vessels in contrast enhanced intracranial MR angiography. *Journal of Magnetic Resonance in Medicine, 40*(6), 873-882.

Rogers, B., & Graham, M. (1979). Motion parallax as an independent cue for depth perception. *Journal of Perception, 8*(2), 125-134.

Rogers, B., & Graham, M. (1982). Similarities between motion parallax and stereopsis in human depth perception. *Journal of Vision Research, 22*(2), 261-270.

ENDNOTE

[1] To view a free, full-color version of this figure, please visit http://www.igi-global.com/vascular_spatial_cognition (PDF viewing software is required.)

Chapter VII
3D Interaction with Scientific Data Through Virtual Reality and Tangible Interfacing

Wen Qi
Eindhoven University of Technology, The Netherlands

Russell M. Taylor II
University of North Carolina–Chapel Hill, USA

Christopher Healey
North Carolina State University, USA

Jean-Bernard Martens
Eindhoven University of Technology, The Netherlands

ABSTRACT

Three-dimensional (3D) interaction with scientific data is still an immature topic. It involves studying visualization methods to faithfully represent data, on the one hand, and designing interfaces that truly assist users in the data analysis process, on the other hand. In this chapter, we study how the human computer interface influences performance in specific scientific visualization tasks. Although a wide range of virtual reality (VR) systems are in use today, there are few guidelines to help system and application developers in selecting the components most appropriate for the domain problem they are investigating. Using the results of an empirical study, we develop guidelines for the choice of display environment for four specific, but common, volume visualization tasks: identification and judgment of the size, shape, density, and connectivity of objects present in a volume. These tasks are derived from data analysis questions being asked by domain specialists studying Cystic Fibrosis (CF). We compared user performance in three different stereo VR systems: (1) a head-mounted display (HMD); (2) a fish tank

VR (fish tank); and (3) a fish tank VR augmented with a haptic device (haptic). HMD participants were placed inside the volume and walked within it to explore its structure. Fish tank and haptic participants saw the entire volume on-screen and rotated it to observe it from different perspectives. Response time and accuracy were used to measure performance. The results show that the fish tank and haptic groups were significantly more accurate at judging the shape, density, and connectivity of objects and completed the tasks significantly faster than the HMD group. Although the fish tank group was itself significantly faster than the haptic group, there were no statistical differences in accuracy between the two. Participants classified the HMD system as an inside-out display (looking outwards from inside the volume), and the fish tank and haptic systems as outside-in displays (looking inwards from outside the volume). Including haptics added an inside-out capability to the fish tank system through the use of touch. We recommend an outside-in system, since it offers both overview and context, two visual properties that are important for the volume visualization tasks we studied. In addition, based on the haptic group's opinion (80% positive) that haptic feedback aided comprehension, we recommend supplementing the outside-in visual display with inside-out haptics when possible. Based on the results from this user study, we further investigated the 3D interaction tasks from the design perspective of tangible interfaces. Since participants using the fish tank VR system performed better than the other groups in terms of time and accuracy, we asked the question whether or not the user performance could be further improved by adding tangible elements to the interface. In particular, we designed tangible interfaces for performing clipping-plane operations. Because of the dense nature of the data, we believe that adding a tangible clipping plane and an intersection image can help the user to better understand the complex data set. The computing platform and tangible interfaces are described to clarify the different design options. An experimental study is planned to quantitatively measure the added value of different aspects of the tangible interface.

INTRODUCTION

When talking about 3D interaction, people often think of 3D input devices, such as a 3D joystick, or 3D output devices, such as 3D stereo shutter glasses. However, 3D interaction should also be concerned about the activities that take place in the context of the 3D space that is being manipulated through these devices. The introduction of 3D interaction was driven by technological opportunities and by our desire to better exploit human familiarity with the 3D world that surrounds us daily. Interacting in 3D space has an intuitive feeling for a wide range of applications. In the early 1960s, Ivan Sutherland (1968) proposed his vision of using an immersive head-mounted-display-based computer system for 3D interaction. His work is generally recognized as the first 3D

interface. Ever since, 3D interfaces and relevant interaction techniques have become increasingly interesting topics to study.

VR is the most popular approach towards 3D human-computer interfaces. Fred Brooks defines a VR experience as "any in which the user is effectively immersed in a responsive virtual world; this implies user dynamics that control the viewpoint" (Brooks, 1999, p.16). VR is an approach towards scientific visualization that makes multi-sensory 3D modeling of scientific data possible. While the emphasis is on visual representation, other senses, such as touch, can potentially complement and enhance what the scientist can visualize.

Although it is difficult to categorize all VR systems, this chapter separates them based on their display technology:

1. Projection-based VR systems, for example, CAVE (Cruz-Neira, 1993) or workbench (Kreuger, 1995).
2. Head-mounted display (HMD) VR systems (Sutherland, 1968).
3. Monitor-based desktop VR systems, for example, fish tank VR (Ware, 1993).

Visualization researchers increasingly use VR interfaces to build applications for domain scientists to display scientific data in 3D using a variety of visualization techniques (Hansen, 2004). However, there are currently few guidelines regarding which type of display system should be used, and even less evidence derived from qualitative and quantitative analysis. This can lead to the development of applications whose design may not use the most effective system to solve domain scientist's problems.

Tangible interfacing is another emerging interface perspective that is highly relevant for designing 3D interactions. One idea of tangible interfaces is that digital spaces have traditionally been manipulated with input devices, such as keyboard and mouse that were developed for traditional (2D) desktop activities. These input devices are ill suited to control and manipulate objects in 3D virtual worlds. Tangible interfaces are introduced to remove/decrease this discrepancy between input and output and are trying to open up new possibilities for interaction that more successfully blend the physical and digital worlds (Ullmer, 2001). Tangible user interfaces emphasize touch and physicality in both input and output. Often tangible user interfaces are coupled to the physical representation of actual objects, such as buildings in an urban planning application (Ishii, 2002), or wooden blocks for manipulation of online media (Ullmer, 1998).

In this chapter, we aim to better understand usability issues in 3D interaction through studying user performance within different 3D interfaces (including different VR systems and tangible interfaces) for four generic visualization tasks. The

discussion of experimental work overlaps with an earlier publication on the use of different VR display systems for visualizing and manipulating volumes (Qi, 2006).

BACKGROUND

Related Work in VR Visualization

There has been a great deal of effort in the VR research community aimed at developing and integrating new devices and technologies to improve the usability of VR systems. Much work has investigated the usability and effectiveness of VR systems for simulating real-world scenarios. The study reported here attempts to validate the usefulness of three VR systems for a set of representative volume visualization tasks.

The case for stereo in scientific visualization is clear. Ware has shown that stereo viewing combined with motion parallax provided improved user performance in the 3D visualization of graphs, which argues for using VR rather than a traditional 2D projected display (Ware, 1996). A study by Arthur also demonstrated the advantages of a fish tank VR system for 3D tasks compared to 2D desktop images (Arthur, 1993). Of interest to us is which type of stereo VR system is most effective for scientific visualization of dense volume scalar fields.

The Effective Virtual Environments (EVE) group at UNC Chapel Hill has conducted presence, locomotion and re-directed walking studies within immersive HMD VR systems (Razzaque, 2001; Meehan, 2002). Immersive versus fish tank VR for searching and labeling has been studied by Demiralp (2003), who compared fish tank VR and CAVE displays for a visual search task. The results of their qualitative study showed that users preferred a fish tank display to the CAVE system for a scientific visualization application because of a perceived higher resolution, brightness, crispness and comfort of use. The results showed users perform an abstract visual search task significantly faster and more accurately in a fish tank environment, compared to the CAVE.

Navigation in HMD versus CAVE has been studied by Bowman (2002). He presented a preliminary experiment comparing human behavior and performance between a HMD and a four-sided spatially immersive display (SID). In particular, he studied users' preferences for real versus virtual turns in the virtual environment. The results indicated that participants have a significant preference for real turns in the HMD and for virtual turns in the SID. The experiment also found that females were more likely to choose real turns than males. This suggests that HMDs are an appropriate choice when users perform frequent turns and require spatial orientation.

Schulze et al. (2005) presented a user study comparing performance across multiple immersive environments for a counting task. They tested three VR displays: a CAVE-like environment, a single-wall display, and a desktop system (fish tank VR). Data they collected "led to four significant findings: (1) in the CAVE the participants preferred medium sized or large spheres over small spheres; (2) when only a few targets have to be marked, larger spheres were marked faster than smaller spheres; (3) large spheres are marked most accurately; and (4) performance for the wall display was not comparable to the fish tank VR display when the spheres were small. Additionally, occlusion and a larger field of view inhibited performance in the CAVE more than in the fish tank display when the task was dominated by visual search."

The scientific visualization community is continually developing better algorithms to represent data in a form suitable for comprehension. Traditional visualization schemes are entirely visually dependent. More and more VR systems for visualization applications incorporate haptic feedback. An early example of haptic representa-

tion of scientific data is found in the work of Brooks (1990). Users are assisted by a force reflective master manipulator during a complex molecular docking task. In this work, a force display is used to drive the system towards a local minimum and indicate tightness of fit. The nanoManipulator (nM) (Taylor, 1997) is a VR system that provides an improved, natural interface to scanning probe microscopy, including scanning tunneling microscopy and atomic force microscopy. The nM couples the microscope to a haptic VR interface that gives the scientist virtual telepresence on the surface, scaled by a factor of up to a million to one. The Visual Haptic Workbench (Brederson, 2000) is another testbed system for conducting research on the synergistic benefits of haptic displays using an integrated, semi-immersive virtual environment.

Several studies have measured the effects of a haptic display on human perception. Studies from Ernst have shown a clear influence of haptics on vision, demonstrating that vision does not necessarily completely capture haptics (Ernst, 2002). The human central nervous system seems to combine visual and haptic information in a fashion that is similar to a maximum-likelihood integrator. Visual dominance occurs only when the variance associated with visual estimation is lower than that associated with haptic estimation. Our study quantitatively investigates differences in user performance due to the presence or absence of haptic feedback for a visualization task.

Kosara (2003) suggested that user studies should be designed to evaluate visualization methods. This also applies to VR systems with visualization capabilities. Previous user studies have offered insight into the appropriate selection of VR systems for universal interaction and manipulation tasks such as rotation, navigation and sparse visual search. Our study extends this work to include several tasks specific to the visualization of dense volumetric data sets.

Related Work in Tangible Interfaces

Interaction in 3D space often requires a user with spatial reasoning and 3D perception skills. Researchers are also trying to tackle this 3D interaction problem from the perspective of interface design. Recent tangible interfaces that are based on more advanced tracking technologies can potentially improve the 3D interaction process, and several studies have already been undertaken to develop better interfaces for 3D interaction. Many of these studies have focused on more generic 3D manipulation tasks (Chen, 1988; Zhai, 1995; Hinckley, 1997).

The Passive Interface Props (PassProps) (Hinckley, 1994) was one of the first 3D interfaces to support continuous clipping interaction in 3D space. The PassProps was developed to allow surgeons to explore a patient's anatomy data by interactively generating cross-sections through the 3D data. The PassProps contains a head prop, a cutting-plane prop for creating intersections, and a pen-like prop for planning trajectories. The six degrees of freedom (DOF) that specify the position (i.e., translation and orientation) of each individual prop are tracked using (wired) magnetic trackers. Visual feedback of the user's actions is provided on a computer display in front of the user. The head prop is used to manipulate the orientation of the patient's anatomy. The rendering of the volumetric data on the screen follows the rotation of the head prop. The rendering is always positioned in the center of the screen, that is, it does not follow the translations of the head prop. The rendering scale (i.e., the zoom factor) is determined by the observer-to-object rendering distance, and is controlled by moving the head prop closer to or further away from the body. The user holds the cutting-plane prop relative to the head prop to specify the location and orientation of the slice through the 3D data. The generated intersection image is presented on the display, next to a (volume) rendering of the 3D model.

De Guzman et al. (2003) presented two tangible devices for navigating a slice through the human body. Interface A consisted of a 30-inch 2D model of a human body, together with a U-shaped fork at the end of an adjustable arm that could be rotated 180 degrees along the device's baseboard. Interface B consisted of a transparent 3D model of the human body and a free-moving hand-held fork. The fork in each case represented the intersection plane (window), and its position and orientation was used to generate an intersection image on a separate display.

The Cubic Mouse (CMouse) (Froehlich, 2000) was developed to support exploration of 3D geological data (seismic data) and car crash analysis data. The CMouse allows users to specify three orthogonal cutting planes and to perform so-called "chair cuts" through the data. The prop is a cube-shaped case with three perpendicular rods passing approximately through the centers of two parallel faces of the case. It is usually held in the non-dominant hand. The rods are used to control three orthogonal slices through the 3D data, that is, by pushing or pulling a rod, usually with the dominant hand, the corresponding intersection plane moves back and forth. The movement of a slice is hence constrained to the direction orthogonal to the slice. There is also a (wired) magnetic tracker embedded in the cube-shaped case. The tracked six DOF are used to translate and orient the data set in the virtual world, relative to the observer. The 3D data set and the orthogonal slices are visualized on a large stereo display in front of the user.

There are some limitations in the above systems that are likely to have an effect on their usability and user acceptance. First, because of the active tracking technology being used in these systems, the interaction elements need to be wired. Such wires obviously will have an effect on the freedom of movement, an effect that is seldom mentioned, let alone evaluated. Alternative techniques such as optical tracking allow for interaction elements that are passive and unwired, and are therefore likely to ameliorate this problem. Second, there is currently little insight into how different aspects of tangible interfaces, such as passive haptic feedback and enhanced perceptual feedback, assist users in their data analysis task in 3D space.

Scientific Problem

There are many medical applications that can benefit from using 3D interaction devices and techniques. For example, surgeons make use of 3D rendering and interaction to plan where to cut a patient because the body is 3D and the location of a tumor has a 3D location that is easier to understand. Our study on 3D interaction starts from the scientific problems asked by domain experts that are studying the structure of human lung mucus in both normal "wild-type" lungs and in the lungs of CF patients. This mucus is made up of a number of long polysaccharide molecules called mucins. It is known that there are a number of different types of mucin present in the mucus, and that the mucus is denser for CF patients than wild-type mucus. What is not known is how the different types of mucin are distributed in the mucus, and how particles can diffuse through it. The mucins may be uniformly distributed, or form distinct domains. There may be web-like superstructures formed by a subset of the mucins which contain clumps of other mucins. There may be large, small, or a variety of different sized water pockets surrounded by thin membranes. There may be continuous water paths within webs of mucins forming a lattice. Researchers are probing this by developing fluorescent dyes that attach differentially to the different mucin types, and by scanning the mucus with a confocal microscope to produce multiple 3D scalar fields, one for each dye. The resulting scalar fields in 3D are displayed to help them estimate sizes, distributions, and shapes of any

resulting voids and structural elements. A virus, bacteria, or bacterial colony would traverse the mucus differently depending on its structure. The motion of such pathogens is of great interest to the study of CF, because lung infections are the source of many CF deaths. Researchers are probing this by placing small beads of various radii into the mucus and tracking the Brownian-driven motion of these beads over time to understand how they move through the mucus matrix. We wish to display the resulting motion paths in the presence of the above mesh structure to help our users correlate structure and density with bead motion paths.

AN EXPERIMENTAL STUDY OF VR SYSTEMS

We have designed different tools to solve the visualization and interaction problems described above with available VR technologies. In particular, we implemented three different VR systems for visualizing and interacting with a simulated data set that shares key properties with the real data. We designed a user study with this simulated data set to help determine which display and interaction system best supports the types of queries researchers are interested in without requiring our participants to be experts in CF. As described already, those experts are performing a diversity of tasks within dense volumetric scalar fields. Connectivity and relative density are of interest in addition to counting, shape, and size analysis. We aimed at providing similar tasks that were as generic as possible, so that the results of the user study could apply to other applications that explore dense 3D scalar fields looking for structure and pathways. We think that oil-field study and tumor segmentation might have similar needs for understanding complex dense data and for studying connectivity between portions of the data (oil reservoirs and blood vessels).

Figure 1. Head-mounted display system: (a) a user in the immersive HMD VR system; (b) head-mounted display with head sensor

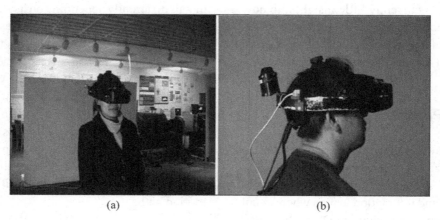

(a)   (b)

VR Systems for Visualization

All three systems display the volumetric data using the Visualization Toolkit (VTK), an open-source library that provides several different rendering algorithms (ray-casting, isosurface and 2D texture mapping) (Levoy, 1988; Schroeder, 2000). To enable real-time interaction, we chose Marching Cubes as the primary algorithm for rendering isosurfaces of the volumetric data. The standard structure of VTK does not provide a mechanism for integration with VR input devices, so we combined the VTK library with VRPN (Virtual Reality Peripheral Network) (Taylor, 2001) and UNC's Vlib (virtual-world library toolkit) to enable access to the visualization capabilities of VTK from our VR setups.

Immersive HMD VR System

The immersive VR system uses a V8 HMD from Virtual Research System. Each LCD provides a color VGA pixel resolution of 640 x 480 at a refresh rate of 60Hz. Head tracking is performed via a 3rdTech HiBall tracking system, a high-performance wide-area optical tracker that incorporates a six DOF sensor. The HMD/head tracking system consists of three main components. The outward-looking HiBall sensor is mounted on the back of the HMD (Figure1). The HiBall observes a subset of fixed-location infrared LEDs embedded in the ceiling. A tracking server coordinates communication and synchronization between the host computer and the HiBall and ceiling LEDs. Tracking data are transmitted through network switched Ethernet from the tracking server to a rendering computer via VRPN. We used a *DELL* Precision 530 (dual 2.8-GHz Xeon with 2GB RDRAM) and an NVidia *Quadro FX 1000* graphics card. The two VGA outputs from the graphics card are connected to the LCDs for each eye in the HMD via a video splitter to provide stereo-offset images. The working space for a user in this VR system is about 4.5 meters wide by 7 meters long by 4 meters tall (15 feet x 23 feet x 13 feet). A calibration procedure is used to calculate a precise transformation matrix between the sensor and the eyes. An additional hand sensor is also available for hand input, although it was not used during our experiments.

Fish-Tank VR

The second VR system is based on the concept of fish tank VR introduced by Colin Ware (1993). The computing platform of this VR system is identical to the HMD system with the following additional components:

1. A 17' CRT monitor with resolution of 1024 x 768 and a refresh rate of 100Hz to support stereo display, together with an infrared emitter and shutter stereo glasses from StereoGraphics Inc.
2. A PHANTOM Desktop™ haptic device for precise 6-DOF positioning and high fidelity 3-DOF force feedback output at 1kHz. In fish tank VR mode, the PHANTOM was used to rotate the volume around its center (additional operations were available during fish tank VR with haptics, as described below).
3. A DynaSight 3D optical tracker for measuring the 3D position of a target (reflective disc) attached to the front of the stereo glasses. When dynamic perspective is combined with stereoscopic viewing, a real-time 3D display appears that provides a virtual window into the computer-generated environment. Dynamic perspective eliminates the perceived image warping associated with static stereoscopic displays. An additional benefit of using the head to tune the perspective is that the hands are free to control the object being visualized, in our case with the PHANTOM.

The hardware components are organized to enable accurate and easy calibration. The tracker's control box is placed above the monitor on a metal plate supported by an arm (Figure 2). The arm's height guarantees continuous detection of the tracking and stereo signals. A cable between the infrared emitter for the stereo glasses and the control box for the head tracker synchronizes the devices. The real setup is shown in Figure 3.

Figure 2. A diagram of the fish tank VR system (with or without haptics)

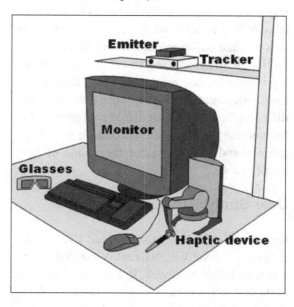

Figure 3. A snap shot of the fish tank VR system

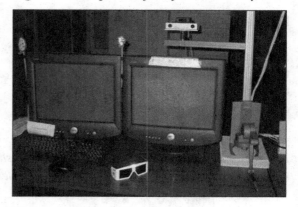

Fish Tank with Haptics

Haptic visualization techniques have been developed for force feedback systems such as the PHANTOM. The fish tank VR with haptics prototype uses the same hardware setup as the fish tank VR system, except that the PHANTOM also provides force feedback, specifically a single point of haptic response, which is sufficient for our tasks. Although the stylus where force is applied is not visually located within the display volume (as compared to the Visual Haptic Workbench or the *ReachIn* systems), no users complained about the cognitive effort required to move the hand in one location while viewing another. An axis-aligned on-screen icon followed the stylus's motion in 3D, producing an effort similar to using a mouse to control the on-screen cursor. The haptic presentation of volumetric data employed different force models for different objects within the volume: viewers felt the outside surface of spheres and ellipsoids, but the inside of long curved tubes.

User Study

Our user study compares the three VR systems described above: VR, fish tank VR and fish tank VR with haptic feedback. Relative performance of these systems is measured over tasks involving the visualization of volumetric data.

Data and Task

Simulated volumetric data are generated to act as trials during our studies. A random number of two to four types of differently-shaped objects (sphere, ellipsoid, cylinder, and curved tube) are inserted

with random positions (Figure 4). These objects may overlap with each other. The objects' properties (size, shape, and density) form experimental conditions that vary between trials. The bounding box of the volume is uniformly subdivided into eight sub-regions (a 2 x 2 x 2 array in the x, y, and z directions) within which object density may differ. Sub-regions are labeled with unique numbers (1 through 8) to enable participants to describe the paths of curved tubes within a volume and to indicate regions with the highest density.

There are always spheres and at least one curved tube within every volume. Trials may also contain ellipsoids, cylinders, and up to two additional curved tubes. Sphere sizes may vary between four possible radii ranging from six to twelve units. The density of objects within each sub-region is controlled to be sparse, medium, or dense. A single dense region (the "densest" region) exists within each volume. Sparse regions contain between 10%-60% of the number of objects in the dense region, while medium regions contain between 60%-90% of this number.

Participants are asked to complete fours tasks within each trial. Each task involves judging the properties of a specific object or of the overall volume, specifically:

Figure 4. An example trial from our experiment, showing a top-down view on a simulated volume with different experiment conditions like shape, size, density, and connectivity highlighted

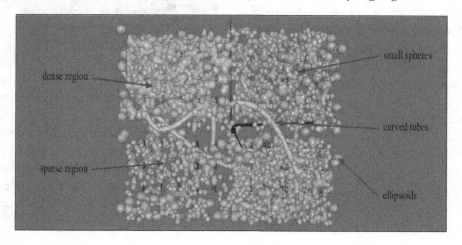

1. **Shape task:** Participants identify the number of differently-shaped objects within the volume and name the objects.
2. **Size task:** Participants report how many different sizes of spheres exist
3. **Density task:** Participants identify the densest sub-region in the volume
4. **Connectivity task:** Participants report how many curved tubes exist in the volume, and then determine which sub-region(s) the longest curved tube passes through. For example, Figure 4 shows two curved tubes

Participants are asked to give their answers as accurately as possible and to minimize response time. The size, density, and curve counting questions are presented in a multiple choice format. Participants are asked to describe the name of each kind of object for the shape question and all the sub-region numbers for the tube tracking question.

Experimental Procedure

A between-subject design was used, with VR system type as an independent factor: HMD, fish tank VR, and fish tank VR with haptics. Participants were randomly assigned into one of three groups. The HMD group wore the HMD and walked around within the tracked environment to observe the volumetric data as seen in Figure 5a. The fish tank group used the fish tank VR system and wore stereo shutter glasses to interact with volumetric data through the stylus of the PHANTOM as seen in Figure 5b. Although the stylus was tracked and displayed as an icon on the monitor, no force feedback was provided to this group. The haptics group added force feedback to the basic fish tank VR system.

Participants completed several steps during the experiment. As part of an initial interview session, they signed a consent form, answered basic demographic questions (age, gender, and occupation or major field of study), and identified their frequency of computer use and prior experience with any kind of VR system. A training session introduced the equipment and described the tasks to be performed. Next, the formal experiment session was conducted. Each experiment included 20 trials, with each trial containing a single volumetric data set. These twenty data sets were completely different from one another, and varied by object property (type,

Figure 5. Two views of volume data from an example experiment trial, (a) as seen in the HMD system, and (b) as seen in the fish tank and fish tank with haptics systems on the right.

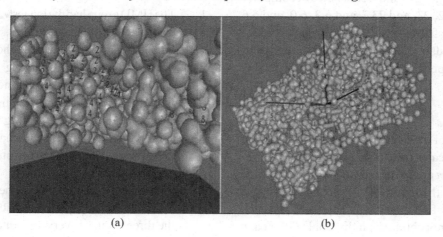

(a)   (b)

size, position, and density). However, the same set of trials (20 data sets) in the same order was used for all three groups (HMD, fish tank, and fish tank with haptics).

Two dependent variables, the time taken to respond for each trial and the participant's accuracy (i.e., percentage correct) for each task were recorded. A short break was provided every half hour or whenever a participant asked for one. After completing the last trial in the formal experiment session, participants filled out a questionnaire describing their opinion about the system, any suggestions they had on how to improve the system, and so on (see Appendix). The study ended with a short debriefing during which the experimenter summarized the study goals. The participants were paid $9 for their participation.

Results

Forty participants volunteered for our experiment, 33 males and 7 females. The participants were randomly assigned into one of the three display system groups: 14 participants (12 males and 2 females) for the HMD group, 13 participants (11 males and 2 females) for the fish tank group, and 13 participants (10 males and 3 females) for the haptic group. The age of each participant and the frequency of computer use (on a scale from one to seven) were recorded before the experiment began. Average ages and frequencies of computer use were 23.2, 23, and 23.7, and 6.3, 6.0, and 5.6 for the HMD, fish tank and haptic groups, respectively. These data suggest we had similar ages and computer experience within each group.

Summary

Two kinds of measures of performance were derived for each trial a subject completed: response time rt and error rates P_e. A single rt value representing the total time in seconds needed to complete all four tasks was captured for each trial. We did not obtain the individual rt's for each

subtask since it was too difficult to record these separately. Four separate P_e values for the four tasks subjects completed were also obtained.

For the shape, size and density tasks, subjects' answers were coded as 1 for correct and 0 for incorrect. Then error rate P_e is defined as the proportion of wrong answers among all the answers. For the connectivity task, subjects' answers were coded in two observed parameters: the *false negative* and the *false positive,* as used in a Receiver Operating Characteristic curve (ROC).

For rt statistics, trials were divided by display system (HMD, fish tank, or fish tank with haptics). For P_e statistics, trials were divided by display system (HMD, fish tank, or fish tank with haptics) and task (shape, size, density, or connectivity). At times, more in-depth analyses on the data were performed when results obviously depended on other task parameters, such as in the case of counting sphere sizes, where performance obviously depended on the number of sizes present.

The shifts across conditions in average values of the logarithm of rt were studies using Analysis of Variance (*ANOVA*). A discussion on why analysis of lg(rt) should be preferred over analysis of rt itself can be found in a recent publication (Martens et al., 2007). The differences in error rates P_e were studied using chi-squared statistics.

In summary, the following significant differences in performance were identified:

1. The HMD group had the longest rt, followed by the fish tank with haptic groups. The fish tank group without haptics had the shortest rt.
2. For the shape task (counting the number of different shapes), the connectivity task (counting the number of curved tubes) and the density task (finding the densest subregion), the HMD group had higher P_e, compared to both fish tank groups (with and without haptics).
3. In the size task (counting the number of different sizes of spherical objects), none of the three groups is very accurate. The HMD

group made significantly more errors than both fish tank groups when only one size of sphere was present. This might be due to higher perspective distortion in the HMD case. When more than one size was present, subjects in all three groups tended to underestimate the number of different sizes.

4. In the connectivity task (identifying the sub-regions that the longest curved tube passes through), the HMD group produced more false negatives (missing the right sub-regions) and false positives (misjudging the wrong sub-regions) compared to both fish tank groups.

Detailed Analysis of Results

Performance Times

The response time rt needed to complete all four tasks during each trial was recorded during the

formal experiment session. Subjects in the HMD group had significantly longer rt compared to the fish tank and the haptic groups. The *ANOVA* for the logarithm of rt was significant, $F(2, 165) = 40.058; p < 0.001$ (Figure 6). Post-hoc paired comparisons showed that the fish tank group was also significantly faster than the haptic group ($p < 0.001$). Overall, the HMD group spent 43% more time compared to the fish tank group, and the haptic group spent 23% more time compared to the fish tank group. Because of the high rt for the HMD group, we were forced to reduce the total number of trials for this system to 16. Because each trial tests all four tasks, this did not unbalance the experiment to favor certain conditions. Although subjects in the other two groups were able to finish all 20 trials within reasonable time, to maintain consistency we analyzed only the first 16 trials completed by each group.

Accuracy in the Density Task

For the density task, the answers for every pairwise combination of groups are compared through a Chi-Squared test to find out whether or not there is an association between the error rates of finding the densest sub-region within a volume and the VR system used. The results are shown in Table 1 (The significant results where $p < 0.05$ are displayed in **boldface**, a convention that will also be used in the following tables) and can be summarized as follows.

The users in the HMD group produced significantly more errors then the users in both fish tank groups, while there was no significant difference between the two latter groups. In absolute terms, none of the three groups demonstrated very high accuracy, with $P_e = 0.62$, 0.38 and 0.43 for the

Figure 6. Mean lg(rt) for the different experiment conditions, all results are divided by display system (HMD, fish tank, fish tank with haptics), error bars represent 95% confidence intervals.

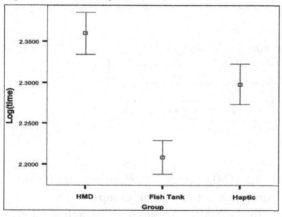

Table 1. Results of the Chi-squared analyses of overall error rate in the density task

	HMD	fish tank
fish tank	$\chi^2 = 25.002; df = 1; p = 0.00 < 0.05$	-
haptic	$\chi^2 = 15.278; df = 1; p = 0.00 < 0.05$	$\chi^2 = 1.206; df = 1; p = 0.272 > 0.05$

Figure 7. Mean Pe *values for the different experiment conditions, all results are divided by display system (HMD, fish tank, fish tank with haptics), error bars represent 95% confidence intervals: (a) mean* Pe *for the density task; (b) mean* Pe *for the shape task; (c) mean* Pe *for the size task; (d) mean* Pe *for counting the number of curved tubes in the connectivity task*

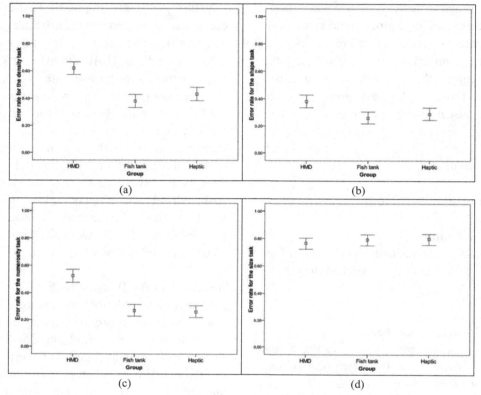

(a) (b)

(c) (d)

Table 2. Results of Chi-Square analyses of overall error rate in the shape task

	HMD	**fish tank**
fish tank	$\chi^2 = 7.277$; $df = 1$; $p = 0.007 < 0.05$	-
haptic	$\chi^2 = 4.143$; $df = 1$; $p = 0.042 < 0.05$	$\chi^2 = 0.435$; $df = 1$; $p = 0.510 > 0.05$

HMD, fish tank, and haptic groups, respectively (Figure 7a).

Accuracy in the Shape Task

The results of the Chi-Squared analysis for the shape task are shown in Table 2 and the conclusions as to the relative performance of all three systems are identical as in the case of the density task, that

is, the HMD group is performing significantly worse than both fish tank groups.

In absolute terms, all three groups had reasonable accuracy, with $P_e = 0.38$, 0.26 and 0.29 for the HMD, fish tank, and haptic groups, respectively (Figure 7b). Further analysis indicated that the user performances of all three groups differed depending on the number of shapes present in a

Figure 8. Mean P_e with 95% confidence intervals for the shape task based on the number of shapes

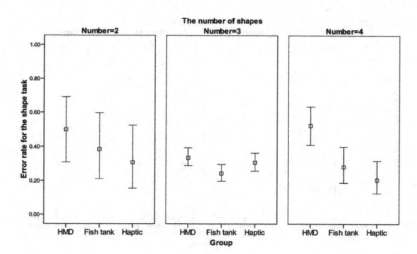

Table 3. Results of Chi-Squared analyses of overall error rate in the size task

	HMD	fish tank
fish tank	$\chi^2 = 0.438$; $df = 1$; $p = 0.508 > 0.05$	-
Haptic	$\chi^2 = 0.617$; $df = 1$; $p = 0.432 > 0.05$	$\chi^2 = 0.015$; $df = 1$; $p = 0.903 > 0.05$

displayed volume (Figure 8). When there are only two (sphere and curved tube) or all four kinds of shapes, the haptic group is more accurate than the other two groups (only the difference between HMD and haptic for the four shapes situation is statistically significant, though). The fish tank group is the most accurate when three kinds of shapes are presented (sphere, ellipsoid and curved tube or sphere, ellipsoid and cylinder or sphere, curved tube and cylinder). Regardless of the number of the shapes, the error rate is always the highest for the HMD group.

Accuracy in the Size Task

The results of the Chi-Squared analysis for the size task are shown in Table 3. No significant differences could be observed between the performances in the three groups.

In absolute terms, none of the three groups was accurate, with $P_e = 0.76, 0.79$ and 0.80 for the HMD, fish tank, and haptic groups, respectively. The error rates were all above 70%, although slightly fewer errors were made in the HMD group (Figure 7c). Further analysis based on the number of sizes showed that performance differences between systems varied (Figure 9).

When there is only one size or when there are two sizes of spheres, the haptic group is more accurate than the other two groups (although only the difference in case of one size between the HMD group and the haptics group is statistically significant). When there are three or four sphere sizes, the HMD group is somewhat more accurate than the other two groups (although this is only statistically significant in the case of four sizes). The only case where the error rate is below 50% (for all three groups) is when there is one size of sphere present. The chance of estimating the number of sizes correctly is even lower than guessing in case of the three- or four-sized condi-

Figure 9. Mean P_e for the size task based on the number of sizes

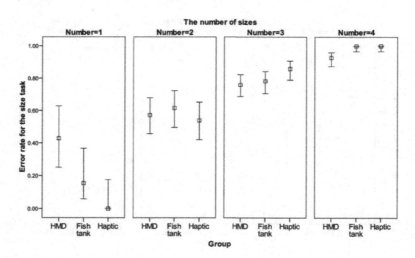

Table 4. Results of Chi-Squared analyses for the size task (including sign of estimation error)

	HMD	fish tank
fish tank	$\chi^2 = 8.713$; $df = 2$; $p = 0.013 < 0.05$	-
haptic	$\chi^2 = 14.777$; $df = 2$; $p = 0.001 < 0.05$	$\chi^2 = 1.347$; $df = 2$; $p = 0.51 > 0.05$

tion, which indicates that subjects significantly underestimate the number of different sizes in these latter cases.

In the previous analysis, user performance is based on the error rate, that is, the proportion of completely wrong answers among all the answers. When performing the size task, three cases can arise. The number of sizes can be estimated correctly, overestimated or underestimated. The resulting Chi-Squared analyses, based on three instead of two (right or wrong) categories, are reported in Table 4.

This more refined analysis reveals a significant difference between the HMD condition and the two fish tank conditions. In absolute terms, the proportion of underestimation was above 65% in all cases, although the proportion was lower during the HMD trials, with 0.68, 0.77 and 0.79 for the HMD, fish tank, and haptic groups, respectively. This reflects the fact that mistakes mainly originate from an underestimation of the number

of different sizes for sphere objects, which is illustrated graphically in Figure 10.

Accuracy in the Connectivity Task

In the connectivity task, subjects answered two questions: the total number of curved tubes in a volume (numerosity question), and which subregions of the volume the longest tube passed through (spatial region question). The results of the accuracy analysis in case of the numerosity question are reported in Table 5. Similarly as in the above tasks, the HMD condition differed significantly in terms of accuracy from the two fish tank conditions, while the two latter conditions performed similarly.

In absolute terms, the accuracies were $P_e = 0.52$, 0.27 and 0.26 for the HMD, fish tank, and haptic groups, respectively (Figure 7d). Further analysis based on the task condition, that is, the number of curved tubes present, provides more insight into the performance differences (Figure

Figure 10. Proportions of answers in the size task, separated according to over- and underestimation

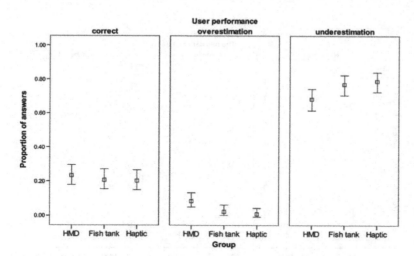

Table 5. Results of Chi-Squared analyses for counting the total number of curved tubes

	HMD	**fish tank**
fish tank	$\chi^2 = 29.224$; $df = 1$; $p = 0.000 < 0.05$	-
haptic	$\chi^2 = 31.187$; $df = 1$; $p = 0.000 < 0.05$	$\chi^2 = 0.037$; $df = 1$; $p = 0.847 > 0.05$

11). The users in the HMD group obviously have more problems distinguishing whether or not the perceived tubes are connected.

For the spatial region question, the answers of all three groups are analyzed using Receiver Operator Curve (ROC) statistics. ROC is a graphical plot of the *sensitivity* versus *1-specificity* for a binary classifier system. The ROC can also be represented by plotting the fraction of *true positive* (TP) versus the fraction of *false positive* (FP). In the context of this user study, there are four possible combinations of whether or not a sub-region is passed through by the longest curved tube in a trial, on the one hand, and a subject's answer based on his/her own judgment, on the other hand (see Table 6).

A *true positive* situation is that the longest curved tube in a trial passes through a sub-region, and a subject does recognize this fact correctly. A *false positive* situation is that the longest curved tube in a trial does not actually passes through

one sub-region, but a subject thinks it does by mistake. The other two situations can be described similarly. From these situations, we can derive several statistics to describe the user performance. The fraction of *false negative* P_{FN} (also known as the chance of missing P_M) is defined as $P_{FN} = FN / NP$, while the fraction of *false positive* P_{FP} (also known as the fraction of false alarm P_F) is defined as $P_{FP} = FP/NE$. Both probabilities can be analyzed as a function of the experimental conditions using Chi-Squared statistics.

The analyses for the false negatives are summarized in Table 7. The fish tank system performs significantly different from the other two systems. In absolute term, the fish tank group is more accurate than the other two groups, with P_{FN} equal to 0.39, 0.31 and 0.39 for the HMD, fish tank, and haptic groups, respectively. This is also reflected in Figure 12.

The analyses for the false positives are summarized in Table 8. In this case, only the differ-

Figure 11. Mean P_e for counting during the connectivity task divided according to the number of curved tubes

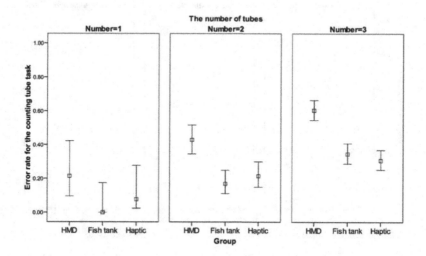

Table 6. Four situations in judging whether the longest tube passes through a sub-region

	pass (real situation)	no pass (real situation)
pass (subjects' answer)	*true positive* (TP)	*false positive* (FP)
no pass (subjects' answer)	*false negative* (FN)	*true negative* (TN)
sum	*number_of_pass* (NP=TP+FN)	*number_of_empty* (NE=FP+TN)

Table 7. Results of Chi-Squared analyses for P_{FN}

	HMD	fish tank
fish tank	$\chi^2 = 10.896$; $df = 1$; $p = 0.001 < 0.05$	-
haptic	$\chi^2 = 0.021$; $df = 1$; $p = 0.884 > 0.05$	$\chi^2 = 11.474$; $df = 1$; $p = 0.001 < 0.05$

ence between the HMD condition and the fish tank condition without haptics is shown to be statistically significant. In absolute terms, the HMD group is less accurate then the two other groups, with P_{FP} equal to 0.20, 0.17 and 0.17 for the HMD, fish tank, and haptic groups, respectively. This is reflected in Figure 12.

The overall performance can be quantified by attributing costs to both the false negatives P_{FN} (misses) and the false positive P_{FP} (false alarm).

In summary, the fish tank (without haptics) group has the best performance. The HMD group is least accurate in both finding the sub-regions the longest curved tube passes through and ignoring the regions that the longest curved tube does not pass through. The haptic group has intermediate performance, with almost the same frequency of false negatives as the HMD group but slightly lower frequency of false positives.

Figure 12. Mean P_{FN} and P_{FP} values for the different experimental conditions, all results are divided by display system (HMD, fish tank, fish tank with haptics), error bars represent 95% confidence intervals: P_{FN} and P_{FP} values for locating the longest curved tube during the connectivity task.

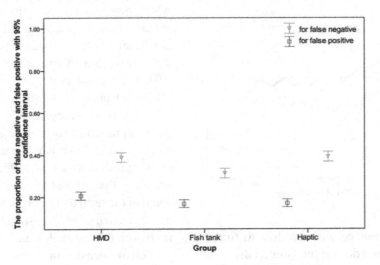

Table 8. Results of Chi-Squared analyses for P_{FP}

	HMD	**fish tank**
fish tank	$\chi^2 = 4.123$; $df = 1$; $p = 0.042 < 0.05$	-
haptic	$\chi^2 = 3.604$; $df = 1$; $p = 0.058 > 0.05$	$\chi^2 = 0.017$; $df = 1$; $p = 0.896 > 0.05$

Interpretation of Results

The time needed to complete tasks in the HMD system was significantly longer, compared to both the fish tank and the fish tank with haptics systems. One explanation is that the HMD system requires participants to walk around within the tracking space, which takes more time to explore compared to moving hands and head in the fish tank systems. Another critical issue was the reported inability of HMD participants to remember where they had previously seen target items within the volume because of the high density of data sets. They would often have to re-search the volume for objects they had previously located, but had "lost" as they walked into a different region. Finally, participants may simply be more familiar with a standard desktop system.

The fish tank group was also significantly faster than the haptic group. When touch was available, participants often spent more time "feeling" inside the volume to confirm their decisions, even when a correct answer could be derived from visual evidence alone.

A curve of the time spent on each trial indicates a similar learning effect for all three groups. Time decreases as the participants complete more tasks (Figure 13). The first five trials show the strongest learning tendency. After the first five trials, time spent on each trial still varies mainly due to the different difficulty of each trial, which is caused mainly by the density of the data set for that trial. The learning effect did not affect our ability to draw conclusions because the three groups shared the same learning pattern. For users who have become familiar with the task and equipment,

Figure 13. A time curve for each VR system, in the order that participants completed the trials

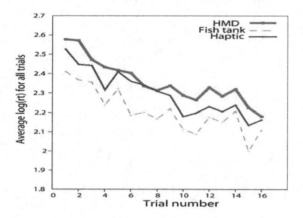

we believe performance will stabilize to times similar to those seen during the later trials.

The HMD group was significantly less accurate than the fish tank and haptic groups in the shape task. Error results showed that participants from all three groups found it relatively easy to identify the sphere object. The HMD group made more mistakes in identifying cylinders than the other two groups. It is difficult to judge the number of shapes for the HMD group when all four shapes exist. The accuracy of the haptic group consistently increases as the number of shapes increases, and gets the best performance among three groups when all four shapes of objects are present. It indicates that touch does help the participants for the shape tasks. Finally, participants from all three groups sometimes misjudged the curved tube as a cylinder. This was also mentioned in the post-experiment feedback from the participants.

Although there were no significant differences in accuracy during the size task, absolute performance was poor across all three groups. Not surprisingly, when there was only one size of sphere, the responses were quite accurate (P_e = 0.43, 0.15, and 0.0 for HMD, fish tank, and haptic, respectively). When two sizes of sphere with a large difference in radii were presented, the participants from all groups also did well.

The haptic group performed best in the cases of one or two sizes. However, when the radius difference between the two spheres was small, or when there were three or four different sizes of sphere, all participants had difficulty determining how many different sizes there were (P_e = 0.76, 0.78, and 0.96 with three sizes of sphere, and P_e = 0.93, 1.0, and 1.0 with four sizes of sphere for the HMD, fish tank, and haptic groups, respectively). The average accuracy of each group is even lower than the probability of guessing in the three or four sizes situation. The participants with the HMD system produced the best performance when there are more than two sizes. This suggests that: (1) some of the radii differences were too small to be distinguished reliably; (2) touch did not help much in distinguishing such small differences.

For the density task, the HMD participants were significantly less accurate than the fish tank and haptic participants. None of the three groups had high accuracies, however. The reason might be both the characteristics of high-density and slight-density differences between adjacent sub-regions. There was no significant difference between the fish tank and haptic groups, implying that haptic feedback did, again, not assist in identifying spatial regions with different densities of objects, particularly in high-density situations. The errors for all three groups were spread out across the trials, and showed no learning effects. This suggests that identifying regions of varying density (especially small differences) within a 3D volume is a difficult task, that none of these three display systems fully supports.

In the connectivity task, participants are asked to count the number of curved tubes in the volume, then locate the longest curved tube and identify which sub-regions of the volume it passed through. For the numerosity question, the HMD participants were significantly less accurate than the fish tank and haptic participants. Identifying that only one tube exists does not present a challenge for any of the participants. When more than one tube is present, the average accuracies for all three groups decrease as the number of tubes increases. However, the ability to "feel" along the inside of the tubes helped the haptic group provide slightly more accurate counts of the number of unique tubes when there are three or more. It indicates that touch can be useful in such a situation. The lack of overview of the volume for the HMD group and the absence of clear complete view of the path of every tube for all three groups create the major difficulty for all participants to judge whether different segments they saw belonged to the same tube or not.

For the spatial region question in the connectivity task, the HMD group was significantly less accurate than the fish tank and haptic groups. The fish tank group was slightly more accurate than the haptic group. Task analysis for this question revealed that participants first had to identify which tube was the longest one by comparing the lengths of all tubes, before continuing with determining which sub-regions this target tube passed through. If the wrong tube was identified as longest, the answer on the second question was obviously also wrong (apart from the cases where the wrong tube crossed the same sub-regions as the longest one). In the HMD system, participants often misjudged a tube to be the longest one. For the fish tank and haptic systems, when the length differences among the tubes were large, haptic feedback helped participants locate the longest tube by touch. They could then correctly identify the sub-regions containing the tube. When the length differences were small, however, the haptic system provided insufficient assistance. This explains the slightly different error rates between the fish tank and the haptic systems. Our results match the findings of Ernst and Banks (2002): when visual and haptic feedbacks are present and haptic feedback can add a definite assistance for a task or judgment, it will be used. Otherwise, visual feedback is still the dominant sensory input.

In addition to statistical results, a number of interesting anecdotal findings were made, point-

ing to: (1) the desire for an overview display in the HMD system; (2) the desire for immersion in the fish tank VR systems; (3) fatigue in the HMD system; and (4) the preference for including touch in the haptic system.

Several HMD users spontaneously suggested adding the ability to see a high-level overview (which might be provided through a button press, Mine's head-butt zoom, or a worlds-in-miniature interface). One casual user was tall enough that he stood above the data, enabling him to get an overview in the HMD system, which he reported to be useful. This matches our later analysis as well as issues related to the effects of memory on participants' results. Some participants in the fish tank and haptic groups wanted to zoom in and see the volume from the inside (some tried to do this by moving their head near the screen). We concluded that both overview and immersion are helpful for performing our tasks. Anecdotal and formal results indicate that a system designed for the study of dense volumes should include both capabilities.

Most participants said that the HMD and haptic systems were "cool" or "neat" upon initial exposure. Several participants mentioned without being asked that they liked the HMD VR system or the haptic system. However, participants in the HMD group requested more breaks after five trials and sometimes asked "How many trials do I still have?" after around ten trials, indicating heavy workload and a dissatisfaction with the system. We believe this is due to physical or mental fatigue. The increased number of breaks requested did not happen in the fish tank or the haptic cases.

Subjective Results

Subjective measurements were obtained through analysis of the post-experiment questionnaires (see Appendix). Most questions used a standard seven point rating scale (some used a five-point rating scale). The answers indicated that overall, participants preferred the haptic and HMD VR systems due to perceived ease of use, presence, and immersion. We summarize our findings over the following categories of questions we asked.

Perception of the VR Systems

The first category of questions addressed perception properties and characteristics of VR systems, including immersion, presence, depth cues, and spatial relationships. For the question: "the extent that you felt you were within a virtual environment" the HMD system ranked significantly higher than the fish tank with hap-

tics systems, $F(2, 37) = 5.481$, $p = 0.008$, with a post-hoc comparison between HMD and haptic of $p = 0.006$, and absolute rankings of 6.0, 5.4, and 4.4 for HMD, fish tank, and haptic, respectively (Figure 14a). There was also a significant difference on the question: "the extent you had a sense of acting in the virtual space, rather than operating something from outside." The HMD system ranked significantly higher than the other two systems, $F(2, 37) = 15.666$, $p = 0.001$, with scores of 5.9, 3.1, and 4.4 for HMD, fish tank, and haptic, respectively (Figure 14b). Further post-hoc comparison showed the fish tank with

Figure 14. Mean values for the different questions about the perception of VR systems, all results are divided by display system (HMD, fish tank, fish tank with haptics), error bars represent 95% confidence interval: (a) mean rank for the presence question; (b) mean rank for the question of acting inside VR space; (c) mean rank for the question of VR surrounding the subject; (d) mean rank for the immersion question.

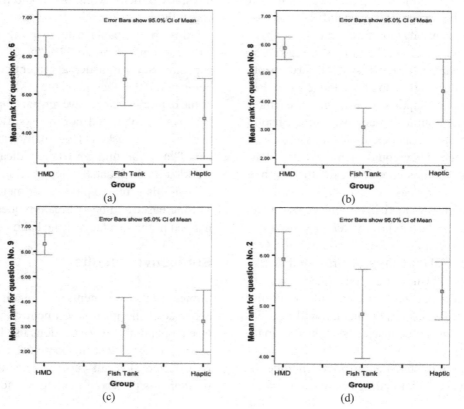

haptics system ranked significantly higher than fish tank alone due to the existence of touch ($p = 0.03$), indicating that haptic feedback does add an inside-out property to a fish tank display. For the question: "the extent you felt that the virtual environment surrounded you", the HMD group again ranked higher than the other two groups, $F(2, 37) = 16.464$, $p = 0.001$, with scores of 6.3, 3.0, and 3.2 for HMD, fish tank, and haptics, respectively (Figure 14c). This suggests that HMD participants felt more strongly that they were acting within a virtual environment. We found no notable statistics differences on the questions: "a sense of being there," "a sense of immersion," "difficulty of understanding the spatial relationships," "the quality of multiple view points," or "the quality of depth cues," although the HMD system did rank slightly higher in absolute terms in the immersion (Figure 14d), presence, multiple viewpoints and depth cues questions.

Usability of the VR Systems

The ease of learning and using a VR system is the main focus of this category of questions. Answers to the question: "how much consistency did you experience in the VR system compared with a real world experience" were similar for participants from each group, indicating the act of moving from place to place was judged to be relatively natural and easy. There were no obvious differences on the question about system delay, although HMD participants reported a slightly shorter perceived delay. No participant from any group complained about the resolution, frame rate or delay; these parameters did not seem to bother them. The haptic system ranked higher than the other two systems for identifying the shape and location of individual objects, and the shape of the global topology. Although participants from all three groups felt their system was easy to use,

Figure 15. Mean values for the different questions about usability issues of VR systems, all results are divided by display system (HMD, fish tank, fish tank with haptics), error bars represent 95% confidence interval: (a) mean rank for the level of demand on the participants' memory; (b) mean rank for the level of confidence in the answers.

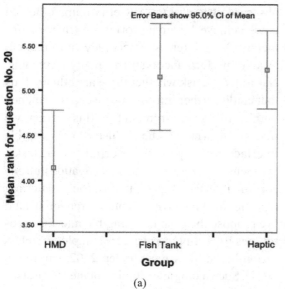

(a)

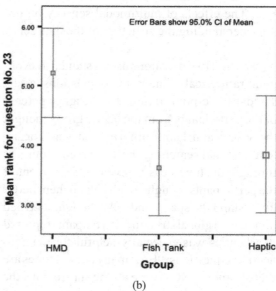

(b)

the HMD group ranked highest for the perceived difficulty in carrying out their tasks. Moreover, HMD participants reported a significantly higher demand for memorizing than the other two groups, $F(2, 37) = 5.017$, $p = 0.012$, with scores of 5.2, 3.6, and 3.8 for HMD, fish tank, and haptics, respectively (Figure 15a). Finally, HMD participants were less confident about the accuracy of their answers, $F(2, 37) = 5.521$, $p = 0.008$, with scores of 4.1, 5.2, and 5.2 for HMD, fish tank, and haptics, respectively (Figure 15b).

The "Added Value" of Haptics

The use of haptics requires participants to employ multiple sensory modalities to perform tasks. Most participants in the haptic group were excited about the additional functionality, and claimed that haptic feedback did help in some way. Participants in the haptics group were asked four questions that related to their experiences:

- Consistency of the information from multiple senses
- Ease of searching within the virtual environment through touch
- The effects of multimodal sensory on understanding the space
- The effects of multimodal sensory on understanding the structure of the data set

The first two questions used a standard seven-point rating scale. The last two questions used a standard five-point rating scale. Eighty percent of the participants from the haptic group thought the visual and haptic information was consistent, and that searching the virtual environment through touch was easy. Seventy-five percent of the participants thought touch helped them better understand the space, and 80% thought it helped understand global structure. Participants reported that haptics was especially helpful for the connectivity questions: "How many curved tubes are there?" and "Please name all the sub-regions the

longest tube crosses" since the tubes are hidden behind other objects.

TANGIBLE INTERFACE FOR CLIPPING PLANE

Spatial reasoning and 3D perception skills are very important for interacting with volumetric data in 3D space. Currently, the dominant interface for 3D manipulation with volumetric data is the computer desktop with a graphical user interface that is controlled by a mouse and keyboard. As described earlier, recent developments within 3D interfaces that add tangible elements to the interface have the potential of improving the 3D interaction process for the purpose of data analysis. However, previous studies have focused on more generic 3D manipulation tasks, such as selection, positioning, and so forth (Chen, 1988; Zhai, 1995; Hinckley, 1997).

The user study in the previous section has indicated that an immersive VR environment without overview capability does not help users with most of the selected tasks (identifying data structure and properties), which was surprising to us. On the other hand, the dense nature of our data sets may explain the low task performances observed. The desktop VR environment helped users achieve better performance (than in immersive VR) in terms of accuracy and time, but absolute performance is still not really acceptable. Naturally, we ask whether there are other means that could further improve the user performance within such an environment. In this section, we investigate whether the inclusion of a tangible interface can help users performing those tasks. We focus on a more in-depth investigation into one specific interface aspect, that is, the positioning of a clipping plane within volume-rendered data. We propose the design of tangible interface prototypes for a clipping plane that employ wireless vision-based tracking (Mulder, 2002; van Liere, 2003). Such a tangible clipping plane can assist a user in exploring the inside of a dense volumetric data set through creating 3D and two-dimensional (2D) intersection images. By varying the design, these prototypes allow us to study and compare different user interface strategies for performing the clipping plane interaction task. A user evaluation is being planned with these prototypes for measuring their effectiveness.

Design Practice of Tangible Interfaces

Positioning of a clipping plane is a common but complex operation in volume visualization for data analysis. Such a plane cuts through a 3D data set in order to explore its interior structure. The common method of controlling the 5 (or 6) DOF of the virtual clipping plane, that is, its position (3 DOF) and orientation (2 DOF in case of a plane, or 3 DOF in case of a window), is by means of a 2 DOF control device such as a mouse. In order to accomplish this, the positioning task needs to be decomposed in at least three subtasks that require at most two DOF at a time. Despite the fact that such a 2D interface (in principle) allows users to perform the task, it is often difficult to obtain enough awareness of the spatial relationships to manipulate the data efficiently. This is due to the fact that the 2D interaction is unrelated to the natural interaction process in 3D space. We therefore propose alternative interface designs for the clipping plane task that make use of 3D (tangible) interaction devices. Our goal is to combine current knowledge and understanding of 3D user interface design (Bowman, 2004) with new technical possibilities to create clipping interfaces for more demanding and realistic tasks. The principles that we adhere to in the design of these interfaces are the following:

1. **Easy to use:** The interface should not distract the user from the actual clipping task.
2. **Easy to learn:** The interaction should be natural and intuitive, requiring little explanation and training.
3. **Adequate perceptual feedback:** The interface should provide (passive) tactile and visual cues that assist in the interaction.
4. **Low-cost setup:** The interface and system should be created using off-the-shelf and inexpensive technology.
5. **Real-time interaction:** The interface should work in real time while still generating volume rendering of realistic high-resolution data.

In order to achieve real-time performance, the hardware setup is organized around two *DELL* graphics workstations with different interface components.

The first workstation is mainly used for tracking the tangible interface and consists of the following components:

*   One *DELL* workstation Precision 530 (Pentium IV, 2.4 GHz, 512 MB RAM with ATI *FireGL 4* graphics card coupled to an infrared emitter from StereoGraphics Inc.
*   Two analog Leutron Vision LV-8500 progressive scan CCD cameras (720x576 pixels, 50Hz frame rate) with COSMICAR/PENTAX lenses with a focal length of 12mm and infrared transparent filters (that block visible light); these cameras are connected to two synchronized Leutron Vision PictPort H4D frame grabbers.
*   A 15' LCD display from *DELL*.

The second workstation includes the following components:

*   One *DELL* workstation Precision 670 (Intel Xeon, Dual CPU, 3.2 GHz, 2.0 GB RAM with NVidia *Quadro FX 4500* graphics card)
*   A 14' CRT monitor from *DELL* with a vertical refresh rate up to 120Hz, so that stereoscopic images can be viewed with the help of active liquid crystal shutter glasses (CrystalEyes 3)

- A 15' LCD display from *DELL*, used for showing intersection images

The separation of tracking and 3D rendering across two different machines enables us to achieve better performance for 3D interaction with a large data set. A wooden chassis has been constructed for integrating the different components and creating a workspace for the users. The two infrared cameras are mounted on the upper layer of the wooden chassis (Figure 16). A silver mirror mounted on a wooden slab is hung in front of the chassis at an angle of 45 degrees to reflect an image of the user's hands with the tangible devices to the cameras. The use of the wooden cabinet with the cameras makes the system set-up stable and allows for easy transportation. In the current prototype there are no provisions for tracking the user's head (which might be useful for also providing motion parallax feedback in the displayed image).

Due to the hardware difference in graphics cards, the volume rendering algorithm used in previous study has been modified to provide direct volume rendering. The rendering engine uses hardware-supported 3D texture mapping in OpenGL, rather than a Marching Cubes algorithm. The algorithm to render the non-polygonal isosurfaces in the data is based on the approach presented by Westermann and Ertl (1998). In a pre-processing step, the gradient vector is computed for each voxel of data set using the central differences method. The three components of the normalized gradient vector together with the original scalar value of the data set are stored as RGBA quadruplets in a 3D texture.

The vector components must be normalized, scaled and biased to adjust their signed range [-1; 1] to the unsigned range [0; 1] of the color components. The alpha test discards incoming fragments conditional on the outcome of a comparison of the incoming alpha value with a user-specified reference value. In our case the alpha channel contains the scalar intensity value and the alpha test is used to discard all fragments that do not belong to the isosurface specified by the reference alpha value. The setup for the OpenGL alpha test is:

```
glDisable(GL_BLEND);
// Enable Alpha Test for isosurface
glEnable(GL_ALPHA_TEST);
glAlphaFunc(GL_EQUAL, fIsoValue);
```

Within the prototype interfaces, the user is given a wooden cube that can be tracked by the system. This cube can be rotated to control the orientation of the virtual cube, with its associated volumetric data, and moved towards or away from the user's body to control the zoom factor (see Figure 17). The image on the display, which is the result of volume rendering for a fixed camera position that is optimized according to the observer's actual viewpoint (the size of objects observed is comfortable to users), changes in accordance with the movement of the tangible cube. The cube can also be placed on a small (physical) pedestal in case the user prefers to perform clipping operations

Figure 16. The diagram of the system setup

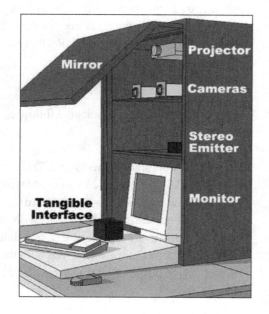

Figure 17. 3D manipulation of volumetric data with tangible cube

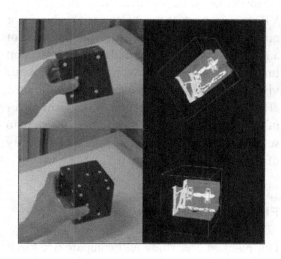

with one hand. Although the data set remains in a fixed position in such a case, its orientation can still be varied discretely in a very simple way, that is, by changing the side of the cube that is resting on the pedestal.

Together with the cube, a square-shaped metal frame is used to control the clipping plane. Five infrared-reflecting stripes on three of its sides form

a unique planar pattern as shown in Figure 19. The six DOF of the frame (three DOF for position and three DOF for rotation) are monitored continuously by the vision-based tracking algorithm. The appearance of this device makes its purpose very obvious. While using this prototype, the user positions the cube with his non-dominant hand, and grasps the frame with his dominant hand on the side that has no dots on it. The physical cube intersects with the physical frame in a way that agrees one-to-one with the intersection of their virtual counterparts on the screen. As a result, even though all six DOF are enabled when moving the plane, the interface does not seem difficult to control.

The clipping plane interface can operate in two modes: the slice mode and the opaque clipping mode. In slice mode only the planar intersection image is displayed in 3D space, as shown in Figure 18a. In the opaque clipping mode, the part of the volume data that is in front of the clipping plane is made transparent, as shown in Figure 18b.

Tangible Devices for 3D Interaction

Considering ease of use, we pursue a further design by adding different handles to the frame. Three different types of handles have been designed in

Figure 18. (a) the slice mode for the 3D intersection interaction; (b) the opaque clipping mode for the 3D intersection interaction

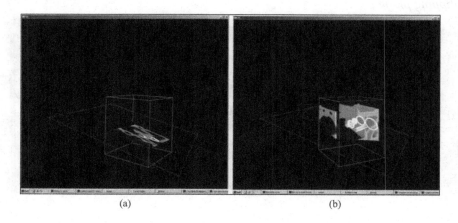

(a)   (b)

order to find an effective solution. First, paper mockups of three handles are constructed to give an impression of the final look of the physical objects. Three wooden plane frames with different handles are made for further comparison as Figure 19a shows.

We have asked several colleagues from our department to try out the different prototypes and give informal feedback. The tangible clipping interfaces have received many positive feedbacks. Further survey among the users indicated that there is no difference in the preference of the shape of the handle, which means it will not be a major factor within future user experiments. The final design of the clipping plane frame is shown in Figure 19b.

With these interfaces, the next logical step is to undertake a more structured and formalized experiment with the different prototypes. We adopt the tasks performed in the previous section as a starting point since the systems in the previous experiment did not have a constantly satisfying user performance. More specifically, the experimental goal is to ask users to cut through 3D simulation data with a clipping plane in different forms and to answer the same questions regarding data properties as were asked in the previous experiment. By repeating that experiment with new interface

prototypes, we plan to establish the relationship between our tangible prototypes and the absolute performance (time and accuracy) for a desktop VR environment. We can also verify whether or not the observed preference for the presence of a tangible clipping plane and a 2D intersection image holds in terms of user performance for our visualization tasks. Moreover, we can study the effect of two-handedness and of the form factor of the interaction device. In addition, we want to see how performance relates to the spatial ability of our individual subjects.

FUTURE WORK

Our planned user study will compare five kinds of setups within one baseline system: non-immersive VR, with fixed virtual clipping or a tangible clipping frame and with/without a 2D intersection image. The relative performance of these configurations will be compared for the four generic tasks that were applied in the earlier experiment. The rendering paradigms are only tested in their most common configuration: outside-in for non-immersive VR. A between-subject design is planned, with interface type as an independent factor:

Figure 19. (a) the wooden model of three handles; (b) the final design of the plane-like tangible interface for virtual clipping plane

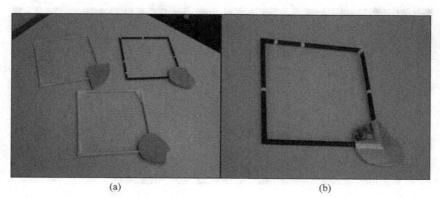

(a)   (b)

- **Condition 1 (abbreviated as cube or C):** Baseline system is a non-immersive VR system with a tangible cube to orient the data set. The visual feedback is only a 3D image of the data set (Figure 20);
- **Condition 2 (abbreviated as fixed-plane or CF):** Baseline system with a fixed virtual clipping plane. A user can manipulate the cube and cut through the data with a fixed clipping plane (Figure 21a);
- **Condition 3 (abbreviated as tangible-frame or CT):** Baseline system with a tangible frame in the shape of a clipping plane. The movement of the visual clipping plane corresponds to the physical plane-shaped object. The visual feedback is a 3D representation of the data set and the virtual clipping plane on the screen (Figure 22a);
- **Condition 4 (abbreviated as fixed-intersection or CFI):** The interaction devices are the same as in condition 2. However, the visual feedback consists of both a 3D rendering result and a synchronized 2D intersection image in another window (Figure 21a and b);
- **Condition 5 (abbreviated as tangible-intersection or CTI):** The interaction devices are the same as in condition 3. However, the visual feedback consists of both a 3D rendering result and a synchronized 2D intersection image in another window (Figure 22a and b).

Participants will be randomly assigned into one of five groups. The first group will use only the baseline system, which contains a tangible wooden cube within the tracked environment to explore the volumetric data. The second group will use the same baseline system, together with a virtual plane on the screen in a fixed position. The participants in this group can manipulate the cube and intersect the virtual cube with the fixed virtual plane, so that part of the 3D data can be made transparent. The third group will use a tangible frame to position the virtual clipping plane and cut through the data. The fourth group will use the same setup as the second group plus an additional 2D intersection image for a fixed clipping plane. The fifth group will use a tangible frame to generate both a 3D rendered result and an additional 2D intersection image presented in a separate window to help participants observe the intersection result.

CONCLUSION

This chapter presents two main results. The first is an empirical evaluation comparing human performance using different VR systems for four generic volume visualization tasks. The second is the design of alternative tangible interfaces for performing a clipping plane operation. The tasks in the first experiment were derived from data

Figure 20. Condition 1 in the planned experiment

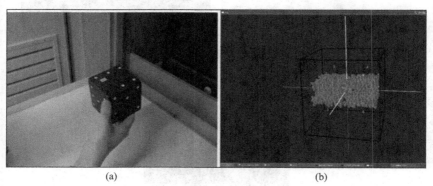

(a)   (b)

Figure 21. The diagram of condition 2 and condition 4: condition 2 includes (a); condition 4 includes the intersection image (b) as well

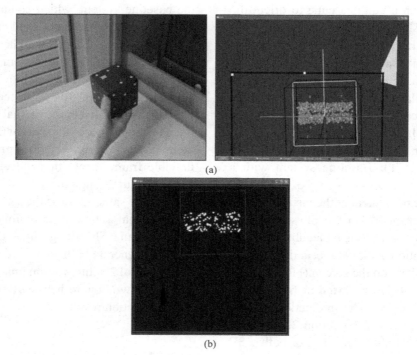

(a)

(b)

Figure 22. The diagram of condition 3 and condition 5: condition 3 includes (a); condition 5 includes the intersection image (b) as well

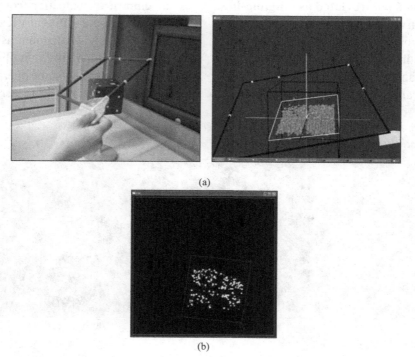

(a)

(b)

with characteristics and questions being asked by researchers studying mucuciliary clearance in CF. Results showed that the haptic system offered participants both an inside-out and an outside-in perspective on a volume, a property that was identified as important to completing our tasks. Participants using the HMD VR system were significantly slower than participants from the other two systems, and were less accurate for the shape, density, counting, and spatial tracking questions. Finally, none of the systems allowed for accurate judgment of different sizes of objects, or of which regions of a volume had the densest spatial packing.

The speed difference for the HMD system was not unexpected, but the inferior task performance was quite surprising. Participants' responses to questionnaires and anecdotal comments reveal that memory load was a significant factor. In the absence of an overview capability, participants were forced to make an internal representation of the total volume; the dense nature of the data removed visible landmarks that can normally provide such a frame of reference. It is believed that a future planned system that includes both an overview and an inside-out capability within the HMD would produce a system whose performance is at or above the level of the haptic-enabled system for some tasks. Furthermore, the poor performance of the HMD VR system for this data visualization task does not mean it is not appropriate for other tasks or applications. The lack of reference of the frame does not exist for other applications, for example, gaming or architecture.

The design of a multimodal interface asks the designer to consider how the brain combines and integrates different sources of information in order to make the interface truly helpful. Correct combination and integration of multiple sources of sensory information, for example vision and touch, is the key to create a robust perception and judgment for search tasks in a multi-modal interaction situation. Combination does not only mean the presence of two modalities, but

an integration and coordination that match the user's physiological senses. We can observe from the experimental results that the haptic system has different effects on the user's performance for different tasks or different conditions of the same task. For some tasks, the presence of haptics maximizes the information received from both modalities (vision and touch). It also reduces the variance of the sensory estimation to increase its reliability. For some tasks, it does not.

Based on the experience of the VR study and its results, we proposed the design of tangible interfaces, particularly a tangible clipping plane for improving task performance. The detailed design strategy for such interfaces was described and the planned further user study will give us the opportunity to quantitatively measure the benefits brought by the tangible objects for the same tasks studied in our original experiment.

FUTURE RESEARCH DIRECTIONS

3D interaction through AR, VR or tangible interfaces continues to be an interesting field for interface experiments. Currently, 3D interaction itself is still an experience, instead of a routine. Practically, though, there still lacks enough evidence that 3D interfaces may improve the speed of interaction, or give the user a better understanding of the observed data. It is argued that current 3D interfaces are simply not right for simulated 3D environments yet. It is also difficult to control a 3D space with the interaction techniques that are currently in use, since they were designed for 2D manipulation (dragging, scrolling) or derived from 2D manipulation.

So regarding 3D interfaces and interactions, the future work should, in our view, concentrate on the following:

- Advancing technology: technology advances can solve part of the existing problems in 3D interaction. A new generation of 3D LCD displays already can be found in the market in terms of hardware development.

- Improving the ergonomics of 3D interfaces: one factor that can lead to frustration with 3D interfaces is the poor ergonomic design of 3D interfaces (devices). For example, it takes time until a user gets used to the heavy goggles, sometimes too long for acceptance.

- Further understanding the perceptual and cognitive issues behind 3D interfaces: Navigating through a 3D space can be natural and attractive in the beginning, but after a while such space and way of interaction may become an obstacle for a user. Although bad ergonomic design may be one of the reasons, further study on perceptual and cognitive issues may uncover additional facts.

- Proposing better evaluation methods and collecting experimental evidences: The novelty and the limitless possibilities of 3D user interfaces and interaction research have resulted in a practice where researchers mostly focus on developing new devices, interaction techniques, and user interface metaphors. Evaluations have not been used much to actively influence the design process. At the same time, although there are several evaluation methods in HCI, customized evaluation methods for 3D interaction are still in their infancy. Proposing customized evaluation methods and carrying out more systematic evaluations should be important future work so that more experimental evidence can be collected to guide the design of 3D interaction.

So with the future development of technology and more understanding of the principles behind 3D interaction, 3D interface will undoubtedly become more useful for data analysis by scientists and professionals.

REFERENCES

Arthur, K., Booth, K., & Ware, C. (1993). Evaluating 3D task performance for fish tank virtual worlds. *ACM Trans. Inf. Syst, 11*(3), 239-265.

Bowman, D., Kruijff, E., LaViola, J., Jr., & Poupyrev, I. (2001). An introduction to 3D user interface design. *Presence, 10*(1), 96-108.

Bowman, D., Datey, A., Ryu, Y., Farooq, U., & Vasnaik, O. (2002). Empirical comparison of human behavior and performance with different display devices for virtual environments. *Proceedings of the Human Factors and Ergonomics Society Annual Meeting,* (pp. 2134-2138).

Brederson, J., Ikits, M., Johnson, C., & Hansen, C. (2000). The visual haptic workbench. *Proceedings of PHANToM Users Group Workshop,* (pp. 46-49).

Brooks, F. (1999). What's real about virtual reality?. *IEEE Computer Graphics and Applications, 9,* 16-27.

Brooks, F., Ouh-Young, M., Batter, J., & Kilpatrick, P. (1990). Project GROPE- haptic displays for scientific visualization. *Computer Graphics, 24*(4), 177-185.

Chen, M., Mountford, S., & Sellen, A. (1988). A study in interactive 3D rotation using 2D control devices. *Computer Graphics, 22*(4), 121-129.

Cruz-Neira, C., Sandin, D., & DeFanti, T. (1993). Surround-screen projection-based virtual reality: The design and implementation of the CAVE. *ACM Computer Graphics, 27*(2), 135-142.

Demiralp, C., Laidlaw, D., Jackson, C., Keefe, D., & Zhang, S. (2003). Subjective usefulness of CAVE and fish tank VR display systems for a scientific visualization application. *Proceedings of IEEE Visualization.* Seattle, WA.

De Guzman, E., Ho-Ching, F., Matthews, T., Rattenbury, T., Back, M., & Harrison, S. (2003).

Eewww!: Tangible instruments for navigating into the human body. *Extended Abstracts of CHI 2003,* 806-807.

Ernst, M., & Banks, M. (2002). Humans integrate visual and haptic information in a statistically optimal fashion. *Nature, 415*(6870), 429-433.

Froehlich, B., & Plate, J. (2000). The cubic mouse: A new device for three-dimensional input. *Proceedings of the SIGCHI conference on Human factors in computing systems,* (pp. 526-531).

Hansen, C., & Johnson, C. (2004). *The visualization handbook.* MA: Elsevier Butterworth Heinemann.

Hinckley, K., Tullio, J., Pausch, R., Profftt, D., & Kassell, N. (1997). Usability analysis of 3D rotation techniques. *Proceedings of the 10th Annual ACM Symposium on User Interface Software and Technology,* (pp. 1-10).

Hinckley, K., Pausch, R., Kassell, N., & Goble, J. (1994). A three-dimensional user interface for neurosurgical visualization. *The SPIE Conf. on Medical Imaging,* (pp. 126-136).

Ishii, H., Ben-Joseph, E., Underkoer, J., Yeung, L., Chak, D., Kanji, Z., & Piper, B. (2002). Augmented urban planning workbench: Overlaying drawings, physical models and digital simulation. *ISMAR '02: Proceedings of the International Symposium on Mixed and Augmented Reality (ISMAR'02),* (pp. 203). Washington, D.C.: IEEE Computer Society.

Kosara, R., Healey, C., Interrante, V., Laidlaw, D., & Ware, C. (2003). User studies: Why, how, and when?. *IEEE Computer Graphics and Applications,* (pp. 20-25).

Kreuger, W., Bohn, C., Froehlich, B., Schueth, Strauss, H., & Wesche, G. (1995). The responsive workbench: A virtual work environment. *IEEE Computer, 28*(7), 42-48.

Levoy, M. (1998). Display of surfaces from volume data. *IEEE Computer Graphics and Applications, 8*(5), 29-37.

Martens, J., van Liere, R., & Kok, A. (2007). Widget manipulation revisited: A case study in modeling interactions between experimental conditions. *IPT-EGVE 2007.* The Eurographics Association.

Meehan, M., Whitton, M., & Brooks, F., Jr. (2002). Physiological measures of presence in stressful virtual environments. *Proceedings of ACM SIGGRAPH2002, 21,* (pp. 645-652).

Mulder, J., & van Liere, R. (2002). The personal space station: Bringing interaction within reach. *Proceedings of VRIC 2002 Conference* (pp. 73-81).

Qi, W., Taylor, R., Healey, C., & Martens, J. (2006). A comparison of immersive HMD, fish tank VR and fish tank with haptics displays for volume visualization. *Proceedings of the 3rd symposium on Applied perception in graphics and visualization 2006,* (pp. 51-58).

Razzaque, S., & Whitton, M. (2001). Redirected walking. *Proceedings of Eurographics 2001,* (pp. 289-294).

Schroeder, W., Avila, L., & Hoffman, W. (2000). Visualizing with VTK: A tutorial. *IEEE Comput. Graph. App., 20*(5), 20-27.

Schulze, J., Zeleznik, J., Forsberg, A., & Laidlaw, D. (2005). Characterizing the effect of level of immersion on a 3D marking task. *Proceedings of HCI International,* (pp. 447-452). HCI International.

Sutherland, I. (1968). A head-mounted three-dimensional display. *Proceeding of the Fall Joint Computer Conference,* (pp. 757-764).

Taylor, R., Chen, J., Okimoto, S., Llopis-Artime, N., Chi, V., Brooks, F., et al. (1997). Pearls found on the way to the ideal interface for scanned-probe microscopes. *Proceedings of Proceedings of IEEE Visualization,* (pp. 467-470).

Taylor, R., Hudson, T., Seeger, A., Weber, H., Juliano, J., & Helser, A. (2001). VRPN: A device-independent, network-transparent VR peripheral system. *VRST'01: Proceedings of the ACM symposium on Virtual reality software and technology,* (pp. 55-61).

Ullmer, B., Ishii, H., & Glas, D. (1998). Media-blocks: Physical containers, transports, and controls for online media. *Proceedings of SIGGRAPH '98,* (pp. 379-386).

Ullmer, B., & Ishii, H. (2001). Emerging frameworks for tangible user interfaces. In: J. Carroll (Ed.), *Human-computer interaction in the new millennium,* (pp. 579-601). Addison-Wesley.

van Liere, R., & Mulder, J. (2003). Optical tracking using projective invariant marker pattern properties. *Proceedings of the IEEE Virtual Reality Conference 2003,* (pp. 191-198).

Ware, C., Arthur, K., & Booth, K. (1993). Fish tank virtual reality. *Proceedings of CHI 93,* (pp. 37-42).

Ware, C., & Franck, G. (1996). Evaluating stereo and motion cues for visualizing information nets in three dimensions. *ACM Trans. Graph., 15*(2), 121-140.

Westermann, R., & Ertl, T. (1998). Using graphics hardware in volume rendering applications. *Proceedings of SIGGRAPH'98,* (pp. 169-178).

Zhai, S. (1995). *Human performance in six degrees of freedom input control.* Doctoral Thesis, University of Toronto, Toronto.

ADDITIONAL READINGS

Card, S., Mackinlay, J., & Robertson, G. (1990). The design space of input devices. *Proceedings of the 1990 ACM Conference on Human Factors in Computing Systems (CHI'90)* (pp. 117-124). ACM Press.

Card, S., Moran, T. & Newell, A. (1986). The model human processor. In: K. Boff, L. Kaufman, & J. Thomas (Eds.), *Handbook of perception and human performance* (vol. 1, pp. 451-455). John Wiley & Sons.

Card, S., Moran, T., & Newell, A. (1983). *The psychology of human-computer interaction.* Lawrence Erlbaum Associates.

Fitts, P. (1954). The information capacity of the human motor system in controlling the amplitude of movement. *Journal of Experimental Psychology, 47,* 381-391.

Gabbard, J., Hix, D., & Swan, J. (1999). User-centered design and evaluation of virtual environments. *IEEE Computer Graphics & Applications, 19*(6), 51-59.

Hix, D., & Hartson, H. (1993). *Developing user interfaces: Ensuring usability through product & process.* John Wiley and Sons.

Jacob, R. (1996). Input devices and techniques. In: A. Tucker (Ed.), *The computer science and engineering handbook,* (pp. 1494-1511). CRC Press.

LaViola, J. (2000a). A discussion of cybersickness in virtual environments. *SIGCHI Bulletin, 32*(1), 47-56.

Mine, M., Brooks, F., & Sequin, C. (1997). Moving objects in space: Exploiting proprioception in virtual environment interaction. *Proceedings of SIGGRAPH'97,* (pp. 19-26). ACM Press.

Milgram, P., & Kishino, F. (1994). A taxonomy of mixed reality visual displays. *IECE Transactions on Information and System, E77-D*(12), 1321-1329.

Preece, J., Rogers, Y., & Sharp, H. (2002). *Interaction design: Beyond human-computer interaction.* John Wiley and Sons.

Shneiderman, B. (1998). *Designing the user interface: Strategies for effective human-computer interaction,* (3rd ed.). Addison Wesley.

State, A., Livingston, M., Hirota, G., Garrett, W., Whitton, M., Fuchs, H., & Pisano, E. (1996). Technologies for augmented reality systems: Realizing ultrasound-guided needle biopsies. *Proceedings of SIGGRAPH'96,* (pp. 439-446). ACM Press.

Stanney, K., Mourant, R., & Kennedy, R. (1998). Human factors issues in virtual environments: A review of the literature. *Presence: Teleoperators and Virtual Environments, 7*(4), 327-351.

Srinivasan, M., & Chen, J. (1993). Human performance in controlling normal forces of contact with rigid objects. *Advances in Robotics, Mechatronics, annd Haptic Interfaces, ASME,* (pp. 119-125).

Simon, A., & Fröhlich, B. (2003). The yoyo: A handheld device combining elastic and istonic input. *Proceedings of INTERACT 2003,* (pp. 303-310). Zurich: IOS Press.

Usoh, M., Catena, E., Arman, S., & Slater, M. (2000). Using presence questionnaires in reality. *Presence: Teleoperators and Virtual Environments, 9*(5), 497-503.

Usoh, M., Arthur, K., Whitton, M., Bastos, R., Steed, A., Slater, M., & Brooks, F., Jr. (1999). Walking > Walking-in-Place > Flying in Virtual Environments. *Proceedings of SIGGRAPH '99,* (pp. 359-364). ACM Press.

van Dam, A., Forsberg, A., Laidlaw, D., LaViola, J., & Simpson, R. (2000). Immersive VR for scientific visualization: A progress report. *IEEE Computer Graphics & Applications, 20*(6), 26-52.

van Dam, A. (1997). Post-WIMP user interfaces: The human connection. *Communication of the ACM, 40*(2), 63-67.

Welch, G., Bishop, G., Vicci, L., Brumback, S., Keller, K., & Colucci, D. (1999). The hiball tracker: High-performance wide-area tracking for virtual and augmented environments. *Proceedings of the 1999 ACM Symposium on Virtual Reality Software and Technology (VRST'99),* (pp. 1-10). ACM Press.

Welch, R., & Warren, D. (1986). Intersensory interactions. In: K. Boff, L. Kaufman, & J. Thomas (Eds.), *Handbook of perception and human performance,* (vol. 2, pp. 251- 256). John Wiley & Sons.

Ware, C. (2000). *Information visualisation: Perception for design.* San Francisco, CA: Morgan Kaufman.

APPENDIX: POST-EXPERIMENT QUESTIONNAIRE

Participant ID:_____

The following questions relate to the Virtual Reality (VR) system you have experienced during the experiment. Please select the correct one:

- ○ **Immersive HMD VR**
- ○ **Fish tank VR**
- ○ **Fish tank with Force-feedback (haptic)**

1. Please rate your sense of being in the virtual environment that has the simulation data on the following scale from 1 to 7, where 7 represents your normal experience of being in a place.
    I had a sense of being in the virtual environment containing the simulation data:

    (Not at all) 1 2 3 4 5 6 7 (Very much)

2. Please rate any sense of immersion you experienced when looking into the dataset.
    The sense of immersion I experienced was...

    (Not at all) 1 2 3 4 5 6 7 (Very much)

3. How difficult or straightforward was it for you to understand spatial relationships between objects in the virtual environment while working with the system?
    The spatial relation was...

    (Very difficult) 1 2 3 4 5 6 7 (Very straightforward)

4. Did you find it relatively simple or relatively complicated to move through the virtual environment and the simulation data?
    To move through the virtual environment was...

    (Very complicated) 1 2 3 4 5 6 7 (Very simple)

5. The act of moving from place to place in the virtual environment can seem to be relatively natural or relatively unnatural. Please rate your experience of this.
    The act of moving from place to place seemed to be...

    (Very unnatural) 1 2 3 4 5 6 7 (Very natural)

6. How often did you to feel you were in virtual environment when observing the simulation data and searching for the required structure?
    I felt I was in virtual environment...

    (Very few) 1 2 3 4 5 6 7 (Very often)

7. To what extent were there times during the experience when you felt dissatisfied with the interface?

continued on following page

There were times during the experience I felt dissatisfied...

(At no time) 1 2 3 4 5 6 7 (Almost all of the time)

8. To what extent did you have a sense of acting in the virtual space, rather than operating something from outside?

(Not at all) 1 2 3 4 5 6 7 (Very much)

9. To what extent did you feel that the virtual environment surrounded you?

(Not at all) 1 2 3 4 5 6 7 (Very much)

10. To what extent did you feel like you just perceived pictures?

(Not at all) 1 2 3 4 5 6 7 (Very much)

11. How much did your experience in the virtual environment seem consistent with your real-world experience?

(Not at all) 1 2 3 4 5 6 7 (Very much)

12. To what extent do you think the virtual reality system you experienced helped you identify the structure within the volumetric simulation data?
I thought the virtual environment helps me...

(Not at all) 1 2 3 4 5 6 7 (Very much)

13. How easy to use was this virtual reality system?

(Hard to use) 1 2 3 4 5 6 7 (Very easy)

14. How effective do you feel you were when working with the virtual reality system compared with a traditional desktop system?

(No difference) 1 2 3 4 5 6 7 (Very effective)

15. How helpful were the depth cues in this virtual reality system compared to the traditional desktop system?

(No difference) 1 2 3 4 5 6 7 (Very much)

16. Rate the degree of difficulty in carrying out the task, for the virtual reality system you experienced:

(Not difficult at all) 1 2 3 4 5 6 7 (Very difficult indeed)

17. How well could you examine objects from multiple viewpoints?

(Very difficult) 1 2 3 4 5 6 7 (Very easy)

continued on following page

18. How much delay did you experience between your actions and expected outcomes?

(None at all) 1 2 3 4 5 6 7 (Very much)

19. When exploring the virtual space, did the objects appear too compressed or too magnified?

(Not at all) 1 2 3 4 5 6 7 (Very compressed)

(Not at all) 1 2 3 4 5 6 7 (Very magnified)

20. During the experiment, your general level of confidence in the accuracy of your answers was:

(Just guessing) 1 2 3 4 5 6 7 (Very sure)

21. During the task, identifying the individual shape and location of an object within the environment was:

(Difficult) 1 2 3 4 5 6 7 (Easy)

22. During the task, identifying the global topology of the simulation data was through the VR system:

(Difficult) 1 2 3 4 5 6 7 (Easy)

23. During the task, what was the level of demand on your memory?

(Small) 1 2 3 4 5 6 7 (Large)

24. How effective was the sense of perspective (further objects appeared the correct size compared to nearer objects)?

(Ineffective) 1 2 3 4 5 6 7 (Effective)

25. Did you think that the VR system you experienced changes the way you observe and analyze the data, in comparison to traditional media?

- ○ **Didn't change at all**
- ○ **Changed just a little bit**
- ○ **Changed slightly**
- ○ **Changed quite some**
- ○ **Changed radically**

Answer the following questions if you experienced fish tank VR with haptic device

1. How consistent or inconsistent was the information coming from your various senses (visual and haptic feedback)?

(Inconsistent) 1 2 3 4 5 6 7 (Very Consistent)

continued on following page

2. How well could you actively survey or search within the virtual environment using touch? Searching within the virtual environment through touch was

(Very difficult) 1 2 3 4 5 6 7 (Very easy)

3. Do you think the addition of multimodal sensory stimulation (haptics) would help you?

A)   Create a better understanding of space:
- O   **Not at all**
- O   **Small chance**
- O   **Possibly**
- O   **Likely**
- O   **Very likely**

B)   Create better understanding the structure and topology of the data:
- O   **Not at all**
- O   **Small chance**
- O   **Possibly**
- O   **Likely**
- O   **Very likely**

Chapter VIII
Automated Overlay of Infrared and Visual Medical Images

G. Schaefer
Aston University, UK

R. Tait
Nottingham Trent University, UK

K. Howell
Royal Free Hospital, UK

A. Hopgood
De Montford University, UK

P. Woo
Great Ormond Street Hospital, London, UK

J. Harper
Great Ormond Street Hospital, London, UK

ABSTRACT

Medical infrared imaging captures the temperature distribution of the human skin and is employed in various medical applications. Often it is useful to cross-reference the resulting thermograms with visual images of the patient, either to see which part of the anatomy is affected by a certain disease or to judge the efficacy of the treatment. In this chapter, we show that image registration techniques can be effectively used to generate an overlay of visual and thermal images and provide a useful diagnostic visualisation for the clinician.

INTRODUCTION

Medical infrared imaging captures the natural thermal radiation generated by an object at a temperature above absolute zero. It is non-invasive, non-contact, passive, radiation-free and complementary to anatomical investigations based on x-rays and three-dimensional scanning techniques such as CT and MRI, and often reveals problems when the anatomy is otherwise normal. Often, visual and infrared images of the patient are taken to relate inflamed skin areas to the human anatomy which in turn is useful for medial diagnosis as well as for assessing the efficacy of any treatment. Currently, this process requires great expertise and is subject to the individual clinician's ability to mentally map the two distinctly different images.

Image registration is one of the most important medical image processing techniques and is used to geometrically align or overlay two images taken from different sensors, viewpoints or instances in time. Both images are typically aligned through a combination of scaling, translation and rotation. Registration is often used to monitor growth, verify the effects of treatment and make comparisons of patient data with anatomically normal subjects.

In this chapter, we show how image registration can be effectively used to overlay medical infrared images and visual images of a patient in order to relate areas that are of interest due to their thermal pattern to the human anatomy. After capturing both thermal and visual images, the visual image is pre-processed with a skin detection technique to separate the patient from the background. Using an intensity-based registration algorithm which requires no user interaction, visual and infrared images are then superimposed and the generated overlay presented to the user for visualisation purpose. The generated system is currently in use at Royal Free and Great Ormond Street hospitals to assess patients suffering from morphea.

BACKGROUND

Thermal Infrared Imaging

Advances in camera technologies and reduced equipment costs are among the factors that have led to an increased interest in the application of thermal imaging in the medical fields (Jones, 1998). Thermal medical imaging (or medical infrared imaging) uses cameras with sensitivities in the infrared to provide a picture of the temperature distribution of the human body or parts thereof. It is a non-invasive, non-contact, passive, radiation-free technique that is often being used in combination with anatomical investigations based on x-rays and three-dimensional scanning techniques such as CT and MRI and often reveals problems when the anatomy is otherwise normal. It is well known that the radiance from human skin is an exponential function of the surface temperature which in turn is influenced by the level of blood perfusion in the skin. Thermal imaging is hence well suited to pick up changes in blood perfusion which might occur due to inflammation, angiogenesis or other causes. Asymmetrical temperature distributions as well as the presence of hot and cold spots are known to be strong indicators of an underlying dysfunction (Uematsu, 1985). Computerized image processing and pattern recognition techniques have been used in acquiring and evaluating medical thermal images (Plassmann & Ring, 1997; Wiecek, Zwolenik, Jung, & Zuber, 1999) and proved to be important tools for clinical diagnostics. Thermal imaging has been successfully employed in, among others, detecting breast cancer (Head, Wang, Lipari, & Elliott, 2000; Anbar et al., 2001), diagnosing Raynaud's phenomenon (Merla et al., 2002), and local scleroderma (morphea) (Black et al., 2002).

Image Registration

Image registration is a method used to geometrically align or overlay two images taken from different sensors, viewpoints or instances in time. Both reference (fixed) and sensed (moving) images are typically aligned through a combination of scaling, translation and rotation although a universal registration method is not possible due to the wide variety of noise and geometric deformations caused by the diverse methods of image capture available. Registration is often used to monitor growth, verify the effects of treatment and make comparisons of patient data with anatomically normal subjects (Maintz & Viergever, 1998).

While there is a wealth of registration techniques available, most of them can be divided into two categories: landmark-based and intensity-based algorithms (Zitova & Flusser, 2003). Landmark-based methods rely on a selection of several corresponding control points in both images and then seek the best image transform between these landmark pairs. Obviously, registration accuracy is determined by the selection of the landmarks. While manual selection might provide good registration results it is a cumbersome method that relies heavily on the user. On the other hand, automatic control point detection and extraction methods are difficult to derive and typically depend on certain image characteristics. In contrast, intensity-based registration approaches do not require identification of landmarks, rather they utilize the image data directly. Additional masking can be introduced to emphasize special features. The basic intensity approach consists of transform optimization, image re-sampling and feature-matching stages. Feature matching is the most fundamental stage and is achieved through the use of a similarity metric in which a degree of likeness between corresponding images is calculated. These steps are iteratively repeated until a good enough match between the two images is achieved.

In multi-modal image registration applications, the data to be registered stem from two different capturing devices, as opposed to single-modal tasks where images are retrieved using the same sensor type. The measure of alignment between images of differing modality can be based on the assumption that although different in value, regions of similar intensity in the fixed image will correspond to regions of similar intensity in the moving image (Woods, Mazziotta, & Cherry, 1993). Also, for all pixels in corresponding regions, the ratio of their intensities should vary only slightly. As a consequence, alignment is achieved when the average variance of this ratio is minimized. Crucially, this idea can be realized through the construction of a feature space also commonly referred to as a joint probability distribution (Hill, Hawkes, Harrison, & Ru, 1993). The joint probability distribution represents a two-dimensional plot containing combinations of intensities taken from corresponding coordinates in both images. Instead of identifying regions of similar intensity directly within the images, combinations of intensities are analyzed using the joint probability distribution.

During the registration process, a variation in alignment between the images causes changes in appearance of the joint probability distribution. When correctly aligned, corresponding structures in both images overlap causing a clustering of intensities combinations. In contrast, misalignment causes structures in the fixed image to overlap with structures in the moving image which are not their counterpart. This results in the dispersal of intensity combinations within the joint probability distribution. Pluim, Maintz, and Viergever (2003) have demonstrated the effects of registering an image with itself using varying degrees of translation and rotation. Based on the changing regions within the joint probability distribution, measures of dispersion which guide the registration process have been proposed and successfully implemented (Maes, Collignon, Vandermeulen, Marchal, & Suetens, 1997; Viola & Wells, 1997).

Importantly, the concept of mutual information which appears low when intensity combinations are dispersed and high when intensity combinations are clustered, is a well recognized and accepted method of similarity calculation. The main advantage of employing mutual information is that the type of dependency between two variables does not have to be specified and as a result complex mappings can be modeled.

As no assumptions about the nature of the capture device need to be made, image registration algorithm can be generalized and applied to data representing a variety of modalities.

METHODS

Our system is designed to provide an overlay of visual and thermal images to be presented to a clinician. Superimposing both image types allows relating areas of certain thermal patterns to the anatomy of the person as well as monitor efficacy of any treatment. After pre-processing both images to segment the patient from the background, an intensity-based registration algorithm with mutual information similarity metric is employed to geometrically align the two images. This is realized using a series of intelligent agents collaborating on a blackboard architecture to provide an efficient and effective framework for image registration. Superimposed images are presented to the user for visualization. The user can adjust the relative importance of the individual modalities in an interactive manner.

Image Pre-Processing and Segmentation

As the overlay is achieved through application of an intensity-based image registration algorithm, and as the background of thermal images taken in a temperature controlled lab is typically in stark contrast to the patient's body heat, the same

contrast must be achieved for the visual image. That is, the background needs to be separated from the foreground (i.e., the patient). In our approach, we make use the fact that thermal imaging picks up the skin temperature and hence employ a skin detection technique on the visual image (Schaefer, Tait, & Zhu, 2006). We adopt, with some variations, a computationally simple method introduced in (Fleck, Forsyth, & Bregler, 1996) which is based on the fact that the hues of human skin occupy only a small region in color space. The algorithm which operates on the visual (RGB) image proceeds in the following steps:

1. The R, G, and B values at each pixel are transformed into a log-opponent color representation by

$$\begin{pmatrix} I \\ R_g \\ B_y \end{pmatrix} = \begin{pmatrix} L(G) \\ L(R) - L(G) \\ L(B) - \dfrac{L(G) - L(R)}{2} \end{pmatrix} \quad (1)$$

with

$$L(C) = 105 \log_{10}(C + 1 + n) \quad C = \{R, G, B\} \quad (2)$$

where n represents some random noise (in the range $(0;1)$) to prevent banding artifacts in dark regions.

2. A measure of texture amplitude T is then derived from the intensity channel by building a difference image of the original image and a median filtered version of it. The resulting texture channel is then again median filtered as are the chromaticity components (at a finer scale compared to the texture channel).

3. Next, hue H and saturation S are calculated as:

$$H = \tan^{-1}\left(\frac{R_g}{B_y}\right)$$

$$S = \sqrt{R_g^2 + B_g^2} \quad (3)$$

4. Pixels that fall within a certain hue-saturation range and do not exceed a texture threshold are identified. In particular, all pixels that fall within

$$\{T<5 \text{ and } 110<H<155 \text{ and } 5<S<60\}$$

or

$$\{T<5 \text{ and } 130<H<170 \text{ and } 30<S<130\}$$

are marked as skin pixels.

5. Using morphological operations holes are filled and edges smoothed to provide the final output of the skin detector.

Registration

Using the detector described above regions in the visual image are identified that correspond to skin colors and hence to the patient. Non-skin areas are removed by setting their pixel values to 0 (black). In the thermal images, patients are usually well separated from the background in controlled lab conditions so little pre-processing is required. If necessary, an adaptive thresholding algorithm can be applied to improve the separation of patient from non-patient areas.

Once both image types have been prepared, the image registration process is initiated. As we are interested in a fully automatic method that should be applicable on a wide range of different images (different patients, poses, etc.) we adopted an intensity-based approach to registering the two images. In intensity-based techniques pixel information is utilized and the best alignment is derived as that which optimises a pre-defined similarity metric between the registered images. The steps involved are transform optimization, image re-sampling and similarity computation which are applied in an iterative manner until the process has converged. We employ a gradient-decent optimizer, B-spline interpolation for the re-sampling and a mutual information measure as similarity metric.

The similarity computation stage is complex and represents a considerable performance bottleneck when employed in an iterative registration process. Based on a worker/manager model, a distributed blackboard system is employed to spread computational workload between a number of intelligent agents and improve performance of the algorithm (Tait, Schaefer, Hopgood, & Nolle, 2006).

The alignment process begins with partitioning of visual and thermal images into segments; regions of interest and initial transform parameters are also added to the blackboard. On addition of transform parameters, for each sample point in the visual segment a corresponding intensity in the thermal segment is calculated. Importantly, interpolation with a B-spline basis function is used to calculate intensities at non-grid positions. A local joint probability distribution realized as a Parzen histogram is then generated from retrieved intensities by a worker process and placed onto the blackboard. As histograms are progressively generated for all image segments, worker processes become inactive.

Deactivation of all worker processes triggers the manager process to construct a global Parzen histogram from local histograms stored on the blackboard. By estimating the density distribution of the global histogram, an entropy value in the form of a gradient is then calculated. Regular step gradient descent optimization is employed by the manager process to advance transform parameters in the direction of the gradient. In each iteration of the optimization process, the step length through the transform search space is calculated using a bipartition scheme. Once updated, transform parameters are propagated to all worker processes and the procedure is repeated. The algorithm converges when the step length fails to exceed a threshold, or a maximum number of iterations have been reached. On convergence, image segments are accumulated by the manager process and a registered image is assembled.

The framework is flexible in nature and can be employed to either distribute the registration of single images as outlined above or to distribute the processing of many images in batch mode.

Although the system by default performs intensity-based registration to provide a fully automated system, in certain cases intensity-based approaches do not produce an accurate overlay. In such instances the user has the possibility to switch to a landmark-based algorithm. Corresponding control points then need to be specified by the user before an accurate overlay is generated.

Once an appropriate transform has been found and image registration performed (typically the visual image is selected as reference and the thermal one as sensed image), a composite image is created. This is simply performed by computing a weighted sum of the respective pixel values of the original visual image and the thresholded thermogram. Equal weights will generate an aver-

age of the two images whereas different weight factors will put more emphasis on one of the two modalities. The actual weightings between the two modalities can be determined by the user and can be controlled interactively.

RESULTS

We have used a set of thermal-visual image pairs to evaluate our proposed method. Two examples are provided in Figures 1 and 2, each of which shows the original visual image, the thermogram, the visual image segmented based on the output of the skin detection step, and the final overlaid image. In both cases, the final image was weighted as 80% visual and 20% thermal. As can be seen, in both cases an accurate overlay of the two image types is achieved.

Figure 1. Example 1 of thermal-visual overlay: Original visual image, thermogram, segmented visual image, composite image (from left to right, top to bottom)

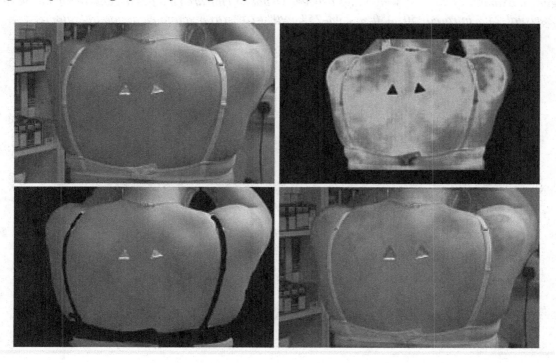

Figure 2. Example 2 of thermal-visual overlay: Original visual image, thermogram, segmented visual image, composite image (from left to right, top to bottom)

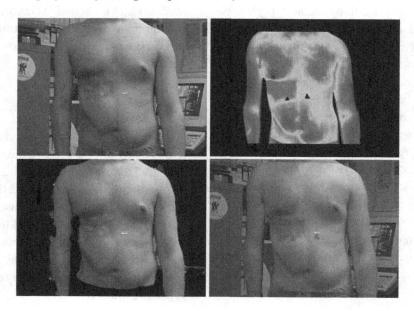

Figure 3. Example of different weightings between visual and infrared images in generating the overlay: 75% visual-25% infrared; 50%-50%; 25%-75%; 90%-10% (from left to right, top to bottom)

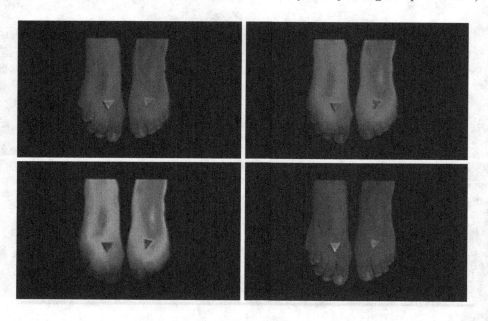

Figure 4. Example of landmark-based registration. Control points have been set for the visual image and copied over to the infrared image.

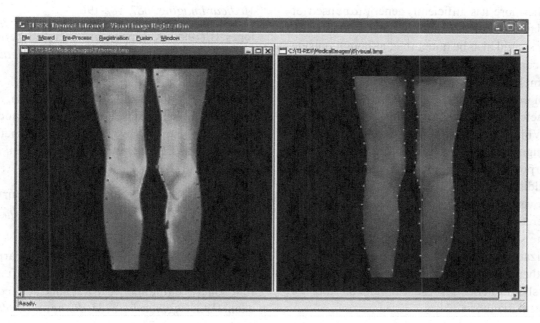

The generated images are currently being used in the assessment of morphea (localized scleroderma) patients. In Figure 2, the warmer area of the chest overlay indicates the distribution of a morphea lesion.

In Figure 3, we show how the weights between the two image modalities can be set so as to put more or less emphasis on one of the original images.

Finally, Figure 4 gives an example of the application where the user is performing a landmark- rather than an intensity-based registration. Control points are placed in one of the modalities which can then be copied to the other image. Control points can be adjusted as a complete set through rotation, translation and scaling operations or individually. If control points are placed correctly, landmark-based registration provides high accuracy overlay images.

CONCLUSION

In this chapter, we have shown how image registration can be employed to perform multi-modal medical image visualization and overlay. In particular we have demonstrated its application to overlay thermal and visual images for medical diagnosis. Following a pre-processing step based on skin detection to perform background segmentation, intensity-based multi-modal registration is performed through a set of intelligent agents communicating via a blackboard structure.

Future Research Directions

The system is currently in use at Royal Free and Great Ormond Street hospitals where it is used in the diagnosis and treatment of morphea (local scleroderma) patients. The methods described can however be used in any scenario where overlay of infrared and visual images is deemed useful. Furthermore, it is sufficiently generic to be used for overlaying medical images of other modalities.

It should also be noted that, although outside the scope of this chapter, the framework can also be employed for registering 3D volume datasets in an equally efficient and effective way (Tait, Schaefer, Hopgood, Zhu, 2006).

While currently the application is restricted to aligning static images, future versions will incorporate superimposed dynamic sequences. In addition, we are currently working at providing overlays of images that have been taken at different times, typically many months apart, of the same patient. These should provide a visualization of how a disease is developing and whether the current treatment shows any effects, and should hence represent a valuable tool for medical diagnosis.

REFERENCES

Anbar, N., Milescu, L., Naumov, A., Brown, C., Button, T., Carly, C., & AlDulaimi, K. (2001). Detection of cancerous breasts by dynamic area telethermometry. *IEEE Engineering in Medicine and Biology Magazine, 20*(5), 80-91.

Black, C., Murray, K., Howell, K., Harper, J., Atherton, D., Woo, P., et al. (2002). Juvenile-onset localized scleroderma activity detection by infrared thermography. *Rheumatology, 41*(10), 1178-1182.

Fleck, M., Forsyth, D., & Bregler, C. (1996). Finding naked people. *4ᵗʰ European Conference on Computer Vision, 2,* 593-602.

Head, J., Wang, F., Lipari, C., & Elliott, R. (2000). The important role of infrared imaging in breast cancer. *IEEE Engineering in Medicine and Biology Magazine, 19,* 52-57.

Hill, D., Hawkes, D., Harrison, N., & Ru, C. (1993). A strategy for automated multi-modal image reg-istration incorporating anatomical knowledge and imager characteristics. *Information Processing in Medical Imaging, 687,* 182-196.

Jones, B. (1998). A reappraisal of infrared thermal image analysis for medicine. *IEEE Trans. Medical Imaging, 17*(6), 1019-1027.

Maes, F., Collignon, A., Vandermeulen, D., Marchal, G., & Suetens, P. (1997). Multi-modality image registration by maximization of mutual information. *IEEE Transactions on Medical Imaging, 16,* 187-198.

Maintz, J., & Viergever, A. (1998). A survey of medical image registration. *Medical Image Analysis, 2,* 1-36.

Merla, A., Di Donato, L., Di Luzio, S., Farina, G., Pisarri, S., Proietti, M., et al. (2002). Infrared functional imaging applied to Raynaud's phenomenon. *IEEE Engineering in Medicine and Biology Magazine, 21*(6), 73-79.

Plassmann, P., & Ring, E. (1997). An open system for the acquisition and evaluation of medical thermological images. *European Journal of Thermology, 7,* 216-220.

Pluim, J., Maintz, J., & Viergever, M. (2003). Mutual information-based registration of medical images: A survey. *IEEE Transactions on Medical Imaging, 22,* 986-1004.

Schaefer, G., Tait, R., & Zhu, S. (2006). Overlay of thermal and visual medical images using skin detection and image registration. *28ᵗʰ IEEE Int. Conference Engineering in Medicine and Biology,* (pp. 965-967).

Tait, R., Schaefer, G., Hopgood, A., & Nolle, L. (2006). Automated visual inspection using a distributed blackboard architecture. *Int. Journal of Simulation: Systems, Science & Technology, 7*(3), 12-20.

Tait, R., Schaefer, G., Hopgood, A., & Zhu, S. (2006). Efficient 3-D medical image registration using a distributed blackboard system. *28ᵗʰ IEEE*

Int. Conference Engineering in Medicine and Biology, (pp. 3045-3048).

Uematsu, S. (1985). Symmetry of skin temperature comparing one side of the body to the other. *Thermology, 1,* 4-7.

Viola, P., & Wells, W. (1997). Alignment by maximization of mutual information, *International Journal of Computer Vision, 24,* 137-154.

Wiecek, B., Zwolenik, S., Jung, A., & Zuber, J. (1999). Advanced thermal, visual and radiological image processing for clinical diagnostics. *21st IEEE Int. Conference on Engineering in Medicine and Biology,* (p. 1108).

Woods, R., Mazziotta, J., & Cherry, S. (1993). MRI-PET registration with an automated algorithm. *Journal of Computer Assisted Tomography, 17,* 536-546.

Zitova, B., & Flusser, J. (2003). Image registration methods: A survey. *Image and Vision Computing, 21,* 977-1000.

Additional Reading

Allen, R., Ansell, B., Clark, R., Goff, M., Waller, R., & Williamson, S. (1987). Localized scleroderma: Treatment response measured by infrared thermography. *Thermology, 2,* 550-553.

Bankman, I. (2000). *Handbook of medical imaging.* Academic Press.

Birdi, N., Shore, A., Rush, P., Laxer, R., Silverman, E., & Krafchik, B. (1992). Childhood linear scleroderma: A possible role of thermography for evaluation. *Journal of Rheumatology, 19,* 968-973.

Black, C. (1999). Scleroderma in children. *Advances in Experimental Medicine and Biology, 455,* 35-48.

Brown, L. (1992). A survey of image registration techniques. *ACM Computing Surveys,* 325-376.

Diakides, N., & Bronzino, J. (Eds.). (2007). *Medical infrared imaging.* CRC Press.

Hill, D., Hawkes, D., Harrison, N., & Ru, C. (1993). A strategy for automated multi-modal image registration incorporating anatomical knowledge and imager characteristics. *Information Processing in Medical Imaging, 687,* 182-196.

Jeongtae, K., & Fessler, J. (2004). Intensity-based image registration using robust correlation coefficients. *IEEE Transactions on Medical Imaging, 23,* 1430-1444.

Kakumanu, P., Makrogiannis, S., & Bourbakis, N. A survey of skin-color modeling and detection methods. *Pattern Recognition, 3,* 1106-1122.

Martini, G., Murray, K., Howell, K., Harper, J., Atherton, D., Woo, P., et al. (2002). Juvenile-onset localized scleroderma activity detection by infrared thermography. *Rheumathology, 41,* 1178-1182.

Mattes, D., Haynor, D., Vesselle, H., Lewellen, T., & Eubank, W. (2001). Non-rigid multi-modality image registration. *Medical Imaging 2001: Image Processing,* (pp. 1609-1620).

Nolle, L., Wong, K., & Hopgood, A. (2001). DARBS: A distributed blackboard system. *Research and Development in Intelligent Systems, 18,* 161-70.

Pratt, W. (1974). Correlation techniques of image registration. *IEEE Transactions on Aerospace and Electronic Systems, 10,* 353-358.

Ring, E., & Ammer, K. (2000). The technique of infrared imaging in medicine. *Thermology International, 10,* 7-14.

Roche, A., Malandain, G., Ayache, N., & Prima, S. (1999). Towards better comprehension of similarity measures used in medical image registration. *Lecture Notes in Computer Science, 1679,* 555-566.

Chapter IX
Software Framework of Medical Visualization Algorithms

Ronghua Liang
Zhejiang University of Technology, China

ABSTRACT

Real-time visualization algorithms which are fully integrated into software framework are of importance for the rapid development of medical visualization applications. This chapter gives an overview of different software frameworks for real-time visualization algorithms. These algorithms are fully integrated into some open-source freely-available software frameworks. First, we introduce the famous Visualization Toolkit (VTK), and we then describe some other specialized toolkits, for example, for image registration and segmentation, MAF (Multimod Application Framework) supported by an EC-funded project MULTIMOD. We discuss the majority of algorithms available that can be easily combined for rapid construction of visualization applications. Finally, we place emphasis on exploiting the characteristics of medical datasets for further utilizing the hardware-accelerated capabilities of modern graphics cards.

INTRODUCTION

Over the past three decades, computer graphics and visualization have played a growing role in adding value to a wide variety of medical applications. The earliest examples were reported in the mid 1970s when three-dimensional visualizations of computerized tomography (CT) data were first reported (Mccloy, 2001). Today, a variety of imaging modalities (e.g., RX, CT, MRI, PET, endoscopy) are in common use by the medical profession for diagnostic purposes, and these modalities provide a rich source of data

for further processing using computer graphics techniques. Applications include medical diagnosis, procedures training, pre-operative planning, telemedicine, and many more (Robb, 1974). The researchers; use of new media technology demonstrates well how far the state-of-the-art has progressed since the early work in medical visualization, for several off-the-shelf surface and volume rendering techniques are available. Some typical medical visualization algorithms include surface rendering (e.g., Marching cubes iso-surface rendering), Volume Rendering, transfer function. However, researchers have to re-develop or integrate some medical visualization algorithms for a specific medical application. Therefore, visualization algorithms which are fully integrated into software framework are of importance for the rapid development of medical visualization applications.

We can also find some open-source, freely-available software frameworks, and the main frameworks can be classified into five following categories:

1. The *Visualization Tool Kit* (VTK) (vtk, 2007), a visualization library developed and made available in the public domain by KitWare Ltd. The objective of the library is not for specific medical application, but for general visualization applications.

2. The *Surgical VTK* (SVTK) (svtk, 2007) is a collection of classes extending the VTK library with various new functions developed in the frame of the Multimod Project. It has been integrated in MAF software framework.

3. The *Insight Tool Kit* (ITK) (itk, 2007) is new software library aimed to provide the most extensive support to image registration and segmentation. It is the result of a collaborative effort between various research groups all located in the USA, promoted by the Library of Medicine to increase the exploitation of the visible human datasets.

4. The *Multimod Application Framework* (MAF) (maf, 2007) is the software framework that will be the final product of the Multimod project. Around the term "framework" in the software-engineering context, a document collecting some definitions from the literature is available. These definitions seem quite consistent with what we had in mind when we wrote the proposal, that is, a software infrastructure not aimed to solve a particular problem but rather to allow the rapid development of a variety of applications all within the same application context.

Since a framework is aimed to capture the context-specific intelligence we expect the patterns design approach to play a relevant role in the project.

5. The *Medical Imaging ToolKit* (MITK) (mitk, 2007), a C++ library for integrated medical image processing and analyzing developed by the Medical Image Processing Group, Key Laboratory of Complex Systems and Intelligence Science, Institute of Automation, the Chinese Academy of Sciences.

Below, we survey the history and development of the use of software frameworks, pay more concentration on MAF, and highlight the major medical visualization algorithms (e.g., volume rendering) that have been fully integrated into the software frameworks to date.

SOFTWARE FRAMEWORK OF MEDICAL VISUALIZATION ALGORITHMS

In this section, we will discuss the four software frameworks, and SVTK will be introduced in MAF section, for SVTK have been fully integrated into MAF framework.

VTK

The Visualization ToolKit (VTK) is an open-source, freely-available software system for 3D computer graphics, image processing, and visualization used by thousands of researchers and developers around the world. VTK consists of a C++ class library, and several interpreted interface layers including TCL/Tk, Java, and Python. Professional support and products for VTK are provided by Kitware, Inc. VTK supports a wide variety of visualization algorithms including scalar, vector, tensor, texture, and volumetric methods; and advanced modeling techniques such as implicit modeling, polygon reduction, mesh smoothing, cutting, contouring, and Delaunay triangulation. In addition, dozens of imaging algorithms have been directly integrated to allow the user to mix 2D imaging or 3D graphics algorithms and data. The design and implementation of the library has been strongly influenced by object-oriented principles. VTK has been installed and tested on nearly every Unix-based platform, PCs (Windows 98/ME/NT/2000/XP), and Mac OSX Jaguar or later.

System Architecture

With VTK, building large, monolithic systems is detrimental to software flexibility. As a result, we wanted to create a sharply focused object library that we could easily embed and distribute into our applications. Figure 1(a) illustrates the basic idea. Toolkits enable complex applications to be built from small pieces. The key here is that the pieces must be well defined with simple interfaces.

Figure 1. System architecture

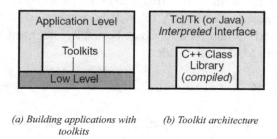

(a) Building applications with toolkits

(b) Toolkit architecture

Figure 2. Inheritance diagram for the base class

In this way, they can be readily assembled into larger systems.

Class Hierarchy

Object-oriented (OO) methods are now widely recognized as effective software design and implementation tools. Design methodologies from such researchers as Rumbaugh and Booch are receiving widespread attention, while C++, SmallTalk, and other object- oriented languages have become widely successful software tools. Also, a variety of class libraries are available, ranging from standard data structures to mathematics and numerical equation solvers. These trends have only recently converged (in the last half-decade) into object-oriented tools for 3D graphics and visualization. They have influenced commercial systems which exhibit object-oriented features such as modular and extensible components. The VTK is built with C++ as an object-oriented toolkit for 3D graphics and visualization. Below, we list some basic classes in VTK.

vtkObjectBase is the base class for all reference counted classes in the VTK; Figure 2(a) shows the Inheritance diagram of the class. vtkObject is the base class for most objects in the visualization toolkit, and vtkCommand is an implementation of the observer/command design pattern. In this design pattern, any instance of vtkObject can be "observed" for any events it might invoke.

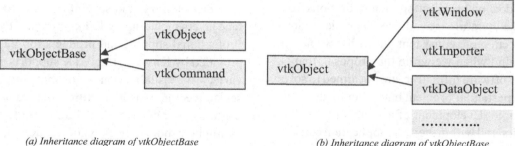

(a) Inheritance diagram of vtkObjectBase

(b) Inheritance diagram of vtkObjectBase

The Graphics and Visualization Pipeline

The graphics model captures the essential features of a 3D graphics system in a form that is easy to understand and use. To render a 3D object in VTK, the pipeline is shown in Figure 3 and the whole graphics model is shown in Figure 4.

There are nine basic objects in the model:

1. **Render Master:** Coordinates device-independent methods and creates rendering windows

2. **Render Window:** Manages a window on the display device. One or more renderers draw into a render window to generate a scene (i.e., final image).

3. **Renderer:** Coordinates the rendering of lights, cameras, and actors

4. **Light:** Illuminates the actors in a scene

5. **Camera:** Defines the view position, focal point, and other camera characteristics

6. **Actor:** An object drawn by a renderer in the scene. Actors are defined in terms of mapper, property, and a transform objects.

7. **Property:** Represents the rendered attributes of an actor including object color, lighting (e.g., specular, ambient, diffuse), texture map, drawing style (e.g., wireframe or shaded); and shading style.

8. **Mapper:** Represents the geometric definition of an actor and maps the object through a lookup table. More than one actor may refer to the same mapper.

9. **Transform:** An object that consists of a 4 x 4 transformation matrix and methods to modify the matrix. It specifies the position and orientation of actors, cameras, and lights.

The visualization model consists of two basic types of objects: process objects and data objects. Process objects are the modules, or algorithmic

Figure 3. Pipeline of rendering

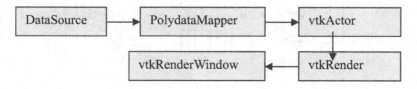

Figure 4. Graphics model

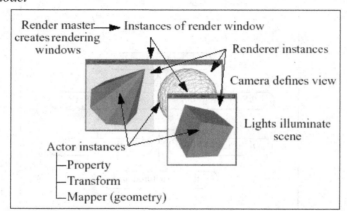

portions of the visualization network, and most visualization algorithms are incorporated here which are refereed as filters. Data objects, also referred to as datasets, represent and enable operations on the data that flows through the network. In our toolkit we initially selected five types of data as shown in Figure 5. As indicated by this figure, an abstract interface to data is specified by the dataset object. Sub-classes of dataset include polygonal data (corresponding to the graphics data vertices, lines, polygons, and triangle strips), structured points (representing both 2D images and 3D volumes), and structured and unstructured grids (e.g., finite difference grids and finite element meshes). In addition, it was convenient to define another abstract object, point set, which is a superclass of objects with explicit point coordinate representation. The fifth data type, unstructured points, was not implemented because it could be represented by one or more of the other types. (Unstructured points are point locations without a topological relationship to one another.)

An Example for Medical Visualization

In the next example we show a portion of a network used to read 16-bit medical data and generate iso-surfaces (Lorensen, 1985), and we implemented it using TCL script language (see Box 1).

The result is as shown in Figure 6.

ITK

The ITK is the National Library of Medicine Insight Segmentation and Registration Toolkit, an open-source software toolkit for performing registration and segmentation. *Segmentation* is the process of identifying and classifying data

Figure 5. Dataset types: (a) polygonal data, (b) structured points, (c) structured grid, (d) unstructured grid, (e) unstructured points, (f) object diagram

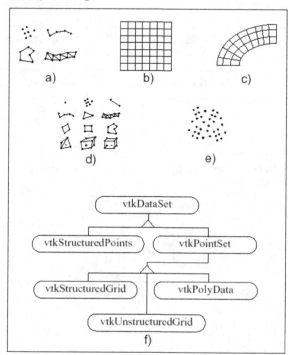

Box 1.

```
vtkVolume16Reader *v16=new vtkVolume16Reader;
v16->SetDataDimensions(64,64);
v16->SwapBytesOn();
v16->SetFilePrefix
("../../../data/headsq/quarter");
v16->SetImageRange(1, 93);
v16->SetDataAspectRatio (3.2, 3.2, 1.5);
// extract the skin
vtkMarchingCubes *skin=new vtkMarchingCubes;
skin->SetInput(v16->GetOutput());
skin->SetValue(0, 500);
....
```

Figure 6. Isosurfaces from medical dataset

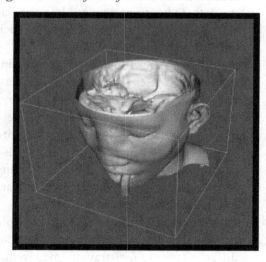

found in a digitally sampled representation. Typically, the sampled representation is an image acquired from such medical instrumentation as CT orMRI scanners. *Registration* is the task of aligning or developing correspondences between data. ITK employs leading-edge segmentation and registration algorithms in two, three, and more dimensions. The Insight Toolkit was developed by six principal organizations, three commercial (Kitware, GE Corporate R&D, and Insightful) and three academic (UNC Chapel Hill, University of Utah, and University of Pennsylvania). Additional team members include Harvard Brigham & Women's Hospital, University of Pittsburgh, and Columbia University. The funding for the project is from the National Library of Medicine at the National Institutes of Health. NLM in turn was supported by member institutions of NIH (see sponsors).

ITK is implemented in C++. It is cross-platform, using a build environment known as CMake (cmake, 2007) (like VTK) to manage the compilation process in a platform-independent way. The system architecture used in ITK is shown in Figure 7.

The ITK consists of several sub-systems. The most important sub-systems is briefly described as follows:

1. **Essential System Concepts:** Like any software system, ITK is built around some core design concepts. Some of the more important

Figure 7. System architecture in ITK application

GUI (MFC, wxWindow)	
ITK toolkit (image processing)	Visualisation (VTK, openGL)

concepts include generic programming, smart pointers for memory management, object factories for adaptable object instantiation, event management using the command/observer design paradigm, and multi-threading support. Generic programming in ITK is implemented in C++ with the *template* programming mechanism and the use of the STL Standard Template Library (Austern, 1999).

2. **Data Representation and Access:** There are two principle types of data represented in ITK: images and meshes which are represented as itk::Image and itk::Mesh classes. In addition, various types of iterators and

containers are used to hold and traverse the data. Other important but less popular classes are also used to represent data such as histograms and BLOX images.

3. **Data Processing Pipeline:** The data representation classes (known as *data objects*) are operated on by *filters* that in turn may be organized into data flow *pipelines*. These pipelines maintain state and therefore execute only when necessary. They also support multi-threading, and are streaming capable (i.e., can operate on pieces of data to minimize the memory footprint).

4. **Registration Framework:** A flexible framework for registration supports four different types of registration: image registration, multi-resolution registration, PDE-based registration, and FEM (finite element method) registration.

5. **FEM Framework:** ITK includes a sub-system for solving general FEM problems, in particular non-rigid registration. The FEM package includes mesh definition (nodes and elements), loads, and boundary conditions.

MAF

MAF is an open-source, freely-available software framework allowing rapid development of medical visualization applications and it is wrapped around the Visualization Toolkit (VTK) (vtk, 1997) and other freely-available biomedical toolkits, for example, for image registration and segmentation, collision detection or numerical computation. The next release of MAF will support multi-modal interaction with tracking devices, for example, two-handed interaction, and integration of multi-sensory control via haptics and speech (see Viceconti et al., 2004 for details).

The MAF Architecture

Different users have their own specific requirement for the software framework; for instance, for a first possible mode of use is that of a *programmer* who wants to use some of the algorithms and functions, and this use suggests a software layer independent for the GUI library, and easy to call from high level programming languages such as TCL or Phyton. The second use is that of an *Application Expert* who wants to develop a specialized computer-aided medicine application targeting a specific medical diagnostic, treatment or rehabilitation service. This user wants to keep focus on the application and do as little as possible in terms of implementation. Ideally there should be a toolbox from which the user can pick only the operations required, specialize such operations by fixing parameters or by combing operations in specialized macro, and add an application-specific user interface.

To meet the needs of different users, the MAF is organized as four-layer framework (see Figure 8). The lowest level (Multimod Foundation Layer, MFL) formed by VTK, SVTK and the specialized libraries, plus the classes defining the collection of Virtual Medical Entities (VME), hereinafter called VMETree. The second level (Abstraction Layer) is that were the operations and the applications services are implemented, with the support of a GUI library (WxWindows). The third level (High Abstraction Layer) is where the totality of the data structure, operations and services made available by the framework are customized toward specialized applications. The last level is that of the specific application aimed to support a particular biomedical activity (diagnosis, treatment of rehabilitation). It also contains the Multimod Data Manager, an application the technician should use to prepare the data for the biomedical professional. The interface of Data Manager is shown in Figure 9, and most applications under MAF have the similar interface as Data manager.

Visualization Library in MAF

Most visualization algorithms are in the lowest level, and are built on VTK, SVTK and specialized

Figure 8. A snapshot of DataManager

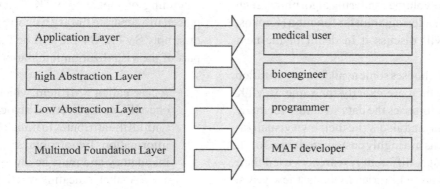

Figure 9. System architecture for MAF

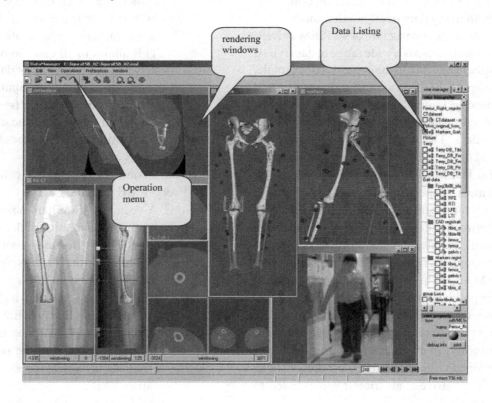

libraries. The researchers of MAF also improve some popular volume rendering algorithms, such iso-surface rendering, transfer function (Krokos, 2004), we will discuss it in detail in the next section.

The MAF chooses some available visualization algorithms which are exactly the same as VTK because they imposes the data structure for many low-level data, and also write their own visualization algorithms in a highly customized way. To our best knowledge, different researchers used their own visualization libraries in the last few years. However, this software, available in sourcecode formed under an open-source license, presents many interesting advantages. It makes available a very wide range of visualization functions combined with many data manipulation tools.

The internal data structure of VTK is very well-designed and supports a wide range of data types, most of them relevant in the context. For example, VTK supports both structured and unstructured grids used in finite element analysis, as well as specialized regular grids typical of diagnostic volume data. The implementation is also quite elegant. The C++ library can be invoked also from Java and TCL. The structure of VTK allows the replacement of specific parts of the library with custom-written software. This allows not only the experimentation of new types of visualization algorithms, but also the possibility in a future of a clean room rewriting the VTK functions used by the MAF, so to fully separate it from VTK. A major problem of VTK is the versioning issue. KitWare, the developer of VTK tends to update the library without ensuring an effective backward compatibility. To avoid this issue, the MAF will be developed targeting a frozen version of VTK. After an extensive evaluation it was decided to adopt version 4.0.

Virtual medical entities (VME) is a collection of MAF objects organized following a pre-defined structure. Such structure should provide an effective abstraction of time and space, the *pose* (position plus orientation)

As mentioned in the above section, the code extending or replacing VTK functions will be placed in a separate library we call Surgical-VTK or simply SVTK. SVTK will be the proprietary part of the visualization foundation:

1. A class called VMEItem, which is formed by one MFL data object and a block of metadata with all the attributes to transform the data in information. Two attributes in particular are mandatory and must be always reported:

    a. A label indicating whether the data are NATURAL (i.e., directly generated by a biomedical sensor such as medical imaging devices or EMG signals recorder) or SYNTHETIC (i.e., produced by any possible numerical elaboration of natural data or of simulation models). This allows in all cases to distinguish between the original raw data and the results of computer manipulations.

    b. A timestamp of creation (synthetic) or collection (natural) of the data block. Such timestamp should be absolute, in terms of date and time.

2. The second SVTK class is called VME. Every VME is formed by:

    a. A vector of VMEItem objects, representing the evolution of the VME over time. The vector may contain single VMEItem if the VME is time-invariant, or is empty to allow the creation of VME group objects, which are mere containers of other VME.

    b. A vector of pose matrices, expressing for each time frame the pose of the VME in the reference system of its father VME.

    c. A block of metadata with all the attributes to transform the data in information. In particular is mandatory and must be always reported the identity of its father VME.

    d. The MFL must make available a mechanism associated to each VME allowing the access to the data as if they were continuous in space and time.

3. Last, the MFL will contain a new class called VMETree, which describes a hierarchical tree of VME objects and a class VMEStorage that provides the mechanisms to make it persistent. The VMETree contains the definition of the Root VME, which is father of all the other VME in the tree. The pose matrix of the Root VME defines the transformation between the absolute space and the application space. The pose of a VME is defined in the reference frame of its father. Thus, to compute the pose of a VME in the application space, it is necessary to pre-multiply all pose matrices of the VME in the branch connecting that VME to the Root VME.

In addition, there are other specialized functions add to our framework. To date, MAF already includes V-Collide, an open-source collision detection library. MAF also completed a preliminary evaluation of the Insight Tool Kit, an open-source library for registration and segmentation of medical imaging data. In the light of the very positive results we obtained, ITK will be integrated in the Foundation Layer, together with VNL, an open-source vector algebra library, which ITK uses. If possible, a SVTK class should abstract such functions. Wrapping external libraries with SVTK classes provides encapsulation, which allows a replacement of any of these libraries without rewriting the upper-level code. This has been done for V-Collide, while it is under study, if it is convenient to take this approach also for ITK, since it provides some built-in methods to integrate VTK classes, which are currently under evaluation.

MITK

The main purpose of MITK is to provide the medical image community a consistent framework to combine the function of medical image segmentation, registration and visualization. As the style of VTK, MITK uses the traditional object-oriented design method, and MITK does not use the generic programming style used by ITK. Therefore, the syntax and interface of MITK is simple and intuitive. Now MITK is a freely-available software and can be used freely for research and education purpose. Main algorithms in MITK contain Surface reconstruction (e.g., improved marching cubes algorithm), Surface rendering, volume rendering (ray casting, texture-based), a variety of segmentation algorithms and registration algorithms, and other hardware accelerated rendering approaches.

System Architecture

The whole framework makes full use of the advantages of VTK and ITK. MITK is developed for medical imaging field, so it is unnecessary to contain many algorithms that can cover almost the fields. For instance, the algorithm of visualization in the MITK only includes the regular data field; the output of image segmentation is binary data field. The MITK is middle scale software framework compared with VTK. The MITK is portable; all code in MITK is written by ANIS C++, so it can run on different operating systems, such as MS Windows, Unix, Linux, and so forth. A main difference among operating systems (Windows, Unix) is the windows interface, they have to re-write the code for the difference systems.

The pipeline in MITK is shown in Figure 10, which is exactly the same as VTK. Most visualization algorithm is filter which only support single entry single exit. Therefore, to deal with a medical object, the MITK firstly transfer the object into a standard dataset, and with the help of many filters, the final target object can be achieved.

Data representation is the core of the data model in the pipeline. The objective of MITK is used for medical objects (medical image), so the data object in MITK can be classified into two

Figure 10. Pipeline in MITK. Process objects A, B, C input and/or output one or more data objects. Data objects represent and provide access to data; process objects operate on the data. Objects A, B, and C are source, filter, and target objects, respectively.

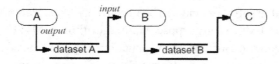

Figure 11. Four filters in MITK

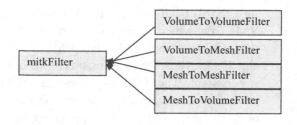

different data objects: volume data and mesh data. Volume is used to represent a dataset of medical image, while mesh is for geometry information of the objects.

There are four filters in MITK, shown in **Figure 11**. For each filters, the input dataset and output dataset can be volume data or mesh data. For example, the input dataset in MeshToVolumeFilter is mesh data while output is volume data.

User Interface

MITK support a rapid development user interface for visual C++ user. **Figure 12** shows a snapshot of the marching cubes reconstruction. The view window is the instance of mitkView in MITK, the reconstruction result is dataset of mitkSurfaceModel for marching cubes iso-surfacing.

Comparisons of the Four Toolkits

Among the four above toolkits, VTK and ITK are the well-known research platforms in visualization and medical image segmentation and registration for the researchers in the world. While MAF and MITK are more specific in medical visualization, registration and segmentation, for both of them, are new. They are used in the relatively small range from the developers to some researchers in some universities. As mentioned in the above section, MAF and MITK are built on VTK and

ITK, or employ the development mechanism of VTK and ITK, so MAF and MITK are more convenient for researchers. What is more, in MAF and MITK, developers improve some visualization algorithms (e.g., marching cubes, volume rendering, transfer function), so the applications under are more efficient than VTK and ITK. ITK pays more attention on medical image segmentation and registration.

The four toolkits are freely-availably used for all researchers (not for commercial purpose), and they can be found in the reference and can be downloaded. Except that MITK is not open-source, the other three toolkits are open-source, which means users in MITK can only invoke the functions and cannot update the core code.

ITK is not good in compatibility in visualization field, for it is necessary for the users to integrate with VTK in order to develop a complete system of medical image process and analysis, for example, we use ITK to implement medical image segmentation and registration, and use VTK to generate the interface for the 3D Visualization, however, the programming language in VTK and ITK—ANSI C++ are not exactly the same; ITK (in 1999) are newer than VTK (in 1998) and some new functions are invoked. In addition, ITK employ the STL, which is not available in some compiler programs, so that ITK only provide the static link library, not dynamic link library. Because of the continuous change in the ANSI C++, it results in the incompatibility in ITK, and most researchers are not familiar with the new property in ANSI.

Figure 12. A snapshot of 3D reconstruction in MITK

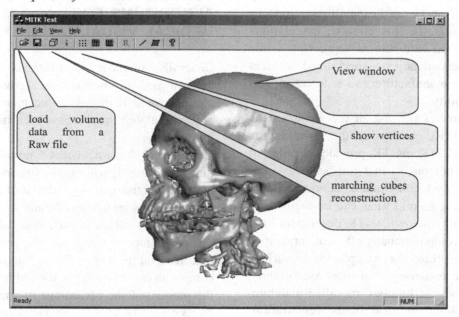

For those reasons mentioned above, nowadays ITK is still only used in a small scale. From this, we can conclude that ITK is much more complicated than the other three toolkits.

VTK tends to solve general visualization problems, and not specially designed for medical visualization field, therefore, some visualization algorithms in VTK are inefficient (e.g., marching cubes). A major problem of VTK is the versioning issue. KitWare, the developer of VTK tends to update the library without ensuring an effective backward compatibility. At least, this has been true so far. But obviously, the internal data structure of VTK is very well designed and supports a wide range of data types, most of them relevant in our context. For example, VTK supports both structured and unstructured grids used in finite element analysis, as well as specialized regular grids typical of diagnostic volume data. The implementation is also quite elegant. Therefore, most special medical software frameworks employ the technology of VTK, and improve its efficiency.

MAF can support the rapid development for the programmers. It uses Wx window interface which can be used in the cross-platform (MS Windows and Unix). Unlike the other three toolkits in which the developers have to develop their own interface, the MAF has implemented it, so users are able to write program under it. A disadvantage of MAF is that the code has a much larger size (up to 200 MB) than the other software frameworks, but the advantage is also obvious. MAF provides a range of high-level components that can be easily combined for rapid construction of visualization applications that support synchronized views. MAF developers have implemented computationally efficient versions of existing algorithms, for example, for surface and volume rendering, and more importantly, developed new techniques, for example, for x-ray rendering and designing volume rendering transfer functions. To achieve interactive rendering, MAF has employed a scheme for space partitioning. The emphasis is on exploiting the characteristics of medical datasets (e.g., density value homogeneity) but further utilizing the hardware-accelerated capabilities of modern graphics cards. In this context, calculations are moved into hardware as appropriate while avoiding dependency on specialized features of particular manufacturers so as to ensure real code portability.

MITK makes full use of the advantage of VTK and ITK, eliminating the disadvantage of VTK and ITK. MITK provides a range of high-level components that can be easily integrated for rapid construction of visualization applications (e.g., mitkView can be easily used for rendering window). MITK developers have performed computationally efficient versions of existing algorithms, for example, for iso-surface and volume rendering, and more importantly, developed new techniques, modified marching cubes, modified medical image registration. Unlike the other three toolkits, the MITK is not open-source, so the end-user of MITK is in the application layer, not for the researcher, which leads to the small user group of it. MITK does not resolve the windows interface in cross-platform, so the viewers of MITK in different platform are completely different. From this, the MITK is also complicated to use.

Finally, we summarize the comparisons of the four toolkits shown in Table 1.

VOLUME RENDERING ALGORITHMS FOR MEDICAL VISUALIZATION

Generally, volume renderer is the centrepiece of modern medical visualization software. In this section, we will discuss some related volume rendering algorithms that have been implemented in MAF.

Figure 13 shows a process diagram of the volume rendering algorithm. The first step in using the volume rendering algorithm is to convert the *input data volume* to a set of *material percentage volumes*. The values in each voxel of the material percentage volumes are the percentage of that material present in that region of space. A composite *color volume* is formed by summing the product of the percentage of each material by its color. An *opacity volume* is computed by assigning each material an opacity value. Boundaries between materials are detected by applying a three-dimensional gradient to a *density* or p *volume*. The gradient is largest where there are sharp transitions between materials with different p's. The direction of the gradient is stored in the *surface normal volume* and is used in shading computations. The *shaded color volume* represents the sum of the light emitted by the volume and scattered by the surfaces. The relative contributions of volume emission and surface scattering

Table 1. comparisons of the four toolkits

Comparison Items	VTK	ITK	MITK	MAF
free-availability	Yes	Yes	Yes	Yes
Open-Source	Yes	Yes	No	Yes
compatibility	Yes	No	Yes	Yes
rapid development of applications	middle-level	middle-level	middle-level	High-level
versioning issue	Yes	No	No	No
Efficient visualization algorithms	N/A	N/A	Yes	Yes

Figure 13. Volume rendering process

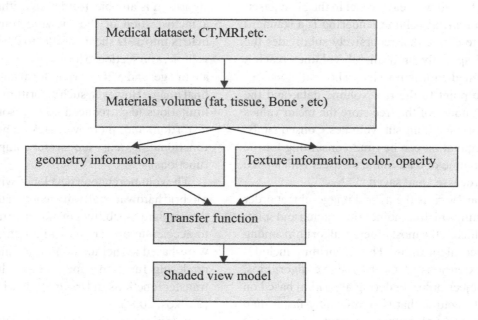

can be varied depending on the application. The reflected component is computed using a surface reflectance function whose inputs are the position and color of the light sources, the position of the eye, the surface normal volume, the surface strength volume, and the color volume. The amount of emitted light is proportional to the percentage of luminous material in the voxel. To form an image, the shaded volume is first transformed and re-sampled so that it lies in the viewing coordinate system.

Volume Rendering

There are three typical volume rendering algorithms with the software technology: ray-tracing (Kajiya, 1984; Westover, 1990; Westermann, 2001), splatting (Laur, 1991; Huang, 2000), and, Shear-Warp (Lacroute, 1994; Schulze, 2003). Ray casting synthesizes image-order space information by computing the ray distribution for every voxel. The ray-tracing volume rendering is to use ray trace volume densities without any viewing or lighting restrictions (Kajiya, 1984). The key to the method is that it separates the rendering procedure into two steps. The first step drives the radiation from light source *i* through a density array $p(x, y, z)$ into an array $Ii(x, y, z)$ which holds the contribution of each light source to the brightness of each point in space. The second step occurs once per ray trace. Each ray is first culled against a bounding rectangular prism as an extent. The brightness of a ray sums the contribution of each volume element. According to the integral, there are two remaining steps which must be done. The first is to compute the integrated optical path length along a particular ray. This is done by simply bilinearly sampling and summing the density array along the ray. The second step is to compute and sum the actual brightness integral. Note that each of the integral terms has been pre-computed so that a point sampling is all that is needed to compute the brightness term.

Splatting is to use the object-order space information to deal with each voxel in the 3D dataset; the hierarchical volume rendering is a standard complete octree that recursively subdivides the volume spatially until all sub-volumes reach a pre-defined minimum size. The leaf nodes of the tree point to the raw volume data, and the internal nodes of the tree store the mean values of the corresponding sub-volumes. Consequently, the computation can be time-consuming for the large volume of data in the datasets which need to be processed and saved.

Shear Warp is the hybrid image-object order algorithm, which combines ray-tracing and splatting, which is the most efficient algorithm among the three algorithms. This algorithm includes three extensions of the two above algorithms. First, object-order rendering algorithm based on the factorization that is significantly faster than the above two algorithms without loss of image quality is presented. The algorithm achieves its speed by exploiting coherence in the volume data and the intermediate image. The shear-warp factorization permits us to traverse both the volume and the intermediate image data structures in synchrony during rendering, using both types of coherence to reduce work. The second extension is a derivation of the factorization for perspective viewing transformations. Third, a data structure for encoding spatial coherence in unclassified volumes (i.e., scalar fields with no pre-computed opacity) is introduced. The algorithms employ run-length encoding, min-max pyramids, and multi-dimensional summed area tables. The method extends readily to support mixed volumes and geometry.

Due to the large amounts of data that volume renderers have to deal with, the approach has previously made them slow and thus impractical. Numerous researchers, such as Guthe et al. (2002), have tackled this problem by developing hardware-based algorithms to render volumes interactively. The new multi-processor algorithm is a parallelization of the serial rendering algorithm

described in VolumePro (2007). The rendering algorithm is an object-order algorithm based on a factorization of the viewing transformation matrix into a 3D shear parallel to the slices of the volume, a projection to form a distorted intermediate image, and a 2D warp to form an undistorted final image. However, such algorithms have many limitations (e.g., reduced color resolution, high distortion) and, moreover, lack some important functionalities (e.g., support for complex transfer functions).

The volume renderer developed within MAF is a hybrid hardware/software renderer that employs the standard capabilities of modern graphics cards to accelerate operations while retaining a software-based kernel to support advanced volume rendering functions, for example, lighting, 2D transfer functions and tri-linear data interpolation (Krokos, 2004).

Additionally, this renderer employs various software optimizations that allow us to achieve interactive frame rates. Among these are: multi-resolution data sampling, adaptive pixel sampling, render caching and efficient Bresenham-like volume traversals. A detailed discussion of these concepts is outside the scope of this chapter. This volume renderer replaces the shear-warp method by Dong et al. (2000) used initially, and offers improved rendering quality with only minor speed compromises.

Another aspect of the volume renderer is hybrid rendering, that is, visualization of volumetric data using both geometric (surface-based) and volumetric methods within the same image. Hybrid rendering plays an important role within the MAF. For example, showing the position and orientation of cut planes can significantly improve the viewer's understanding of a volumetric dataset. For orthopaedic operation planning, this functionality is an indispensable tool for depicting surgical instruments, or prostheses, together with the volumetric data for a particular limb position, thus allowing surgeons to see their instruments in relation to important structures within a volume of interest. For example, a surgeon has the ability to define the anatomically correct position and orientation of the femoral and pelvic components of an implant and to determine its optimal size.

Geometric rendering may not necessarily be confined to medical instruments or implants, it can also include tissue, for example, a skin iso-surface or a soft tissue model.

Iso-Surface Rendering

The surface renderer employs a significantly enhanced version of the marching-cubes iso-surface rendering algorithm (Lorensen, 1985) in conjunction with multi-resolution to produce surface models within a region of interest in a volume dataset.

The standard marching cubes approach suffers from two significant drawbacks: surface extraction is very slow (a typical time for extracting a surface from a standard size CT dataset is in the region of tens of seconds) and resulting surface models generally contain large numbers of very small triangles. When trying to manipulate such large polygonal models interactively, computational performance can be considerably degraded even on high-end, graphics-supported workstations.

The iso-surface rendering algorithm tackles these problems by employing a number of optimisation techniques such as multi-resolution, min-max blocks, point caching and multi-threading.

Multi-resolution allows us to generate light-weight preview models simply by skipping pixels at regular intervals. Min-max blocks essentially pre-compute minimum and maximum values for data blocks, thus allowing the rendering algorithms to skip irrelevant blocks of data (i.e., with values below or above the iso-surface threshold) very quickly. Point caching ensures that vertices on a polygonal model are computed only once.

The speed improvement of iso-surface rendering in MAF compared to standard VTK iso-surface rendering is normally in the range of 30-100

times faster (even without multi-resolution). This performance gives users the ability to select an optimal iso-surface threshold interactively, an impossible task with the standard implementation. See Van Sint Jan (2004) for discussion of the use of this algorithm in practice.

Transfer Functions

Perhaps one of the most common problems that prohibits the effective use of volume rendering techniques is the difficulty in specifying a transfer function (TF). A transfer function assigns optical properties, for example, opacity/color, to data values in a dataset. A "good" transfer function can make a vast difference in rendered image quality, but automatic derivation of such a function is difficult as it is heavily dependent upon the semantics of the dataset to be visualized.

The most common scheme for TF specification is by trial and error. This involves manually editing a typically linear function by manipulating "control points" and periodically checking the resulting volume rendering. Even if specialized hardware support is available, for example, a VolumePro board (VolumePro, 2007), this method can be very laborious and time-consuming. The problem lies in the lack of a precise correspondence between control point manipulation and its effects on the rendered images.

Another scheme based on the design galleries paradigm of Marks et al. (1994) generates a large number of volume renderings simultaneously, each resulting from a different transfer function. The user then selects renderings satisfying individual requirements, thus implicitly optimizing the transfer function. The challenges are automatically to generate different transfer functions that produce a sufficiently wide spread of dissimilar output renderings and to present these renderings in an effective way. A typical session may involve hundreds of renderings. To ensure interactivity, real-time hardware volume rendering functionality is essential.

The contour spectrum algorithm computes metrics over the data values of a dataset and the resulting spectrum is displayed within the user interface as a collection of signature curves, each representing a different attribute (Bajaj, 1997). Such curves offer an alternative concise way of revealing global characteristics of datasets and can be very helpful in creating transfer functions.

Edge detection concepts for locating boundaries are employed by a method based on distance maps originated by Kindlmann and Durkin (1998). A computationally inexpensive pre-processing step requiring minimal user intervention is performed to construct a 3D volume histogram of data value against first/second derivatives. A distance map is afterwards produced to record the relationship between data value and boundary proximity. Using the distance map, users can interactively experiment with a variety of settings but the transfer functions are always usefully constrained by the boundary information measured in a given dataset.

Based on the previous method, multi-dimensional transfer functions introduced recently by Kniss et al. (2002) provide an effective way to extract materials and their boundaries that is applicable not only to scalar but also to multi-variate datasets. Multi-dimensional transfer functions allow voxel classification based on a combination of values, thus increasing the probability that a feature can be uniquely isolated in the transfer function domain. An unavoidable drawback is, of course, the increased memory consumption that is necessary to store all relevant transfer function variables at a voxel sample point.

The transfer function design interface currently employed in MAF is founded on the aforementioned method and employs 2D functions. The end-user interacts with a set of direct manipulation widgets (triangles and rectangles). Each widget precisely corresponds to a different material and widgets are blended automatically to compute an overall transfer function.

Figure 14. Transfer function design using 2D widgets

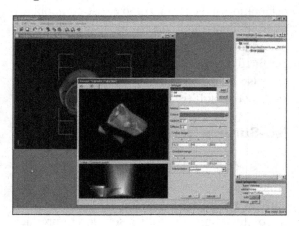

This interaction process allows users without specialized graphics knowledge to specify, quickly and intuitively, appropriate transfer functions for informative volume rendering. Nevertheless, as pointed out in Kniss (2002), novice users will typically need to pass through a training period to learn to appreciate the information provided by the widgets. As this may not be an easy or desirable process for medical professionals who have traditionally employed only 2D views, MAF allows meaningful and fast visual feedback through a 2D slice preview of the actual volume rendering appropriately superimposed on a slice-based view of the data being rendered, as in Botha and Post (2002). This greatly facilitates the correlation of structures in the volume rendering with their recognizable counterparts in a traditional 2D view. Also, it is easier to quantify the impact of small changes being made to the transfer function widgets.

Initial feedback based on early MAF demonstrators suggests that transfer function specification using 2D functions constitutes a far superior tool for correctly assigning color and opacity. Our tests indicate that, compared to traditional techniques, for example, 1D linear ramps, the overall specification process takes a fraction of the time. Figure 14 shows a transfer function for a 100MB CT dataset. Three widgets are shown (one rectangular and two triangular) for bones muscles and skin. The overall process lasted less than 10 minutes for a user previously unfamiliar with the system.

CONCLUSION

In medical software framework, there also exist other algorithms, such as surface rendering, image processing, but in all the visualization modules, the volume rendering is the centerpiece. Over the last few years, the sizes of medical datasets have continued to increase steadily as a result of improved resolution of the imaging devices and they may nowadays even be measured in gigabytes. Meanwhile, the memory of an average-specification workstation has only recently become sufficiently large to store a "standard" size dataset, so providing appropriate visualization tools continues to produce many challenges. Several off-the-shelf surface and volume rendering techniques are available within the standard libraries incorporated into the software framework. However, they are often either slow or too general. Future researches have moved as much as possible of the algorithmic execution into the hardware for fast rendering for specialized users. To achieve interactive rates under all possible circumstances, some image quality may have to be traded for speed; this is achieved through extensive use of lower LODs and sub-sampling. Therefore, all the software frameworks of medical visualization have to be designed open to allow to add new algorithm in them.

Future Research Directions

Software framework of medical visualization algorithms is essential for the rapid development of medical applications. Therefore, the architecture of the software framework is of importance for the further development under it. The future research on the architecture is as follows:

1. Cross-platform. To support multi-platform development environment is always the objective of the software framework for medical visualization algorithms, for most medical applications running under different operating systems (e.g., MS windows, Linux). To meet the needs of cross-platform, the software frameworks should be implemented under C++ or Java. To our best knowledge, the programming language used in the existed frameworks is C++, because the code in C++ is more efficient more that in Java.

2. Open System architecture. As mentioned in the previous sections, the medical visualization algorithms have always been improving these years. For example, Marching Cubes for iso-surface rendering which was proposed in 1987 is running at a very slow rate, and the current modified Marching Cubes is hundreds of times faster than the old one. It is the same case for the other volume rendering algorithms. To meet the requirements of improved visualization algorithms, the software frameworks should be open and easily upgraded.

3. Easy-to-use development platform. Future architecture will support rapid prototyping development of medical applications, so the software framework provides not only integrated medical algorithms but also user interface. The MAF architecture aforementioned is one of the representatives of the future directions, in which data storage format, service in different layers, graphics user interface implemented by WxWindows are integrated in the platform, and the programmer will only concentrate on the applications, so the programming time will be greatly shortened.

Finally, in the software framework of the visualization alogrithms, the volume rendering is the centerpiece. Though volume data provides much richer information than 3D surface meshes, the rendering time is much more consuming. Even the 256 x 256 x 256 voxels in a volume data cannot be rendered in real time on the ordinary PC. The efficiency of volume rendering has been a challenging issue for many years. The pure software technology of rendering cannot completely resolve the problem, and the future research directions should be the hybrid rendering using both software and hardware technology. Of course other algorithms such as extensive use of LODs and sub-sampling can also achieve it.

REFERENCES

Austern, M. (1999). *Generic programming and the STL: Professional computing series*. Addison-Wesley.

Bajaj, C., Pascucci, V., & Schikore, D. (1997). The contour spectrum. *Proceedings of IEEE Visualization 1997,* (pp. 167-173).

Botha C., & Post, F. (2002). New technique for transfer function specification in direct volume rendering using real-time visual feedback. *Proceedings of SPIE Symposium on Medical Imaging, 4681,* 349-356.

cmake software introduction. (2007). http://www.cmake.org/HTML/Index.html.

Dong, F., Krokos, M., & Clapworthy, G. (2000). Fast volume rendering and data classification using multi-resolution min-max octrees. *Computer Graphics Forum, 19*(3), 359-368.

Guthe, S., Wand, M., Gosner, J., & Straßer, W. (2002). Interactive rendering of large volume data sets. *Proceedings of IEEE Visualization 2002,* (pp. 53-60).

Huang, J., Mueller, K., Shareef, N., et al. (2000). FastSplats: Optimized splatting on rectilinear grids. *Proceedings of IEEE Visualization 2000,* (pp. 219-226).

ITK insight segmentation and registration toolkit. (2007). http://www.itk.org.

Kajiya, J., & Herzen, B. (1984). Ray tracing volume densities. *Computer Graphics, 18*(3), 165-174.

Kindlmann, G., & Durkin, J. (1998). Semi-automatic generation of transfer functions for direct volume rendering. *Proceedings of IEEE Symp. Volume Visualization,* (pp. 79-86).

Kniss, J., Kindlmann, G.., & Hansen, C. (2002). Multi-dimensional transfer functions for interactive volume rendering. *IEEE Trans. on Visualization. & Comp. Graphics, 8*(3), 270-285.

Krokos, M., Savenko, A., Clapworthy G.., et al. (2004). Real-time visualisation within the multimod application framework. *Proceedings of Information Visualization 04,* (pp. 21-26). IEEE Computer Society Press.

Lacroute, P., & Levoy, M. (1994). Fast volume rendering using a shear-warp factorization of the viewing transformation. *Proc. ACM SIGGRAPH 1994, Computer Graphics, 28*(4), 451-458.

Laur, D., & Hanrahan, P. (1991). Hierarchical splating: A progressive refinement algorithm for volume rendering, *Proceedings of ACM SIGGRAPH 1991,* (pp. 285-287).

Lorensen, W., & Cline, H. (1985). Marching cubes: A high resolution 3D surface construction algorithm. *Computer Graphics, 21*(4),163-169.

MAF—Multimod Project introduction. (2007). http://www.tecno.ior.it/multimod/.

Marks, J., Andalman, B., Beardsley, P., et al. (1997). Design galleries: A general approach to setting parameters for computer graphics and animation. *ACM Comp. Graphics (SIGGRAPH '94),* (pp. 389-400).

Mccloy, R., & Stone, R. (2001). Virtual reality in surgery. *British Medical Journal, 323,* 912-915.

MITK—The Medical Imaging ToolKit. (2007). http://www.mitk.net.

Robb, R., Greenleaf, J., Ritman, E., et al. (1974). Three-dimensional visualization of the intact thorax and contents: A technique for cross-sectional reconstruction from multi-planar x-ray views. *Comput. Biomedl Res, 7,* 395-419.

Schulze, J., Kraus, M., Lang, U., et al. (2003). Integrating pre-integration into the Shear-Warp Algorithm. *Proceedings of the 3rd International Workshop on Volume Graphics,* (pp. 109-118).

Van Sint Jan, S., Viceconti, M., & Clapworthy, G. (2004). Modern visualisation tools for research and education in biomechanics. *Proceedings of Information Visualization 04,* (pp. 9-14). IEEE Computer Society Press.

Viceconti, M., Leardini, A., Zannoni, C., et al. (2004). The multi-mod application framework. *Proceedings of Information Visualization 04,* (pp. 15-20). IEEE Computer Society Press.

VolumePro. (2007). http://www.terarecon.com.

VTK—the visualization toolkit. (2007). http://public.kitware.com/VTK/index.php.

Westover, L. (1990). Footprint evaluation for volume rendering. *Computer Graphics, 24*(4), 367-376.

Westermann, R., & Sevenich, B. (2001). Accelerated volume ray-casting using texture mapping. *Proceedings of IEEE Visualization 2001,* (pp. 271- 278).

Additional Reading

Ackerman, M. (1998). The visible human project. *Proceedings of the IEEE, 86*(3), 504-511.

Ackerman, M., Yoo, T., & Jenkins, D. (2000). The visible human project: From data to knowledge.

In: H. Lemke et al., (Eds.), *Computer-assisted radiology and surgery* (pp. 11-16) *(Proceedings of CARS2000).* Amsterdam: Elsevier.

Bacon, J., Tardella, N., Pratt, J., & English, J. (2006). The surgical simulation and training markup language: An XML-based language for medical simulation. *Proceedings of MMVR,* (pp. 37-42).

Bruckner, S., & Gröller, M. (2007). Style transfer functions for illustrative volume rendering. *Computer Graphics Forum, 26*(3).

Bruckner, S., & Gröller, M. (2007). Exploded views for volume data. *IEEE Transactions on Visualization and Computer Graphics, 12*(5), 1077-1084.

Callahan, S., & Comba, J. (2005). Hardware-assisted visibility sorting for unstructured volume rendering. *IEEE Transactions on Visualization and Computer Graphics, 11*(3), 285-295.

Cavusoglu, M., Goktekin, T., & Tendick, F. (2006). GiPSi: A framework for open source/open architecture software development for organ level surgical simulation. *IEEE Transactions on Information Technology in Biomedicine, 10*(2), 312-322.

Goktekin, T., Cenk Cavusoglu, M., & Tendick Gipsi, F. (2004). An open source software development framework for surgical simulation. *International Symposium on Medical Simulation,* (pp. 240-248).

Huamin, Q. (2007). *Information graphics and visualization.* Reported in Department of Computer Science and Engineering, The Hong Kong University of Science and Technology.

Jansen, T., Krol, Z., & Keeve, E. (2001). JULIUS—an extendable application framework for medical visualization and surgical planning. *CARS, 6,* 27-30.

Keeve, E., Jansen, T., et al. (2003). An open software framework for medical applications.

International Symposium on Surgery Simulation and Soft Tissue Modeling IS4TM, (p. 302-310).

Kelly, H., Bassingthwaighte, J., et al. (2001). *Open source software framework for organ modeling & simulation.* http://www.fas.org/dh/conferences/proceedings2001.php.

Kraus, M. (2003). *Direct volume visualization of geometrically unpleasant meshes.* Unpublished doctoral dissertation, Universit at Stuttgart.

Kraus, M., Strengert, M., Klein, T., & Ertl, T. (2007). Adaptive sampling in three dimensions for volume rendering on GPUs. *Proceedings APVIS 2007.*

Ljung, P., Lundstrom, C., Ynnerman, A., & Museth, K. (2004). Transfer function-based adaptive decompression for volume rendering of large medical data sets. *IEEE Symposium on Volume Visualization and Graphics,* (pp. 25- 32).

Lum, E., & Ma, K. (2004). Lighting transfer functions for direct volume rendering. *Proceedings of the IEEE Visualization 2004.*

Manssour, I., Furuie, S., et al. (2000). A multimodal visualization framework for medical data. *Proceedings XIII Brazilian Symposium on Computer Graphics and Image Processing,* (p. 356).

Phillips, P., Manning, D., et al. (2005). A software framework for diagnostic medical image perception with feedback, and a novel perception visualization technique. *Medical Imaging 2005, Proceedings of the SPIE, 5749,* (pp. 572-580).

Rezk-Salama, C., & Kolb, A. (2006). Opacity peeling for direct volume rendering. *Computer Graphics Forum (Proceedings of Eurographics), 25*(3), 597-606.

Rymon-Lipinski, B., Jansen, T., Hanssen, N., Lievin, M., & Keeve, E. (2002). A software framework for medical visualization. *Proceedings of IEEE Visualization '02.* Boston, MA.

Sarni, S., Maciel, A., Boulic, R., & Thalmann, D. (2005). A spreadsheet framework for visual exploration of biomedical datasets. *18th IEEE Symposium on Computer-Based Medical Systems,* (pp. 159-164).

Schroeder, W., Avila, L., & Hoffman, W. (2000). Visualizing with VTK: A tutorial. *IEEE Trans. on Computer Graphics and Applications, 20*(5), 20-27.

Sielhorst, T., Feuerstein, M., Traub, J., et al. (2006). CAMPAR: A software framework guaranteeing quality for medical augmented reality. *International Journal of Computer Assisted Radiology and Surgery, 1*(Suppl. 1), 29-30.

Tani, B., Nobrega, T., Santos, T., & Wangenheim, A. (2006). Generic visualization and manipulation framework for three-dimensional medical environments. *Proceedings of the 19th IEEE Symposium on Computer-Based Medical System*s, (pp. 27-31).

Udupa, J., & Herman, G. (2000). *3D imaging in medicine.* Boca Raton, FL: CRC.

Vollrath, J., Weiskopf, D., & Ertl, T. (2005). A generic software framework for the GPU volume rendering pipeline. *Vision, Modeling, and Visualization VMV '05 Conference,* (pp. 391-398).

Wang, W., Sun, H., & Wu, E. (2005). Projective volume rendering by excluding occluded voxels. *International Journal of Image and Graphics, 5*(2), 413-431.

Yoo, T., Ackerman, M., Lorensen, W., et al. (2002). Engineering and algorithm design for an image processing API: A technical report on ITK—the insight toolkit. In: J. Westwood, et al. (Eds.), *Medicine meets virtual reality* (pp. 582-592). Amsterdam: IOS Press.

Yoo, T., Michael, J., & Ackerman, M. (2005). Open source software for medical image processing and visualization. *Communications of the ACM, 48*(2), 55-59.

3DSlicer. (2007). http://www.slicer.org/.

Chapter X
Navigation in Computer Assisted Orthopaedic Surgery

Elena De Momi
Politecnico di Milano, Italy

Pietro Cerveri
Politecnico di Milano, Italy

Giancarlo Ferrigno
Politecnico di Milano, Italy

ABSTRACT

Originally developed for neurosurgery procedures, since late nineties Computer Assisted Surgery (CAS) systems have been used in orthopaedic interventions. Such systems assist the surgeon during the pre-operative or the intra-operative planning phase from diagnostic data, during the intra-operative phases of registration and navigation. They provide quantitative information of the overall surgical outcome and allow controlling range of accuracy and repeatability. Despite recognized advance in introducing the computer in the orthopaedic operative room (OR), several aspects are still debated such as operative time prolongation, information provided to the surgeon and user interface management. The chapter is aimed at reviewing main navigation systems as far as the visual and interactive aspects are concerned and at suggesting useful tools in order to enhance the surgeon usability of a navigation system. We developed modules for Total Knee Replacement (TKR) and Total Hip Replacement (THR), named KneeLab and HipLab respectively. In the two applications, we coped with two main aspects of the navigation in knee and hip replacement combining new visualization methods and new working methods. In the chapter, the reader can find a detailed description of the solution proposed to overcome problems commonly found with navigation systems in orthopaedics. We introduced innovative methods and algorithms, new modality of vocal interface, fully 3D graphics, recovery session from file system. The development aimed at the fulfilment of the critical user requirements of the operating room, by providing the user with a tightly guided procedure and an immediate graphical virtual environment.

INTRODUCTION

Computer Assisted Surgery (CAS), also known as navigated surgery, refers to computer-enabled technologies including medical robotics, image guided surgery, computer-integrated advanced orthopaedics, stereotactic guidance and computer assisted medical interventions. Any CAS system is principally aimed at providing quantitative evaluation of single operation acts and of the overall surgical outcome. Secondly, surgeons can take advantage by the use of assistive instruments integrated in or even monitored and controlled by the CAS system. Thirdly, measurements and surgical evaluations are provided within controlled range of accuracy and repeatability. Besides enhancing the accuracy and the repeatability, CAS systems improve surgeon's 3D perception of the surgical scenario and surgeon's skill in performing highly demanding procedures (Martelli, 2003). All these features improve surgical performance and clinical outcomes (Delp, 1998). In general, non-contact

measure technologies, real-time computer feedback and augmented 3D visualization constitute the main facilities within CAS systems. In particular, 3D localization equipments (exploiting different physical principles as electromagnetic fields or video camera-based sensors) are utilized to obtain the intra-operative registration of the surgical site with the pre-operative diagnostic data. In addition, such equipments allow measuring indirectly the position and orientation of surgical instruments, implants and anatomical regions by directly tracking small rigid bodies are attached to them (Jaramaz, 1998; Zheng, 2002; Tria, 2006). The great advantage of such equipments rests in the ability to get measurements in real-time within a sufficient range of acquisition frequency which allows the acquisition of location of surgical instruments in motion.

The most general approach of CAS systems includes first a pre-operative step where diagnostic data are used to indicate the surgical planning (Figure 1). CAS systems can assist the surgeon

Figure 1. Typical CAS system flowchart

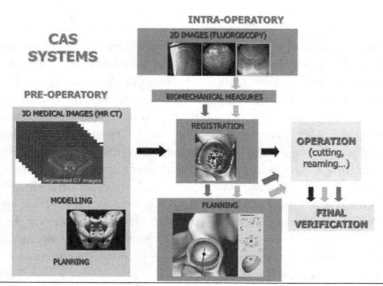

Coloured arrows indicate possibility of intervention (black arrows is the path followed in case of pre-operative planning availability, light gray arrows indicate the intra-operative images acquisition while dark gray arrows indicate the image-free navigation modality).

in the realization of such planning. At the initial step of the navigated intervention, the registration stage requires the measure of specific anatomical landmarks and surface regions so that the coordinate system located at the surgical site is coherent with the coordinate system of the planning expressed in the diagnostic (virtual) environment. Also, the registration allows the pre-operatory planning to be improved. After intra-operative planning definition, the navigation takes place and the surgeon can get quantitative measures of the location of the surgical instruments with respect to the anatomical site represented within a 3D visualization environment according to the planning. These indications allow a quantitative control of each step of the operation.

In orthopaedics, several surgical interventions can benefit from CAS systems: ligaments reconstruction, spine screw insertion, osteotomies and joint replacement (arthroplasty). Along this chapter, we will focused on describing how the computer and localization technologies can be

useful during total knee replacement (TKR) and total hip replacement (THR), where joints are replaced with artificial articulating surfaces. As far as the knee is concerned, alignments of the prosthesis components in the coronal, axial and sagittal plane have to be considered. Bone cuts of both the femur and the tibia have to result perpendicular to the mechanical axis of the two bones in order to assure the positive clinical outcome of the intervention (Confalonieri, 2005). Target outcome of plus or minus 3° of varus valgus in the coronal plane is considered clinically acceptable (Jeffery, 1991). For hip replacement, inclination and anteversion of the acetabular cup have to be within the "safe zone" (Lewinnek, 1978) to assess avoiding the risk of dislocation or impingements between bones or prosthesis components. Navigation of the traditional reamer and of the traditional wrench is then considered. The sketch in Figure 2 shows the general operational flowchart during navigated TKR or THR. Information buffer coming from camera sensors (2) enters the PC via

Figure 2. Example of a possible snapshot of interactions during computer assisted total knee replacement

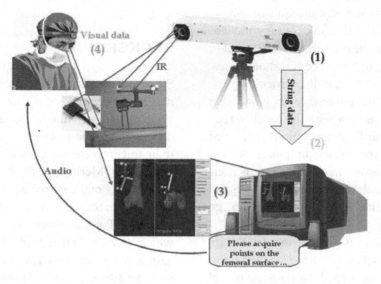

(1) Data coming from localization system enter (2) the computer. information is visualized on the monitor (3). The surgeon (4) receives vocal commands from the navigation system.

serial cable and is processed by the computer in real time. Object movement is displayed on the monitor (3), as long as information about current visibility and current computation accuracy. The surgeon channels of communication (4) is audio (information coming from the system), visual (towards the monitor and the operating table) and tactile (towards the system).

Despite clear advantage in introducing the computer in the operative room (OR) for TKR (Stoeckl, 2004; Haaker, 2005) and THR (Di Gioia, 1998), several aspects are still debated. Navigation systems not always offer statistically relevance in better the operation outcome, but it is demonstrated that outliers are reduced (Anderson, 2005). Surgical procedures must not be prolonged in time since the patient is suffering from the haemostasis string. Additional time required for the extra surgeon manoeuvres needed by the navigation system can vary from 15 to 30 minutes (Ilsar, 2006). This is approximately the maximum additional time amount currently allowed to the surgical orthopaedic procedure. The surgeon needs to know which could be the error implied on relying on the indication provided by the navigation system. It is consequently necessary to provide the user with accuracy indexes and information on the risks that could be met in accepting the system tolerance threshold. Interaction with the system is another crucial aspect: surgeon's gloves are covered with blood that prevents easy interaction with the touch-screen or with the keyboard, on the contrary, allowed interaction tools are voice commands or foot pedals. For this reason, the possible interactions between the user and the system in each surgical step have to be limited (for example: go back, go ahead and exit).

Aim of this chapter is twofold: to review main navigation systems as far as the visual and interactive aspects are concerned, and suggest useful tools in order to enhance the surgeon usability of a navigation system. We refer to our particular experience with navigation system (De Momi,

2006). In the framework of a national funded project for enterprise development in cooperation with Lima-Lto (Udine, Italy), a prototype for navigation of knee total arthroplasty and hip total arthroplasty was developed by our group at Bio-engineering Department - Politecnico di Milano University (Milano, Italy). With respect to already available systems on the market (VectorVision – BrainLab, Feldkirchen, Germany; StealthStation – Medtronic Inc., Minneapolis, MN, US; Surgigate – Praxim Medivision, Grenoble, France; Stryker, Kalamazoo, MI, US), the prototype presents innovative methods and algorithms, new modality of vocal interface, fully 3D graphics, recovery session from file system. It is based on an opto-electronic localiser (Polaris by Northern Digital - NDI, Canada) and on a purposely designed software. The development aimed at the fulfilment of the critical user requirements of the operating room, by providing the user with a tightly guided procedure and an immediate graphical virtual environment. In the chapter, the reader can find a detailed description of the solution proposed to overcome problems commonly found with navigation systems in orthopaedics.

BACKGROUND

Since late nineties, research centres and companies have been putting on the market navigation systems to assist the orthopaedic surgeons in different surgical tasks (from joint replacement, to ligaments reconstruction and bone screws implantation) (Merlotz, 1998; Picard, 2001). As far as the TKR (total knee replacement) is concerned, except from Stryker system (which uses cameras from FlashPoint, Boulder, CO, US) and Medtronic, which recently introduced electromagnetic localization system in knee joint replacement, all systems are based on video-based marker detection (usually provided by NDI), whether based on active or passive communication (Ferrigno, 1985) between the markers and the sensors. Active markers are IR LED detected by the camera sensors, while passive markers are retro reflective sphere lightened by camera IR flashes. High costs of those systems depend on both the hardware components (approximately for the 30% of the total cost) and the software modules (which is the major responsible for the cost).

Differences in hardware components are based on the modification made on the traditional surgical tools in order to fix the rigid bodies in a solid and unique modality. Rigid bodies are made by three or more markers connected in a geometrical shape previously stored in the computer or in the connection cable (in case of active tools). Smart connection systems between rigid bodies and bony parts are based on one or two mono-cortical or bi-cortical screws (Mayr, 2005). BrainLAB tools are based on two mono-cortical pins while Medtronic are even smaller since they have to carry the weight of just electromagnetic sensors.

Systems differ in software components at different levels, from the bottom level, which concerns operative system (Windows OS is used by BrainLab, Orthopilot - Aesculap, Tuttligen, Germany - and Stryker, Linux by Medacta - Lugano, Switzerland), development environment (Visual C++, Borland, Qt), graphic libraries (VTK, OpenGL, ITK) and graphical user interfaces. BrainLab working interface layout is certainly the best structured, but has been criticized by some surgeons since it provides too much information. Also, in the graphic visualization the bone model (specific on the patient or a generic model) could be shown or just the biomechanical axes and angles are displayed. Computations are done on points acquired by landmarks digitization or computed through cinematic acquisition.

At methodological level, the computation of the biomechanical parameters of interest can require different sources of information. As an example, there is no overall agreement on the definition of biomechanical joint centres used for the definition of the mechanical axes. Different algorithms, expressing different performance indexes and computational performances, can be used to compute the joint centres. Galileo (Plus Orthopedics, Rotkreuz, Switzerland) system requires the acquisition of several positions of the rigid body attached to the femur bone pivoting around hip joint in order to compute the hip joint centre, while BrainLAB and Stryker systems fit a sphere with the cloud of acquired points during pivoting movement. Praxim (Stindel, 2005) system minimizes a cost function to approximate the hip joint with the point with the minimum movement during pivoting. Reported errors are about 5mm in the hip joint centre estimation.

Currently available systems display different kind of information during cutting mask alignment: the differences to the target position in terms of angular and translational displacements. It has to be kept in mind that the surgeon needs a constant update on the accuracy of the measurements, i.e. on the errors the system considers acceptable.

Another point often debated between engineers and surgeons consists in the resolution of the presented measure and computation data: the surgeon has to be aware that even if the joint centre is computed with a sub-millimetre resolution, the error chain contains errors coming from the localization system (minimum declared is 0.25mm of accuracy for Optotrack by Northern Digital), from the localization of the target point (West, 2004) with respect the fiducial markers and from mechanical joints which allow relative movements between markers.

MAIN THRUST OF THE CHAPTER

Issues, Controversies, Problems

As general purpose, CAS systems have to be very simple, fast, intuitive and as close as possible to the user's standard working conditions. They benefit from modern medical images acquisition techniques, which allow virtual models reconstruction with increased accuracy. Nevertheless, one of the main issues in computer aided knee and hip replacement is the compromise between the accuracy of the virtual model reconstruction and pre-operative or intra-operative images acquisition, which is time and cost consuming and causes radiation dose to be directed to the patient (and also to the surgical team, in case of intra-operative acquisition). In case of pre-operative CT or MR images acquisition, the 3D virtual model of the patient can be computed and visual accuracy is guaranteed by rigid registration (BrainLAB system in case of CT-based modules). If pre operative session of image acquisition, elaboration and treatment planning has to be avoided, the virtual model necessarily lacks of accuracy, and provides less information for prostheses size automatic positioning and orientation. During the surgery visual information could be totally neglected (Orthopilot) or partially taken into account in case of deformable models adapted to

the patient's morphological situation (BrainLAB system in case of CT-free modules).

During navigation the following reference system are established (Figure 3): *camera reference system* (RS), which collected data by the localization system are referred to, *anatomic reference system*, placed on the bones, decided by the user according the specific geometry of the tools, *bone reference systems* defined by biomechanical and functional axes and *probe reference system*. During acquisition, points coordinates are expressed in the anatomical RS as shown in equation (1), so the cameras can be freely moved during the operation in order to not be an obstacle to the surgeon's movements, as described by following equation:

$$T_{Anatomic}^{ProbeRS} = T_{Camera}^{ProbeRS} \bullet T_{Anatomic}^{Camera} \qquad (1)$$

where $T_{Camera}^{ProbeRS}$ is the transformation matrix of the calibrated probe in the camera RS, while

Figure 3. Used reference frames in navigation camera reference system (RS), to which collected data are referred, anatomic reference system decided by the user according the specific geometry of the tools, bone reference systems defined by biomechanical and functional axes and the probe reference system

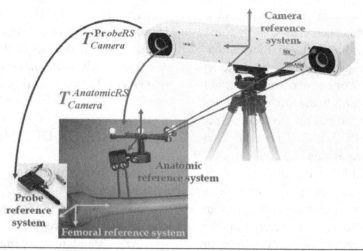

Acquired coordinates are expressed in the camera reference frame. In order to free camera movements in the OR, computations are referred to anatomical reference frames fixed on the bones.

$T_{Anatomic}^{Camera}$ is the inverse transformation matrix of the anatomic reference frame in the camera RS $(T_{Anatomic}^{Camera} = (T_{Camera}^{Anatomic})^{-1})$ and, finally, $T_{Anatomic}^{ProbeRS}$ is the transformation matrix of the probe in the anatomic tool RS.

As far as interfaces are concerned, some surgeons complains about the virtual environment displayed on the screen, which has ever some limitation in reproducing real bones since the approximations due to medical images acquisition (Viceconti, 1999) or to the bone morphing technique (Fleute, 1999). They want to navigate the operation by aligning cutting planes (current plane with the desired one) with plane projections on the monitor. Other surgeons rather claim that the virtual clinical environment resembles as much as possible the real one. In general, each navigation system must compromise between virtual models resolution and time required for models loading and visualization.

Currently available systems are not customizable on the single user. They were designed by the company developers and users have limited access to settings, in particular as far as the decision on the views on the anatomy are concerned. On the contrary, such systems usually let the user choose the preferred sequence of operation (femur first or tibia first) and there is always the possibility to repeat points digitization if the user is not satisfied with the resulting accuracy of the computation. Finally, there is always the chance to quit the application and to continue with traditional technique since navigation strictly follows traditional surgical steps. Ideally a completely customable system should allow the surgeon to save his/her personal settings regarding sequence of surgical steps, landmarks points to be digitized and views of the anatomy.

Interaction with the system, before and during the surgery takes place, should not require the help of a technician, so that the system had to be conceived for a direct dialogue with the surgeon. Even though, the learning curve could be long and company's engineers assist the surgeon during the training period (Daubresse, 2005). Results and indications on the ongoing operation should be presented in many modalities, such as voice commands, sound and visual signals.

Attention should be paid in reducing time needed for setting up the surgical field according to navigation requirements (tools visibility verification and camera field of view corresponding to the operation table). Also measurement tasks (joint centre computation, surface registration and surface morphing) must be performed with surgically compatible time.

Solutions and Recommendations

We developed modules for TKR and THR, named *KneeLab* and *HipLab* respectively. In the two applications, we coped with two main aspects of the navigation in knee and hip replacement combining new visualization methods and new working methods.

Developed Graphics Environment

In our opinion, graphical aspects are crucial, clear information have to be provided to the surgeon in a good-looking graphical user interface. Information has to be organized in a well explained manner: the so called human factor has to be considered in order to enhance surgeon's 3D perception of the operative scenario and "surgeon-based" criteria have to be considered.

We decided to put in a fix dialogue bar all the information and buttons on the right of the screen and two or more views of the same patient's objects in the virtual environment on the right, which comprises about 70% of the screen. Buttons on the right are labelled with self-explanatory commands and corresponding buttons remains the same in all the phases (for instance, the EXIT button is placed in the right bottom corner in each navigation step). Anatomical objects, surgical tools and prostheses are represented as 3D surface meshes. The user can interact with the virtual environment through the mouse. In this way, views of the anatomy (whether anterior posterior, medial lateral or cranial caudal views) are selected by the user at the beginning of the surgical procedure. Subsequent accesses to the module will load previously stored user-dependent configuration. In femur prosthesis size planning, coronal and sagittal views are displayed, while in tibia prosthesis size planning, coronal and axial views are displayed. During hip acetabular component planning, the acetabular area is zoomed in: sagittal and coronal views are displayed. Displayed bone models represent a compromise between details resolution and time required for data loading and management. Even if we used a 3.2GHz Xeon processor and 3DLabs Wildcat Realizm 800 graphic card, our virtual models were limited in the number of triangles, however holding details in the clinically significant sub-regions, resulting in *.stl* files of 1.5 Mb size each. The system never overloads the user with too much information in order to reduce complexity and make it more fast and intuitive.

Special attention is devoted to the user friendliness of the interface. The use in surgical room is in fact a demanding requirement for man-machine interface, as an example, vocal commands and colour changes of represented items (tools, bones, prostheses) in function of correct execution of the procedure are used. Our applications are build in a way that allows minimal interference between the system and the surgeon and maximum navigating possibility. Output commands are imposed to the surgeon through audio files that were previously synthesized, in such a way the surgeon does not need to divert the attention from the knee joint while waiting for the next command. Output information is displayed on the screen in a font clearly visible at the distance the surgeon usually stays during the operation. Real images and virtual environment, as long as quantitative measures and results, shown in the monitor, have to be clearly visible from the distance the surgeon usually operates, not requiring

additional movement towards the system or the help of an assistant in interpreting data shown on the screen. Also, differently coloured or dimensioned objects give immediate qualitative perception. In order to provide the surgeon with multi modality communication channel, sound signals were also added: for example in order to indicate the end of an acquisition procedure or the non visibility of a tool. On the other way, input information is sent to the system via foot pedal which comprises three different buttons: next, previous and enter (see Figure 1).

In the Microsoft Visual Studio environment, we used Microsoft Foundation Classis (MFC). We used *The Visualization Toolkit* (VTK, Kitware) Libraries to load and move surface models, set camera views and display arrows, labels and numbers on the screen. VTK are high level (object-oriented) graphics utilities where 3D *source geometries* (data) are visualized on the screen by the *renderer* object and managed in terms of graphical properties (visual appearance) by the *actor* object. The interactor object manage messages from the user interface (keyboard and mouse control).

New Methods and Tools

Clinically, two radiographic images both in TKR and in THR are acquired for computing prostheses optimal size, position and orientation. Navigation systems, currently available on the market, do not require any pre-operative medical image and compute joint biomechanics by landmarks acquired intra-operatively with a calibrated pointer. The presented system is characterised by modular navigation software: the surgeon is allowed to choose whether he/she wants to acquire and process CT or MR images or if he/she wants to proceed with intra-operative planning. The surgeon is also allowed to choose the sequence of the procedural steps (start cutting femur or tibia, dislocating the femur before or after anterior pelvic plane computation), the landmarks to be selected in order to perform registration and to compute biomechanical axes. Sorted procedural steps correspond to the expected user actions. The sequence is clinically meaningful from the user point of view, reflecting the steps of the surgical technique and making interaction simple and intuitive.

As far as the usability is concerned, the system allows saving intermediate data and possibly going back automatically to the saved configuration. This could be useful in case of sudden interruption of the procedure, so that the surgeon can re-start skipping already performed procedures thanks to stored computed data. Furthermore many analytical controls are provided in order to check for possible errors in the execution of localisation and calibration procedures. Some extra points are required for performing such controls and provide the surgeon with an evaluation of the quality of the procedure. After each computation procedure the user is allowed to verify accuracy of the result. Implicit verification is always present and errors are eventually communicated to the user, while explicit verification is not mandatory. User requirements fulfilling represents the main result of the development. Guided procedure and complete virtual environment for the representation of bones, tools and prostheses in virtual environment are a must for the user friendliness required in operating room.

From an algorithmic point of view the effort has been focused on a better estimate of the hip joint rotation centre that is used for computing the femur mechanical axis (Figure 4). Based on the acquired transformations of the anatomic RS fixed on the femur, the algorithm gives a least square approximation of the hip joint centre (HJC) location (Siston, 2006). In order to overcome the limitation in the pelvis movement (occurring during surgeon's clinical manoeuvres) hypothesized by the pivoting algorithm, we proposed data filtering in order to delete data outliers and to give a better estimation of the HJC true location in the femoral reference frame. In order to

evaluate filtered hip rotation centre algorithm, we tested the new algorithm by a simulated dataset. Several variations on the motion pattern were applied to the simulation linkage, including altered directions of motion, ranges of motion, and trial duration trying to reproduce the clinical scenario. The proposed algorithm proved to give significantly better results both in case of a small amount of axial displacement up to cases in which the amount of data spread required a larger data filtering (De Momi, 2006).

In case the pre-operative images acquisition phase is avoided, deformable distal bone models of femur, tibia and acetabular cup are adapted on the specific patient with bone morphing (Fleute, 1999). This latter is used both for the localisation and graphic representation of the bones (femur, tibia and acetabular cup) and for plan prosthesis size by automatically superimposing CAD models of the prosthesis to bone 3D representation. Morphing is based on the recording of several points on the surface of the surgically exposed part of bones that must be cut or reamed in order to insert prosthesis components (as can be seen in Figure 5).

Quality of bone morphing algorithm was evaluated computing the median and the standard deviation values of the Euclidean distance between the reconstructed surface patch (deformed model) and the reference shape. Preliminary results are comparable with literature.

Following the specific prosthesis company indications we developed an automatic planning of the best prostheses size, position and orientation. If the surgeon is not satisfied with the proposed plan, he/she can change the size and the rotation and the translation parameters of the prostheses components updating the transformation matrix (Figures 6 and 7). The size is automatically computed according the specific virtual model of the patient, obtained after the morphing of the deformable model. On the dialogue bar the prosthesis ideal dimension is displayed in the range of the lower and the bigger size.

Figure 4. Hip Joint Centre (HJC) computation during TKR

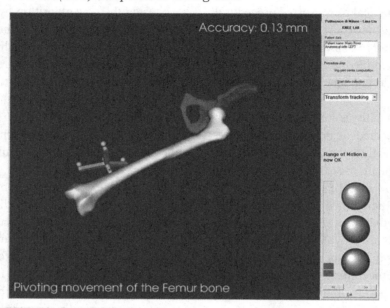

The femur is pivoted around the hip with a circumduction movement. Accuracy index is displayed in the upper right corner; information about the range of motion is displayed on the dialogue bar.

Figure 5. Realtime visualization of the acquired points through calibrated pointer

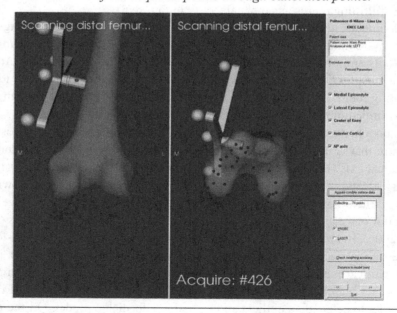

In the bottom right corner the number of remaining points to be acquired is displayed.

Figure 6. Tibia prosthesis automatic planning (sizing, positioning and orientation)

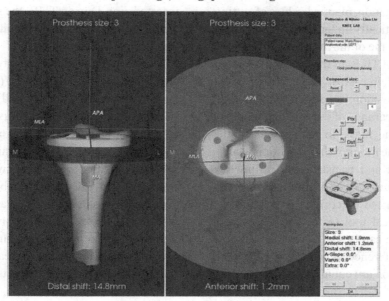

The prosthesis size, automatically computed, can be increased or decreased by the surgeon pressing the arrows buttons. The prosthesis component is automatically aligned in the tibia reference frame. Adjustment buttons (for rotation and translation respect the prosthesis reference frame) are displayed on the dialogue bar.

Figure 7. Acetabular prosthesis automatic positioning and orientation

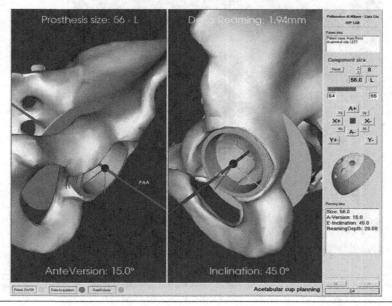

The prosthesis size, automatically computed, can be varied by the surgeon pressing the arrows buttons. The prosthesis component is automatically aligned in the acetabular reference frame. Adjustment buttons (for rotation and translation respect the prosthesis reference frame) are displayed on the dialogue bar. The yellow displayed plane represents the upper limit in the acetabular axis dimension. It is useful for the surgeon to have the visual perception of the upper limit position of the prosthesis.

After the surgeon agreed with the prostheses position and orientation, planned values of cutting planes are automatically updated. In order to navigate the cutting plane of the mask (equipped with markers), in case of TKR, or the axis of the reamer and of the wrench, in case of THR, to their target orientation and position, we specifically studied the graphical appearance of the working window. While keeping the mask in his/her hands, the surgeon sees on the monitor the correction values. Rotational angles and translational millimetres (as shown in Figures 8 and 9) are expressed as clinical parameters to be corrected. In this way, moving the surgical tool in the physical space, the target position can be easily reached. In case of TKR, once difference values between desired and current position are equal to zero, the cutting

mask has to be fixed on the bones through drill inserted pins. During THR, the surgeon looks the feedback indications on the monitor while handling the reamer or the wrench.

Developed navigation prototype was validated during experimental session (Figure 10). The system proved to be a valid and robust to failure. In case of landmark data acquisition, the system automatically performed a consistency test in respecting geometrical constraints and asked to repeat acquisition when errors were detect in real time (during acquisition) or in batch mode (when acquisition was stopped). Also, acquisitions had to be repeated if variance of acquired data distribution overcame a pre-defined threshold value.

Surgical instruments were easily navigated by the user to their planned target position.

Figure 8. Femoral cutting mask alignment graphical interface

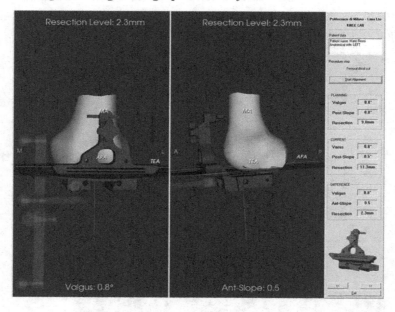

On the dialogue bar on the right planned and current cutting values are displayed, as long as the corrections needed to reach the target. In the virtual environment on the right, localization tool fixed to the cutting mask is shown in transparency. Deformable femoral bone model was adapted to the patient's anatomy thanks to the intra-operative acquired surface points. Axes of the plotted reference system (trans-epicondylar –TEA-, anterior-posterior –APA- and femoral mechanical axis, not visible in the Figure), were computed on the basis of kinematics acquisition and landmarks digitization.

Figure 9. Acetabular reamer alignment graphical interface

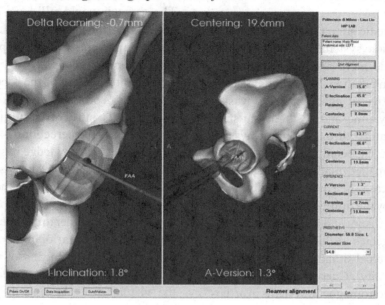

On the dialogue bar on the right planned and current cutting values are displayed, as long as the corrections needed to reach the target. Deformable acetabular model was adapted to the patient's anatomy thanks to the intra-operative acquired surface points. The navigated reamer is shown in transparency in order to facilitate alignment of the surgical instrument axis with the target position and orientation.

Figure 10. Experimental validation of the HipLab application

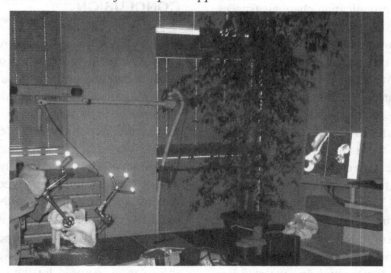

A rigid body is attached to the pelvis (iliac crest) and a rigid body is fixed into the navigated wrench. On the right the monitor displays quantitative information about the tracked movement facilitating the alignment procedure of the wrench to the target planned position.

FUTURE RESEARCH DIRECTIONS

Certainly orthopaedic surgery will benefit from low cost navigation systems in the OR since they could provide more accurate outcome of the prostheses implantation. Surgical navigation has proven effective at enabling less invasive surgery. Recovery time and aesthetic satisfaction could be obtained through a mini-invasive surgical approach, especially in case of lateral approach in the so called quad-sparing technique (Alan, 2006). In case the surgeon's visibility of bones is reduced by the limited surgical aperture, electromagnetic sensors and localization system enhances the surgeon's visibility and perception of the patient's clinical situation (bone morphology and functionality). Current obstacles to the introduction of electromagnetic systems in orthopaedic surgery are represented by the high cost of the specific surgical instrumentation (titanium instead of iron), by the wires connecting the sensors and by the limited accuracy respect optically guided surgery. As for optoelectronic systems, human factor of this systems usability would be related to graphical user interface and improved man-machine communication channels (speech recognition tools, for example).

Another step towards minimally invasiveness is represented by ultrasound intra-operative images acquisition. At present A-mode (Heger, 2005) and B-mode (Barratt, 2006) ultrasonic signal acquisition is used for automatically register the patient with the virtual model obtained previously through CT data acquisition. Further step is to automatically detect the specific virtual model of the patient during the surgery through ultrasound probe acquisition. This image acquisition modality allows enhancing the surgeon field of view on the patient in a harmless and non invasive way.

In order to avoid the loss of accuracy during cutting guides fixation through drill inserted pins could be solved thanks to free-hand smart cutting tools. Provided with markers, those tools would let the surgeon cut only planned parts of bones. The surgeon would still have the perception of performing the cutting by himself, but surgical errors are prevented by the computer programmed cutting tools.

The introduction of the robot in orthopaedic has not given promising results so far. If the robot has the total control of the surgical operation, the surgeon loses the perception of what is going on and this lack of knowledge has prevented robots entrance in the OR. New robots would have to be passive systems which guide the surgeon's hands in being more precise in cuts performing.

In the end, in order to enhance surgeon perception about the scenario, immersive environment can be created by means of wearable display glasses. In this case, the surgeon perceives only the virtual scene loosing the real appearance of the scene. Differently, solutions augmented reality approach, based on the superimposition of virtual details to the real scenario perception, allow the surgeons to quantitatively deal with a single integrated scenario.

CONCLUSION

Devices for orthopaedic CAS represent a strong challenge for Medical Visualisation systems in terms of user requirements, safety and reliability. Surgical room has its own requirements in terms of sterile and non sterile areas, of constraints to the operator movements and of completeness and simplicity of graphical information conveyed to the surgeon. The procedures must be accurate, in order to guarantee a correct positioning of the prosthesis fulfilling the orthopaedic requirements (varus-valgus angle, tibial slope, femoral external rotation) robust to operator errors and must provide, in the simplest way, the minimum information required for the execution and assessment of the steps. This has been attained by a real user friendly interface and by designing and implementing mathematical algorithms for the estimate of the data needed for the implant. Navigation in orthopaedic has to keep perception-based engineering aim into account in order to integrate into the design of engineering systems the ways in which people perceive and are affected by machinery outputs such as images and sound.

Keeping OR constraints, surgeon demands and hardware limitations into account, we developed our applications for assist TKR and THR, named KneeLab and HipLab, respectively. Differently from other systems on the market (Orthopilot), our graphical user interface was studied in order to provide the surgeon with a virtual scene on the screen as close as possible to the real situation, thanks to the adaptation of a deformable model to the patient anatomy. It is fundamental to inform the user of the degree of approximation of the virtual bone models displayed on the monitor. Quantitative data, clinically significant, are also computed and displayed on the monitor. Communication with the surgeon involves different modalities in order to have redundant information outputs. In order to meet surgeon requests, the system allows high specialization: the user can choose preferred views of patient virtual anatomy in each surgical step and store the values for subsequent employments of the system. Customization is a crucial aspect in order to take human factor into account. Also, new methods for joint centres computation, bone meshes morphing and prostheses size, position and orientation automatic planning were developed and validated. Our developed navigation prototype could also find application for surgical training, navigating knee and hip prostheses implantation on phantoms.

ACKNOWLEDGMENT

Authors thank Lima-Lto (Udine, Italy) for technical and financial support.

REFERENCES

Alan, R., & Tria, A. (2006). Quadriceps-sparing total knee arthroplasty using the posterior stabilized TKA design. *The journal of knee surgery, 19*(1), 71-76.

Anderson, K., Buehler, K., & Markel, D. (2005). Computer-assisted navigation in total knee arthroplasty. *The Journal of Arthroplasty, 20*(7), 132-138.

Barratt, D., Penney, G., Chan, C., Slomczykowski, M., Carter, T., Edwards, P., & Hawkes, D. (2006). Self-calibrating 3D-ultrasound-based bone registration for minimally invasive orthopedic surgery. *IEEE transactions on medical imaging, 25*(3), 312-323.

Confalonieri, N., Manzotti, A., Pullen, C., & Ragone, V. (2005). Computer-assisted technique versus intramedullary and extramedullary alignment system in total knee replacement: A radiological comparison. *Acta orthopaedica Belgica, 71,* 703-709.

Daubresse, F., Vajeu, C., & Loquet, J. (2005). Total knee arthroplasty with conventional or navigated technique: comparison of the learning curves in a community hospital. *Acta orthopaedica Belgica, 71*(6), 710-713.

Delp, S., Stulberg, S., Davies, B., Picard, F., & Leitner, F. (1998). Computer-assisted knee replacement. *Clinical Orthopaedics, 354,* 49-56.

De Momi, E., Cerveri, P., Audrito, M., Facchini, A., Ferrigno G. (2006). A new Algorithm for hip joint center computation in TKR. In: F. Langlotz, B. Davies, & R. Ellis (Eds.), 6th Annual Meeting of CAOS-International. *Computer-Assisted Orthopaedic Surgery* (pp. 119-122).

De Momi, E., Cerveri, P., Audrito, M., Facchini, A., & Ferrigno G. (2006). 3D shape iterative reconstruction method based on statistical models. In: F. Langlotz, B. Davies, & R. Ellis (Eds.), 6th Annual Meeting of CAOS-International. *Computer Assisted Orthopaedic Surgery* (pp. 123-126).

DiGioia, A., Jaramaz, B., Blackwell, M., Simon, D., Morgan, F., Moody, J., et al. (1998). Image-guided navigation system to measure intraoperatively acetabular implant alignment. *Clinical orthopaedics and related research, 355,* 8-22.

Ferrigno, G., & Pedotti, A. (1985). ELITE: A digital dedicated hardware system for movement analysis via real-time TV-signal processing. *IEEE Transaction on Biomedical Engineering, 32,* 943-950.

Fleute, M., Lavallee, S., & Julliard, R. (1999). Incorporating a statistically-based shape model into a system for computer-assisted anterior cruciate ligament surgery. *Medical Image Analysis, 3*(3), 209-222.

Haaker, R., Stockheim, M., Kamp, M., Proff, G., Breitenfelder, J., & Ottersbach, A. (2005). Computer-assisted navigation increases precision of component placement in total knee arthroplasty. *Clinical Orthopaedics and Related Research, 433,* 152-159.

Heger, S., Portheine, F., Ohnsorge, J., Schkommodau, E., & Radermacher, K. (2005). *IEEE engineering in medicine and biology magazine, 24*(2), 85-95.

Ilsar, I., Joskowicz, L., Kandel, L., Matan, Y., & Liebergall, M. (2006). Navigated total knee replacement—a comprehensive clinical state of the art study. In: F. Langlotz, B. Davies, & R. Ellis (Eds.), 6th Annual Meeting of CAOS-International. *Computer-Assisted Orthopaedic Surgery* (pp. 229-231).

Jaramaz, B., DiGioia, A., Blackwell, M., & Nikou, C. (1998). Computer-assisted measurement of cup placement in total hip replacement. *Clinical orthopaedics and related research, 354,* 70-81.

Jeffery, R., Morris, R., & Denham, R. (1991). Coronal alignment after total knee replacement.

The Journal of bone and joint surgery. British volume, 73(5), 709-714.

Lewinnek, G., Lewis, J., Tarr, R., Compere, C., & Zimmerman, J. (1978). Dislocations after total hip-replacement arthroplasties. *The Journal of bone and joint surgery. American volume, 60,* 217-220.

Mayr, E., Moctezuma de la Barrera, J., Krismer, M., & Nogler, M. (2005). The impact of fixation type and location on tracker stability in navigated THA—a cadaver study. In: F. Langlotz, B. Davies, & R. Ellis (Eds.), 5th Annual Meeting of CAOS-International. *Computer-Assisted Orthopaedic Surgery* (pp. 314-315).

Martelli, S., Nofrini, L., Vendruscolo, P., & Visani, A. (2003). Criteria of interface evaluation for computer-assisted surgery systems. *International Journal of Medical Informatics, 72,* 35-45.

Merloz, P., Tonetti, J., Pittet, L., Coulomb, M., Lavallee, S., Troccaz, J., et al. (1998). Computer-assisted spine surgery. *Comput-Aided Surgery, 3*(6), 297-305.

Picard, F., DiGioia, A., Moody, J., Martinek, V., Fu, F., Rytel, M., et al. (2001). Accuracy in tunnel placement for ACL reconstruction. Comparison of traditional arthroscopic and computer-assisted navigation techniques. *Comput-Aided Surgery, 6*(5), 279-89

Siston, R., & Delp, S. (2006). Evaluation of a new algorithm to determine the hip joint center. *Journal of Biomechanics, 39,* 125-130.

Stindel, E., Gil, D., Briard, J., Merloz, P., Dubrana, F., & Lefevre, C. (2005). Detection of the center of the hip joint in computer-assisted surgery: An evaluation study of the Surgetics algorithm. *Computer-Aided Surgery, 10*(3), 133-139.

Stoeckl, B., Nogler, M., Rosiek, R., Fischer, M., Krismer, M., & Kessler, O. (2004). Navigation improves accuracy of rotational alignment in total knee arthroplasty. *Clinical Orthopaedics and Related Research, 426,* 180-186.

Tria, A. (2006). The evolving role of navigation in minimally invasive total knee arthroplasty. *The American journal of orthopedics, 35*(7), 18-22.

Viceconti, M., Zannoni, C., Testi, D., & Cappello, A. (1999). CT data sets surface extraction for biomechanical modeling of long bones. *Computer Methods and Programs in Biomedicine, 59,* 159-166.

West, J., & Maurer, C. (2004). Designing optically tracked instruments for image-guided surgery. *IEEE Transactions on Medical Imaging, 23*(5), 533-545.

Zheng, G., Marx, A., Langlotz, U., Widmer, K., Buttaro, M., & Nolte, L. (2002). A hybrid CT-free navigation system for total hip arthroplasty. *Computer-Aided Surgery, 7*(3), 129-145.

Additional Reading

Baroni, G., Ferrigno, G., Orecchia, R. & Pedotti, A. (2000). Real-time opto-electronic verification of patient position in breast cancer radiotherapy. *Computer-Aided Surgery, 5,* 296-306.

Barratt, D.C., Penney, G.P., Chan, C.S.K., Slomczykowski, M., Carter, T.J,. Edwards, P.J. & Hawkes, D. (2006). Self-calibrating 3D-ultrasound-based bone registration for minimally invasive orthopedic surgery. *IEEE Trans Med Imaging 25*(3), 312-323.

Besl, P. & McKay, N.D. (1992). A method for registration of 3-D shapes. IEEE Trans Pattern Anal Machine Intell 14, 239-256

Camomilla, V., Cereatti, A., Vannozzi, G. & Cappozzo, A. (2006). An optimized protocol for hip joint centre determination using the functional method. J Biomech. 39(6), 1096-106

Cerveri P., Pedotti A. & Ferrigno G. (2003). Model-based approach and extended Kalman filters for accurate human motion estimation, Human Movement Science, 22(3), 377-404

Cerveri, P., Pedotti, A. & Ferrigno G., (2004). Evolutionary optimization for robust hierarchical computation of the rotation centres of kinematical chains from reduced ranges of motion: the lower spine case. Journal of Biomechanics, 37(12), 1881-1890

Cootes, T., Taylor, C., Cooper, D. & Graham, J. (1995) Active shape models—Their training and application," Comput. Vis Imag. Understand 61 (1), 38–59

De Momi, E., Chapuis, J., Pappas, I., Ferrigno, G., Hallermann, W., Schramm, A. & Caversaccio M. (2006) Automatic Extraction of the Mid-facial Plane for Cranio-Maxillofacial Surgery Planning, Int. J of Oral and Maxillofacial Surgery, 35(7), 636-42

Delp, S.L., Stulberg, S.D. & Davies, B. (1998). Computer assisted knee replacement. Clin Orthop Relat Res 354, 49-56

Frosio, I., Spadea, M., De Momi, E., Riboldi, M., Baroni, G., Ferrigno, G., Orecchia, R., Pedotti, A. (2006). A neural network based method for optical patient set-up registration in breast radiotherapy. Ann Biomed Eng. 34(4), 677-86

Haaker, R.G., Stockheim, M., Kamp, M., Proff, G., Breitenfelder, J. & Ottersbach, A. (2005). Computer-Assisted Navigation Increases Precision of Component Placement in Total Knee Arthroplasty, Clin Orthop Rel Res (433), 152–159

Heckbert, P. & Garland, M. (1999). Optimal Triangulation and Quadric-Based Surface Simplification. J. Computational Geometry: Theory and Applications 14 (1), 49-65

Heger S, Mumme T, Sellei R, De La Fuente M, Wirtz DC, Radermacher K. (2007). A-mode ultrasound-based intra-femoral bone cement detection and 3D reconstruction in RTHR. Computer-aided Surg. 12(3), 168-75

Heger, S., Portheine, F., Ohnsorge, J.A.K., Schkommodau, E. & Radermacher, K. (2005). User-Interactive Registration of Bone with A-Mode Ultrasound IEEE Eng Med Biol Magazine, 24(2), 85-95

Jaramaz, B., DiGioia, A.M. III, Blackwell & M., Nikou, C. (1998). Computer assisted measurement of cup placement in total hip replacement. Clin Orthop 354 70-81

Langlotz, F., Berlemann, U., Ganz, R. &Nolte, L.P. (2000). Computer-Assisted Periacetabular Osteotomy Operative Techniques in Orthopaedics, 10(1) 14-19

Piazza, S. & Delp, S. (2001). Three-Dimensional Dynamic Simulation of Total Knee Replacement Motion During a Step-Up Task, Journal of Biomechanical Engineering, 123, 99-606

Pluim, J.P.W., Maintz, J.B.A. & Viergever, M.A. (2003) Mutual-Information-Based Registration of Medical Images: A Survey, IEEE Trans. Med. Imag., 22(8), 986-1004

Rodriguez, F., Harris, S., Jakopec, M., Barrett, A., Gomes, P., Henckel, J., Cobb, J., Davies, B. (2005) Robotic clinical trials of uni-condylar arthroplasty. Int J Med Robot. 1(4), 20-8.

Shoham, M., Lieberman, I.H., Benzel, E.C., Togawa, D., Zehavi, E., Zilberstein, B., Roffman, M., Bruskin, A., Fridlander, A., Joskowicz, L., Brink-Danan, S. & Knoller, N. (2007). Robotic assisted spinal surgery-from concept to clinical practice. Computer-aided Surg. 12(2),105-15

Siston, R.A., Giori, N.J., Goodman, S.B. & Delp, S.L. (2007) Surgical navigation for total knee arthroplasty: a perspective. J Biomech. 40(4), 728-35.

Siston, R.A., Patel, J.J., Goodman, S.B., Delp, S.L., Giori, N.J. (2005). The variability of femoral rotational alignment in total knee arthroplasty. J Bone Joint Surg Am. 87(10), 2276-80.

Szekely, G., Kelemen, A., Brechbuhler, C. & Gerig, G., Segmentation of 2-D and 3-D objects constrained elastic deformations of flexible Fourier contour and from MRI volume data using surface models, Medical Image Analysis (1996) volume 1, number 1, pp 19–34

Tria, A.J. Jr. (2006). The evolving role of navigation in minimally invasive total knee arthroplasty. Am J Orthop. 35(7 Suppl), 18-22

Wolf, A., Jaramaz, B., Lisien, B. & DiGioia, A.M. (200). MBARS: mini bone-attached robotic system for joint arthroplasty. Int J Med Robot., 1(2), 101-21.

Yau, W.P., Leung, A., Chiu, K.Y., Tang, W.M., T.P. Ng TP, (2005). Intraobserver errors in obtaining visually selected anatomic landmarks during registration process in nonimage-based navigation-assisted total knee arthroplasty: a cadaveric experiment, J Arthroplasty. 20 (5), 591-601

Zheng, G., Tannast, M., Anderegg, C., Siebenrock, K.A. & Langlotz, F. (2007). Hip(2)Norm: An object-oriented cross-platform program for 3D analysis of hip joint morphology using 2D pelvic radiographs .Comput Methods Programs Biomed.87(1), 36-45

Chapter XI
Multi–Dimensional Transfer Functions Design

Hai Lin
Zhejiang University, China

ABSTRACT

Transfer function design is one of the most important procedures in volume rendering. Transfer function maps, which is a function mapping relationship, data values to display attributes, such as color and opacity. This chapter introduces region growing- based multi-dimensional transfer function design method, which can improve the effect of the multi-dimensional transfer function design, and help the users save the time used in the interactive design and decrease the difficult. In order to use the spatial information as independent variable, we combine spatial information to generate multi-dimensional transfer function. This chapter discusses the GPU-based transfer function lookup method and illumination parameter setting problems. In the last part of this chapter, we discuss the data layout of large scale volume data set and its volume rendering methods.

INTRODUCTION

Direct volume rendering is an effective method for data visualization. Transfer function design is one of the most important procedures in volume rendering. Transfer function maps, which is a function mapping relationship, data values to display attributes, such as color and opacity. According to the domain of the transfer function, there is one-dimensional transfer function and multi-dimensional transfer function. Transfer functions design has an important effect on the result of the volume rendering. Effective trans-

fer function can distinguish visually different materials and different structures in an original data set, and remove the unimportant information while displaying the important structure in which people are interested. In the simplest type of transfer function, the domain of the transfer function is 1D, representing a scalar data value. Usually, one-dimensional transfer function can be designed through the gray histogram. One-dimensional transfer function can be designed easily, but it is difficult to identify the difference between materials. For example, CT data or MRT data may contain many materials and complex boundaries between different materials. When a scalar value relates to many materials, only using scalar data value is impossible to distinguish it.

Because of the limitation of the one-dimensional transfer function, people consider using other information to distinguish different structures and materials, and multi-dimensional transfer function is brought. While adding the gradient magnitude and other information, multi-dimensional transfer function can work better for distinguishing different materials. But multi-dimensional transfer function brings higher request for the interactive design. How to use the information of the original data set to design effective transfer function is our goal. This chapter introduces region growing-based multi-dimensional transfer function design method, which can improve the effect of the multi-dimensional transfer function design, and help the users save the time used in the interactive design and decrease the difficulty.

Transfer function design's other difficulty is that it does not use the spatial information as an independent variable, so it is difficult to classify the volume data, as the other region may contain the same scalar value. To solve this problem, this chapter combines spatial information to generate multi-dimensional transfer function.

In the last part of the chapter, we discuss the GPU-based transfer function lookup method and illumination parameter setting problems.

REGION GROWING-BASED METHOD OF AUTOMATICALLY GENERATED TRANSFER FUNCTION

The Multi-Dimensional Transfer Function

Multi-dimensional transfer function uses multi-information for classify volume data, not just only the scalar value. Using multi-information of the data can increase the opportunity of separating the attributes of materials and express the differ-ence between different structures of the original dataset effectively. This data information can be regarded as coordinates of the transfer function domain (Kindlmann, 1998; Pfister, 2001).

We can use gradient magnitude as the second dimension of the transfer function while using the scalar value as the first dimension (Kindlmann, 2002). For scalar data, gradient can be retrieved from the first order derivative. As a vector, it denotes the largest variety direction. Normalized gradient are always used as normal in surface-based volume rendering. The magnitude of the gradient is a scalar value; it denotes the change ratio in the scalar value. In this chapter we use f representing the gradient magnitude of function f, and f is the function representing the scalar value of the data. We note:

$$f' = \| \nabla f \|$$

Using this value as a coordinate of the transfer function is useful. Within the same material, the scalar values are almost the same, so according to the attributes of the gradient, the magnitude of the gradient is small. On the boundaries of different materials, the scalar value is changing very quickly, and the magnitude of the gradient will be large. So we can use the gradient magnitude to distinguish the internal regions of the materials and the boundaries of different materials.

Because the data set is discrete, we need an approximate method to compute gradient.

For the internal points, we can use center derivative to compute the gradient of the point (i, j, k):

$$\nabla F_{i,j,k} = \begin{bmatrix} F_x(x_i, y_j, z_k) \\ F_y(x_i, y_j, z_k) \\ F_z(x_i, y_j, z_k) \end{bmatrix} = \begin{bmatrix} \dfrac{F_{i+1,j,k} - F_{i-1,j,k}}{2\nabla x} \\ \dfrac{F_{i,j+1,k} - F_{i,j-1,k}}{2\nabla y} \\ \dfrac{F_{i,j,k+1} - F_{i-1,j,k-1}}{2\nabla z} \end{bmatrix}$$

Figure 1. The relationship of the arcs in the transfer function and the boundaries of materials

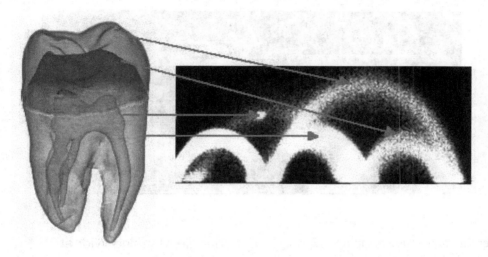

For the points on the boundaries, we can use frontward derivative or backward derivative to calculate the gradient. If the request for precision is high, we can use second order derivative or thrice strip method to compute gradient.

We use the scalar value as the x-axis in the transfer function domain and gradient magnitude as the y-axis. By going through all the points of the data set, and projecting them to the transfer function domain, we can get a set of arcs. Each arc represents a kind of material. In the top of the arc, the gradient magnitude is large, so this part represents the boundary and two ends of the arc represent two different materials. (see Figure 1)

In the actual application, two-dimensional transfer functions' arcs usually overlap each other, because the boundaries between different materials are complex. During this situation, some materials cannot be correctly distinguished. To solve this problem, we can add the second order derivative as the third dimension of transfer function. This method can solve ambiguity. As we know, theoretically, when the first order derivative obtains the largest value, the second order derivative equals 0. So some boundary survey algorism also use the second order derivative whether pass the zero point to determine the boundary.

Here we use a more precise method and it needs more calculation. This method uses the second order derivative along the gradient direction, and includes Hessian matrix. We use f represent first order derivative.

$$f'' = \frac{1}{|\nabla f|^2}(\nabla f)^T H f \nabla f$$

Apply Mapping Widget to Multi-Dimensional Transfer Function Design

Introducing gradient magnitude and second order derivative for the transfer function's second and third dimension increases the freedom of transfer function design. This needs a more flexible, more convenient and more intuitive interactive manner. Kniss introduced a mapping widget-based interactive method (Kniss, 2001; 2002). It uses the scalar value as the x-axis of the transfer function domain and gradient magnitude as the y-axis. All the voxels of the data set are passed through and are projected to the transfer function domain, as the above picture shows. In the previous section, we discuss the meaning of the arc in

Figure 2.Widget-based transfer function design

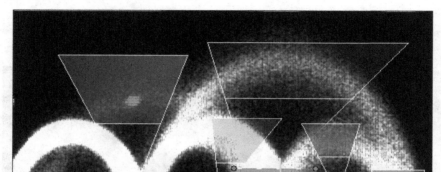

the transfer function. Using mapping widgets, we can distinguish those boundaries and give them different colors and opacities.

We design two different mapping widgets and define their interactive behavior in this paper. Figure 2 is the transfer function of rendering tooth dataset:

Rectangle Mapping Widget

Like the above figure shows, rectangle mapping widget chooses a rectangle region in the transfer function domain. Rectangle mapping widget is suited for mapping the internal region of the materials.

Movement: After choosing the mapping widget, the user puts the mouse in the internal region of the widget and the mouse's shape denotes the move state. The user can move the widget to the appropriate location.

Zoom: After choosing the mapping widget, the user puts the mouse in the four vertexes then the mouse's shape denotes the zoom state. The user can move the vertexes to change the size of the widget.

Adjust the largest opacity point: After choosing the mapping widget, there will appear a yellow line for setting the largest opacity point. It can be moved to the right or left to change the largest opacity point.

Triangle Mapping Widget

Comparing rectangle mapping widget, triangle mapping widget is more flexible, and supplies more interactive control. Like the picture below shows, triangle mapping widget's effect region is within the boundaries. It is suited for control of the gradient magnitude range. Triangle mapping widget is suited for choosing the boundaries part of the materials (the top of the arc). Figure 3 shows the interactive operations of triangle mapping widget.

Zoom: The two control points in the upper line control zooming of the mapping widget. It is based on the center line and is zoomed proportionally.

Movement on the upper boundary: The shape of the mouse will indicate free motion state when the mouse is put around the upper boundary. Dragging the mouse can move the location of the upper boundary, and then the shape of the triangle will change.

Moving horizontally: When choosing the mapping widget, the shape of the mouse will indicate the move state, as the picture above shows. Dragging to the right or left can move the mapping widget. The bottom of the widget is fixed in the x-axis of the transfer function domain and it is allowed only moving horizontally.

Figure 3. Interaction of the triangle widget

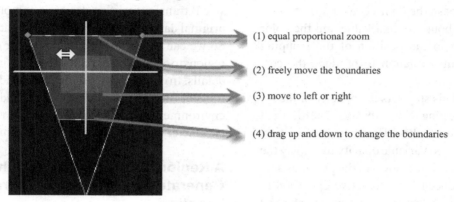

(1) equal proportional zoom

(2) freely move the boundaries

(3) move to left or right

(4) drag up and down to change the boundaries

Fluctuate the boundary: The mapping widget's valid region is determined by the upper boundary and lower boundary. Hold the mouse around the lower boundary, the shape of the mouse will indicate the move state. Dragging the mouse can change the location of the lower boundary.

Adjusting the maximal opacity point is the same with the rectangle widget.

Setting Optics Attributes Based on Mapping Widget

After defining the mapping widget's position in the transfer function, the next step is to set the optics attributes of color, opacity and illumination parameter for each mapping widget. Because the position of the mapping widget has already distinguished the interested region, after setting the optics, attributes for mapping widget the multi-dimensional transfer function design has been completed. This chapter extends the transfer function and adds the illumination parameters to the setting, so different regions distinguished by different mapping widgets can use different illumination parameters to render. In that way, internal information of the data can be more visible. The main configurable attributes of the mapping widget are displayed in Figure 4.

Figure 4. Attributes setting in the mapping widget

Widget Property	
Name	Widget0
Visible	True
Color	(0,127,255)
Opacity	0.80
Ambient	0.50
Diffuse	0.80
Specular	0.20
Interpolation	True
Auto Color	
Enable Auto Color	False
From Color	(0,0,255)
To Color	(255,0,0)

Color: This step sets the color of the region which mapping widgets covers. After all the mappings widgets are set with color, the multi-dimensional transfer function can map the multi-dimensions volume information to color value. But data of different types have different characteristics, some data have the special request to the visible color. For instance, the data in the temperature field of meteorological cloud picture should be based on the temperature to set the color value: The lowest temperature corresponding to blue color, the maximum temperature corresponding to red color, the medial data's color is produced by interpolation. In order to meet this kind of need, we add the automatic function to set color. The user can base the data visible request to set the relations about the data value and the color and according to the position of the mapping widgets, use interpolation to produce the corresponding color.

Opacity: This step sets the opacity of the region which mapping widgets covers. The different material region has the different characteristics; some regions need variable opacity to display the internal information clearer. In the previous section, we introduced the interactive operation in the mapping widget and we can adjust the largest opacity point. This way improves the flexibility and allows us to change the opacity in a specified way. This chapter provides three ways to change opacities: no attenuation, ellipse attenuation way and linear attenuation way. In the no attenuation way, the opacity is the same, and is equal to the setting value. The other two kinds of attenuation ways set the largest opacity point of the setting values, and opacity values of other points are computed by the distance from the largest opacity point. In the ellipse attenuation way, ellipse's axis is set by the proportion of the width and height of the mapping widget. In the linear attenuation way, the opacity value decreases linearly in horizontal direction or the vertical direction.

Illumination parameter: The illumination computation is very important for direct volume rendering. The illumination intensity can show the normal information. Adding the illumination computation to the volume rendering result can reflect the internal structure of the material clearer. Generally, we calculate the environment reflection, diffuse reflection and the specula reflection first, and then combine the three parts' contributions. The computation needs the environment reflection parameter, diffuse reflection parameter and specula reflection parameter. But traditional method can only set the global parameter and cannot act according to the different region to set different illumination parameter. This section introduces the illumination parameter setting method based

on the mapping widget. After the multi-dimensional transfer function design is completed, the original data set is divided into different regions. So we can set different parameters for different regions to emphasize certain important, interested details. In other words, besides color and opacity, transfer function's output values are added to the environment light parameter, diffuse reflection parameter and specula reflection parameter.

A Region Growing-Based Method to Generate Multi-dimensional Transfer Function

We have the interactive design tools in the transfer function domain already, so we can design the transfer function now. But the transfer function domain is not intuitive. We introduce a region growing based method to generate multi-dimensional transfer function automatically. This makes the transfer function designing procedure more easy.

Dual-Domain Interactive Method

In a traditional volume rendering system, the process of setting the transfer function involves moving the control points (in a sequence of linear ramps defining color and opacity), and then observing the resulting rendered image. That is, interaction in the transfer function domain is guided by careful observation of changes in the spatial domain. We prefer a reversal of this process, in which the transfer function is set by direct interaction in the spatial domain, with observation of the transfer function domain. Furthermore, by allowing interaction to happen in both domains simultaneously, the conceptual gap between them is significantly lessened.

We use the term "dual-domain interaction" to describe this approach to transfer function exploration and generation. The data set in x,y,z three directions' slices are used to interact in the spatial domain. Users can select an interested region in the data slice as the seed point to start the region growing. After that, we calculate the data of the result set, and project them to the transfer function domain. Based on this statistic information, a temporary mapping widget will be added to the transfer function domain, and the volume rendering result will be displayed. Now users have already designed a multi-dimensional transfer function through interaction in the spatial domain. And the result of the volume rendering displays a part of the data set which has the same attributes with user's selected region. If the features rendered are of interest, the user can copy the temporary transfer function to the permanent one. If the automatically generated mapping widget is not ideal, the user can change the attributes of the mapping widget. After several dual-domain interactive steps, a transfer function is completed.

Automatically Generated Multi-Dimensional Transfer Function-Based Region Growing

There is a problem in the dual-domain: how to use the data information of the spatial domain to automatically generate the mapping widget and how to set the attributes of the mapping widget. We use the based region growing method to solve the problem.

Algorithm Description

Region growing begins from a seed point. In our system the user picks a seed by interactively slicing through the volume data. Alternatively, the user can specify a line segment instead of a point. A line segment consists of a sequence 3D points. When a point is selected, its 26 neighbors are checked. If its neighbor has satisfied the growing criteria, the neighbor is added as a new seed point. Otherwise it is ignored. This step is repeated until all the seed points are processed and then the region growing is completed.

After the region growing, we can get a data set and we can regard it as the user's interested region. For the next step we base this point set to generate transfer function. We know that the triangular classification widgets are particularly effective for visualizing surfaces in scalar data. Rectangle classification widgets are effective for visualizing the internal region. The data points of the region growing result are mapped to the transfer function domain and their scalar values and standard variances, gradient magnitude values and standard variances are calculated. If the standard variance is very small, it is regarded as internal area and described by the rectangle widget. If the standard variance is very large, it is regarded as surface and described by the triangle widget. The center position of the mapping widget is determined by the average of the scalar value and the gradient magnitude and the size of it are determined by the scalar value and gradient magnitude's standard variance.

It is noticeable that complete region-growing takes time, especially if the region is bigger, the consumed time is longer. But the data values in the same region have some similar attributes. So the completed region growing is unnecessary. Partial region-growing can also pick the attributes of the interested region and we can get the interested region using this information.

Region-Growing Criteria

The data scalar values and the gradient magnitudes are considered in the criteria. The criteria are described by the function below:

$$f_c(p) = \frac{|v - v_s|}{k\sigma_v} p + \frac{|g - g_s|}{k\sigma_g}(1 - p)$$

If the function value is smaller than 1, the current point is considered to have satisfied the criteria and it is determined in the same region with the current point. Otherwise it is not considered to have satisfied the criteria, where v is the data value of the current voxel and g is the gradient magnitude value of the current voxel. v_s is the data value of the seed voxel and g_s is the gradient value of the seed voxel. σ_v is the standard deviation of the values of the 26 neighboring voxels of the seed voxel and σ_g is the standard deviation of the gradient. k is a constant specified by the user. Note that $0 < k$. It is used to control the strictness of the criterion, and its default value is1. p is a weight specified by the user or by the system and $0 \leq p \leq 1$. When p=1,the criteria only consider the data scalar value; when p=0, the criteria only consider the gradient magnitude information. By default, $p = \dfrac{\sigma_g}{(\sigma_v = \sigma_g)}$.

COMBINE SPATIAL INFORMATION IN MULTI-DIMENSIONAL TRANSFER FUNCTION

There will be some problems in the transfer function design. That is because the spatial information is lost in the data set. For example, the bone of the medical data set can be distinguished by the scalar value and the gradient magnitude. But different bones of different position can hardly be distinguished by this method. So we must combine spatial information in the transfer function design.

We apply a transfer function method which combines the spatial information (Roettger, 2005). This method can use the information of spatial domain and the multi-dimensional transfer function domain to generate transfer function automatically.

Box 1.

Classify the Spatial Information

The first step of the spatial transfer function design is to classify the transfer function domain. First, the transfer function domain is divided into several small panes, the size of the pane can be specified; we set it a pixel here, and then, the scalar value is set as the x-axis and the gradient magnitude is set as the y x-axis. All the voxels are projected into the transfer function domain and the arc structure is formed. The spatial information (the coordinates of x,y,z axis) in each pane must be recorded.

We calculate the coordinate of the barycenter and spatial variance for all voxels in each pane. Suppose u,v are the data scalar value, the gradient magnitude, and have been normalized.

So (u,v) corresponding to a pane in the transfer function domain. The number of the voxels in the pane is noted as H(u, v)=n. And the coordinates of corresponding voxels are noted as $P_i(u, v)$.

Then the coordinate of the barycenter of (u,v) is: $barycenter(u,v) = \dfrac{1}{n} \sum_{i=1}^{n} P_i(u,v)$.

And its spatial variance is:

$$\mathrm{var}iance(u,v) = \frac{1}{n} \sum_{i=1}^{n} \| P_i(u,v) - barycenter(u,v) \|$$

Lastly, we classify the panes according to the criteria. In the unclassified pane set, we choose the one which has the largest n as the standard, and it is noted as T_0. For other unclassified pane T, we compute the distance in Box 1.

If $D(T, T_0) < r$, T and T_0 are considered as the same class, and it is deleted from the unclassified class. The process is repeated until the unclassified set is empty.

$$D(T, T_0) = \| barycenter(T) - barycenter(T_0) \| + | \mathrm{var}ivance(T) - \mathrm{var}iance(T_0) |$$

For the same data set, barycenter and variance are just calculated once. The classified distance r is selected by the users. For different data sets, it will be different. We can set a larger r and decrease it gradually until the interested materials are distinguished.

Setting the Color and the Opacity

After using spatial information to classify the transfer function domain, it is needed to set the proper color and opacity for each class. It is easy to set the color: give a unique class color for each class. We set each pane which belongs to that class the color value *classColor* $\times C_c$. Where C_c is the color coefficient. The opacity is set by the gradient magnitude: suppose the global opacity is O_g. Then each pane's opacity is $O_g \times v$. Where v is the normalized gradient magnitude. The boundaries of different materials have large opacity, but in the internal region of the material the gradient magnitude is small; we can enhance the boundary by this method.

Each class can be set with a different parameter: environment reflection parameter, diffuse reflec-

tion parameter and specula reflection parameter. This can improve the flexibility.

The multi-dimensional transfer function which uses the spatial information is completely generated now. When the user selects a certain class, the system will set its color as a smaller coefficient to display the selected class more clearly.

Figure 5 is the result of using automatically generated multi-dimensional transfer function when r=0.2 and classification selection. The dataset is the engine (256x256x128).

FAST LOOKUP OF GPU-BASED TRANSFER FUNCTION

The volume rendering algorithm discussed is primarily based on GPU's three-dimensional texture acceleration method. For each sampling point, we use transfer function to compute corresponding optical attributes such as color value and opacity. In order to boost rendering speed, mapping is done in the GPU's fragment shader. Time consumed by computing is significantly reduced by converting the process of mapping

Figure 5. Rendering result of combined spatial message transfer function

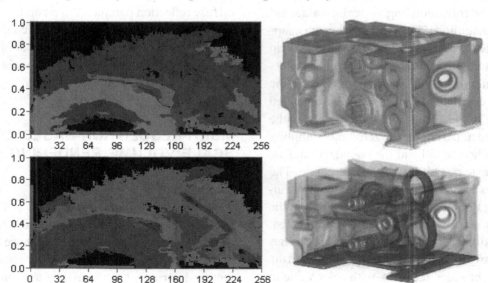

transfer function to the process of looking up for two-dimensional texture (Gelder, 1996; Westermann, 1998). Next, we will introduce the method generating the transfer function texture.

Generation Lookup Texture for Multi-dimensional Transfer Function

It will definitely take a great deal of time if we compute mapping's optical attributes according to transfer function for each sampling point during rendering. We can convert transfer function sampling to lookup a table before rendering. Therefore, in the rendering process, we can just treat independent variables of transfer function as index, then obtain optical attributes such as color value and opacity from lookup table. The process of lookup can be further accelerated by GPU. By loading lookup table as two-dimensional texture into the video memory and searching 2D texture in the fragment shader, we can easily get the mapping value.

Take an example of multi-dimensional transfer function-based on mapping widget. First, we compute its scalar value and gradient magnitude for each sampling point along x axis and y axis according to sampling number in the multi-dimensional transfer function domain. Color value and opacity corresponding to scalar value and gradient magnitude are available by the mapping widget. If several mapping widgets overlap for some sampling points, we blend those colors as the sampling point, with opacity being the weighted coefficient. Opacity can be amended according to the second order derivative. If the second order derivative is zero, the sampling point is indicated to be at the boundary, and we increase opacity. Otherwise, we decrease it. The boundaries among materials become more prominent using three-dimensional information of the transfer function. After sampling is completed, the multi-dimensional transfer function becomes a discrete two-dimensional lookup table. Load the table into the video memory, with color value in

r, g, b components, respectively, and opacity in alpha component. Color and opacity is mapped to the range of 0-255. The corresponding color and opacity can be found in the transfer function texture, with texture coordinates being the current voxel's scalar value and gradient magnitude in the fragment shader. Spatial information combined multi-dimensional transfer texture can be generated by similar method.

Lighting Parameters Textures

As we have mentioned before, for better display of internal structure of materials, we have added lighting parameters configuration to the transfer function, enabling different regions to be rendered by different lighting parameters. Environment reflection parameter, diffuse reflection parameter and specular reflection parameter are also processed using two-dimensional texture lookup table, which has been applied to querying color value and opacity in the previous section.

The process of obtaining lighting parameters for each sampling point is similar to the process of sampling color value and opacity. After changing three lighting parameters to the range [0, 255], we load lighting parameter texture. We store environment reflection parameter to r component, diffuse reflection parameter to g component and specular reflection parameter to b component. During rendering, we query texture value according texture coordinates, with scalar value and gradient value being their value.

MULTI-RESOLUTION-BASED LARGE SCALE VOLUME RENDERING

Background

In recent years, along with science and technology's rapid development, people have higher demand for data; this promotes the science detecting instrument performance and precision.

In many areas like medicine, geology and so on produce more and more data, the data scale has achieved gigabyte and even terabyte magnitude. Some data can even contain the time information, namely the 4D data. This can make the movement information visible, like heart beating, the cloud layer activity and so on. It can be imagined just how astonishing such data quantity is.

Large-scale data has provided rich source materials to the visible work, on the one hand, and on the other hand, it also brings a higher request to the visible technology. This brings a bigger challenge. How to interactively render large-scale data in an ordinary PC machine has become an urgent problem to be solved. In recent years, programmable graph accelerator chip's (GPU) development is extremely rapid; we should certainly fully use it. But the video card's capacity is far smaller than the large- scale data. This must be solved by another technique.

The method of solving the capacity limit is mainly data layout, compression and procedure simulate. The data layout is based on the idea of divides and rule: it divides the large-scale data into small blocks, it can be separately rendered, it finally puts various blocks' rendering results together to be the final picture. Compression uses various technologies, like texture compression based on the wavelet transformation compression and so on. Before storing the data in the memory, it must be compressed. In the volume rendering stage, decompression occurs. This way can save the storage capacity. The procedure simulation method considers the data's characteristics, like the cloud; the boundary's detail shape is extremely complex, so the complete data quantity is inevitably extremely large. We can only store the approximate shape, and re-establishes the detail information by the procedure simulation method. This can greatly decrease the data quantity.

The methods of accelerating the rendering are mainly optimized rendering algorithm, computer cluster parallel rendering and multi- resolution rendering and so on.

Multi-Resolution-Based Large Scale Volume Rendering

We adopt multi-resolution layer structure to manage the original data set and introduce accelerative volume rendering method which is based on transfer function. Large-scale data rendering's bottleneck is mainly the speed of the AGP main line. The multi-resolution technology can eliminate parts of sub-trees and leave nodes and allow low-resolution nodes instead of whole sub-trees under some condition. This saves the memories, decreases the time of switching vide data and supplies flexibility and expansibility.

Based multi-resolution layer structure large-scale volume rendering's main steps are: in the pretreatment stage, according to the establishment rules, to decompose the original data set, and to establish original data set's different display level. The higher the level is, the smaller the data needs. The upper lever data's resolution generally is the lower level data's half. The leaf node's resolution is equal to the original data set's resolution. While volume rendering, spreads calendar this level eight to fork the tree, visit to each pitch point, the lay octree is went through. For each node, the previous established visited rule is applied. The result of application rule has three kinds of possibilities: (1) skip this visited node and its all children node; (2) skip the visited nodes, continue visiting its N children node; (3) apply the direct volume rendering method to render this visited node, and skip its all children nodes (LaMar , 1999).

Multi-Resolution Layer Structure Establishment

Lower resolution data's generation: Before establishing a layer structure of the original data set, multi-resolution data needs to be generated (Boad, 2001). The lay octree's leaf node's resolution is the same with the original data set. The higher the node's layer, the lower the resolution is. Figure 6 uses the one-dimensional schematic

Figure 6. The relationship of various resolution layers

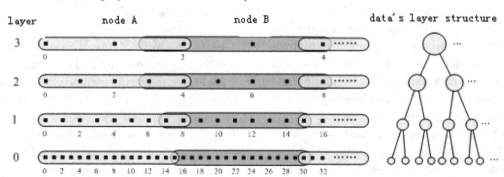

chart to show the relationship of different resolution layer.

Lower resolution data can be generated by average method or two-times sampling method. Suppose A is a linear array of 2n elements, in which the original data has been preserved. B is A's low resolution array, constituted by n elements, $B_i = A_{2i}, i = 0, 1, ..., n - 1$. The average principle calculates the low-resolution data point and neighboring high-resolution data point's average value, and takes the average value as low resolution data. The low-resolution data set generated by this way has fuzzy effect.

From Figure 6 we can see the neighboring node's data overlap; the reason is mainly that while rendering, boundary interpolation cannot be continual.

Lay Octree's establishment: For the sake of solving the problem of capacity, we should use the methods to split the data set by lays to improve the rendering speed, for the permission that we could keep the rendering result. We can manage, store the data and render by splitting the data. When rendering the huge data based on the GPU, we could break the limit of video memory by the means showing above. When coming to the next stage, volume rendering, we could make use of the flexibility rules to effectively travel the structures of the tree. For the permission not to affect the result of the rendering, we could ignore

some nodes or render some low-solution nodes to speed up the rendering.

Figure 7 shows two-dimension sketch maps of the lay structure partition and the multi-resolution rendering.

When coming to three dimensions, every non-leaf nods could at most split into eight child nodes. In the whole tree structure, parent node is higher than the children node. Although the size of the father node is twice the son's, the size of the data is as lager as the children, so the solution is half of the child's. How to produce the low- resolution data has been discussed above.

When building the lay tree, we should build some rules. The rules are to determine whether the node should be split or not. The rule used in this chapter is to check the node data's maximum value and the minimum value. If the maximum and minimum value are almost the same, that means the node is in the interior of the original data set, so we do not need to split the node again.

The other problem in building lay octree is to discuss the size of the leaf nodes. The smaller the size of the leaf node, the finer the partition of the original data base, the smaller the data unit we can manage, the more agile when we travel the tree structure. However, we should need a high tree, so that we should store more low-resolution data. Because such redundancy data is independent of the original data set, it is a waste of the capacity. Besides, in the periods of volume rendering, the

Figure 7. Two-dimension sketch maps of the lay structure and the multi-resolution rendering

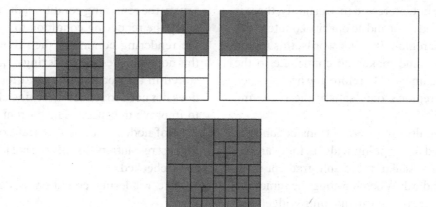

time to travel the lay tree and sort the data block will increase. So we should make a balance in the time or space. The size of leaf node depends on the original data set. In fact, we will control the height of lay tree from 3 to 5, by which we could not only effectively control the tree, but also avoid lager consume of the time and the space.

Besides, when building the lay octree, we should discuss the flatness gliding in the joint, and the texture size must be a number which is a power of 2, and so on. Such things should be discussed in the section about how to implement based by the GPU.

Volume Rendering and Layer Octree's Traversal

After the original data set is divided into a layer structure, we need to traverse this layer Octree. According to the preset conditions, choose the node needed and render them directly in a certain order.

Setting of choosing condition: When you traverse a layer tree and visit each node of it, according to the pre-installed condition on this node, judged what action should be taken on it. Conditions and actions you may choose to take are as following:

1. If the visited node satisfies the removing condition, the node visited at present and all the children nodes will be removed.
2. If the visited node satisfies the condition of rendering, it means this node's resolution has already satisfied the request of rendering. So render the current node only.
3. If the previous two conditions are not met, it means this node's resolution is too low to render, and to check his children nodes recursively.

The removing condition: As mentioned above, when visiting a node, the first application condition is a removing condition. It shows that the impact of the removing condition setting was enormous. So the empty nodes should be removed, obviously. In addition, we define another two rules. The removing condition is satisfied if any rule is satisfied.

Our removing condition is based on multi-dimensional transfer function. In the previous section, we discussed the concepts and application of multi-dimensional transfer function in detail. Multi-dimensional transfer function maps the scalar value, gradient magnitude and second order derivative to the color, opacity and illumination parameters. We will sample the transfer function as a look-up table. Practically, because of the characteristics of data acquisition, most of the region we are not interested in. Certainly, there is no pre-designed color and no opacity counterparts with this data region. In other words, this region is transparent, and makes no contribute to the final rendered image. Therefore, the nodes which include this region's data satisfy the removing condition.

Take the multi-dimensional transfer function which is based on mapping widgets for example. Here, we adopt scalar value and gradient magnitude as standard. When building the removing condition and traversing all mapping widgets, we preserve their scalar value and gradient magnitude range into the removing condition. When applying the removing condition on the node visited, test whether the data scalar value of this node and that already preserved in the removing condition are intersected. If it is intersected, it means this node does not satisfy the removing condition, and reserve the node; then test whether it intersects with the gradient magnitude range, if both of them are not intersected. This node is considered to satisfy the removing condition and remove it. This removing condition can extremely improve the speed of rendering, while it does not affect the quality of rendering completely.

The size of the current node's projection is in the view plane. Every node on the layer tree, not only leaf nodes, but also other nodes, preserve their own geometry information. Generally, it is cuboids of geometry space. We project the corresponding cuboids of the currently visited node in the view plane. If the proportion of the Polygon area after projection and the root node's projection area is smaller than the threshold value which is presented in advance (it is 0.02 in this chapter). This indicates the current node has little affects on the ultimate result of rendering, we can ignore it and all its children nodes, and remove them; otherwise, it means that the node's affect is too obvious to remove.

Rendering condition: If the node does not satisfy the removing condition, the next step is to apply the rendering condition to it. If it satisfies the rendering condition, then the resolution of this node satisfies the rendering request. The data stored in the node can be used for rendering. It does not need to render more fine children nodes to improve the speed. The current node may be the leaf node or not. If it is leaf node, it has the highest resolution. So only the not leaf nodes have to be checked.

The rendering condition is defined as follows:

The calculated the distance between the node and the view point. First, compute the distance between view point and the center of the cuboids. If this distance is larger than the diagonal, the node is considered very far away and its resolution has satisfied the request. Otherwise, it needs to recursively travel to find higher resolution children node.

The rendering procedure: In the image composition stage of direct volume rendering, the color and opacity of the sampling point must be composed in a certain order. Generally, there are back to front composition and front to back composition. No matter which one we use, we must base a certain order to carry on. Because the original data set's lay octree is founded in pre-treatment stage, the structure of it is determined. But along with the change of the view point, children nodes' rendering order is changing. This requires us to sort the children before rendering. This chapter adopts the back to front order to travel the lay octree. If the visited node has satisfied the condition, it will be rendered at once.

Figure 8 shows the complete procedure of travel lay octree and applies the selection condition to volume rendering.

Figure 8. The flow chart of based layer structure multi-dimensional resolution volume rendering

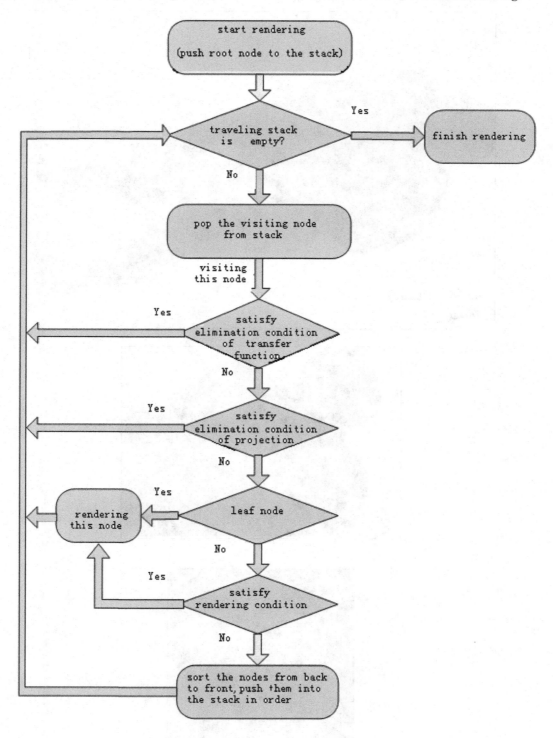

Figure 9. Volume rendering result from visible human (male) data set (1760x1024x1878)

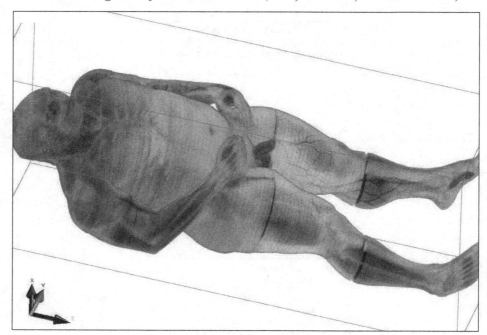

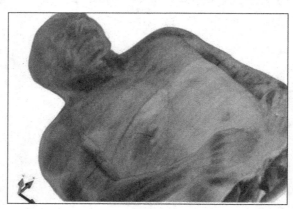

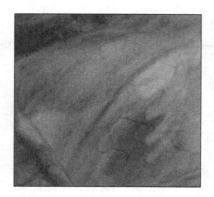

FUTURE RESEARCH DIRECTION

Volume rendering is playing a very important role in volume visualization, especially in medical area. There are several research issues that have been explored and still are the challenges in the field. How to make the visualization system more effective, more intuitive and more effective are always the topics.

The importance of human factors when designing a visualization system has been realized by the visualization community over the past several years. There are some techniques to quantify the effectiveness and errors or uncertainty in volume rendering. In the future, people can design a new visualization system that can automatically or by computer-guidance quantify the effectiveness of the system or tools, and visualize the evaluation to users in an intuitive way.

Some approaches to make visualization more intuitive have already been tackled like automatic transfer function design, viewpoint selection, GPU-based rendering. They are very helpful to improve the efficiency of the visualization systems.

Applying various artificial intelligent techniques to improve the efficiency of visualization procedure, especially for the transfer function design, is a promising research direction. Also, how to use AI techniques to guide the automatic user's viewpoint selection in visualization procedure is another big research issue.

REFERENCES

Boad, I., Navazo, I., & Scopigno, R. (2001). Multi-resolution volume visualization with a texture-based octree. *The Visual Computer, 17,* 185-197.

Gelder, A., & Kim, K. (1996). Direct volume rendering with shading via three-dimensional textures. *Volume Visualization Symposium 96,* (pp. 23-30).

Kindlmann, G., & Durkin, J. (1998). Semi-automatic generation of transfer functions for direct volume rendering. *IEEE Symposium on Volume Visualization,* (pp. 79-86).

Kindlmann, G. (2002). Transfer functions in direct volume rendering: Design, interface, interaction. *Proceedings of SIGGRAPH '02 Course Notes.*

Kniss, J., Kindlmann, G., & Hansen, C. (2001). Interactive volume rendering using multi-dimensional transfer functions and direct manipulation widgets. *Proceedings of IEEE Visualization'01 Conference,* (pp. 255-262).

Kniss, J., Kindlmann, G., & Hansen, C. (2002). Multi-dimensional transfer functions for interactive volume rendering. *IEEE Transactions on Visualization and Computer Graphics, 8*(3), 270-285

LaMar, E., Hamann, B., & Joy, K. (1999). Multi-resolution techniques for interactive texture-based volume visualization. *Proceedings of IEEE Visualization'99,* (pp. 355-361).

Pfister, H., Lorensen, B., Bajaj, C., Kindlmann, G., Schroeder, W., Sobeierajski A., et al. (2001). The transfer function bake-off. *IEEE Computer Graphics and Applications,* 16-22.

Roettger, S., Bauer, M., & Stamminger, M. (2005). Spatialized transfer functions. *Proceedings IEEE/EuroGraphics Symposium on Visualization,* (pp. 271-278).

Westermann, R., & Ertl, T. (1998). Efficiently using graphics hardware in volume rendering applications. *Proceedings of SIGGRAPH 98,* (pp. 169-177).

Additional Reading

Drebin, R., Carpenter, L., & Hanrahan, P. (1998). Volume rendering. *ACM Computer Graphics (SIGGRAPH '88 Proceedings),* pp. 65-74.

Fang, S., Biddlecome, T., & Tuceryan, M. (1998). Image-based transfer function design for data exploration in volume visualization. *Proceedings of IEEE Visualization'98,* (pp. 319-326). IEEE Computer Society.

Fujishiro, I., Azuma, T., & Takeshima, Y. (1999). Automating transfer function design for comprehensible volume rendering based on 3D field topology analysis. *Proceedings IEEE Visualization,* (pp. 467-470,563).

Fujishiro, I., Azuma, T., Yakeshima, Y., & Takahashi, S. (2000). Volume data mining using 3D field topology analysis. *IEEE Computer Graphics and Applications, 20*(5), 46-51.

He, T., Hong, L., Kaufman, A., & Pfister, H. (1996). Generation of transfer functions with stochastic search techniques. *Proceedings Visualization '96,* (pp. 227-234).

Kindlmann, G., Whitaker, R., TTasdizen, T., Möller, T. (2003). Curvature-based transfer functions for direct volume rendering: Methods and applications. *IEEE Visualization,* (pp. 513-520).

Kniss, J., Premoze, S., Ikits, M., Lefohn, A., Hansen, C., Praun, E. (2003). Gaussian transfer functions for multi-field volume visualization. *IEEE Visualization,* (pp. 497-504).

Levoy, M. (1988). Display of surfaces from volume data. *IEEE Computer Graphics & Applications, 8*(5), 29-37.

Lorensen, W., & Cline, H. (1987). Marching cubes: A high-resolution 3D surface construction algorithm. *Computer Graphics, SIGGRAPH'87, 21*(4), 163-169.

Lichtenbelt, B., Crane, R., & Naqvi, S. (1998). *Introduction to volume rendering,* (chap. 4). New Jersey: Prentice-Hall.

Ma, K. (1999). Image graphs—a novel approach to visual data exploration. *Proceedings of IEEE Visualization,* (pp. 81-88,513).

Marks, J., Andalman, B., Beardsley, P., & Pfister, H., et al. (1997). Design galleries: A general approach to setting parameters for computer graphics and animation. *ACM Computer Graphics (SIGGRAPH '97 Proceedings),* (pp. 389-400).

The National Library of Medicine's Visible Human Project. http://www.nlm.nih.gov/research/visible/visible_human.html.

Rodgman, D., & Chen, M. (2001). Refraction in discrete ray tracing. *Proceedings of Volume Graphics 2001,* (pp. 3-17,403).

Takahashi, S., Takeshima, Y., & Fujishiro, I. (2004). Topological volume skeletonization and its application to transfer function design. *Graphical Model, 66*(1), 24-49.

Chapter XII
Graphical Modeling of Human Muscles

X. Ye
Medicsight PLC, UK

F. Dong
Brunel University, UK

ABSTRACT

Muscle simulation is an important component of human modeling. However, there have been few attempts to demonstrate, in an anatomically-correct way, muscle structures and the way in which these change during motion. This chapter proposes a feature-based approach to muscle modeling which attempts to provide models for human musculature based on the real anatomical structures. These models provide a good visual description and form a sound basis for further developments towards medically-accurate simulation of human bodies. Three major problems have been addressed: geometric modeling, deformation and texture. To allow for the wide variety of muscle shapes encountered in the body, the geometric models are based on muscle features identified from radiological data. The results are realistic models with correct anatomical structures, the deformation of these muscle models is fully controlled by, and consistent with, the motion of underlying joint. We suggest a general deformation model that can be adopted for many of our muscle models, but we also model separately the deformation of specific cases for which the general model is not suitable. Interactions between muscles are also taken into account to avoid penetration occurring between adjacent muscles in our model. To provide a suitable visual effect, an algorithm was developed to generate the muscle texture directly on the model surface, rather than by using conventional pattern mapping on to the surface. Some results are presented on the geometric modeling, the deformation and the texture of muscles related to the knee.

INTRODUCTION

Human simulation is an area which has fascinated researchers in computer graphics for many years. The associated problems are very complex, involving the definition of deformable shapes, the calculation of articulated-body motion with complex joints and the overall control of the figure within a dynamic environment.

The multifarious aspects of the problem have been tackled by many researchers, including Cohen (1992), Hodgins and Pollard (1997), Gleicher (1998), Laszlo (1996), Funge et al. (1999), Maurel and Thalmann (1999), Scheepers et al. (1997) and Wilhelms and Gelder (1997). In most of the published work, the authors have adopted very simplified models. While they may have suited the authors' purposes, these simplified models cannot truly be considered to represent the functioning of an actual body.

As technology has improved, the methods adopted to tackle the complex problems involved with body modeling have become increasingly sophisticated, and the flood of publications in this area shows no sign of abating.

A recent example by Savenko et al. (1999) adapted work by Van Sint Jan et al. (1998; 1999) on knee kinematics to create an improved joint model for figure animation that is more in keeping with newly-available biomechanics data.

If the models to be created are to represent, effectively, the full complexity of the human body, then muscle simulation is one of the fundamental areas that has to be addressed.

The structure of even a single muscle is very complex. However, muscles also stretch across joints and are arranged alongside or on top of each other, so there is regular interaction with other moving or deformable parts of the anatomy. In addition, there exists a wide variety of irregular muscle forms.

Any attempt at realistic muscle simulation should address three major problems:

- **Muscle geometry:** It is difficult to find a general graphics primitive for muscle modeling because of the large number of free-form muscle shapes. Although muscles fall into several categories, such as fusi-form, uni-pennate, bi-pennate, multi-pennate, and triangular, muscles within a category may, in fact, be quite different from one another.
- **Muscle deformation:** The form of a muscle could appear shorter and thicker when contracted, and longer and thinner when stretched. In other words, the same muscle should appear differently in different actions and poses.
- **Muscle texture:** Texture is a distinctive feature of each muscle and relates to the orientation of the muscle fibers. The textures appear quite different from one muscle to another, and the model must be capable of faithfully representing these differences.

In fact, muscle structure is so complex that it is unlikely that a general muscle model will succeed. This leads to the motivation of this work.

This chapter proposes an approach to anatomy-based muscle simulation in which the geometry, the deformation and the texture of each muscle is modeled individually according to its features. The main purpose is to bring muscle models one step closer to the real anatomical structure.

The process involved three main steps addressing the three major problems identified above.

Firstly, muscle features were extracted from the Visible Human Data to build geometric models for the muscles. Because it is very difficult to create a general model to describe all types of muscle, each muscle was individually built based on its own features. Secondly, deformation models were developed to describe the deformation of the muscle models produced in the first step. These deformations are fully controlled by the muscle model attachments on the bone, the motion of which follows the extension and flexion of the joint. Interaction between muscle models, which affects the model deformation, was also taken into account.

Thirdly, the muscle texture was generated directly on the surface of the muscle model, using curves to represent the muscle fibers. The technique of line integration through a noise field was used to color the fibers to generate the texture. This contrasts with the conventional approach of mapping a 2D image on to the surface which would be difficult to implement well in this context. The modeling of the muscle fibers in the whole volume will be another interesting, and even more challenging, problem for the future (See section Muscle Texture).

The objective of this modeling approach is to build a graphics model that is closer to the real anatomical structure than previous work. The initial focus has been on the muscle structure of the lower limb and the knee joint. In medical visualization, this is an area that has attracted more attention than any other, apart from the brain. However, the techniques could be applied equally well to modeling any other muscular structures within the body.

The remainder of this chapter is organized as follows. Related Work contains a brief overview of related work in this area. Sections Geometric Modeling and Muscle Deformation describe our work on geometric modeling, deformation and texture mapping, respectively. The results of each part of the work are provided at the end of the respective section. Section Future Research Direction includes a summary of the work and indications of future directions in which it is hoped the work will develop.

RELATED WORK

In many recently published papers, the human figure is represented using a layered model rather than a simple line-segment skeleton. Such a layered model normally has four layers, consisting of a skeleton, muscle, fatty tissue and skin.

This is an important step in the direction of anatomically-based modeling and can be found in the work of, amongst others, Chadwick et al. (1989) who presented a method for layered construction of flexible animated characters, Kalra et al. (1998) who built a single system of simulating a virtual human that allows real-time animation, Gourret et al. (1989) and Turner et al. (1993). However, none of these built each individual model in an anatomically-based way.

Other work includes that of Chen and Zeltzer (1992) who developed a finite element model to simulate the force of a few individual muscles and visualize the deformations, Maurel and Thalmann (1999) who did a case study on human upper limb modeling for dynamic simulation, which performed a biomechanics-based analysis on both skeleton and muscles, Semwal and Hallauer (1994) who modeled human muscles and bones using generalized cylinders, and Ng-Thow-Hing et al. (1998) who attempted to reconstruct muscle fiber architecture using B-spline volumes.

Our work is closer to that of Scheepers et al. (1997) and Wilhelms and Gelder (1997), in which muscles were modeled according to their anatomical structure.

Scheepers's work was motivated by an artistic study of anatomy; it used ellipsoids as the graphical primitives for the muscle belly on which a more sophisticated model was built. However, we argue that, as muscle form varies greatly, the use of any specific kind of primitive will create an artificial effect both in shape and texture.

Wilhelms and Gelder introduced a general muscle primitive, the "deformed cylinder," to model various types of muscle. Human intervention was necessary to alter the default muscle type into the particular form required in each case. The muscle deformation was greatly simplified, as the purpose was mainly to produce good visual effects.

The aim of our work is to develop a model that is not only visually accurate, but is sufficiently robust to demonstrate muscle shape and behavior for a wide variety of movements, while requiring as little intervention as possible.

Thus, while Scheepers and Wilhelms used a muscle-based model to form an inner layer in order to produce a visually-appealing skin surface, we are demanding that our model portrays accurately not only the skin surface, but also the behavior of each individual muscle.

We do not claim that the model we present here is, at the moment, totally anatomically accurate, but we do feel that it represents progress towards such a model.

Other research work relating to muscles has taken place in facial animation by authors including Platt and Badler (1981), Terzopoulos and Waters (1990) and Waters (1987). However, this work has mainly focused on the behavior of the muscle (such as the force produced) rather than its physical presence, and is thus different from our research.

GEOMETRIC MODELING

Normally, a muscle is attached to two locations through tendons on the bones. One attachment is mostly fixed and is called the *origin*, while the other is considered to be the more movable part and is termed the *insertion* (Goldfinger, 1991). For simplicity, most of our muscle models contain both the muscle bodies and their tendons in one geometric surface. This is because, from a geometric viewpoint, the tendons can be regarded as extensions of the main muscle bodies. Thus, we consider that the muscle models are attached directly to the bones.

To create the geometric model, we first find the geometric features of the muscle from well-segmented visible human data and build the models based on these features. Two advantages of this approach are that the resulting shape is very realistic and that little human intervention is required. In this section, we discuss the two key techniques relating to this issue:

- Analyzing and extracting the features from the muscles
- Modeling the muscle geometry via B-spline surfaces

Feature Analysis

We analyze the geometric features of a muscle via its cross-sectional contours in the 2D slices of the data. Within the slice, we shall require the straight line, $p = x \cos\theta + y \sin\theta$, which is defined relative to the local x-y coordinate system within the slice. Here, θ defines the line direction (see Figure 1).

For each contour, we compute the following features:

- **Area, S:** S can be computed as the number of pixels inside the contour.

- **Direction Radius, $R(\theta)$ and Diameter $D(\theta)$:** The Direction Radius $R(\theta)$ and Diameter $D(\theta)$ are, respectively, the radius and diameter along θ. They can be mathematically defined as:

Figure 1. Straight line $p = x \cos\theta + y \sin\theta$, where p is the distance from the origin to the line, θ is the line direction

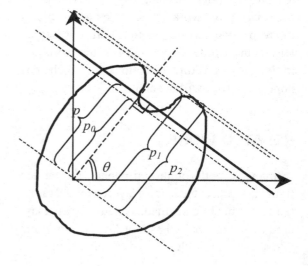

$$R(\theta) = \frac{1}{2} \int_0^\infty n(p,\theta)dp$$

$$D(\theta) = R(\theta) + \frac{1}{2} \int_0^\infty n(p,\pi+\theta)dp$$

where $n(p,\theta)$ is the number of intersections between the contour and the straight line. In this work, $R(\theta)$ is used to calculate the circumference (see below), and $D(\theta)$ in four directions, 0°, 45°, 90°, 135° is used as features.

- **Circumference, *L*:** Once we have $R(\theta)$, then L can be computed as

$$L = \int_0^{2\pi} R(\theta)d\theta$$

Again we did this in a numerical way by computing $R(\theta)d\theta$ at every 5°, and then added them together.

- **Direction Concavity, *Con*(θ):** Direction concavity can be used to measure the concavity along direction θ. If we define:

$$J(\theta) = \int_0^\infty F(p,\theta)dp + \int_0^\infty F(p,\pi+\theta)dp$$

Then:

$$Con(\theta) = D(\theta) / J(\theta)$$

where $F(p,\theta) = 1$ if the straight line intersects the contour, else $F(p,\theta) = 0$. As for $D(\theta)$, we select 4 directions of $Con(\theta)$ 0°, 45°, 90°, 135° as features.

- **General Concavity, *GCon*:** *GCon* is a general measurement of the concavity of the contour

$$GCon = L / \pi J_m$$

$$J_m = \frac{1}{2\pi} \int_0^{2\pi} J(\theta)d\theta$$

These features of a contour form a multi-dimensional vector *[S, D(0), D(45), D(90), D(135), L, Con(0), Con(45), Con(90), Con(135), GCon]*.

Based on the feature vector of each contour, we select some key contours and put them into a set, which is used for the geometric modeling at the next step. The distance between the feature vectors of two successive key contours must be beyond a pre-defined threshold.

B-Spline Expression

The geometric models are represented by cubic B-spline surfaces, the input that are the key contour sets that were built in Feature Analysis.

The problem is then: given several contours, find a B-spline control polygon mesh to fit the data.

Our solution is similar to that of Hoppe et al. (1994) and is based on subdivision. However, we use a B-spline subdivision scheme rather than Loop scheme since our goal is a B-spline representation.

As we know, subdivision can be used to create uniform and non-uniform B-splines: starting from the mesh of control points, we obtain the B-spline surface by subdividing the control mesh repeatedly. This subdivision scheme is used here to fit a B-spline surface to the key contours. The algorithm starts by initializing the mesh of control points to an ellipsoid that approximates the muscle shape, then successively employs the following steps:

- **Subdivision:** For a fixed control-point mesh, compute the B-spline subdivision (we use subdivision level 5 in practice) to produce the points $\{\bar{m}_0 \cdots \bar{m}_i\}$.
- **Matching:** For each data point $\{\bar{c}_0 \cdots \bar{c}_i\}$ on the contours, find the closest point among $\{\bar{m}_0 \cdots \bar{m}_i\}$.
- **Optimization:** Since the subdivision can be seen as a linear combination of control

points, once the contour data points { $\vec{c}_0 \cdots \vec{c}_i$ } are matched to { $\vec{m}_0 \cdots \vec{m}_i$ }, we can set up a system of linear equations, and address the problem using least-squares fitting. This creates a new control-point mesh.

We now return to step 1 and resume the whole procedure. It continues until the distance between the two data sets { $\vec{m}_0 \cdots \vec{m}_i$ } and { $\vec{c}_0 \cdots \vec{c}_i$ } is below a pre-defined threshold.

Figure 2 shows the results of the geometric modeling. Using the algorithm described in previous sections, we produce these muscle models with little human intervention.

By using the B-spline expression, the models are very concise. Table 1 indicates the size of some of the models. Also, from Figure 2 we can see that the muscle shape varies greatly from one to another. It would be very cumbersome to have to produce these manually.

Figure 2. Results of muscle modeling

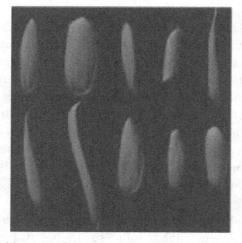

Table 1. Model sizes in terms of control points

Muscle Name	Model Size
Vastus Lateralis	10×20
Rectus Femoris	8×16
Semimembranosus	7×6
Sartorius	36×6
Soleus	10×18

MUSCLE DEFORMATION

In this section, we present the deformation of the muscle models generated in the last section. The way in which each model contracts is based on its anatomical structure, such as its shape and its attachments to the bone. We categorize these model deformations into several types and process each type separately.

Deformation is an important characteristic of a muscle. The contraction and extension of muscles generate the forces that produce the motion of the body. A muscle produces motion by pulling: when a muscle contracts, its two ends are brought closer together and the muscle belly gets shorter and thicker. Effectively, by means of this deformation, a muscle causes the motion of a joint.

However, in computer animation this problem is normally treated the other way around, with the muscle being deformed in accordance with the motion of its attachments to the bones of the joint. Our muscle deformation is also triggered by the joint motion. The flexion and extension of the joint pull the attachments of the muscle and cause it to deform.

The modeling and animation of deformable objects is an active research area in computer graphics. Maintaining precise control of the shape of a deformable object throughout an animation is frequently very challenging.

Free-form deformations (FFDs) were first proposed by Sederberg and Parry (1986), and many variations of these have been produced subsequently by various authors. The shape is controlled via a lattice of control points. An object embedded within the lattice is deformed by defining a mapping from the lattice to the object.

Lazarus et al. (1994) proposed an axial deformation, which provides a compact representation in which a one-dimensional primitive, such as a curve, is used to define a global deformation. Other work by Desbrun and Gascuel (1995), James and Pai (1999) and Noble and Clapworthy (1998) have addressed similar problems. Unfortunately, none of these techniques fulfils our requirements. They are either not suited to the muscle deformation mechanism, or their computation is too expensive for our purposes.

Our deformations are produced by moving and scaling the cross-sectional contours. It is a natural approach since the geometry of the muscle models is also defined via their cross-sectional contours (see section Geometric Modeling). A similar approach was adopted by Kalra et al. (1998), but their work deformed the whole body using the contours, while our work applies the deformation to each muscle individually.

We divide the deformation of our models into a general type and other individual cases. The general model can be applied to most of the Fusiform muscles. Separate models are applied to the muscles *Rectus Femoris, Biceps Femoris Short Head, Vastus Lateralis* and *Vastus Medialis.* The remainder of the section describes the various deformation models that were developed:

- Knee motion in terms of Biomechanics
- Deformation of quadriceps
- Deformation of hamstrings
- Deformation of Gas (Multi-Head case)

Figure 3. Semitendinosus on the skeleton

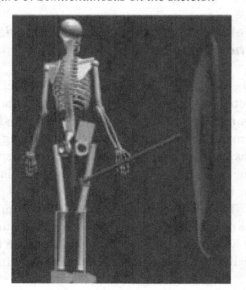

- Interaction between muscles and muscle groups (subject to papers in biomech)

General Deformation Model

For most of our muscle models, the attachments (origin and insertion) are two small areas that can be simplified into two points. We call such muscle models "Point to Point" (PP) models. Figure 3 shows an example—*Semitendinosus(ST)*, which has a long, narrow, fleshy belly. Its origin is at the point on the ischial tuberosity of the pelvis, and the insertion is in the upper part of the medial surface of the shaft of the tibia.

The deformation of a PP model is simple. It bulges when the two points come closer during contraction and becomes thinner when the two points move away during stretching.

We call the central axis of a PP muscle its spine; the curve of the spine starts at the origin and ends at the insertion. In the general deformation of a PP model, the spine curve always remains a straight line.

During deformation, each contour moves along the spine curve and also changes shape. The overall deformation here is basically in accordance with volume conservation, though no precise computation ensuring volume conservation is pursued at this stage. The volume of a muscle model over a set of contours, can be approximately expressed in terms of the areas of the contours:

$$V = \frac{length}{N-1} \times (\frac{S_0 + S_1}{2} + \frac{S_1 + S_2}{2} + \ldots\ldots\ldots)$$

where *length* is the length of the spine curve, N is the number of cross-sections, and $S_0, S_1, S_2 \ldots$ are the areas of the respective cross-sections.

Obviously, if the length increases by a factor k, the area of each cross-section should decrease to keep the volume constant. In our model, this scaling by a factor *1/k* is applied uniformly for all contours; it can be performed by scaling the B-spline control points of the contour.

Figure 4. Muscle fibers on RF surface

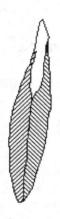

Figure 5. Deformation of the Rectus Femoris Mode:1 (a) Non-uniform deformation of a contour, (b) Deformation of spine curve & rotation of contour

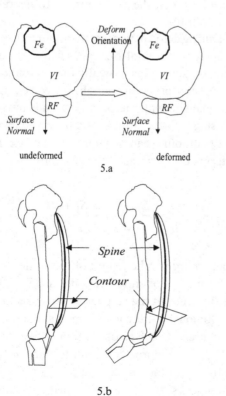

5.a

5.b

Deformation of the *Rectus Femoris* Model

Rectus Femoris (RF) starts at the anterior inferior iliac spine and goes down to the top of the patella. The deformation of RF is different from that of the PP muscles due to the different configuration of its muscle fibers, which run from the central line diagonally to the muscle edges (this is called bipennate in anatomy; see Figure 4). During contraction, they pull the muscle body towards the muscle edges and, ultimately, towards the underlying muscles.

Further, the RF spine does not remain straight when the knee joint flexes. This is because the insertion of the RF, which is at the patella, is pulled by the inelastic patellar ligament while the tibia slides around the surface of the lower end of femur, forcing the spine line to curve, as well.

Correspondingly, our RF model deforms as follows. Firstly, the contours of the RF model are not scaled uniformly during deformation. Scaling occurs only in the direction of the normal to the underlying surface, which is called *Vastus Internus* (see Figure 5a).

Secondly, each cross-sectional contour is given a small rotation due to the curve of the spine line (see Figure 5b).

Deformation of the *Biceps Femoris Short Head* Model

The *Biceps Femoris Short Head* (BFs) model has a unique geometric feature. Its origin is a line on the middle third of the back of the femur. This line remains attached to the bone (femur) during the flexion of the knee joint (see Figure 6). The spine line of the muscle starts from the upper point of the origin and runs to the insertion.

To remain consistent with the above features, we deform the model as follows: for the contours in which the muscle is attached to the origin line on the femur, the scaling pivot points remain on the line, while for the other contours, where the muscle can separate from the bone, the pivot points are on the spine line and thus move during joint action (see Figure 6).

Deformation of the *Vastus Lateralis* (VL) and *Vastus Medialis* (VM) Models

The insertions of the *Vastus Lateralis* (VL) and *Vastus Medialis* (VM) models are on either side of the patella, and their origins are two lines on the back of the femur. When the knee flexes, the patella moves around the end surface of the femur, elongating the VL and VM models. At the same time, there is also a small rotation about their origin lines.

Figure 7 illustrates the deformation of the VL model. The pulling and deformation occur almost simultaneously. We model the deformation of VL and VM models by applying the following two steps incrementally during the motion:

1. Pull the lower end of VL & VM models along the femur.
2. Rotate the VL & VM models around their origin lines.

Results of Model Deformation

Figure 8 shows results of our work on individual muscle models, including deformation of *Semitendinosus*, *Rectus Femoris*, *Biceps Femoris Short Head* and *Vastus Lateralis Models* during the flexion of the knee joint. The deformation of the whole leg will be demonstrated in a future section after further consideration of model interaction.

Interaction Between Muscle Models

The discussion above has concerned only deformations of single muscle models. In fact, the deformation of a muscle model is also affected by its surroundings. In this section, we discuss the

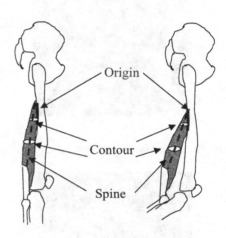

Figure 6. Deformation of the BFs Model. The thick line denotes the line of the origin.

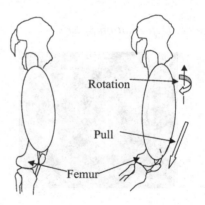

Figure 7. Deformation of the VL model

interaction between muscle models, after which we can put them together to produce a whole leg deformation.

Computing the interaction between muscle models is important, not only for deformation, but also to prevent penetration between models

Figure 8a. Deformation of ST

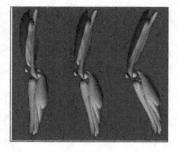

Figure 8b. Deformation of RF

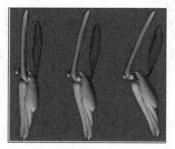

Figure 8c. Deformation of BFs

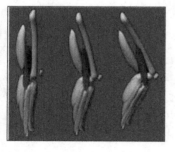

Figure 8d. Deformation of VL

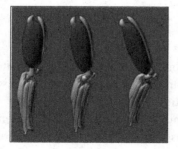

during deformation. The algorithm to compute the interaction is as follows:

After the muscle modeling, we produce a table associating with each vertex V_i on the muscle surface, the following information:

- The identity of the neighboring muscle model
- The face on this neighboring muscle model to which V_i is attached

Figure 9 illustrates two surfaces from neighboring muscle models A and B. V_i from model A is attached to the face f_i of model B. We record model B and face f_i into the table associated with V_i.

The final deformation of a muscle model relies both on its own deformation and the influence from other muscle models. We simulate the interaction between muscle models by scaling transformations.

The detailed procedure is as follows:

- Compute the deformation of all the individual models
- Detect penetration between neighboring models by checking each vertex of the muscles; the information stored at the vertex is used to find which face on which muscle to check
- If there is an interaction between 2 models, scale the models by a pre-defined factor along the primary surface normal[1], then return to the previous step
- If there is no interaction, terminate the algorithm

This approach efficiently describes the interaction between the muscle models and has been proved to work well in practice. Figure 10 is a demonstration of deformation of the whole leg model during knee flexion.

Figure 9. Computing the muscle interaction

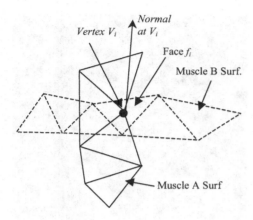

Figure 10. Deformation of leg muscles

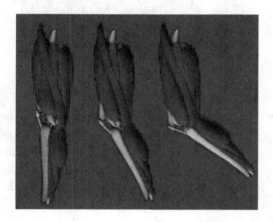

MUSCLE TEXTURE

Each muscle has a unique texture on its surface. This is an important feature, which is formed by the muscle fibers.

We can generate the texture by modeling the fibers on the muscle surface and putting colors on to these fibers. In fact, muscle fibers exist inside the whole muscle body but we model only those on the surface, since we are using surface models. This is quite different from other work on texture mapping, such as those by Bennis et al. (1991), Maillot et al. (1993), and Pedersen (1995), in which the surface is re-parameterized

and a two-dimensional picture is mapped on to it. Here, we find the orientation of the fibers on the surface, then generate the texture directly on the muscle surface. The reminder of this section will discuss:

- How to model the muscle fibers on the surface
- How to color the fibers to produce the texture

Modeling of Muscle Fibers

We model the muscle fibers on the surface using curves. These curves are from a start line and run to an end line. For most of our muscle models, we use the line of the origin as the start and the line of the insertion as the end. But there are several exceptions, such as RF, in which we define the start and end lines manually.

Interpolating curves on a 3D surface remains an active area of research. Many authors have addressed this problem extensively, for instance, Welch and Witkin (1992) and Kimmel et al. (1994). However, most of the methods described are expensive, both to compute and to maintain. Since there are so many fibers on the muscle surface, we sought a quick and efficient algorithm to address this problem. We first obtain a rough estimate and then refine it using the following procedure:

Project the straight line joining the two points (the dashed line P_0P_1 in Figure 11) on to the surface to create an initial curve. The key problem here is to find the faces on to which the line is projected. This is done as follows: we first find the greedy graph path, (see Figure 11, the bold line is the graph path between points P_0 and P_1), then find the projection of P_0P_1 among the faces adjacent to the graph path. For instance, in Figure 11, the projection is found among faces *B, C, D, E, F, I*, which are along the greedy graph path. The result is a curve that consists of a set of successive face points (see black points in Figure 11). This curve is a good guess for the geodesic.

Figure 11. Finding the curve between P_0 and P_1 by projecting the line on to the surface

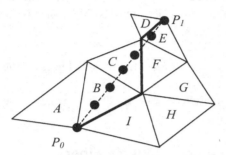

Figure 12. Texture of the leg muscle models

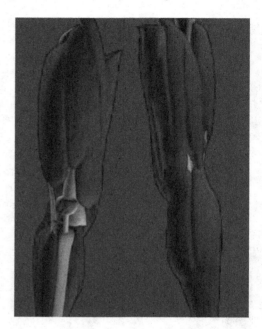

Using the initial sampled geodesic points, find the curve passing through these points that has minimum length. Perform this as follows: for each sample p_i along the curve, the midpoint between two adjacent samples is first projected on to the tangent plane through p_i, and then projected back towards the surface. This is similar to the work of Pedersen (1995), but with the difference that we project the point on to the surface rather than calculate the feedback formula.

Texture Color

To produce the texture using the curves generated above, we use a vector field visualization technique, which performs convolution along the curve over a white noise field. We begin by setting up a white noise field on the muscle surface, then we integrate along the fiber curves over the white noise field. This generates the texture directly on to the muscle surface. The complete algorithm for computing the muscle texture is, as follows:

- Consider N data points on the lines of the start and the end; each point at the start line is to be used as a starting point of a muscle fiber that ends at one point on the end line.
- Generate N curves on the surface connecting corresponding points on the start and end lines using the method described in section Modeling of Muscle Fibers.

- Create a *u-v* iso-parametric grid on the muscle surface and compute the direction of muscle fiber at each grid point by interpolating the tangents of the curves generated in step 2; this results in a vector field on the muscle surface.
- Compute the color for each grid point *(u,v)* by convolution over a white noise field. It starts from the grid point and performs the integration in the vector field produced in step 3. At each step in the integral, re-sample the white noise and sum it. Finally, save the result as the color contributing to point *(u,v)*.

An example of muscle texture produced by this method is shown in Figure 12.

FUTURE RESEARCH DIRECTION

We feel that we are now well placed to extend the work to consider more advanced issues, with particular emphasis on muscle deformation and interaction.

In co-operation with the biomechanicians, we shall extend our current work to the biomechanical context, so as to contribute to motion analysis and understanding. For example, we shall measure the muscle movement on real subjects to compare with our deformation model and, if necessary, we shall update the model to accommodate the new medical evidence. Other muscle functions, such as producing force without joint movement, will also be under investigation.

Work will be undertaken to improve the muscle interaction, for instance, taking the muscle material and dynamics into account, and to speed up the collision testing and response. We also wish to include more medical detail in the rendering of the bones, tendons and muscles.

Reflecting our desire to improve authenticity, we shall also consider replacing the surface muscle models by volumetric muscle models. The main advantage of a volumetric model over a surface model is that it can exhibit a greater variation of muscle-fiber orientations within the muscle volume, which is important for the way in which muscles contract. Also, collision detection is easier under a volumetric scheme.

CONCLUSION

This chapter describes a general approach to human muscle simulation. It is anatomically-based work in which we attempt to deal with each muscle based on its individual anatomical features, so it is representative of the real morphological structure. The purpose of this chapter is not only to achieve a good visual result, but also to provide a good base from which to produce a more comprehensive human model with greater medical accuracy in the future.

Feature-based modeling extracts the features from well-segmented anatomical data to establish the muscle models. This is a simple way to set up realistic muscle models with little human labor; it produces realistic-looking muscle models across the whole range of muscle types and retains the correct anatomical structures for all the muscles.

The work on muscle deformation simulates the model contractions based on their features. The model developed is not simply a general deformation model, but it also takes into account special cases, based on their particular features. We believe that this step is necessary as muscle simulation is too complex for a general model to work well. The effects of interaction between muscles have been included.

Muscle texture is produced directly on the surface by generating curves on the surface and using line integration over a white noise field. This produces a good simulation to the actual muscle texture. Some experimental results have been presented.

We believe that the work in this chapter brings us one step closer to realistic human modeling. We feel that we are now well placed to extend the work to consider more advanced issues, such as volumetric modeling of muscle and tendon fibers, the configuration of which exhibits great variation within the muscle volume amongst the various muscles. This issue is interesting not only because modeling the complicated configuration is a challenge, but also because fiber orientation is important to the way in which a muscle contracts.

REFERENCES

Bennis, C., Vezien, J., & Iglesias, G. (1991). Piecewise surface flattening for non-distorted texture mapping. *Computer Graphics, 25*, 237-246.

Chadwick, J., Haumann, D., & Parent, R. (1989). Layered construction for deformable animated characters. *Computer Graphics, 23*, 243-252.

Chen, D., & Zeltzer, D. (1992). Pump it up: Computer animation of a biomechanically-based model of muscle using the finite element method. *Computer Graphics, 26*(2), 89-98.\

Cohen, M. (1992). Interactive spacetime control for animation. *Computer Graphics Proceedings, 26*(2), 293-302.

Desbrun, M., & Gascuel, M-P. (1995). Animating soft substances with implicit surfaces. *Proceedings of SIGGRAPH'95,* (pp. 287-290).

Funge, J., Tu, X., & Terzopoulos, D. (1999). Cognitive modeling: Knowledge, reasoning and planning for intelligent characters. *Proceedings of SIGGRAPH'99,* (pp. 29-38).

Gleicher, M. (1998). Retargeting motion to new characters. *Proceedings of SIGGRAPH'98,* (pp. 33-42).

Goldfinger, E. (1991). *Human anatomy for artists.* New York, NY, Oxford: Oxford University Press.

Gourret, J., Magnenat Thalmann, N., & Thalmann, D. (1989). Simulation of object and human skin deformations in a grasping task. *Computer Graphics, 23,* 21-30.

Hodgins, J., & Pollard, N. (1997). Adapting simulated behaviors for new characters. *Proceeding of SIGGRAPH'97,* (pp. 153-162).

Hoppe, H., DeRose, T., Duchamp, T., Halstead, M., Jin, H., McDonald, J., et al. (1994). Piecewise smooth surface reconstruction. *Proceedings of SIGGRAPH'94,* (pp. 295-302).

James, D., & Pai, D. (1999). ArtDefo: Accurate real-time deformable objects. *Proceedings of SIGGRAPH'99,* (pp. 65-72).

Kalra, P., Magnenat Thalmann, N., Moccozet, L., Sannier, G., Aubel, A., & Thalmann, D. (1998). Real-time animation of realistic virtual humans. *IEEE Computer Graphics and Applications, 18*(5), 42-55.

Kimmel, R., Amir, A., & Bruckstein, A. (1994). Finding shortest paths on surfaces. In: P-J. Laurent

(Ed.), *Curves and surfaces in geometric design,* (pp. 259-268). Wellesley, MA: A.K. Peters.

Laszlo, J. (1996). Limit cycle control and its application to the animation of balancing and walking. *Proceeding of SIGGRAPH'96,* (pp. 155-162).

Lazarus, F., Coquillart, S., & Jancene, P. (1994). Axial deformations: An intuitive deformation technique. *Computer-Aided Design, 26*(8), 607-613.

Maillot, J., Yahia, H., & Verroust, A. (1993). Interactive texture mapping. *Computer Graphics, 27,* 27-34.

Maurel, W., & Thalmann, D. (1999). A case study analysis on human upper limb modeling for dynamic simulation. *Journal of Computer Methods in Biomechanics and Biomechanical Engineering, 2*(1), 65-82.

Ng-Thow-Hing, V. (1998). Reconstruction of multiple regions of muscle fiber architecture using B-Spline solid models. *Proceedings of NACOB'98,* the Third North American Congress on Biomechanics, (pp. 219-220).

Noble, R., & Clapworthy, G. (1998). Sculpting & animating in a desktop VR environment. *Proceedings of Computer Graphics International '98,* (pp. 187-195). Hanover (Germany), IEEE Computer Society Press.

Pedersen, H. (1995). Decorating implicit surface. *Proceedings of the SIGGRAPH'95,* (pp. 291-300).

Pierrynowski, M. (1995). Analytic representation of muscle line of action and geometry. In: P. Allard, I. Stokes, J. Blanchi, (Eds.), *Three-dimensional analysis of human movement.* Human Kineticss, (chap. 11, pp. 215-256).

Platt, S., & Badler, N. (1981). Animating facial expressions. *Computer Graphics, 15*(3), 245-252.

Savenko, A., Van Sint Jan, S., & Clapworthy, G. (1999). A biomechanics-based model for the animation of human locomotion. *Proceedings of GraphiCon '99,* (pp. 82-87). Moscow: Dialog-MGU Press.

Scheepers, F., Parent, R., Carlson, W., & May, S. (1997). Anatomy-based modeling of the human musculature. *Proceedings of SIGGRAPH'97,* (pp. 163-172).

Sederberg, T., & Parry, S. (1986). Free-form deformation of solid geometric models. *Computer Graphics, 20,* 151-160.

Semwal, S., & Hallauer, J. (1994). Biomechanical modeling: Implementation line-of-action algorithm for human muscles and bones using generalized cylinders. *Computers & Graphics, 18*(1), 105-112.

Terzopoulos, D., & Waters, K. (1990). Physically-based facial modeling, analysis and animation. *Journal of Visualization and Computer Animation, 1*(2), 73-80.

Turner, R., & Thalmann, D. (1993). The Elastic Surface Layer Model for animated character construction. In: N. Magnenat-Thalmann & D. Thalmann, (Eds.), *Communicating with virtual worlds,* (pp. 399-412). Springer Verlag.

Van Sint Jan, S., Clapworthy, G., & Rooze, M. (1998). Visualization of combined motions in human joints. *IEEE Computer Graphics & Applications, 18*(6), 10-14.

Van Sint Jan, S., Salvia, P., Clapworthy, G., & Rooze, M. (1999). Joint-motion visualization using both medical imaging and 3D-electrogoniometry. *Proceedings of the 17th Congress International Society of Biomechanics.* Calgary (Canada).

Waters, K. (1987). A muscle model for animating three-dimensional facial expression. *Computer Graphics, 21*(4), 17-24.

Welch, W., & Witkin, A. (1992). Variational surface modeling. *Computer Graphics, 26,* 157-166

Wilhelms, J., & Gelder, A. (1997). Anatomically-based modeling. *Proceedings of SIGGRAPH'97,* (pp. 173-180).

Additional Reading

Allbeck, J., & Badler, N. (2006). Automated analysis of human factors requirements. *Proceedings of the 2006 Digital Human Modeling for Design and Engineering Conference,* Document 2001-01-2366.

Badler, N., Allbeck, J., Lee, S., Rabbitz, R., Broderick, T., & Mulkern, K. (2005). New behavioral paradigms for virtual human models. *Proceedings of the SAE International Digital Human Modeling for Design and Engineering.*

Badler, N., Allbeck, J., Megahed, A., & Whitmore, M. (2006). RIVET: Rapid interactive visualization for extensible training. *Habitation 2006.* Orlando, FL.

Cavazza, M., Earnshaw, R., Magnenat-Thalmann, N., & Thalmann, D. (1998). Motion control of virtual humans. *IEEE Computer Graphics and Applications, 18*(5), 24-31.

Emering, L., Boulic, R., Molet, T., & Thalmann, D. (2000). Versatile tuning of humanoid agent activity. *Computer Graphics Forum, 19*(4), 231-242.

Gilles, B., Perrin, R., Magnenat-Thalmann, N., & Vallée, J. (2005). Bones motion analysis from dynamic MRI: Acquisition and tracking. *Academic Radiology, 12*(10), 2385-2392.

Gu, E., & Badler, N. (2006). Visual attention and eye gaze during multi-party conversations with distractions. *Lecture Notes in Computer Science,* (vol. 4133, pp. 193-204).

Gu, E., Stocker, C., & Badler, N. (2005). Do you see what eyes see? Implementing inattentional blindness. *Lecture Notes in Computer Science,* (vol. 3661), Intelligent Virtual Agents, (pp. 178-190).

Gu, E., Wang, J., & Badler, N. (2005). Generating sequence of eye fixations using decision-theoretic attention model. *Proceedings of the International Workshop on Attention and Performance in Computational Vision (WAPCV), in conjuction with CVPR*. San Diego, CA.

Molet, T., Boulic, R., Rezzonico, S., & Thalmann, D. (1999). An architecture for immersive evaluation of complex human tasks. *IEEE Transactions on Robotics and Automation, 15*(3), 475-485.

Molet, T., Boulic, R., & Thalmann, D. (1999). Human motion capture driven by orientation measurements. *Presence, MIT, 8*(2), 187-203.

Oh, S., Kim, H., Magnenat-Thalmann, N., & Wohn, K. (2005). Generating unified model for dressed virtual humans. Visual Comput, *21*(8), 522-531.

Pelechano, N., & Badler, N. (2006). Modeling crowd and trained leader behavior during building evacuation. *IEEE Computer Graphics and Applications, 26*(6), 80-86.

Pelechano, N., O'Brien, K., Silverman, B., & Badler, N. (2005). Crowd simulation incorporating agent psychological models, roles and communication. *First International Workshop on Crowd Simulation (V-CROWDS '05)*, (pp. 24-25). Lausanne (Switzerland).

Yahia-Cherif, L., Gilles, B., Molet, T., & Magnenat-Thalmann, T. (2004). Motion capture and visualization of the hip joint with dynamic MRI and optical systems. *Computer Animation and Virtual Worlds, 15*(3-4), 377-385.

Zhang, Y., & Badler, N. (2006). Synthesis of 3D faces using region-based morphing under intuitive control. *Proceedings of the Computer Animation and Social Agents (CASA); Computer Animation and Virtual Worlds (CAVW) Journal.*

Zhao, L., & Badler, N. (2005). Acquiring and validating motion qualities from live limb gestures. *Graphical Models, 67*(1), 1-16.

Zhao, L., Liu, Y., & Badler, N. (2005). Applying empirical data on upper torso movement to real-time collision-free reach tasks. *Proceedings of the SAE International Digital Human Modeling for Design and Engineering.*

Allbeck, J., & Badler, N. (2006). Automated analysis of human factors requirements. *Proceedings of the 2006 Digital Human Modeling for Design and Engineering Conference,* Document 2001-01-2366.

Badler, N., Allbeck, J., Lee, S., Rabbitz, R., Broderick, T., & Mulkern, K. (2005). New behavioral paradigms for virtual human models. *Proceedings of the SAE International Digital Human Modeling for Design and Engineering.*

Badler, N., Allbeck, J., Megahed, A., & Whitmore, M. (2006). RIVET: Rapid interactive visualization for extensible training. *Habitation 2006.* Orlando, FL.

Cavazza, M., Earnshaw, R., Magnenat-Thalmann, N., & Thalmann, D. (1998). Motion control of virtual humans. *IEEE Computer Graphics and Applications, 18*(5), 24-31.

Emering, L., Boulic, R., Molet, T., & Thalmann, D. (2000). Versatile tuning of humanoid agent activity. *Computer Graphics Forum, 19*(4), 231-242.

Gilles, B., Perrin, R., Magnenat-Thalmann, N., & Vallée, J. (2005). Bones motion analysis from dynamic MRI: Acquisition and tracking. *Academic Radiology, 12*(10), 2385-2392.

Gu, E., & Badler, N. (2006). Visual attention and eye gaze during multi-party conversations with distractions. *Lecture Notes in Computer Science,* (vol. 4133, pp. 193-204).

Gu, E., Stocker, C., & Badler, N. (2005). Do you see what eyes see? Implementing inattentional blindness. *Lecture Notes in Computer Science,* (vol. 3661), Intelligent Virtual Agents, (pp. 178-190).

Gu, E., Wang, J., & Badler, N. (2005). Generating sequence of eye fixations using decision-theoretic attention model. *Proceedings of the International Workshop on Attention and Performance in Computational Vision (WAPCV), in conjuction with CVPR*. San Diego, CA.

Molet, T., Boulic, R., Rezzonico, S., & Thalmann, D. (1999). An architecture for immersive evaluation of complex human tasks. *IEEE Transactions on Robotics and Automation, 15*(3), 475-485.

Molet, T., Boulic, R., & Thalmann, D. (1999). Human motion capture driven by orientation measurements. *Presence, MIT, 8*(2), 187-203.

Oh, S., Kim, H., Magnenat-Thalmann, N., & Wohn, K. (2005). Generating unified model for dressed virtual humans. Visual Comput, *21*(8), 522-531.

Pelechano, N., & Badler, N. (2006). Modeling crowd and trained leader behavior during building evacuation. *IEEE Computer Graphics and Applications, 26*(6), 80-86.

Pelechano, N., O'Brien, K., Silverman, B., & Badler, N. (2005). Crowd simulation incorporating agent psychological models, roles and communication. *First International Workshop on Crowd Simulation (V-CROWDS '05)*, (pp. 24-25). Lausanne (Switzerland).

Yahia-Cherif, L., Gilles, B., Molet, T., & Magnenat-Thalmann, T. (2004). Motion capture and visualization of the hip joint with dynamic MRI and optical systems. *Computer Animation and Virtual Worlds, 15*(3-4), 377-385.

Zhang, Y., & Badler, N. (2006). Synthesis of 3D faces using region-based morphing under intuitive control. *Proceedings of the Computer Animation and Social Agents (CASA); Computer Animation and Virtual Worlds (CAVW) Journal*.

Zhao, L., & Badler, N. (2005). Acquiring and validating motion qualities from live limb gestures. *Graphical Models, 67*(1), 1-16.

Zhao, L., Liu, Y., & Badler, N. (2005). Applying empirical data on upper torso movement to real-time collision-free reach tasks. *Proceedings of the SAE International Digital Human Modeling for Design and Engineering*.

ENDNOTE

[1] The primary surface normal is the major direction of the common surface between the two muscles.

Chapter XIII
Image Segmentation

Dongbin Chen
Brunel University, UK

ABSTRACT

This chapter introduces image segment techniques. These techniques, including pixel- based approaches, region-based approaches, classification techniques, deformable model algorithms, artificial neural network approaches and texture-based algorithms are detailed. Color image segmentations and 3D image segment methods are briefly introduced. With developments of computer and medical imaging techniques, there is an increase in demand of new segment algorithms for developing or upgrading medical image systems. Therefore, the author hopes that this chapter not only details the current segment techniques, but also assists researchers in quickly selecting their research directions under their applications, imaging modality, image features and other factors.

INTRODUCTION

Image segmentation is the process that divides an image into regions corresponded to similarly characteristic objects in the scene. Image segmentation is a kind of image representation. Image segmentation is one of the most important methods in image analysis or understanding since interested objects or features are extracted at segmentation.

Image segmentation algorithms can most widely be divided into two classes as pixel- based segment algorithms and region-based segmentation algorithms. Region-based segmentation algorithms assign pixels to a certain region by taking local image properties into account. It is to analyze the neighborhood of a pixel for the occurrence of properties that cluster for a region. Searching regions of similar image properties uses two methods. These are pixel classification and boundary determination. Pixel classification is generally called a region growing process, which method is to select a seed pixel in an of-interest region and then to expand it in all directions until the properties of the image change. The boundary of the image is found implicitly by this method.

The boundary determination is explicitly aimed at locating the boundary of an image initially. Then, the located boundary implicitly determines its region. The two kinds of image segmentation algorithms have their own advantages in different applications. Sometimes, a combined algorithm is most adequate.

In practice, performances of segment algorithms vary depending on the private application, imaging modality, and other factors. General imaging artifacts, such as noise, partial volume effects, and motion, also have significant consequences on the performances of segment algorithms. Furthermore, applications of each imaging modality have its own advantages. There is not any segment method that produces acceptable results for every medical image. Segment algorithms were developed for applying to different kinds of images. However, methods developed for particular applications often achieve better performances, especially when taking into account prior knowledge. It is therefore difficult to select an appropriate segment approach to a kind of image and an application. Analysis of the image features in advance and trials with different algorithms are needed during the select process.

This chapter provides an overview of various segment techniques. Traditional robust methods such as pixel-based approaches, region-based techniques and texture-based segmentations are detailed. Segment algorithms for manipulating medical images, which include classification approaches, artificial neural network techniques, deformable model algorithms and atlas-guided medical image segmentations, are briefly described. These methods only concern to the very commonly radiological modalities, such as magnetic resonance imaging (MRI), x-ray-computed tomography (CT), ultrasound imaging, and x-ray projection radiography. Of course, these algorithms may also be applied to other imaging modalities.

PIXEL-BASED SEGMENTATION

Image segmentation only-based pixel values have different mature approaches. The common and robust algorithms are from selecting the best intensity threshold by an analysis of the grey level histogram. The size of the segmented objects varies with the threshold value. The approaches can give very good results when the background is uniformly illuminated and the objects to be segmented have distinct ranges of intensity. The key of these segmentation algorithms is how to automatically obtain a threshold value from the grey level histogram in an image.

Adapted Threshold Algorithm

Automatic image segmentation algorithm based on an adapted threshold defines the threshold of the pixel values in the image, which hopefully divides the image into two regions, background and foreground. The success of histogram threshold depends entirely on the separability of the grey level bands in the histogram and of the spatial occurrence of the grey levels. Otsu (1979) used a clustered analysis to calculate automatically the threshold from the histogram of the image, and then used this threshold to binary the image. Suppose that the original image is f (x, y), its binary image is g (x, y) and threshold value is T. The automatic image segmentation algorithm based on a histogram threshold consists of the following six steps:

1. Calculates the grey value histogram of f (x, y). It is defined as h (i).
2. Computes the grey level average μ_T.

$$\mu_T = \sum_{i=0}^{255} ih(i) \qquad (1)$$

3. Calculates the zero order moment ω (k) and first order moment μ (k). Here, k is a series of integers from 0 to 255.

$$\omega(k) = \sum_{i=0}^{k} h(i) \qquad (2)$$

$$\mu(k) = \sum_{i=0}^{k} ih(i) \qquad (3)$$

4. Calculates the clustering function σ_B (k) by the equation (4). Here, k is the same as the above k.

$$\sigma_B(k) = \frac{\left[\mu_T\omega(k) - \mu(k)\right]^2}{\omega(k)\left[1 - \omega(k)\right]} \qquad (4)$$

5. Searching the maximum value of σ_B (k). The k that corresponds to the maximum value σ_B (k) is the adapted threshold T in the image.

6. Using the threshold T to binary the image f (x, y). The output segmented image g (x, y) is given by:

$$g(x,y) = 255, f(x,y) \geq T$$
$$g(x,y) = 0, f(x,y) < T \qquad (5)$$

The above procedure is easily generalized as a computer program so that the resulting image of the segment algorithm can be watched and valued.

Optimal Threshold Algorithm

The histogram of an image can be considered as an estimate of the grey level probability density function, p(x). The overall density function is considered as the sum or mixture of two class densities, which one class belongs to the foreground and another class is presented as background in the image. The mixture parameters are, furthermore, proportional to the areas of the image of each grey level. When the form of the densities is known, a threshold can be determined by an optimal process. This threshold then segments the image into two regions.

Suppose that an image has two grey levels combined with additive Gaussian noise. The mixture probability density function is given as:

$$p(x) = p_1 p_1(x) + p_2 p_2(x) \qquad (6)$$

For the Gaussian case, see equation 7 in Box 1.

In equation 7 μ_1 and μ_2 are the mean values of the two grey levels respectively. σ_1 and σ_2 are the standard deviations about these means respectively. p_1 and p_2 are the priori probabilities of the two grey levels. Since the constraint is

$$p_1 + p_2 = 1 \qquad (8)$$

When the five unknown parameters of the mixture density are obtained, the threshold is then determined.

Suppose that a threshold, T, divides the image into background with grey levels below T and foreground with grey levels above T. The probability of classifying a foreground point as a background point by threshold, T, is

$$E_1(T) = \int_{-\infty}^{T} p_2(x) dx \qquad (9)$$

Similarly, the probability of classifying a background point as a foreground point by the threshold, T, is

$$E_2(T) = \int_{T}^{\infty} p_1(x) dx \qquad (10)$$

Therefore, the overall probability of error is detailed by

Box 1.

$$p(x) = \frac{p_1}{\sqrt{2\pi}\sigma_1} \exp\left[-\frac{(x-\mu_1)^2}{2\sigma_1^2}\right] + \frac{p_2}{\sqrt{2\pi}\sigma_{21}} \exp\left[-\frac{(x-\mu_2)^2}{2\sigma_2^2}\right] \qquad (7)$$

$$E(T) = p_2 E_1(T) + p_1 E_2(T) \qquad (11)$$

When this error is minimal, the threshold, T, is considered as the optimal threshold. Therefore the E(T) is differentiated and equates to 0. We have

$$p_1 p_1(T) = p_2 p_2(T) \qquad (12)$$

applying the above result to Gaussian density. After taking logarithms and simplifying, we obtain the following quadratic equation.

$$AT^2 + BT + C = 0 \qquad (13)$$

Here

$$A = \sigma_1^2 - \sigma_2^2 \qquad (14)$$
$$B = 2(\mu_1 \sigma_2^2 - \mu_2 \sigma_1^2)$$
$$C = \mu_2^2 \sigma_1^2 - \mu_1^2 \sigma_2^2 + 2\sigma_1^2 \sigma_2^2 \ln(\frac{\sigma_2 p_1}{\sigma_1 p_2})$$

When the variances are equal, we have

$$\sigma^2 = \sigma_1^2 = \sigma_2^2 \qquad (15)$$

Therefore, the optimal threshold is obtained by

$$T = \frac{\mu_1 + \mu_2}{2} + \frac{\sigma^2}{\mu_1 - \mu_2} \ln(\frac{p_2}{p_1}) \qquad (16)$$

Finally, the optimal threshold, T, segments the image as a binary image.

Discussion of Pixel-Based Segmentation

Figure 1-(a) is an original CT head image. It is selected to test the performances of the introduced algorithms and manual methods. The results are shown from Figure 1-(b) to 1-(f). Generally, manual methods for image segmentations give better segment results than automatic image segmentation algorithms. Depending on the

threshold selected by users, each interested part can be segmented, such as Figure 1-(d), 1-(e) and 1-(f). In practice, automatic image segmentation algorithms are more useful than manual methods. Automatic image segmentation algorithm based on adapted histogram threshold is certainly one of the most reliable when it is feasible. Another advantage is that these algorithms are not too complex.

REGION-BASED SEGMENTATION

Segmentation means that an image is divided into regions, which have similar pixel properties, such as intensity, color or texture. Region-based segmentation techniques use image features to find the regions directly. Since this technique is based on regional features or information, many segment algorithms developed for medical image applications come from the source of the technique.

Region Growing by Pixel Aggregation

Region growing is a procedure that divides either pixels into groups or sub-regions into larger regions. Pixel aggregation technique starts with a set of seed pixels and from these grow regions by appending to each seed pixel those neighboring pixels that have similar properties, such as grey value, color or texture.

The above procedure is simply illustrated below. Consider Figure 2-(a), for example, the synthetic image, size 5×5 pixels, contains nine different grey values. Let the pixels with coordinates (3, 2) and (3, 4) be used as seeds. Using two starting pixels produces to a segmentation consisting of two regions, R_1 and R_2, in which R_1 associates with seed (3, 2) and R_2 associates with seed (3, 4). The property, P, used to include a pixel in either region is that the absolute difference between the grey value of that pixel and the grey

Figure 1. (a) Is an original CT head image; (b) is the segment result by Otsu's algorithm; (c) is the segment result by the optimal threshold algorithm; (d) is the segment result by manual approach with the threshold, 122; (e) is the segment result by manual approach with the threshold,116; (f) is the segment result by manual approach with the threshold, 52

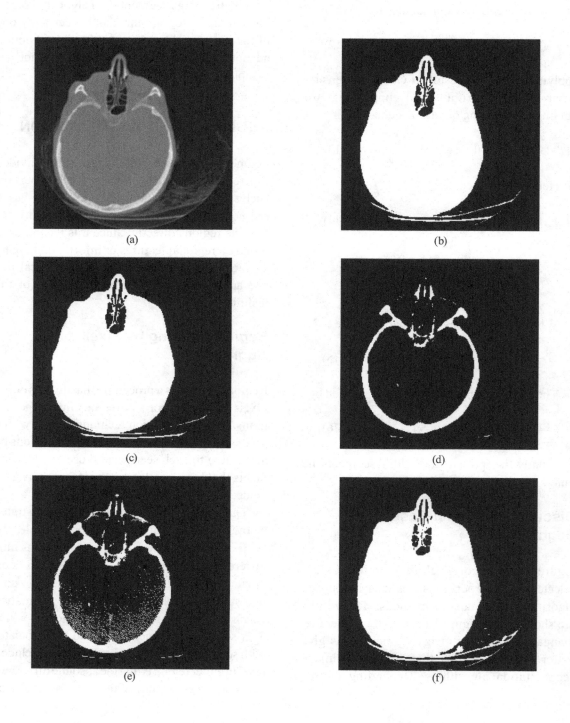

Figure 2. (a) Is an original image; (b) is the segment result with the threshold, 3; (c) is the segment result with the threshold, 8

	1	2	3	4	5
1	0	0	5	6	7
2	1	1	5	8	8
3	1	2	6	7	7
4	1	1	7	5	6
5	0	1	5	7	6

(a)

10	10	20	20	20
10	10	20	20	20
10	10	20	20	20
10	10	20	20	20
10	10	20	20	20

(b)

10	10	10	10	10
10	10	10	10	10
10	10	10	10	10
10	10	10	10	10
10	10	10	10	10

(c)

value of the seed be less than a threshold, T. Any pixel that satisfies this property simultaneously for both seeds is assigned to region R_1. The result obtained using T = 3 is shown in Figure 2-(b). In this case, the segmentation consists of two regions, in which the pixels in R_1 are denoted by 10s and the pixels in R_2 are denoted by 20s. Any starting pixel in either of these two resulting regions yields the same result. Note that it is important to this algorithm that thresholds should be selected properly. Otherwise, this algorithm may segment an unwanted result. For example, if we select a threshold, T = 8, a single region, as shown in Figure 2-(c), results from Figure 2-(a).

The preceding simple example shows us some important problems in region growing. Two critical problems are the selection of initial seeds that properly represent regions of interest, and the selection of suitable properties for including pixels in the various regions during the growing process. Selecting a set of starting pixels can often be based on the nature of the problem. When a priori information is not available, one may proceed, by computing at every pixel, the same set of properties that will ultimately be used to assign pixels to regions during the growing process. If the result of this computation shows clusters of values, the pixels whose properties place them near the centroid of these clusters can then be applied as seeds. For instance, in the example given above, a grey value histogram shows that

pixels with intensity of 1 and 7 are the most predominant.

The selection of similarity criteria is dependent on not only the problem under consideration, but also the type of image features. For example, the analysis of medical CT imagery is mainly dependent on the use of texture. This problem is more difficult to handle by using low-resolution images. Region analysis must use a set of descriptors based on intensity and spatial properties of a single image source, such as moment or texture.

There are typical regional descriptors, topological descriptors, texture descriptors and similarity descriptors. Topological properties are applied to global descriptions of regions in the image plane. It is defined as that topology in the study of properties of a figure that are unaffected by any deformation, as long as there is no tearing or joining of the figure. Another topological property used for region description is the number of connected components. A connected component of a set is a subset of maximal size such that any two of its points can be joined by a connected curve lying entirely within the subset.

An important approach to region description in medical image application is to quantify its texture content. Although no formal definition of texture exists, texture descriptors often come from a measure of properties, such as smoothness, coarseness, orientation, spatial patterns and frequency features. The three principal techniques applied in image processing to describe the texture of a region are statistical, structural and spectral. Statistical approaches produce characterizations of textures as smooth, coarse, grainy and so on. Structural techniques yield the arrangement of image primitives, such as the description of texture based on regularly spaced parallel lines. Spectral approaches are based on properties of the Fourier spectrum and are used primarily to detect global periodicity in an image by identifying high-energy, narrow peaks in the spectrum.

It is important to note that descriptors alone can produce misleading results if connectivity or adjacency information is not used in the region growing process. An illustration of this is visualized by considering a random arrangement of pixels with only three distinct intensity values. Grouping pixels with the same intensity to form a region without paying attention to connectivity would produce a segmentation result that is meaningless in the context.

Another important problem in region growing is the formulation of a stopping rule. Basically, a growing region is stopped when no more pixels satisfy the criteria for inclusion in that region. The criteria such as intensity, texture and color, are local in nature and do not take into account the history of a region growth. Additional criteria can increase the power of a region-growing algorithm, which incorporate the concept size, likeness between the intensity of a candidate pixel and the average intensity of the region, and the shape of a given region being grown. The use of these types of descriptors is based on the assumption that a model of expected results is at least partially available.

CLASSIFICATION APPROACHES

Classification approaches are pattern recognition techniques that search for partition: a feature space derived from the image using data with known labels. A feature space is the range space of any function of the image, which has the most common feature space of the image intensities. For example, a grey value histogram is a typical 1D feature space. Classification techniques are known as supervised methods since they require training data that are manually segmented and then used as references for automatically segmenting new data. There are a number of ways in which training data can be applied in classification methods.

Classifications require clearly marked features to label training data. Classifications then transfer these labels to new data as long as the feature space sufficiently distinguishes each label as well. They can be applied to multi-channel images.

Correlation Techniques

Measures of correlation may be established at various levels of complexity in an image, ranging from the trivial case of comparing two pixels to the highly complex problem of determining in a meaningful way. Once features are identified in both regions, they can be measured using a number of different methods. A simple technique is to compute the correlation between a small window of pixels centered around the feature and a same size window centered around every potential similar feature in the image. The feature with enough correlation is considered as the similarity.

Depending on different applications, many image features can be used in this technique, such as mean, variance, moment, energy, entropy, skewness or kurtosis. Based on the correlation coefficient method, suppose that a kind of image feature is defined as $f_1(x, y)$, and $f_2(x, y)$ represents the same feature of a sample.

The correlation between two features, $f_1(x, y)$ and $f_2(x, y)$ is given by

$$r(m, n) = \sum_{x, y \in s} f_1(x, y) f_2(x - m, y - n) \quad (17)$$

Where s represents the pixels in the window. Typical window sizes range from 3×3 to 15×15

pixels. The size of $f_1(x, y)$ is M × N and the $f_2(x, y)$ is interested sample with the typical window size. When under m = 0,1,2,...,M-1, n = 0,1,2,....,N-1, the $f_2(x, y)$ moves around the $f_1(x, y)$, we obtain the summation of r(m, n). The values of r(m, n) indicates a difference that the feature $f_1(x, y)$ where (x, y) is the similar to $f_2(x, y)$.

Consider features of two positions as an image, f_1, and a sample, f_2. Let the pair of candidate features to be similar have a disparity of (d_x, d_y). Then a measure of similarity between the two positions around the features is given by the correlation coefficient r (d_x, d_y) defined as shown in Box 2.

In Box 2 $\overline{f}_1$ and $\overline{f}_2$ are the average features of the pixels in the two positions being compared and the summations are carried out over all pixels within small windows centered around the feature points.

Using the group of correlation values or correlation coefficients, a classification is curried out by setting a threshold in between them.

Bayesian Classification

From Bayesian theory, it is the minimum of the product between the image prior and the conditional probability of the image given segmentation. Probabilistic segmentation simultaneously addresses the problems of spectral overlap and of mixed pixels, particularly for natural vegetation. When a pixel with feature vector x is given, Bayesian classifiers compute the posterior probability $p(C_i | x)$ for each class C_i (i = 1.. N) by the Bayesian formula, in which the pixel belongs to that class.

$$p(C_i|x) = \frac{p(x|C_i) \times p(C_i)}{p(x)} \qquad (22)$$

Here, the $p(x | C_i)$ is the conditional probability to find feature vector x within class C_i. This probability is estimated by analyzing samples of C_i, pixels that the user designated as belonging to class C_i during the training stage of the classification. The collection of estimates of this probability for each feature vector x determines the probably density function of a class.

The $p(C_i)$ is the prior probability for class C_i, which is the relative area that C_i covers in the image, or in a designated region included in the pixel.

The p(x) is unconditional feature density, the probability that feature vector x occurs in the image or the above mentioned region. The p(x) is often not considered since it is the same for all classes. When the possibility of an unknown class is not considered, p(x) can be replaced by a normalization factor, since the posterior probabilities add up to 1 at the end.

Box 2.

$$r(d_x, d_y) = \frac{r_{f_1f_2}(d_x, d_y)}{\sqrt{r_{f_1}(d_x, d_y) \times r_{f_2}(d_x, d_y)}} \qquad (18)$$

Where

$$r_{f_1f_2}(d_x, d_y) = \sum_{x,y \in s} [f_1(x, y) - \overline{f}_1(d_x, d_y)][f_2(x - d_x, y - d_y) - \overline{f}_2(x, y] \qquad (19)$$

$$r_{f_1}(d_x, d_y) = \sum_{x,y \in s} [f_1(x, y) - \overline{f}_1(d_x, d_y]^2 \qquad (20)$$

$$r_{f_2}(d_x, d_y) = \sum_{x,y \in s} [f_2(x - d_x, y - d_y) - \overline{f}_2(x, y]^2 \qquad (21)$$

Figure 3. (a) Is an optical laser image of human retina; (b) is the segmentation result by Kalitzin's technique

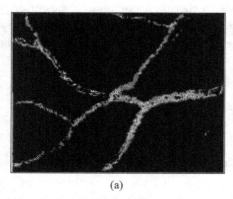

(a)

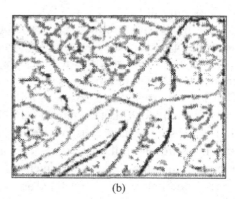

(b)

The probability density function for class C_i is a function of x, denoting the probability that that feature vector occurs in that class. It is estimated on the basis of the training samples for C_i. There is a problem here, with the possibilities for x being more than training samples. A common solution is to assume a parametric distribution, for example a multi-variation normal distribution, and then to estimate the parameters, such as mean vector and covariance matrix. Drawbacks are that this assumption may not be valid. Therefore, non-parametric estimation is often applied, based on an approximate k-nearest neighbor searching algorithm, developed by Arya and Mount (1993).

In the nearest neighbor problem, a set P of data points in d-dimensional space is given. These points are pre-processed into a data structure, so that given any query point q, the nearest (or generally k nearest) points of P to q can be reported efficiently. This algorithm is designed for data sets that are small enough that the search structure can be stored in main memory. The distance between two points can be defined in many ways. This algorithm assumes that distances are measured using any class of distance functions called Minkowski metrics. These include the well-known Euclidean distance, Manhattan distance, and max distance.

In the above description, the feature vector x of a pixel to be classified is used as a query point.

The k-nearest neighbor searching algorithm returns the k nearest training samples, after which it is possible to distribute these according to their classes, which yields a sequence of numbers k_i, i = 1... N. To transfer these neighbors-per-class counts k_i into class probability densities $p(x \mid C_i)$, the number of samples S_i per class has to be taken into account as well. Otherwise, the probability densities would be biased towards classes with more training samples. It can be shown that unbiased estimates are obtained by taking $p(x \mid C_i)$ proportional to k_i / S_i.

For applications of the Bayesian technique, this approach is able to compute within each segment the class proportions, in an iterative procedure. Note that in many regions only a single class may be present. By using the class proportions as prior probabilities, posterior probabilities are computed for each class in each pixel during the same procedure, as in fuzzy classification. The input for the iterative procedure consists of the probability densities, as computed from the training samples using a k-nearest neighbor technique. An implicit assumption is that probability densities within a class are global, independent of image segmentations.

Kalitzin, Staal, Romeny, and Viergever (2000) developed an algorithm to manipulate blood vessel images. Their technique selects subsets of local image primitives and uses a Bayesian formulation to associate to each of the subsets a solution for a prior model. Figure 3 shows an example of how they applied their technique to manipulate an optical laser image of human retina.

Relaxation Segmentation Algorithm

Relaxation technique has been applied to resolve many problems in image processing, from edge segment to image matching. Relaxation image segmentation algorithm assigns the pixels to a segment in such a way that neighboring pixels are assigned in a compatible way. This algorithm takes, as input, a set of probabilities that each pixel belongs to each possible class, in which probabilities are updated by an iterative technique. The updating is based on the possible segment assignments of the neighboring pixels, the associated probabilities of these assignments, the measuring compatibility of the neighbor's class assignments and the central pixel's class assignments.

It is a key element of relaxation image segmentation algorithm that a set of compatibility measures $c(k, s:l, t)$ to give the compatibility of assigning pixel k to class s and the neighboring pixel l to class t. The $c(k, s:l, t)$ is assumed to be in the range $(-1, +1)$ where -1 denotes a strong incompatibility, $+1$ means a strong compatibility, and 0 implies neutral. Suppose that $f^0(k, s)$ is an initial estimate of the probability that pixel k belongs to class s for all pixels k and all classes s. At the same time, let n be the number of neighbors considered for each pixel, such as 4 or 8. To simplify the notation, only one subscript k or l in the formulas is used to denote pixel location. A series of estimates $f^j(k, s)$ is calculated iteratively as:

Step 1. Calculating the neighboring compatibility between ls possible class assignments and ks possible class assignments for each neighbor l of pixel k.

$$c'_l(k,s) = \sum_t c(k,s:l,t) f^{j-1}(l,t) \quad (23)$$

Where the sum is calculated over all possible classes t.

Step 2. Searching the average neighbor compatibility for pixel k assigned to class s:

$$a(k,s) = (\frac{1}{n})\sum_l c'_l(k,s) \quad (24)$$

This summation is over all of the neighbors of l.

Step 3. Repeating the step 1 and step 2 to calculate a (k, s) for each class s.

Step 4. For each class s, updating the probability $f^{j+1}(k, s)$ as:

$$f^{j+1}(k,s) = \frac{f^j(k,s)(1+a(k,s))}{\sum_s f^j(k,s)(1+a(k,s))} \quad (25)$$

Step 5. Repeating from step 1 to step 4 for all pixels k.

When the process is iterated, these probabilities tend to converge to 0 or 1 so that pixels may be assigned to the class for which $f^j(k, s) = 1$. The formulas given above for $c'_l(k, s)$, $a(k, s)$ and $f^{j+1}(k, s)$ were only stated and not derived. Others are possible. These were chosen to obey the following three heuristic guidelines:

1. The pixels with high compatibility tend to reinforce each other. The pixels with low compatibility tend to discourage each other.
2. A neighbor's degree of reinforcing or discouraging is proportional to its own probability of assignment for each class.
3. The probabilities $f^j(k, s)$ are in the range (0, 1) and sum to 1.

Figure 3. (a) Is the segment result of Figure 1-(a) by the relaxation image segmentation algorithm; (b) is the segment result of Figure 1-(a) by the relaxation image segmentation algorithm based on the background model histogram after a 3 × 3 Gaussain filter removes its noise

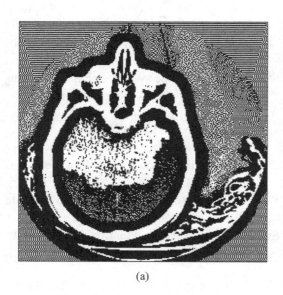

(a)

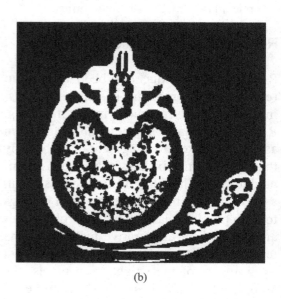

(b)

For example, suppose that the technique is applied to identify the foreground and the background in images. Therefore, there is only $f(k, 1)$ and $f(k, 2)$ for each pixel k so that the mathematics are simplified because of $f(k, 2) = 1 - f(k, 1)$. Another simplification is to set $c(k, 1{:}l, 2) = c(k, 2{:}l, 1)$, which means that the compatibility of class 1 being a neighbor of class 2 is the same as the compatibility of class 2 being a neighbor of class 1. In practice, consider all neighbors equally, therefore $c(k, s{:}l, t) = c(s, t)$.

The compatibilities reduce to the set: $c(1, 1)$ equal to the compatibility of class 1 neighboring class 1; $c(1, 2)$ equal to $c(2, 1)$, and equal to the compatibility of class 1 neighboring class 2, and equal to the compatibility of class 2 neighboring class 1; and $c(2, 2)$ equal to the compatibility of class 2 neighboring class 2. Another simplification in the application is to assign a positive constant to compatibilities for similar classes and a negative number for different classes.

Relaxation image segmentation algorithm is based on two properties, such as every pixel value and probabilities derived directly from pixel val-

ues, which are calculated over some small local area. In real-world images, these conditions are rarely met but the method is sometimes successfully applied after corrections have been made for both background intensity variations and noise. Figure 3-(a) where the global relaxation approach is applied does not give a good result. If it is hoped that the relaxation segment technique produces adequate results from real-world images, typically involving texture features, multimodal histograms or more complicated methods must be applied. Figure 3-(b) shows the segment result by the relaxation segment algorithm involved in the background model histogram after a 3 × 3 Gaussain filter removes its noise. Therefore Figure 3-(b) displays a better result than the Figure 3-(a).

DEFORMABLE MODEL APPROACHES

Deformable models are originally developed for application to computer vision and computer graphics. It has been known that 2D and 3D deformable models have been used to segment images. Deformable models are also named as snakes, which are generally represented as parametric curves that evolve in the plane of a grayscale image. Manual curve initialization is followed by curve evolution until the snake settles into a low energy state, at which point it is expected to enclose the structure of interest in the image. Deformable models carry out delineating region boundaries using parametric curves or surfaces that deform under the influence of internal and external forces. To delineate an object boundary in an image, a closed curve or surface must first be placed near the desired boundary and then allowed to undergo an iterative relaxation process.

Energy Minimizing Deformable Models

The premise of the energy minimizing formulation of deformable models is to find parameterized contours that minimize the weighted sum of internal energy and potential energy. The internal energy specifies the tension or the smoothness of the contours. The potential energy is defined over the image domain and typically possesses local minima at the image intensity edges occurring at object boundaries. Minimizing the total energy yields internal forces and potential forces. Internal forces hold the contours together and keep it from bending too much. External forces attract the contours toward the desired object boundaries. To find the object boundary, parametric contours are initialized within the image domain, and are forced to move toward the potential energy minima under the influence of both these forces.

The two dimensional deformable model is a parametric contour embedded in the image plane $(x, y) \in R^2$. The contour is represented as $v(s) = (x(s), y(s))^T$, where x and y are the coordinate functions and $s \in [0, 1]$ is the parametric domain. The shape of the contour subject to an image $I(x; y)$ is dictated by the functional

$$E(v) = S(v) + P(v) \qquad (26)$$

The functional can be viewed as a representation of the energy of the contour and the final shape of the contour corresponds to the minimum of this energy. The first term of the functional,

$$S(v) = \int_0^1 (\omega_1(s) \left| \frac{\partial v}{\partial s} \right|^2 + \omega_2 \left| \frac{\partial^2 v}{\partial s^2} \right|^2) ds \qquad (27)$$

is the internal deformation energy. It characterizes the deformation of a stretchy, flexible contour. Two physical parameter functions dictate the simulated physical characteristics of the contour: $\omega_1(s)$ controls the "tension" of the contour while $\omega_2(s)$ controls its "rigidity". The second term in equation (26) couples the snake to the image. Traditionally,

$$P(v) = \int_0^1 P(v(s)) ds \qquad (28)$$

where P(x, y) denotes a scalar potential function defined on the image plane. To apply snakes to images, external potentials are designed whose local minima coincide with intensity extrema, edges, and other image features of interest. For example, the contour will be attracted to intensity edges in an image I(x, y) by choosing a potential P(x; y) as:

$$P(x, y) = -c \left| \nabla [G_s \times I(x, y)] \right| \qquad (29)$$

where c controls the magnitude of the potential, ∇ is the gradient operator, and $G_\sigma \times I$ denotes the image convolved with a Gaussian smoothing filter whose characteristic width σ controls the spatial extent of the local minima of P(x, y).

In accordance with the calculus of variations, the contour v(s) which minimizes the energy E(v) must satisfy the Euler-Lagrange equation

$$-\frac{\partial}{\partial s}(\omega_1 \frac{\partial v}{\partial s}) + \frac{\partial^2}{\partial s^2}(\omega_2 \frac{\partial^2 v}{\partial s^2}) + \nabla P(v(s,t)) = 0$$

$$(30)$$

This vector-valued partial differential equation expresses the balance of internal and external forces when the contour rests at equilibrium. The first two terms represent the internal stretching and bending forces, respectively, while the third term represents the external forces to the image data. The usual approach to solve equation (30) is through the application of numerical algorithms detailed in section Numerical Simulation.

Dynamic Deformable Models

Energy minimization technique is used to solve a static problem. A potent approach to compute the local minima of a functional is from the equation (26). This equation constructs a dynamical system that is governed by the functional, and allows the system to evolve to equilibrium. The system may be constructed by applying the principles of Lagrangian mechanics. This leads to dynamic deformable models that unify the description of shape and motion, making it possible to quantify not just static shape, but also shape evolution through time. Dynamic models are valuable for medical image analysis, since most anatomical structures are deformable and continually undergo adapted motion. Moreover, dynamic models exhibit intuitively meaningful physical behaviors, making their evolution amenable to interactive guidance from a user.

Suppose that a dynamic snake is represented by a time varying contour v(s, t):

$$v(s,t) = (x(s,t)\ y(s,t))^{T} \qquad (31)$$

Here v(s, t) is with a mass density μ(s) and a damping density γ(s). The Lagrange equations of motion for a snake with the internal energy given by

equation (27) and external energy given by equation (28) is shown by equation (32) in Box 3.

The first two terms on the left hand side of this partial differential equation (32) represent inertial and damping forces. Referring to equation (30), the remaining terms represent the internal stretching and bending forces, while the right-hand side represents the external forces. Equilibrium is achieved when the internal and external forces balance and the contour comes to rest. Therefore we have

$$\frac{\partial v}{\partial t} = \frac{\partial^2 v}{\partial t^2} = 0 \qquad (33)$$

Equation (33) yields the equilibrium condition equation (30).

Numerical Simulation

For numerically computing a minimum energy solution, the energy E(v) is represented as a discrete form. The usual approach represents the continuous geometric model v in terms of linear combinations of local-support or global-support basis functions. The continuous model v(s) is represented in discrete form by a vector u of shape parameters associated with the basis functions. The discrete form of energies E(v) for the snake is written as

$$E(u) = \frac{1}{2} u^{T} K u + p(u) \qquad (34)$$

where K is called the stiffness matrix, and p(u) is the discrete version of the external potential. The minimum energy solution results from setting the gradient of equation (34) to 0, which is equivalent to solving the set of algebraic equations

Box 3.

$$\mu \frac{\partial^2 v}{\partial t^2} + \gamma \frac{\partial v}{\partial t} - \frac{\partial}{\partial s}(\omega_1 \frac{\partial v}{\partial s}) + \frac{\partial^2}{\partial s^2}(\omega_2 \frac{\partial^2 v}{\partial s^2}) = -\nabla p(v(s,t)) \qquad (32)$$

$$Ku = -\nabla p = f \qquad (35)$$

where f is the generalized external force vector.

The discrete version of the Lagrangian dynamics equation (30) is written as a set of second order ordinary differential equations for

$$M\ddot{u} + C\dot{u} + Ku = f \qquad (36)$$

where M is the mass matrix and C is a damping matrix. The time derivatives in equation (30) are approximated by finite differences and explicit or implicit numerical time integration methods are applied to simulate the resulting system of ordinary differential equations in the shape parameters u.

Discussion of Deformable Models

Figure 4 shows the results of a deformable model algorithm developed by Poon and Braun (1997). In their algorithm, a contour is represented by a polygon with node points at its vertices. Continuity and curvature at each node point are evaluated using the finite difference approximation. Figure 4 demonstrates the results of their model for a single contour, which the boundary of the left ventricle in a MR cardiac image is outlined at

Figure 4. (a) is the result of the contour from a 0 iteration, which is around a user-supplied seed point; (b) is the result of the contour from 10 iterations; (c) is the result of the contour from 20 iterations; (d) is the result of the contour from 42 iterations.

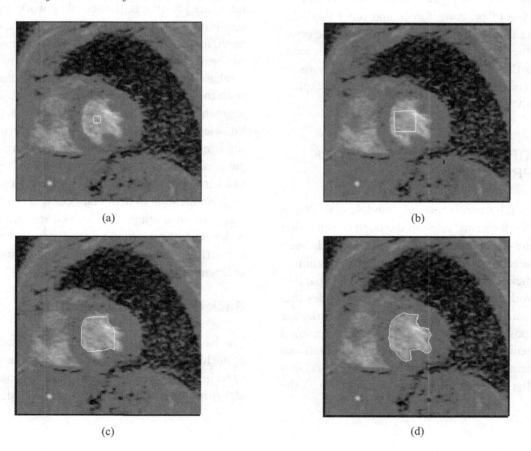

(a)

(b)

(c)

(d)

different iterations. The weights for the internal energies are made weak relative to the image forces to allow the contour to conform to the irregular boundary of the ventricle. Figure 4-(a) shows the evolution of the contour from an initial estimate, a small square around a user-supplied seed point. Figure 4-(b), 4-(c) and 4-(d) display the evolution of the contour from 10 time iterations, 20 time iterations and 42 iterations, respectively.

The main advantages of deformable models are their ability to directly generate closed parametric curves or surfaces from images and their incorporation of a smoothness constraint that provides robustness to noise and spurious edges. A disadvantage is that the techniques require manual interaction to place an initial model and choose appropriate parameters. Reducing sensitivity to initialization can improve performances of the techniques. Standard deformable models can also exhibit poor convergence to concave boundaries. The use of pressure forces and other modified external force models can improve on the error. Another important extension of deformable models is the adaptability of model topology using an implicit representation rather than an explicit parameterization.

ARTIFICIAL NEURAL NETWORK APPROACHES

Artificial neural network models have been studied for many years in the hope of achieving human-like performance in several fields such as speech processing and image understanding. Artificial neural networks are massively parallel networks of processing elements or nodes that simulate biological learning. The networks are composed of many nonlinear computational elements operating in parallel. Computational elements or nodes are connected in several layers that are input, hidden and output through the

Figure 5. A two-layer neural network

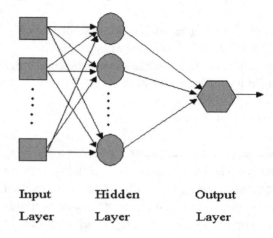

Input   Hidden   Output
Layer   Layer   Layer

adaptation of weights assigned to the connections between nodes.

For applications of image segmentation, an interesting feature is that neural networks permit accounting for spatial information. On the other hand, in most kind of networks, the final number of segments within an image must be known beforehand and run a preliminary learning phase to train the network to recognize patterns. Usually segmentations are derived with some a priori knowledge about the problem or in a pre-processing stage. Artificial neural networks represent a paradigm for machine learning and can be used in a variety of ways for image segmentation. The wide application of artificial neural networks in image segmentations is as a classifier, where the weights are determined using training data, and the artificial neural networks are then used to segment new data.

Back Propagation Algorithm

The back propagation technique is an extension of the least mean square algorithm that is applied to train multi-layer networks. Back propagation algorithm is an approximate steepest descent technique that minimizes squared error. The back propagation algorithm uses the chain rule in order to compute the derivatives of the squared error with respect to the weights and biases in the hidden layers. It is called back propagation since the derivatives are computed first at the last layer of the network, and then propagated backward through the network, using the chain rule, to compute the derivatives in the hidden layers. For a multi-layer network, the output of one layer becomes the input of the following layer. A typical two-layer neural network is described in Figure 5. It schematizes the neural network with one node in the output layer since two class labels is applied to the example.

The example of the neural network consists of three layers: an input layer, a hidden one and an output layer. The number of nodes in the input layer is equal to the number of elements existing in one transaction in the database. In the example, the input layer had 80 nodes. Ten nodes are selected for the hidden layer while the output layer consists of one node. The node of the output layer is the one that produces the classification for an image as normal or abnormal. Due to the many interconnections used in the neural network, spatial information is easily incorporated into its classification procedures.

The internal weights of the neural network are adjusted according to the transactions used in the learning process. For each learning transaction the neural network receives in addition the expected output. This allows the modification of the weights as an adaptation. In the next step, the trained neural network is used to classify new data.

When the selected features are merged and put in the transactional database, the neural network algorithm is applied to find the association rules in the database constrained by these features and the category. Once the association rules are found, they are used to construct a classification system that categorizes the data as malign, normal or benign. This classification works when the number of rules extracted for each class is balanced.

TEXTURE-BASED SEGMENTATIONS

Texture is an important property used in **image segmentation**. Texture provides useful information about shape, orientation and depth of objects. Generally, texture is together with size, tone, shape and pattern. It is hardly to present a universally accepted formal definition of texture. Texture can be defined as a function of the spatial variation in pixel intensities, its coarseness, contrast, density, orientation, frequency, repetitiveness of spatial patterns. Typically repetition of some basic pattern is included. The usual approach to texture segmentation involves extracting texture features from two or more classes of texture images to train a classifier or filter. The features and classifier or filter can then be used on new images. Currently, algorithms for representing texture features are developed by human intuition and analysis. Texture segmentation is a significant tool and has been applied in many domains, for example, remote sensing, automatic inspection, medical image processing, pattern recognition and document processing.

Co-Occurrence Matrix

This technique segments an image into regions of similar surface texture. Co-occurrence matrix applied in image texture segmentation is the two-dimensional matrix of joint probabilities $P_{d,r}(i,j)$ between pairs of pixels, separated by a distance, d, in a given direction, r. It is popular in texture description and based on the repeated occurrence of some grey value configuration in the texture.

Texture is a variation of pixel values in a small region. The variation is regular and repetitive. The variance of the pixel values of a small region is a measure for the variation. Obtaining texture features from pixel value co-occurrence matrix are on the following measurements:

1. Angular second moment:

Figure 6. (a) Is an original synthetic image; (b) is the co-occurrence matrix of (a); (c) is the neighboring pixels of (a) by chain code 7

3	3	3	3	3	3	3	3
1	3	3	3	3	3	3	2
1	1	3	3	3	3	2	2
1	1	1	3	3	2	2	2
1	1	1	0	0	2	2	2
1	1	0	0	0	0	2	2
1	0	0	0	0	0	0	2
0	0	0	0	0	0	0	0

(a)

16	0	3	0
3	6	0	3
0	0	6	0
0	0	3	16

(b)

10	0	0	0
5	8	0	0
0	0	6	0
1	0	4	15

(c)

$$\sum_i \sum_j P_{d,r}(i,j)^2 \qquad (37)$$

2. Entropy:

$$\sum_i \sum_j P_{d,r}(i,j) Log P_{d,r}(i,j) \qquad (38)$$

3. Contrast:

$$\sum_i \sum_j |i-j|^2 P_{d,r}(i,j) \qquad (39)$$

4. Homogeneity:

$$\sum_i \sum_j \frac{P_{d,r}(i,j)}{|i-j|} \qquad (40)$$

Another measure for texture feature is the frequency of grey value pairs occurring in predefined spatial patterns. For example, an image seen in Figure 6-(a), size 8×8 pixels, has four different grey values. The dimension of the co-occurrence matrix is equal to the number of the above four grey values. The spatial pattern is characterized by the position of a pixel with respect to the center pixel. Following the chain code pattern, the direct neighbor to the right has the number 0, the diagonal neighbors up and down the numbers 1 and 7, respectively. The determination of the co-occurrence matrix involves counting the pixel combination $g_n(i,j)$; $g_m(i',j')$, $n = 0, ..., g_{max}$, $m = 0, ..., g_{max}$ where (i,j) is the pixel location of the pixel under consideration and (i',j') is the pixel location determined by the spatial relationship. For example, with the relationship 0, we obtain $i' = i$, $j' = j + 1$.

It is found that there are four different grey values in the image. The co-occurrence matrix in Figure 6-(b) shows the occurrence of grey value combinations between a pixel and its direct right neighbor (chain code = 0). The neighboring pixels are related to chain code 7 in Figure 6-(c). The co-occurrence matrices have dimensions of $n \times n$ with n the number of grey values in the original image.

Gabor Filters

Gabor filters are effective tools for texture segmentation. Two-dimensional Gabor functions are attractive in texture analysis since they perform in a fashion that is remarkably similar to the human visual system. In fact Gabor functions can be conceived as hypothetical structures of receptive fields in the visual cortex. The two-dimensional Gabor function is defined by a complex sinusoidal, and modulated by a Gaussian,

$$g(x, y) = \frac{1}{2\pi\sigma_x\sigma_y} e^{-(\frac{x^2}{2\sigma_x} + \frac{y^2}{2\sigma_y})} e^{2\pi i(Ux+Vy)} \qquad (41)$$

with σ_x and σ_y the standard deviations with respect to the x axis and y axis, and U = Fcosθ, V = Fsinθ, where θ = actan(V/U). Since the retinal receptive fields in human vision have unity aspect ratio, we have $\sigma = \sigma_x = \sigma_y$ and simplify the above equation as

$$g(x, y) = e^{-(\frac{x^2+y^2}{2\sigma^2})} \sin(\omega(x\cos\theta - y\sin\theta) + \varphi)$$

$$(42)$$

where the angular frequency is ω = 2πF and φ denotes the phase shift. Parameters of Gabor filters are:

1. σ is the standard deviation of the Gaussian envelope.
2. ω is the spatial frequency.
3. θ is the orientation.
4. φ is the phase.

These four parameters characterize texture patterns. Therefore, depending on the choice of the parameters, Gabor filters extract different texture primitives. It is noted that extraction of useful texture information from images requires a variety of parameters.

It is the most crucial step for applications of Gabor filters to select appropriate filter parameters. An image is divided into regions that are as an initial segmentation at a first step. This may be yielded by determining the entropy. Entropy measures the degree of randomness of the grey values in an image. The parameters of Gabor filters are independently determined in each subdivision.

Orientation: The underlying assumption is that texture is a dominant local orientation in each subdivision. A straightforward approach used to determine the dominant orientation, θ, is to compute the weighted average of the gradient vectors at every pixel with in the region.

$$\theta_{ij} = \arctan\frac{G_y(i, j)}{G_x(i, j)} \qquad (43)$$

$$l_{ij} = \sqrt{G_x^2(i, j) + G_y^2(i, j)}$$

$$\theta = \frac{\sum_{i=0}^{m-1}\sum_{j=0}^{n-1}\theta_{ij}l_{ij}}{\sum_{i=0}^{m-1}\sum_{j=0}^{n-1}l_{ij}}$$

where $G_x(i, j)$ and $G_y(i, j)$ are the components of the gradient vector respectively along x and y directions at pixel (i, j). The window size is m × n. The standard deviation of the estimated orientation in equation (6-39) serves as an indication for the significance of the local orientation.

Spatial frequency: The local spatial frequency is defined as ω = 2π/T, which the wavelength, T, is considered an average local dimension of the texture elements within the subdivision. Since the spatial frequency must be determined with respect to the dominant orientation, it stands to reason to compute the orientation first.

Filter size: The standard deviation of the Gaussian envelope controls the Gabor filter size. The selection of an appropriate filter size depends on the image content, scale and resolution. In addition, the entropy determines a proper size for every subdivision.

OTHER TECHNIQUES

Color image segmentations are applied to medical image processing more and more. Color images obviously contain much information than grey scale images. Therefore color image segment techniques have their own advantages, and may obtain more reliable results than grey scale images. Fortunately, most approaches described in this chapter can be extended to carry out color image segmentations, such as pixel-based approaches, region-based algorithms, texture-based techniques and classification approaches.

Three dimensional image segmentations are used to identify either 3D geometrical objects from 3D images or 2D interested regions from a group of sliced images. The techniques to classify 2D interested regions from a group of sliced images are named as atlas-guided approaches since a standard atlas or template is available in a medical imaging system. The atlas is generated by compiling information, and then used as a reference frame for segmenting new images. Due to that, atlas-guided approaches are to search 2D interested regions with similar features from a group of sliced images, the approaches consider segmentation as a registration problem when image features and samples are determined. Depending on different segmentation approaches, atlas-guided techniques have been applied to MR imaging systems by Davatzikos, Vaillant, Resnick, Prince, Letovsky, and Bryan (1996), and Thompson and Toga (1997).

FUTURE RESEARCH DIRECTIONS

There is a steady increase in demand for medical imaging systems, along with pressures to improve the quality and automation of segmentations. The medical imaging segmentations are a very important stage for developing or upgrading various medical imaging systems. Improvements in new medical image segment techniques should combine high levels of segment accuracy with rapid, and more robust to segment interested regions from a class of images. However, it very much depends on the application to select an adequate segment algorithm. Therefore, not only the advantages and disadvantages of each class of segment techniques, but also the image features should be known before you choose your segment algorithms.

Segment accuracy can be improved by applying sub-pixel segment techniques, incorporating prior knowledge within algorithms and employing continuous-based segment approaches. It is aimed that automatic segment techniques will replace human to interfere segmentations. Future segment algorithms may be reliable and robust. They may also have adaptability and learning ability.

With developments of computer and medical imaging technology, color image segmentations likely become crucial and popular. It is obvious that color images carry on much information than grey scale images. Based on the advantage, some effective color image segment algorithms may be developed in the future.

No matter which segment technique is used, it is crucial for every segment algorithm to obtain unique image features. If new unique image features are found from medical images and represented by accurately mathematical formulas, new effective segment algorithms are certainly produced. Based on prior knowledge and multi-features, some new segment algorithms may be developed.

ACKNOWLEDGMENT

This work was supported by grant No. EP/C006623/1 from the Engineering and Physical Sciences Research Council of the UK.

REFERENCES

Arya, S., & Mount, D. (1993). Approximate nearest neighbor searching. *Proceedings of ACM-SIAM Symposium on Discrete Algorithms (SODA'93)*, (pp. 271-280).

Chen, K., Lin, J., & Moa, C. (1996). The applications of competitive Hopfield neural network to medical image segmentation. *IEEE Transactions on Medical Imaging, 15*(4), 560-567.

Davatzikos, C., Vaillant, M., Resnick, S., Prince, J., Letovsky, S., & Bryan, R. (1996). A computerized method for morphological analysis of the corpus callosum. *Journal of Computer-Assisted Tomography, 20,* 88-97.

Gorte, B., & Stein, A. (1998). Bayesian classification and class area estimation of satellite images using stratification. *Trans.GeoRS, 36*(3), 803-812.

Jain A., et al. (1992). Text segmentation using Gabor filters for automatic document processing. *Machine Vision and Applications, 5,* 169-184.

Kalitzin, S., Staal, J., Romeny, B., & Viergever, M. (2000). Image segmentation and object recognition by Bayesian grouping. *IEEE Image Processing, Proceedings 2000 International Conference, 3,* 580-583.

Najarian, K. (2006). *Biomedical signal and image processing.* CRC.

Nixon, M. (2002). Feature extraction and image processing. Newnes.

Otsu, N. (1979). A threshold selection method from gray-level histograms. *IEEE Trans. Systems, Man, and Cybernetics, 9*(1), 62-66.

Petrou, M. (2006). *Image processing: Dealing with texture.* John Wiley and sons Ltd.

Pham, D., Xu, C., & Prince, J. (1999). *A survey of current methods in medical image segmentation.* Technical Report JHU/ECE 99-01, Department of Electrical and Computer Engineering, John Hopkins University, Baltimore, MD. Retrieved May 16, 2007, from http://www.rfai.li.univtours. fr/webrfai/chercheurs/rousselle/Docu -m/pdf /p124r.pdf.

Poon, C., & Braun, M. (1997). Image segmentation by a deformable contour model incorporating region analysis. *Physics in Medicine and Biology, 42,* 1833-1841.

Additional Reading

Atkins, M., Siu, K., Law, B., Orchard, J., & Rosenbaum, W. (2002). Difficulties of T1 brain image segmentation. *Proceedings of SPIE Conference on Medical Imaging,* (pp. 1837-1844).

Behiels, G., Maes, F., Vandermeulen, D., & Suetens, P. (2002). Evaluation of image features and search strategies for segmentation of bone structures in radiographs using Active Shape Models. *Medical Image Analysis, 6*(1), 47-62.

Betke, M., & Ko, J. (1999). Detection of pulmonary nodules on CT and volumetric assessment over time. *Proceedings of the International Conference on Medical Image Computing and Computer-Assisted Intervention,* (pp. 245-252). Cambridge, UK.

Blond, P., Bennardo, A., Satalino, G., Pasquariello, G., De Blasi, R., & Milella, D. (1996). *Fuzzy neural network-based segmentation of multi-spectral magnetic resonance brain images.* Applications of Fuzzy Logic Technology III, B.

Chan, T., & Vese, L. (2001). Active contours without edges. *IEEE Trans. Image Proc., 10,* 266-277.

Choi, S., Lee, J., Kim, J., & Kim, M. (1997). Volumetric objection reconstruction using the 3D-MRF model-based segmentation. *IEEE T. Med. Imag., 16,* 887-892.

Clarke, L., Velthuizen, R., Camacho, M., Heine, J., Vaidyanathan, M., Hall, L., et al. (1995). MRI segmentation: Methods and applications. *Magnetic Resonance Imaging, 13*(3), 343-368.

Harvey, N., Levenson, R., & Rimm, D. (2003). Investigation of automated feature extraction techniques for applications in cancer detection from multi-spectral histopathology images. *Proc. of SPIE 2003, 5032,* 557-566.

Huib de Ridder. (1992). Minkowski metrics as a combination rule for digital image coding impairments. *SPIE Human Vision Visual Processing and Digital Display III 1666,* pp. 16-26.

Jain, R., Katsuri, R., & Schunck, B. (1995). *Machine vision.* McGraw-Hill International Editions.

Kshirsagar, A., Robson, M., Watson, P., Herrod, N., Tyler, J., & Hall, L. (1996). Computer analysis of MR images of human knee joints to measure femoral cartilage thickness. *Engineering in Medicine and Biology Society, 1996.* Bridging Disciplines for Biomedicine. *18th Annual International Conference of the IEEE, 2,* 746-747.

Kulkarni, A. (1994). *Artificial neural networks for image understanding.* Van Nostrand Reinhold.

Pemmaraju, S., Mitra, S., Shieh, Y., & Roberson, G. (1995). Multi-resolution wavelet decomposition and neuro-fuzzy clustering for segmentation of radiographic images. *Proceedings of the 1995 IEEE Computer-Based Medical Systems Conference (CBMS '95).*

Petrakis, E., & Faloutsos, C. (1997). Similarity searching in medical image databases. *IEEE Transactions on Knowledge and Data Engineering, 9*(3), 435-447.

Pien, H., Desai, M., & Shah, J. (1997). Segmentation of MR images using curve evolution and prior information. *Int. J. Patt. Rec. Art. Intel., 11,* 1233-1245.

Pohl, K., Fisher, J., Grimson, W., Kikinis, R., & Wells, W. (2006). A Bayesian model for joint segmentation and registration. *NeuroImage, 31*(1), 228-239.

Pohl, K., Wells, W., Guimond, A., Kasai, K., Shenton, M., Kikinis, R., et al. (2002). Incorporating non-rigid registration into expectation maximization algorithm to segment MR images. *Proceedings of MICCAI'2002: Fifth International Conference on Medical Image Computing and*

Computer-Assisted Intervention, (pp. 564-572).

Pohlman, S., Powell, K., Obuchowski, N., Chilcote, W, & Grundfest-Broniatowski, S. (1996). Quantitative classification of breast tumors in digitized mammograms. *Med. Phys., 23,* 1337-1345.

Rajapakse, J., Giedd, J., & Rapoport, J. (1997). Statistical approach to segmentation of single-channel cerebral MR images. *IEEE T. Med. Imag., 16,* 176-186.

Rajapakse, J., & Kruggel, F. (1998). Segmentation of MR images with intensity in homogeneities. *Im. Vis. Comp., 16,* 165-180.

Reddick, W., Glass, J., Cook, E., Elkin, T., & Deaton, R. (1997). Automated segmentation and classification of multi-spectral magnetic resonance images of brain using artificial neural networks. *IEEE T. Med. Imag., 16,* 911-918.

Stephanakis, I., Anastassopoulos, G., Karayiannakisl, A., & Sirnopoulos, C. (2003). Enhancement of medical images using a fuzzy model for segment dependent local equalization. *Proceedings of the 3rd Intesnetional Syinposiurn on Image and Signal Processing and Analysis,* (pp. 970-975).

Storvik, G. (1994). A Bayesian approach to dynamic contours through stochastic sampling and simulated annealing. *IEEE Trans. Pattern Anal. Machine Intell., 16,* 976-986.

Thompson, P., & Toga, A. (1997). Detection, visualization and animation of abnormal anatomic structure with a probabilistic brain atlas based on random vector field transformations. *Medical Image Analysis, 1,* 271-294.

Tsai, A., Yezzi, A., Wells, W., Tempany, C., Tucker, D., Fan, A., et al. (2003). A shape-based approach to the segmentation of medical imagery using level sets. *IEEE Trans. on Medical Imaging, 22,* 137-154.

Tsai, A., Wells, W., Warfield, S., & Willsky, A. (2005). An EM algorithm for shape classification based on level sets. *Medical Image Analysis, 9*(5), 491-502.

Umbaugh, S. (2005). *Computer imaging: Digital image analysis and processing.* CRC, Taylor and Francis.

Vadis, Q. (2006). Medical image segmentation. *Computer Methods and Programs in Biomedicine, 84*(2-3), 63-65.

Vese, L., & Chan, T. (2002). A multi-phase level set framework for image segmentation using the Mumford and Shah model. *Intl. J. Computer Vision, 50*(3), 271-293.

Woo, C. (1998). Image segmentation of MRI images using wavelet transform and artificial neural network. *Proceedings of the 7th JSPS-VCC Seminar in Integrated Engineering,* (pp. 32-27). University of Malaya.

Zabih, R., & Kolmogorov, V. (2004). Spatially coherent clustering with graph cuts. *IEEE Conference on Computer Vision and Pattern Recognition.*

Zhang, Y., Brady, M., & Smith, S. (2000). A hidden Markov random field model for segmentation of brain MR images. *Proceedings of SPIE Medical Imaging 2000 (SPIE Proceedings 3979,* (pp. 1126-1137). San Diego, CA.

Selected Readings

Chapter XIV
A Content–Based Approach to Medical Image Database Retrieval

Chia-Hung Wei
University of Warwick, UK

Chang-Tsun Li
University of Warwick, UK

Roland Wilson
University of Warwick, UK

ABSTRACT

Content-based image retrieval (CBIR) makes use of image features, such as color and texture, to index images with minimal human intervention. Content-based image retrieval can be used to locate medical images in large databases. This chapter introduces a content-based approach to medical image retrieval. Fundamentals of the key components of content-based image retrieval systems are introduced first to give an overview of this area. A case study, which describes the methodology of a CBIR system for retrieving digital mammogram database, is then presented. This chapter is intended to disseminate the knowledge of the CBIR approach to the applications of medical image management and to attract greater interest from various research communities to rapidly advance research in this field.

INTRODUCTION

John Doe, a radiologist in a university hospital, takes X-rays and MRI scans for patients producing hundreds of digital images each day. In order to facilitate easy access in the future, he registers each image in a medical image database based on the modality, region, and orientation of the image. One day Alice Smith, a surgeon, comes to discuss a case with John Doe as she suspects there is a tumor on the patient's brain according to the brain MRI. However, she cannot easily judge if it is a benign or malign tumor from the MRI scan, and would like to compare with previous cases to decide if this patient requires a dangerous operation. Understanding Alice's needs, John helps Alice find similar-looking tumors from the previous MRI images. He uses the query-by-example mode of the medical image database, delineates the tumor area in the MRI image, and then requests the database to return the brain MRI images most similar to this one. Alice finds eleven similar images and their accompanying reports after reviewing the search results. Alice compares those cases and verifies the pattern of the tumor. Later on, she tells her patient that it is a benign tumor and the operation is unnecessary unless the tumor grows.

This scenario briefly describes the creation of medical images, categorization of medical images, and a content-based access approach. Although a mature content-based access technology has not appeared yet, this field is developing actively. In the last decade, a large number of digital medical images have been produced in hospitals. Large-scale image databases collect various images, including X-ray, computed tomography (CT), magnetic resonance imaging (MRI), ultrasound (US), nuclear medical imaging, endoscopy, microscopy, and scanning laser ophtalmoscopy (SLO). The most important aspect of image database management is how to effectively retrieve the desired images using a description of image content. This approach of searching images is known as content-based image retrieval (CBIR), which refers to the retrieval of images from a database using information directly derived from the content of images themselves, rather than from accompanying text or annotation (El-Naqa, Yang, Galatsanos, Nishikawa, & Wernick , 2004; Wei & Li, in press).

The main purpose of this chapter is to disseminate the knowledge of the CBIR approach to the applications of medical image retrieval and to attract greater interest from various research communities to rapidly advance research in this field. The rest of the chapter is organized as follows: The second section addresses the problems and challenges of medical image retrieval and describes potential applications of medical

CBIR. The third section reviews the existing medical CBIR systems. The fourth section provides greater details on the key components of content-based image retrieval systems for medical imaging applications. The fifth section presents a case study, which describes the methodology of CBIR systems for digital mammograms. The sixth section discusses potential research issues in the future research agenda. The last section concludes this chapter.

MEDICAL IMAGE DATABASE RETRIEVAL

This section will discuss the problems of image retrieval using the conventional text-based method and addresses the challenges of the CBIR approach. Potential applications of the CBIR approach will also be discussed.

Challenges in Medical Image Retrieval

Before the emergence of content-based retrieval, medical images were annotated with text, allowing the images to be accessed by text-based searching (Feng, Siu, & Zhang, 2003). Through textual description, medical images can be managed based on the classification of imaging modalities, regions, and orientation. This hierarchical structure allows users to easily navigate and browse the database. Searching is mainly carried out through standard Boolean queries.

However, with the emergence of massive image databases, the traditional text-based search suffers from the following limitations (Shah et al., 2004; Wei & Li, 2005):

- Manual annotations require too much time and are expensive to implement. As the number of images in a database grows, the difficulty in finding desired images increases. Muller, Michous, Bandon, and Geissbuhler

(2004a) reported that the University Hospital of Geneva produced approximately 12,000 medical images per day. It is not feasible to manually annotate all attributes of the image content for this number of images.

- Manual annotations fail to deal with the discrepancy of subjective perception. The phrase, "an image says more than a thousand words," implies that the textual description is not sufficient for depicting subjective perception. Typically, a medical image usually contains several objects, which convey specific information. Nevertheless, different interpretations for a pathological area can be made by different radiologists. To capture all knowledge, concepts, thoughts, and feelings for the content of any images is almost impossible.

- The contents of medical images are difficult to be concretely described in words. For example, irregular organic shapes cannot easily be expressed in textual form, but people may expect to search for images with similar contents based on the examples they provide.

These problems limit the feasibility of text-based search for medical image retrieval. In an attempt to overcome these difficulties, content-based retrieval has been proposed to automatically access images with minimal human intervention (Eakins, 2002; Feng et al., 2003). However, due to the nature of medical images, content-based retrieval for medical images is still faced with challenges:

- Low resolution and strong noise are two common characteristics in most medical images (Glatard, Montagnat, & Magnin, 2004). With these characteristics, medical images cannot be precisely segmented and extracted for the visual content of their features. In addition, medical images obtained from different scanning devices may display different features, though some approaches to image correction and normalization have been proposed (Buhler, Just, Will, Kotzerke, & van den Hoff, 2004);

- Medical images are digitally represented in a multitude of formats based on their modality and the scanning device used (Wong & Hoo, 2002). Another characteristic of medical images is that many images are represented in gray level rather than color. Even with the change of intensity, monochrome may fail to clearly display the actual circumstance of lesion area.

Medical Applications of Content-Based Image Retrieval

Content-based image retrieval has frequently been proposed for various applications. This section will discuss three potential applications of medical CBIR.

PACS/Health Database Management

Content-based image retrieval has been proposed by the medical community for inclusion into picture archiving and communication systems (PACS) (Lehmann, Wein, & Greenspan, 2003). The idea of PACS is to integrate imaging modalities and interfaces with hospital and departmental information systems in order to manage the storage and distribution of images to radiologists, physicians, specialists, clinics, and imaging centers (Huang, 2003). A crucial point in PACS is to provide an efficient search function to access desired images. Image search in the digital imaging and communication in medicine (DICOM) protocol is currently carried out according to the alphanumerical order of textual attributes of images. However, the information which users are interested in is the visual content of medical images rather than that residing in alphanumerical format (Lehmann et al., 2003). The content of images is a powerful and direct query which can be used to search for other images containing similar content. Hence, content-based access approaches are expected to have a great impact on PACS and health database management. In addition to PACS, medical imaging databases that are unconnected to the PACS can also obtain benefits from CBIR technology.

Computer-Aided Diagnosis

Computer-aided diagnosis has been proposed to support clinical decision making. One clinical decision-making technique is case-based reasoning, which searches for previous, already- solved problems similar to the current one and tries to apply those solutions to the current problem (Hsu & Ho, 2004; Schmidt, Montani, Bellazzi, Portinale, & Gierl, 2001). This technique has a strong need to search for previous medical images with similar pathological areas, scrutinize the histories of these cases which are valuable for supporting certain diagnoses, and then reason the current case (Chang et al., 2004).

Medical Research, Education, and Training

CBIR technology can benefit any work that requires the finding of images or collections of images with similar contents. In medical research, researchers can use CBIR to find images with similar pathological areas and investigate their association. In medical education, lecturers can easily find images with particular pathological attributes, as those attributes can imply particular diseases. In addition, CBIR can be used to collect images for medical books, reports, papers, and CD-ROMs based on the educational atlas of medical cells, where typical specimens are collected according to the similarity of their features, and the most typical ones are selected from each group to compose a set of practical calibrators.

EXISTING MEDICAL CBIR SYSTEMS

Although content-based image retrieval has frequently been proposed for use in medical image management, only a few content-based retrieval systems have been developed specifically for medical images. These research-oriented systems are usually constructed in research institutes and continue to be improved, developed, and evaluated over time. This section will introduce several major medical content-based retrieval systems.

ASSERT (Automatic Search and Selection Engine with Retrieval Tools)

- **Developers:** Purdue University, Indiana University, and University of Wisconsin Hospital, USA.
- **Image Database:** High-Resolution Computed Tomography (HRCT) of lung.
- **Selected References:** Shyu, Brodley, Kak, Kosaka, Aisen, and Broderick (1999), and Brodley, Kak, Dy, Shyu, Aisen, and Broderick, (1999).
- **Web site:** http://rvl2.ecn.purdue.edu/ ~cbirdev/WWW/CBIRmain.html

Main Characteristics:

- The ASSERT system uses a physician-in-the-loop approach to retrieving images of HRCT of the lung. This approach requires users to delineate the pathology-bearing regions and identify certain anatomical landmarks for each image;
- This system extracts 255 features of texture, shape, edges, and gray-scale properties in pathology-bearing regions;
- A multi-dimensional hash table is constructed to index the HRCT images.

CasImage

- **Developer:** University Hospital of Geneva, Switzerland.
- **Image Database:** A variety of images from CT, MRI, and radiographs, to color photos.
- **Selected References:** Muller, Rosset, Vallee, and Geissbuhler (2004b), and Rosset, Ratib, Geissbuhler, and Vallee (2002).
- **Web site:** http://www.casimage.com/

Main Characteristics:

- The CasImage system, which has been integrated into a PACS environment, contains a teaching and reference database, and the med-GIFT retrieval system, which is adapted from the open-source GIFT (GNU Image Finding Tool) (Squire, Muller, Muller, Marchand-Maillet, & Pun, 2001);
- The medGIFT retrieval system extracts global and regional color and texture features, including 166 colors in the HSV color space, and Gabor filter responses in four directions each at three different scales;
- Combinations of textual labels and visual features are used for medical image retrieval.

IRMA (Image Retrieval in Medical Applications)

- **Developer:** Aachen University of Technology, Germany.
- **Image Database:** Various imaging modalities.
- **Selected References:** Lehmann, Guld, Keysers, Deselaers, Schubert, Wein, and Spitzer (2004a), and Lehmann, Guld, Thies, Plodowski, Keysers, Ott, and Schubert (2004b).
- **Web site:** http://libra.imib.rwth-aachen.de/irma/

Main Characteristics:

- The IRMA system is implemented as a platform for content-based image retrieval in medical applications;
- This system splits the image retrieval process into seven consecutive steps, including categorization, registration, feature extraction, feature selection, indexing, identification, and retrieval.

NHANES II (The Second National Health and Nutrition Examination Survey)

- **Developer:** National Library of Medicine, USA.
- **Image Database:** 17,000 cervical and lumbar spine X-ray images.
- **Selected References:** Antani, Lee, Long, and Thoma (2004a), and Antani, Xu, Long, and Thoma (2004b).
- **Web site:** http://archive.nlm.nih.gov/proj/dxpnet/nhanes/nhanes.php

Main Characteristics:

- This system contains the Active Contour Segmentation (ACS) tool, which allows the users to create a template by marking points around the vertebra. If the segmentation of a template is accepted, the ACS tool will estimate the location of the next vertebra, place the template on the image, and then segment it;
- In data representation, a polygon approximation process is applied for eliminating insignificant shape features and reducing the number of data points. The data obtained in the polygon approximation process represent the shape of vertebra. Then, the approximated curve of vertebra is converted to tangent space for similarity measurement.

CONTENT-BASED RETRIEVAL SYSTEMS

Content-based retrieval uses the contents of images to represent and access the images (Wei & Li, in press). A typical content-based retrieval system is divided into *off-line feature extraction* and *online image retrieval*. A conceptual framework for content-based image retrieval is illustrated in Figure 1. In off-line feature extraction, the contents of the images in the database are extracted and described with a multi-dimensional feature vector, also called descriptor. The feature vectors of the image constitute a feature dataset stored in the database. In online image retrieval, the user can submit a query example to the retrieval system in search of desired images. The system represents this example with a feature vector. The distances (i.e., similarities) between the feature vectors of the query example and those of the media in the feature dataset are then computed and ranked. Retrieval is conducted by applying an indexing

scheme to provide an efficient way of searching the image database. Finally, the system ranks the search results and then returns the results that are most similar to the query examples. If the user is not satisfied with the search results, the user can provide relevance feedback to the retrieval system, which contains a mechanism to learn the user's information needs. The following sections will clearly introduce each component in the system.

Feature Extraction

Representation of images needs to consider which features are most useful for representing the contents of images and which approaches can effectively code the attributes of the images. Feature extraction of the image in the database is typically conducted off-line so computation complexity is not a significant issue. This section will introduce two features—texture and color—which are used most often to extract the features of an image.

Figure 1. A conceptual framework for content-based image retrieval

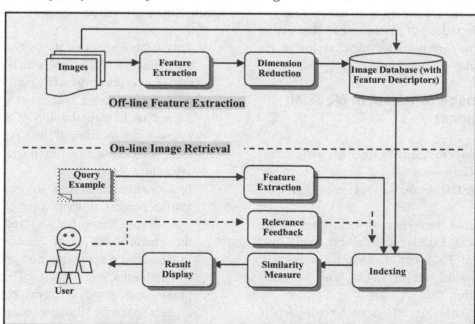

Color

Color is a powerful descriptor that simplifies object identification (Gonzalez & Woods, 2002) and is one of the most frequently used visual features for content-based image retrieval. To extract the color features from the content of an image, a proper color space and an effective color descriptor have to be determined.

The purpose of a color space is to facilitate the specification of colors. Each color in the color space is a single point represented in a coordinate system. Several color spaces, such as *RGB, HSV, CIE L*a*b, and CIE L*u*v,* have been developed for different purposes. Although there is no agreement on which color space is the best for CBIR, an appropriate color system is required to ensure perceptual uniformity. Therefore, the *RGB* color space, a widely used system for representing color images, is not suitable for CBIR because it is a perceptually non-uniform and device-dependent system (Gevers, 2001).

The most frequently used technique is to convert color representations from the *RGB* color space to the *HSV,* CIE *L*u*v,* or CIE *L*a*b* color spaces with perceptual uniformity (Li & Yuen, 2000). The *HSV* color space is an intuitive system, which describes a specific color by its hue, saturation and brightness value. This color system is very useful in interactive color selection and manipulation; The CIE *L*u*v* and CIE *L*a*b* color spaces are both perceptually uniform systems, which provide easy use of similar metrics for comparing color (Haeghen, Naeyaert, Lemahieu, & Philips, 2000).

After selecting a color space, an effective color descriptor should be developed in order to represent the color of the global or regional areas. Several color descriptors have been developed from various representation schemes, such as color histograms (Quyang & Tan, 2002), color moments (Yu et al., 2002), color edge (Gevers & Stokman, 2003), color texture (Guan & Wada, 2002), and color correlograms (Moghaddam,

Khajoie, & Rouhi, 2003). For example, color histogram, which represents the distribution of the number of pixels for each quantized color bin, is an effective representation of the color content of an image. The color histogram can not only easily characterize the global and regional distribution of colors in an image, but also be invariant to rotation about the view axis.

For the retrieval of medical images, color allows images to reveal many pathological characteristics (Tamai, 1999). Color also plays an important role in morphological diagnosis (Nishibori, Tsumura, & Miyake, 2004). Color medical images are usually produced in different departments and by various devices. For example, color endoscopic images are taken by a camera that is put into the hollow organs of the body such as stomachs and lungs. A common characteristic in such kind of images is that most colors are made of various stains, though fine variations of natural colors are crucial for diagnosis. Nishibori (2000) pointed out that problems in color medical images include inaccurate color reproduction, rough gradations of color, and insufficient density of pixels. Therefore, effective use of the various color information in images includes absolute color values, ratios of each tristimulus color, differences in colors against adjacent areas, and estimated illumination data. In addition, many medical images are represented in gray level. For this kind of gray level images, CBIR can only regard color as secondary features because gray levels provide limited information about the content of an image. For specific purposes, some gray level images have pseudo-color added to enhance specific areas instead of gray level presentation. Such processing increases difficulties in retrieval.

Texture

Texture in CBIR can be used for at least two purposes (Sebe & Lew, 2002). First, an image can be considered to be a mosaic that consists of different texture regions. These regions can be used as examples to search and retrieve similar areas. Second, texture can be employed for automatically annotating the content of an image. For example, the texture of an infected skin region can be used for annotating regions with the same infection.

Textural representation approaches can be classified into statistical approaches and structural approaches (Li, 1998). Statistical approaches analyze textural characteristics according to the statistical distribution of image intensity. Approaches in this category include gray level co-occurrence matrix, fractal model, Tamura feature, Wold decomposition, and so on (Feng et al., 2003). Structural approaches characterize texture by identifying a set of structural primitives and certain placement rules.

If medical images are represented in gray level, texture becomes a crucial feature, which provides indications about scenic depth, the spatial distribution of tonal variations, and surface orientation (Tourassi, 1999). For example, abnormal symptoms on female breasts include calcification, architectural distortion, asymmetry, masses, and so forth. All of those reveal specific textural patterns on the mammograms. However, selection of texture features for specifying textural structure should take account of the influence from the modulation transfer function on texture (Veenland, Grashuis, Weinans, Ding, & Vrooman, 2002). As the intensifying screens are used to enhance the radiographs, the blurring effect also changes texture features, that is, spatial resolution, contrast, and sharpness are all reduced in the output. Low resolution and contrast result in difficulties in measuring the pattern of tissue and structure of organs (Majumdar, Kothari, Augat, Newitt, Link, Lin, & Lang, 1998).

Dimension Reduction

In an attempt to capture useful contents of an image and to facilitate effective querying of an image database, a CBIR system may extract a large number of features from the content of an image. Feature set of high dimensionality causes the "curse of dimension" problem in which the complexity and computational cost of the query increase exponentially with the number of dimensions (Egecioglu, Ferhatosmanoglu, & Ogras, 2004).

To reduce the dimensionality of a large feature set, the most widely-used technique in image retrieval is principal component analysis (PCA). The goal of principal component analysis is to specify as much variance as possible with the smallest number of variables (Partridge & Calvo, 1998). Principal component analysis involves transforming the original data into a new coordinate system with low dimension, thus creating a new set of data. The new coordinate system removes the redundant data, and the new set of data may better represent the essential information. However, there is a trade-off between the efficiency obtained through dimension reduction and the completeness of the information extracted. As data is represented lower dimensions, the speed of retrieval is increased, but some important information may be lost in the process of data transformation. In the research of medical CBIR, Sinha and Kangarloo (2002) demonstrated the PCA application to the image classification of 100 axial brain images.

Similarity Measure

Selection of similarity metrics has a direct impact on the performance of content-based image retrieval. The kind of feature vectors selected determines the kind of measurement that will be used to compare their similarity (Smeulders, Worring, Santini, Gupta, & Jain, 2000). If the features extracted from the images are presented as multi-dimensional points, the distances between corresponding multi-dimensional points can be calculated. Euclidean distance is the most common metric used to measure the distance between two points in multi-dimensional space (Qian, Sural, Gu, & Pramanik, 2004). For other kinds of features such as color histogram, Euclidean distance may not be an ideal similarity metric or may not be compatible with the human-perceived similarity. Histogram intersection was proposed by Swain and Ballard (1991) to find known objects within images using color histograms. A number of other metrics, such as Mahalanobis Distance, Minkowski-Form Distance, Earth Mover's Distance, and Proportional Transportation Distance, have been proposed for specific purposes. Antani, Long, Thoma, and Lee (2003) used several approaches to code the shape features for different classes of spine X-rays. Each class used a specific similarity metric to compare the distance between two feature vectors.

Multi-Dimensional Indexing

Retrieval of an image is usually based not only on the value of certain features, but also on the location of a feature vector in the multi-dimensional space (Fonseca & Jorge, 2003). A retrieval query on a database of multimedia with multi-dimensional feature vectors usually requires fast execution of search operations. To support such search operations, an appropriate multi-dimensional access method has to be used for indexing the reduced but still high dimensional feature set. Popular multi-dimensional indexing methods include the R-tree (Guttman, 1984) and the R*-tree (Beckmann, Kriegel, Schneider, & Seeger, 1990).

The R-tree, which is a tree-like data structure, is mainly used for indexing multi-dimensional data. Each node of an R-tree has a variable number of entries. Each entry within a non-leaf node can have two pieces of data. The goal of the R-tree is to organize the spatial data in such a way that a search will visit as few spatial objects as possible. The decision on which nodes to visit is made based on the evaluation of spatial predicates. Hence, the R-tree must be able to hold some sort of spatial data on all nodes. The R*-tree, an improved version of the R-tree, applies more complex criteria for

the distribution of minimal-bounding rectangles through the nodes of the tree, such as: The overlap between the minimal-bounding rectangles of the inner nodes should be minimized; the perimeter of a directory rectangles should be minimized; and storage utilization should be maximized. Both techniques perform well in low-dimensional features-space with a limit of up to 20 dimensions. For high-dimensional features-space, it is necessary to reduce the dimensionality using statistic multi-variate analysis techniques such as the aforementioned principal component analysis.

With regard to medical CBIR research, Shyu et al. (1999) successfully applied multi-dimensional indexing in the ASSERT system. In this system, lobular feature sets (LFS) on HRCT images are translated into an index for archiving and retrieval. A multi-dimensional hash table for the LFS classes is constructed for the system. A decision tree algorithm is used to construct a minimum-entropy partition of the feature space where the LFS classes reside. After translating a decision tree to a hash table, the system prunes the set of retrieved LFS classes and candidate images.

Relevance Feedback

Relevance feedback was originally developed for improving the effectiveness of information retrieval systems. The main idea of relevance feedback is for the retrieval system to understand the user's information needs. For a given query, the retrieval system returns initial results based on pre-defined similarity metrics. Then, the user is required to identify the positive examples by labeling those that are relevant to the query. The system subsequently analyzes the user's feedback using a learning algorithm and returns refined results.

A typical relevance feedback mechanism contains a learning component and a dispensing component. The learning component uses the feedback data to estimate the target of the user. The approach taken to learn feedback data is key to the relevance feedback mechanism. In addition to Rocchio's (1971) and Rui and Huang's (2002) learning algorithms, recent work has reported that support vector machine (SVM) is a useful learning approach in relevance feedback (Ferecatu, Crucianu, & Boujemaa, 2004a; Hoi, Chan, Huang, Lyu, & King, 2004; Tao & Tang, 2004). The dispensing component should provide the most appropriate images after obtaining feedback from the user. However, the dispensing component has two conflicting goals during each feedback round. On the one hand, the dispensing component has to provide as many relevant images as possible. On the other hand, the dispensing component, based on the information needs of the user, has to investigate the images of unknown relevance to the target (Ferecatu, Crucianu, & Boujemaa, 2004b). As the dispensing component returns more relevant images to the user, it has fewer images to mine the needs of the user at each round, and vice versa. A sensible strategy also plays an important role in relevance feedback. Hence, approaches to learning user feedbacks and dispensing strategies for returning the results both determine the performance of relevance feedback mechanisms.

Medical images have a unique characteristic in that their contents always reflect pathological attributes or symptoms for specific diseases. Image classification is often used to group the similar features based on their contents. With this characteristic, relevance feedback is expected to assist in mining the common features of relevant images and finding a specific class where the query example should reside. Those images grouped in the same class have the same semantics and are likely to be target images. El-Naqa, Yang, Galatsanos, and Wernick (2003) proposed a relevance feedback approach based on incremental learning for mammogram retrieval. They adapted support vector machines (SVM) to develop an online learning procedure for similarity learning. The approach they proposed was implemented using clustered micro-calcifications images. They reported that the approach significantly improves

the retrieval effectiveness. In addition, El-Naqa et al. (2004) also demonstrated a hierarchical two-stage learning network, which consists of a cascade of a binary classifier and a regression module. Relevance feedback is incorporated into this framework to effectively improve precision based on online interaction with users.

CASE STUDY

This section will propose a general CBIR framework and its application to mammogram retrieval, and demonstrate its method. Breast cancer continues to be a serious disease across the world. Mammography is a reliable method for detection of breast cancer. There are an enormous number of mammograms generated in hospitals. How to effectively retrieve a desired image from mammogram databases is a challenging problem. This study concentrates on textural analysis based on gray level co-occurrence matrices for the content-based retrieval of mammograms. The objectives of this study are as follows:

1. To analyze and examine the textural features present in the ROI (Region of Interest) of abnormal breast tissue as compared to the same information presented in normal tissue;
2. To develop the optimal mammographic descriptor generated from gray level co-occurrence matrices; and
3. To evaluate the effectiveness of the CBIR system using descriptors with different unit pixel distances.

The method in this work contains two major stages — *image analysis* and *image retrieval*. The objective of the image analysis stage is to examine the textural features of mammograms, and then test the statistical significance of the differences between normal and abnormal mammograms. These discriminating features are selected to construct a textural descriptor of mammograms. The descriptor constructed in the image analysis stage is embedded into the CBIR system. The feature descriptor is extracted from the query image in order to retrieve the mammograms relevant to the query image. The performance of the CBIR system is then evaluated. The detailed steps and components of the experiment are described in the following sections.

Mammogram Dataset

Mammograms were obtained from the database of the Mammographic Images Analysis Society (MIAS) (Suckling, Parker, Dance, Astley, Hutt, Boggis, Ricketts, Stamatakis, Cerneaz, Kok, Taylor, Betal, & Savage, 1994). The size of each image was 1024×1024 pixels. All of the images have been annotated for class, severity and location of abnormality, character of background tissue, and radius of circle enclosing the abnormality. Abnormalities are classified into calcifications architectural distortions, asymmetries, circum-

scribed masses, speculated masses, and ill-defined masses. Sub-images of size 200×200 pixels were cropped as ROIs from each mammogram. One hundred and twenty-two sample ROIs (including 29 images in calcification class, 19 in architectural distortion class, 15 in asymmetry class, 25 in circumscribed masses class, 19 in speculated masses class, and 15 in other or ill-defined masses class) were selected deliberately from abnormal tissues. Another 207 ROIs were obtained arbitrarily from normal tissues. These 329 ROIs were used to analyze their textural features based on gray level co-occurrence matrices.

Feature Analysis

The presence of a breast lesion may cause a disturbance in the homogeneity of tissues, and result in architectural distortions in the surrounding parenchyma (Cheng & Cui, 2004). Therefore, the textures of digital images contain a lot of valuable information for further research and application. This

Figure 2. Abnormal mammograms are classified into calcification, architectural distortion, asymmetry, circumscribed masses, speculated masses, and ill-defined masses

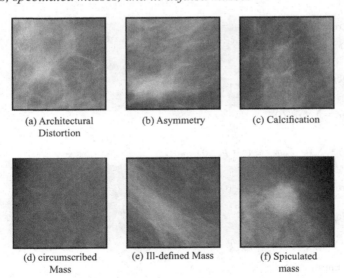

(a) Architectural Distortion (b) Asymmetry (c) Calcification

(d) circumscribed Mass (e) Ill-defined Mass (f) Spiculated mass

study applies gray level co-occurrence matrices, a statistical textural method, to analyze the textural features of mammograms and develop descriptors for content-based image retrieval. Gray level co-occurrence matrices will be introduced in the following section.

Gray Level Co-Occurrence Matrices

Gray level co-occurrence matrix (GLCM) is a statistical method for computing the co-occurrence probability of textural features (Haralick, 1979). Given an image $f(x, y)$ of size $L_r \times L_c$ with

a set of N_g gray levels, define the matrix $p(i, j, d, \theta)$ as shown in Box 1.

Mammogram Analysis Using GLCM

In order to develop the tailored descriptors described in the next section, it is necessary to analyze the features of the mammogram. In this study, 12 GLCMs are constructed in order to compute each ROI in the 0°, 45°, 90°, and 135° directions, each with unit pixel distances of 1, 3, and 5, respectively. The 11 features described earlier are computed for the 12 GLCMs, thus resulting in a total of 132 texture features for each ROI.

Box 1.

$$P(i, j, d, \theta) = card\{((x_1, y_1), (x_2, y_2)) \in (L_r \times L_c)(L_r \times L_c)|$$
$$(x_2, y_2) = (x_1, y_1) + (d\cos\theta, d\sin\theta),$$
$$f(x_1, y_1) = i, f(x_2, y_2) = j, 0 \le i, j < N_g\} \tag{1}$$

where d denotes the distance between pixels (x_1, y_1) and (x_2, y_2) in the image, θ denotes the orientation aligning (x_1, y_1) and (x_2, y_2), and card $\{\cdot\}$ denotes the number of elements in the set. Texture features that can be extracted from gray level co-occurrence matrices (Haralick, Shanmugan, & Dinstein, 1973) are:

$$\text{Angular Second Moment (ASM)} = \sum_i \sum_j \{p(i, j)\}^2 \tag{2}$$

$$\text{Contrast} = \sum_{n=0}^{Ng-1} n^2 \left\{ \sum_{i=1}^{Ng} \sum_{\substack{j=1 \\ |i-j|=n}}^{Ng} p(i, j) \right\} \tag{3}$$

$$\text{Correlation} = \frac{\sum_i \sum_j (ij) p(i, j) - \mu_x \mu_y}{\sigma_x \sigma_y} \tag{4}$$

$$\text{Variance} = \sum_i \sum_j (i - j)^2 p(i, j) \tag{5}$$

$$\text{Inverse Difference Moment (ID\_Mom)} = \sum_i \sum_j \frac{1}{1 + (i - j)^2} p(i, j) \tag{6}$$

$$\text{Sum Average (Sum\_Aver)} = \sum_{i=2}^{2Ng} i p_{x+y}(i) \tag{7}$$

$$\text{Sum Variance (Sum\_Var)} = \sum_{i=2}^{2Ng} (i - Sum\_Entro)^2 p_{x+y}(i) \tag{8}$$

$$\text{Sum Entropy (Sum\_Entro)} = \sum_{i=2}^{2Ng} p_{x+y}(i) \log\{p_{x+y}(i)\} \tag{9}$$

$$\text{Entropy} = -\sum_i \sum_j p(i, j) \log p(i, j) \tag{10}$$

$$\text{Different Variance (Diff\_Vari)} = \text{variance of } p_{x-y} \tag{11}$$

$$\text{Different Entropy (Diff\_Entro)} = -\sum_{i=0}^{Ng-1} p_{x-y}(i) \log\{p_{x-y}(i)\} \tag{12}$$

Feature Selection for Image Retrieval

At the stage of feature analysis, 132 texture features are generated for each ROI. We obtain 5,148 texture feature sample images from 20 normal and 19 abnormal images. To select the most discriminant features, a statistical multivariate t-test is used to assess the significance of the difference between the means of two sample set A and B, which are independent of each other in the obvious sense, that is, the individual measures in set A are in no way related to any of the individual measures in set B. The value of the t-test is obtained as follows (Serdobolskii, 2000):

$$D_a = \sum (A_i - \mu_a)^2 \qquad (13)$$

$$D_b = \sum (B_i - \mu_b)^2 \qquad (14)$$

$$V = \frac{D_a + D_b}{(n_a - 1) + (n_b - 1)} \qquad (15)$$

$$\sigma = \sqrt{\frac{V}{n_a} + \frac{V}{n_b}} \qquad (16)$$

$$t = \frac{\mu_a - \mu_b}{\sigma} \qquad (17)$$

where A_i and B_i in equations (13) and (14) are the ith element of the set A and B, while μ_a and μ_b are the means of the set A and B, respectively. D_a and D_b in the equations (13) and (14) are the sum of squared deviates of *the* set A and B. V in equation (15) is the estimated variance of the source population. σ in equation (16) is the standard deviation of the sampling distribution of sample-mean differences. t in equation (17) is the value of the t-test. The degree of freedom (d.f.) is $(n_a - 1) + (n_b - 1)$.

In our case study with 20 normal images (set A) and 19 abnormal images (set B), the degree of freedom (d.f.) is 37. According to the Table of Critical Values of t (Rencher, 1998), the t value for 37 degrees of freedom (d.f.) is 1.305. When the value t obtained in this experiment is greater than 1.305, it means that there is a significant mean difference between normal and abnormal mammograms with regard to the given feature.

The descriptor is composed of features with significant differences in the t statistic. Individual descriptors were developed for three distances (d = 1, 3, and 5) in the gray level co-occurrence matrices.

Data Normalization

The purpose of normalization in this experiment is to assign a weight to all features in order to measure their similarity on the same basis. The technique used was to project each feature onto a unit sphere. However, a potential problem exists — if a few elements in a feature space are extremely large, other elements may be dominated by these large ones after normalization.

To solve this problem, the value located at the point of the top 95% of the distribution is taken as the nominal maximum. All features greater than

Figure 3. Process of normalization

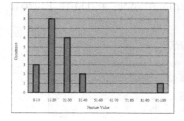 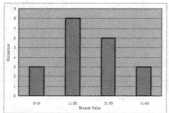 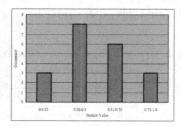

(a) The original distribution.   (b) The trimmed distribution.   (c) The normalized distribution.

the nominal minimum in the feature space were clipped to the nominal maximal value, that is, the top 5% of distribution are trimmed. Then all values are divided by the maximal values. An example is given to illustrate the use of this approach to normalization. Figure 3a shows the original distribution of feature values in a feature vector. The results of trimming the top 5% and normalization are illustrated in Figures 3b and 3c.

Similarity Measure

The similarity measure of two images I_a and I_b is the distance between their descriptors f_a and f_a. In this work, L_2 norm was adopted to measure the similarity between the query image and each ROI. L_2 is defined as follows:

$$\| d_{ab} \|_2 = | f_a - f_b |^2 = \sqrt{\sum_{i=1}^{n} | f_{a,i} - f_{b,i} |^2}$$ (18)

where d_{ab} is the similarity distance between descriptors f_a and f_b, $f_{a,i}$ and $f_{b,i}$ are the ith element of f_a and f_a, respectively, and n is the number of elements of the descriptors. The smaller the distance is, the more similar the two images are. After calculating the distance, our CBIR system ranks similarity in descending order and then returns the top five images that are most similar to the query image.

Performance Evaluation

Relevance judgment is a vital part of performance evaluation. The relevance criteria described in Table 1 were developed and used in this work. For example, suppose the query image belongs to the calcification class, the retrieved image would score

0.5 if it belongs to any of the following abnormal classes: ill-defined masses, circumscribed masses, speculated masses, architectural distortion, and asymmetry.

Precision and recall are basic measures used in evaluating the effectiveness of an information retrieval system. Precision is the ratio of the number of relevant records retrieved to the total number of irrelevant and relevant records retrieved (Baeza-Yates, & Ribeiro-Neto, 1999). It indicates the subject score assigned to each of the top five images in this experiment. The formula is expressed as follows:

$$p = \frac{\sum_{i=1}^{n} S_i}{N}$$ (19)

where S_i is the score assigned to the ith hit, N is the number of top hits retrieved.

Recall is the ratio of the number of relevant records retrieved to the total number of relevant records in the database (Baeza-Yates & Ribeiro-Neto, 1999). It is defined as follows:

$$R = \frac{R_n}{T_n}$$ (20)

where R_n is the number of retrieved relevant hits, and T_n is the total number of relevant images in the database.

Results of *t*-Test

Table 2 presents the results of the t statistic for d = 1 of gray level co-occurrence matrices. From the results, it can be seen that the differences between the mean values of ASM, Correlation, Sum_Var (sum variance), and Diff_Entro (differ-

Table 1. Criteria for measurement of performance evaluation of CBIR

Score	Criteria
1.0	The retrieved image belongs to the class of query image.
0.5	The retrieved image belongs to one of the abnormal classes, but not the class of query image.
0	The retrieved image does not belong to any abnormal class.

Table 2. Comparison of mean values obtained by co-occurrence matrices with the distance of 1

Feature	Normal		Abnormal		t (37 .d.f.)
	μ_a	D_a	μ_b	D_b	
ASM	1.7721	0.6127	1.3890	0.5542	1.6042
Contrast	5.8209	2.2742	5.6187	3.7038	0.3755
Correlation	-0.3392	0.0742	-0.6135	0.5345	1.6071
Variance	0.2413	0.0768	1.5446	1.9193	-4.2257
ID_Mom	2.9460	0.0671	3.0654	0.1442	-1.1812
Sum_Aver	2.1943	0.3391	2.6984	1.2137	-1.8444
Sum_Var	3.2636	2.2970	0.7699	1.3261	5.9097
Sum_Entro	-6.7253	2.7305	-0.7922	0.1327	-15.6895
Entropy	-4.0729	0.1476	-3.8611	0.3262	-1.3995
Diff_Vari	5.2007	2.3020	6.7532	1.4977	-3.5953
Diff_Entro	-1.7865	0.0332	-1.9603	0.0141	3.5986

Table 3. Comparison of mean values obtained by co-occurrence matrices with the distance of 3

Feature	Normal		Abnormal		t (37 .d.f.)
	μ_a	D_a	μ_b	D_b	
ASM	1.2846	0.3212	1.0075	0.2905	1.6046
Contrast	1.3822	0.2398	1.6247	0.4604	-1.3191
Correlation	0.8311	0.0402	3.6871	15.2704	-3.3534
Variance	1.5943	3.4598	1.1012	0.9300	1.0584
ID_Mom	1.465	0.0518	1.5281	0.1695	-0.6123
Sum_Aver	1.6135	0.1835	1.9774	0.6539	-1.8161
Sum_Entro	-4.9365	1.4720	-0.5789	0.0708	-15.7084
Entropy	-2.6801	0.1052	-2.4949	0.4599	-1.1262
Diff_Vari	4.1858	1.2969	5.3510	0.8446	-3.5984
Diff_Entro	-1.6118	0.0184	1.7424	0.0088	-91.7379
Diff_Entro	-1.7865	0.0332	-1.9603	0.0141	3.5986

ence entropy) of the normal and abnormal ROIs are significant ($t > 1.305$). As a result, these four features are selected to construct the descriptor. Table 3 shows that ASM is the only feature with significant discriminating power for two groups of ROIs when $d = 3$. The descriptor with $d = 3$ contains only ASM.

Table 4 shows that Sum_Var (sum-variance) is the only feature with significant discriminating power for two groups of ROIs when $d = 5$. The descriptor with $d = 5$ contains only Sum_Var.

Results of Performance Evaluation

Precision can be used to describe the accuracy of the proposed CBIR system in finding only relevant images on a search for query images. Table 5 shows that precision rates for the three descriptors ($d = 1, 3,$ and 5) are 47%, 50%, and 51%, respectively. The descriptor with $d = 5$ obtained the highest value in precision and the smallest values in standard deviation. This indicates that the performance of the descriptor ($d = 5$) is more

Table 4. Comparison of mean values obtained by co-occurrence matrices with the distance of 5

Feature	Normal		Abnormal		
	μ_a	D_a	μ_b	D_b	t (37 .d.f.)
ASM	1.2466	0.3019	0.9784	0.2730	0.7924
Contrast	2.1675	0.8227	2.9725	2.0665	-1.5708
Correlation	0.8822	0.0387	4.6453	14.6955	-7.1316
Variance	1.4357	2.8461	1.0654	0.8467	1.0316
ID_Mom	1.2008	0.0497	1.227	0.1625	-0.0742
Sum_Aver	1.5855	0.1775	1.9376	0.6293	-0.8292
Sum_Var	2.3006	2.6245	0.5359	0.6438	4.5870
Sum_Entro	-4.8432	1.4197	-0.5657	0.0677	-8.0337
Entropy	-2.5128	0.1179	-2.3037	0.2179	-0.4203
Diff_Vari	4.1858	1.2969	5.3510	0.8446	-1.6684
Diff_Entro	-1.6118	0.0184	-1.7424	0.0088	0.3150

Table 5. Precision for the 3 descriptors

	CALC	CIRC	SPIC	MISC	ARCH	ASYM	Mean	Std
d=1	42%	44%	54%	44%	46%	54%	47%	5.32%
d=3	57%	43%	54%	42%	54%	51%	50%	6.24%
d=5	48%	53%	54%	50%	50%	48%	51%	2.51%

Table 6. Recall for the 3 descriptors

	CALC	CIRC	SPIC	MISC	ARCH	ASYM	Mean	Std
d=1	10.69%	12.80%	20.53%	18.67%	16.84%	26.00%	17.59%	5.51%
d=3	13.45%	11.60%	20.00%	20.00%	18.42%	25.33%	18.13%	4.97%
d=5	12.07%	15.20%	21.05%	24.00%	20.00%	22.00%	19.05%	4.51%

Note: CALC = calcification; CIRC = circumscribed masses, SPIC = speculated masses; ARCH = architectural distortion; ASYM = asymmetry; MISC = other or ill-defined masses.

stable. On the whole, about half of the results retrieved by these three descriptors are relevant to the query images.

Recall measures how well the CBIR system finds all relevant images in a search for a query image. Table 6 indicates that the descriptor with $d = 5$ outperforms the other two. However, the recall values are very close. The largest difference is only 1.5%. The three descriptors can retrieve, on average, about 18% of relevant images in the database. In theory, as precision goes up, recall goes down. The relationship explains why the three recall values are low.

The experimental results also show that the descriptor with the largest distance ($d = 5$) has the best performance in both precision and recall. The descriptor with $d = 3$ outperforms the descriptor with $d = 1$ in both measures. Although the larger distance has better performance in this experiment, it is still too early to make any conclusions.

The main contribution of this work is to present a sound CBIR methodology for mammograms. The methodology is divided into image analysis and image retrieval stages. The purpose of the image analysis is to collect samples from the database, obtain the image signature, and then apply it for the feature extraction in the image retrieval stage. A complete CBIR system based on gray level co-occurrence matrices was implemented. A technique was also proposed to improve the effectiveness of normalization. Three descriptors were evaluated by query images to retrieve the ROIs for the mammogram dataset consisting of 122 images of six sub-classes from abnormal class, and 207 images from normal class. The best precision rate of 51% and recall rate of 19% were achieved with the descriptor using gray level co-occurrence matrices with the pixel distance of 5.

RESEARCH ISSUES

Content-based retrieval for medical images is still in its infancy. There are many challenging research issues. This section identifies and addresses some issues in the future research agenda.

Bridging the Semantic Gap

An ideal medical CBIR system from a user perspective would involve semantic retrieval, in which the user submits a query like "find MRIs of brain with tumor". This kind of open-ended query is very difficult for the current CBIR systems to distinguish brain MRI's from spine MRIs even though the two types of images are visually different. Current medical CBIR systems mainly rely on low-level features like texture, color, and shape.

Systems Integration

Most medical retrieval systems are designed for one particular type of medical image, such as

mammogram or MRIs of spine. Specific techniques and modalities are developed based on the characteristics of these highly homogeneous images in their databases. However, medical image databases across different medical institutions have been expected to connect through PACS. With PACS, a user may make a request to search for medical images among different databases, where images display different characteristics such as degree of resolution, degree of noise, use of color, shape of object, and texture of background. In other words, PACS can be seen as a single retrieval system with distributed image databases, which collect medical images with various modalities. Therefore, systems capable of finding images across heterogeneous image databases are desirable.

Human-Computer Interaction and Usability

Current research on medical CBIR concentrates on the effectiveness of the system, rarely evolving the relationship between CBIR and user interface design. However, innovative retrieval systems alone may not obtain user acceptance as users of medical CBIR systems may include radiologists, surgeons, nurses, or other users without specific knowledge of these systems. The user's experience, or how the user experiences the system, is the key to acceptance. Good user interface design is usually required for the end user to easily learn and use the system. Also, empirical usability testing permits naïve users to provide information about the usability of individual system functions and components.

Performance Evaluation

The National Institute of Standards and Technology (NIST) has developed TREC (Text REtrieval Conference) as the standard test-bed and evaluation paradigm for the information retrieval community (Smeaton, 2003). The image retrieval community still awaits the construction and implementation of a scientifically-valid evaluation framework and standard test bed. To construct a test bed for medical CBIR, imaging modalities, regions, and orientations of images should be taken into account. Due to the complexity of medical images, how to construct a common test bed for medical CBIR is a research issue.

CONCLUSION

The goal of medical image databases is to provide an effective means for organizing, searching, and indexing large collections of medical images. This requires intelligent systems that have the ability to recognize, capture, and understand the complex content of medical images. Content-based retrieval is a promising approach to achieve these tasks and has developed a number of techniques used in medical images. Despite recent developments, medical content-based image retrieval still has a long way to go and more efforts are expected to be devoted to this area. Ultimately, a well-organized image database, accompanied by an intelligent retrieval mechanism, can support clinical treatment, and provide a basis for better medical research and education.

REFERENCES

Antani, S., Lee, D. J., Long, L. R., & Thoma, G. R. (2004a). Evaluation of shape similarity measurement methods for spine X-ray images. *Journal of Visual Communication and Image Representation, 15*(3), 285-302.

Antani, S., Long, L. R., Thoma, G. R., & Lee, D. J. (2003). Evaluation of shape indexing methods for content-based retrieval of X-ray images. In *Proceedings of IS&T/SPIE 15th Annual Symposium on Electronic Imaging, Storage, and Retrieval for Media Databases* (pp. 405-416). Santa Clara, CA: SPIE.

Antani, S., Xu, X., Long, L. R., & Thoma, G. R. (2004b). Partial shape matching for CBIR of spine X-ray images. In *Proceedings of IS&T/SPIE Electronic Imaging — Storage and Retrieval Methods and Applications for Multimedia 2004* (pp. 1-8). San Jose, CA: SPIE.

Baeza-Yates, R., & Ribeiro-Neto, B. (Eds.). (1999). *Modern information retrieval.* Boston: Addison-Wesley.

Beckmann, N., Kriegel, H.-P., Schneider, R., & Seeger, B. (1990). The R*-tree: An efficient and robust access method for points and rectangles. In *Proceedings of ACM SIGMOD International Conference on Management of Data* (pp. 322-331). Atlantic City, NJ: ACM Press.

Brodley, C. E., Kak, A, Dy, J., Shyu, C. R., Aisen, A., & Broderick, L. (1999). Content-based retrieval from medical image database: A synergy of human interaction, machine learning, and computer vision. In *Proceedings of the Sixteenth National Conference on Artificial Intelligence* (pp. 760-767). Orlando, FL: AAAI Press / MIT Press.

Buhler, P., Just, U., Will, E., Kotzerke, J., & van den Hoff, J. (2004). An accurate method for correction of head movement in PET. *IEEE Transactions on Medical Imaging, 23*(9), 1176-1185.

Chang, C.-L., Cheng, B.-W., & Su, J.-L. (2004). Using case-based reasoning to establish a continuing care information system of discharge planning. *Expert Systems with Applications, 26*(4), 601-613.

Cheng, H. D., & Cui, M. (2004). Mass lesion detection with a fuzzy neural network. *Pattern Recognition, 37*(6), 1189-1200.

Eakins, J. P. (2002). Towards in intelligent image retrieval. *Pattern Recognition, 35*(1), 3-14.

Egecioglu, O., Ferhatosmanoglu, H., & Ogras, U. (2004). Dimensionality reduction and similarity computation by inner-product approximations. *IEEE Transactions on Knowledge and Data Engineering, 16*(6), 714-726.

El-Naqa, I., Yang, Y., Galatsanos, N. P., & Wernick, M. N. (2003). Relevance feedback based on incremental learning for mammogram retrieval. In *Proceedings of the International Conference of Image Processing 2003* (pp. 729-732). Barcelona, Spain: IEEE Press.

El-Naqa, I., Yang, Y., Galatsanos, N. P., Nishikawa, R. M., & Wernick, M. N. (2004). A similarity learning approach to content-based image retrieval: Application to digital mammography. *IEEE Transactions on Medical Imaging, 23*(10), 1233-1244.

Feng, D., Siu, W. C., & Zhang, H. J. (Eds.). (2003). *Multimedia information retrieval and management: Technological fundamentals and applications.* Berlin: Springer.

Ferecatu, M., Crucianu, M., & Boujemaa, N. (2004a). Retrieval of difficult image classes using SVM-based relevance feedback. In *Proceedings of the 6th ACM SIGMM International Workshop on Multimedia Information Retrieval* (pp. 23-30). New York: ACM Press.

Ferecatu, M., Crucianu, M., & Boujemaa, N. (2004b). Sample selection strategies for relevance feedback in region-based image retrieval. In *Pacific-Rim Conference on Multimedia 2004* (pp. 497-504). Tokyo, Japan: IEEE Press.

Fonseca, M. J., & Jorge, J. A. (2003). Indexing high-dimensional data for content-based retrieval in large database. In *Proceedings of the Eighth International Conference on Database Systems for Advanced Applications* (pp. 267-274). Kyoto, Japan: IEEE Press.

Gevers, T., (2001). Color-based retrieval. In M. S. Lew (Ed.), *Principles of visual information retrieval* (pp. 11-49). London: Springer.

Gevers, T., & Stokman, H. (2003). Classifying color edges in video into shadow-geometry, highlight, or material transitions. *IEEE Transactions on Multimedia, 5*(2), 237-243.

Glatard, T., Montagnat, J., & Magnin, I. E. (2004). Texture based medical image indexing and retrieval: Application to cardiac imaging. In *Proceedings of the ACM SIGMM International Workshop on Multimedia Information Retrieval* (pp. 135-142). New York: ACM Press.

Gonzalez, R. C., & Woods, R. E. (2002). *Digital image processing.* Upper Saddle River, NJ: Prentice Hall.

Guan, H. & Wada, S. (2002). Flexible color texture retrieval method using multi-resolution mosaic for image classification. In *Proceedings of the 6th International Conference on Signal Processing: Vol. 1* (pp. 612-615). Beijing, China: IEEE Press.

Guttman, A. (1984). R-trees: A dynamic index structure for spatial searching. In *Proceedings of ACM SIGMOD International Conference on Management of Data* (pp. 47-54). New York: ACM Press.

Haeghen, Y. V., Naeyaert, J. M. A. D., Lemahieu, I., & Philips, W. (2000). An imaging system with calibrated color image acquisition for use in dermatology. *IEEE Transaction on Medical Imaging, 19*(7), 722-730.

Haralick, R. M. (1979). Statistical and structural approaches to texture. In *Proceedings of the IEEE, 67*(5), 786-804.

Haralick, R. M., Shanmugan, K., & Dinstein, I. (1973). Textural features for image classification. *IEEE Transactions on Systems, Man and Cybernetics, 3*(6), 610-621.

Hoi, C.-H., Chan, C.-H., Huang, K., Lyu, M. R., & King, I. (2004). Biased support vector machine for relevance feedback in image retrieval. In *Proceedings of International Joint Conference on Neural Networks* (pp. 3189-3194). Budapest, Hungary: IEEE Press.

Hsu, C.-C., & Ho, C.-S. (2004). A new hybrid case-based architecture for medical diagnosis. *Information Sciences, 166*(1-4), 231-247.

Huang, H. K. (2003). PACS, image management, and imaging informatics. In D. Feng, W. C. Siu, & H. J. Zhang (Eds.), *Multimedia information retrieval and management: Technological fundamentals and applications* (pp.347-365). New York: Springer.

Lehmann, T. M., Guld, M. O., Keysers, D, Deselaers, T., Schubert, H., Wein B. B., & Spitzer, K. (2004a). Similarity of medical images computed from global feature vectors for content-based retrieval. *Lecture Notes in Artificial Intelligence* (pp. 989-995).

Lehmann, T. M., Guld, M. O., Thies, C., Plodowski, B., Keysers, D., Ott, B., & Schubert, H. (2004b). IRMA—Content-based image retrieval in medical applications. In *Proceedings of the 14th World Congress on Medical Informatics* (pp. 842-848).

Lehmann, T. M., Wein, B. B., & Greenspan, H. (2003). Integration of content-based image retrieval to picture archiving and communication systems. In *Proceedings of Medical Informatics Europe*. Amsterdam, The Netherlands: IOS Press.

Li, C. H., & Yuen, P. C. (2000). Regularized color clustering in medical image database. *IEEE Transaction on Medical Imaging, 19*(11), 1150-1155.

Li, C.-T. (1998). *Unsupervised texture segmentation using multi-resolution Markov random fields*. Doctoral dissertation, University of Warwick, Coventry, UK.

Majumdar, S., Kothari, M., Augat, P., Newitt, D. C., Link, T. M., Lin, J. C., & Lang, T. (1998). High-resolution magnetic resonance imaging: Three-dimensional trabecular bone architecture and biomechanical properties. *Bone, 22*, 445-454.

Moghaddam, H. A., Khajoie, T. T., & Rouhi, A. H. (2003). A new algorithm for image indexing and retrieval using wavelet correlogram. In *Proceedings of the International Conference on Image*

Processing 2003: Vol. 3 (pp. 497-500). Barcelona, Catalonia, Spain: IEEE Press.

Muller, H., Michous, N., Bandon, D., & Geissbuhler, A. (2004a). A review of content-based image retrieval systems in medical applications — Clinical benefits and future directions. *International Journal of Medical Informatics, 73*(1), 1-23.

Muller, H., Rosset, A. Vallee, J.-P., & Geissbuhler, A. (2004b). Comparing features sets for content-based image retrieval in a medical-case database. In *Proceedings of IS&T/SPIE Medical Imaging 2004: PACS and Imaging Informatics* (pp. 99-109).

Nishibori, M. (2000). Problems and solutions in medical color imaging. In *Proceedings of the Second International Symposium on Multi-Spectral Imaging and High Accurate Color Reproduction* (pp. 9-17). Chiba, Japan: SPIE.

Nishibori, M., Tsumura, N., & Miyake, Y. (2004). Why multi-spectral imaging in medicine? *Journal of Imaging Science and Technology, 48*(2), 125-129.

Partridge, M., & Calvo, R. A. (1998). Fast dimensionality reduction and simple PCA. *Intelligent Data Analysis, 2*(1-4), 203-214.

Ouyang, A., & Tan, Y. P (2002). A novel multi-scale spatial-color descriptor for content-based image retrieval. In *Proceedings of the 7th International Conference on Control, Automation, Robotics and Vision: Vol. 3* (pp. 1204-1209).

Qian, G.., Sural, S., Gu, Y., & Pramanik, S. (2004). Similarity between Euclidean and cosine angle distance for nearest neighbor queries. In *Proceedings of 2004 ACM Symposium on Applied Computing* (pp. 1232-1237). Nicosia, Cyprus: ACM Press.

Rencher, A. C. (1998). *Multi-variate statistical inference and applications*. New York: John Wiley & Sons.

Rocchio, J. J. (1971). Relevance feedback in information retrieval. In G. Salton (Ed.), *The SMART retrieval system-experiments in automatic document processing* (pp.313-323). Englewood Cliffs, NJ: Prentice Hall.

Rosset, A., Ratib, O., Geissbuhler, A., & Vallee, J. P. (2002). Integration of a multimedia teaching and reference database in a PACS environment. *Radiographics, 22*(6), 1567-1577.

Rui, Y., & Huang, T. (2002). Learning based relevance feedback in image retrieval. In A. C. Bovik, C. W. Chen, & D. Goldfof (Eds.), *Advances in image processing and understanding: A festschrift for Thomas S. Huang* (pp. 163-182). New York: World Scientific Publishing.

Schmidt, R., Montani, S., Bellazzi, R., Portinale, L., & Gierl, L. (2001). Cased-based reasoning for medical knowledge-based systems. *International Journal of Medical Informatics, 64*(2-3), 355-367.

Sebe, N., & Lew, M. S. (2002). Texture features for content-based retrieval. In M. S. Lew (Ed.), *Principles of visual information retrieval* (pp.51-85), London: Springer.

Serdobolskii, V. (2000). *Multivariate statistical analysis: A high-dimensional approach.* London: Kluwer Academic Publishers.

Shah, B., Raghavan, V., & Dhatric, P. (2004). Efficient and effective content-based image retrieval using space transformation. *Proceedings of the 10th International Multimedia Modelling Conferenc* (p. 279). Brisbane, Australia. IEEE Press.

Shyu, C., Brodley, C., Kak, A., Kosaka, A., Aisen, A., & Broderick, L. (1999). ASSERT: A physician-in-the-loop content-based image retrieval system for HRCT image databases. *Computer Vision and Image Understanding, 75*(1/2), 111-132.

Shyu, C.-R., Pavlopoulou, C., Kak, A. C., Brodly, C. E., & Broderick, L. (2002). Using human perceptual categories for content-based retrieval from a medical image database. *Computer Vision and Image Understanding, 88*(3), 119-151.

Smeaton, A. F., & Over, P. (2003). TRECVID: Benchmarking the effectiveness of information retrieval tasks on digital video. In *International Conference on Image and Video Retrieval*, 18-27.

Smeulders, A. W. M., Worring, M., Santini, S., Gupta, A., & Jain, R. (2000). Content-based image retrieval at the end of the early years. *IEEE Transactions on Pattern Analysis and Machine Intelligence, 22*(12), 1349-1380.

Sinha, U., & Kangarloo, H. (2002). Principal component analysis for content-based image retrieval. *RadioGraphics, 22*, 1271-1289.

Squire, D. M., Muller, H., Muller, W., Marchand-Maillet, S., & Pun, T. (2001). Design and evaluation of a content-based image retrieval system. In S. M. Rahman (Ed.), *Design and management of multimedia information systems: Opportunities and challenges* (pp. 125-151). Hershey, PA: Idea Group Publishing.

Squire, D. M., Muller, W., Muller, H., & Pun, T. (2000). Content-based query of image databases: inspirations from text retrieval, *Pattern Recognition Letters, 21*(13-14), 1193-1198.

Suckling, J., Parker, J., Dance, D. R., Astley, S., Hutt, I., Boggis, C. R. M., Ricketts, I., Stamatakis, E., Cerneaz, N., Kok, S.-L., Taylor, P., Betal, D., & Savage, J. (1994). The mammographic image analysis society digital mammogram database. In *Proceedings of the 2nd International Workshop on Digital Mammography*, 375-378.

Swain, M. J., & Ballard, D. H. (1991). Color Indexing. *International Journal of Computer Vision, 7*(1), 11-32.

Tamai, S. (1999). The color of digital imaging in pathology and cytology. *Proceedings of the First Symposium of the "Color" of Digital Imaging in Medicine.* Tokyo, Japan: SPIE.

Tao, D., & Tang, X. (2004). Random sampling based SVM for relevance feedback image retrieval. In *The IEEE Computer Society Conference on Computer Vision and Pattern Recognition 2004*, 647-652. Washington, DC: IEEE Press.

Tourassi, G. D. (1999). Journey toward computer-aided diagnosis: Role of image texture analysis. *Radiology*, 317-320.

Veenland, J. F., Grashuis, J. L., Weinans, H., Ding, M., & Vrooman, H. A. (2002). Suitability of texture features to assess changes in trabecular bone architecture. *Pattern Recognition Letters, 23*(4), 395-403.

Veltkamp, R. C., & Hagedoorn, M. (2002). State of the art in shape matching. In M. S. Lew (Ed.), *Principles of visual information retrieval* (pp.87-119), London: Springer.

Wei, C.-H, & Li, C.-T. (2005). Design of content-based multimedia retrieval. In M. Pagani (Ed.), *Encyclopedia of multimedia technology and networking* (pp. 116-122). Hershey, PA: Idea Group Reference.

Wong, S., & Hoo, K. S. (2002). Medical imagery. In V. Castelli, & L. D. Bergman (Eds.), *Image databases: Search and retrieval of digital imagery* (pp. 83-105). New York: John Wiley & Sons.

Wong, S. T. C. (1998). CBIR in medicine: Still a long way to go. In *Proceedings of the IEEE Workshop on Content-Based Access of Image and Video Libraries*, 114. Santa Barbara, CA: IEEE Press.

Yu, H., Li, M., Zhang, H.-J., & Feng, J. (2002). Color texture moments for content-based image retrieval. In *Proceedings of the International Conference on Image Processing 2002: Vol. 3* (pp. 929-932).

This work was previously published in Database Modeling for Industrial Data Management: Emerging Technologies and Applications, edited by Z. M. Ma, pp. 258-292, copyright 2006 by Information Science Publishing (an imprint of IGI Global).

Chapter XV
Methods and Applications for Segmenting 3D Medical Image Data

Hong Shen
Siemens Corporate Research, USA

ABSTRACT

In this chapter, we will give an intuitive introduction to the general problem of 3D medical image segmentation. We will give an overview of the popular and relevant methods that may be applicable, with a discussion about their advantages and limits. Specifically, we will discuss the issue of incorporating prior knowledge into the segmentation of anatomic structures and describe in detail the concept and issues of knowledge-based segmentation. Typical sample applications will accompany the discussions throughout this chapter. We hope this will help an application developer to improve insights in the understanding and application of various computer vision approaches to solve real-world problems of medical image segmentation.

INTRODUCTION

The advances in medical imaging equipment have brought efficiency and high capability to the screening, diagnosis and surgery of various diseases. The 3D imaging modalities, such as multi-slice computer tomography (CT), magnetic resonance imaging (MRI) and ultrasound scanners, produce large amounts of digital data that are difficult and tedious to interpret merely by physicians. Computer aided diagnosis (CAD) systems will therefore play a critical role, especially in the visualization, segmentation, detection,

registration and reporting of medical pathologies. Among these functions, the segmentation of objects, mainly anatomies and pathologies from large 3D volume data, is more fundamental, since the results often become the basis of all other quantitative analysis tasks.

The segmentation of medical data poses a challenging problem. One difficulty lies in the large volume of the data involved and the on-time requirement of medical applications. The time constraints vary among applications, ranging from several tens of milliseconds for online surgical monitoring, to seconds for interactive volumetric measures, to minutes or hours for off-line processing on a PACS server. Depending on the application, this puts a limit on the types of methods that may be used. Another major hurdle is the high variation of image properties in the data, making it hard to construct a general model. The variations come from several aspects. First, the complexity of various anatomies maps to the large variation of their images in the medical data. Second, the age, gender, pose and other conditions of the patient lead to high inter-patient variability. Last, but not the least, are the almost infinite variations in an anatomy due to pathology or in the pathological structures. On the other hand, medical applications usually have a strong requirement of robustness over all variations. Beside the above challenges, system issues exist for the major modalities, such as noise, partial volume effects, non-isotropic voxel, variation in scanning protocols, and so forth. These all lead to more difficulties for the medical segmentation problem.

Knowledge-Based Segmentation

Medical image segmentation has the advantage of knowing beforehand what is contained in the image. We also know about the range of size, shape, and so forth, which is extracted from expert statements. In other fields of computer vision, such as satellite image analysis, the task of segmentation sometimes contains a recognition step. Bottom-up strategy is usually used, which starts with the low-level detection of the primitives that form the object boundaries, followed by merging. One sophisticated development is Perceptual Organization (Sarkar & Boyer, 1994; Guy & Medioni, 1996; Mohan & Nevatia, 1989), which attempts to organize detected primitives into structures. It is regarded as the "middle ground" between low-level and high-level processing. In 3D medical data, grouping is much more difficult due to the complexity of medical shapes. Because of this, top-down strategies prevail in 3D medical image analysis.

Knowledge-based segmentation makes strong assumptions about the content of the image. We use prior knowledge to find and tailor a general segmentation method to the specific application. Global priors are applied when the local information is incomplete or of low quality. It is a top-down strategy that starts with knowledge or models about high-level object features and attentively searches for their image counterparts.

The past several decades witnessed dramatic advances in the fields of computer vision and image analysis, from which the area of medical image analysis is derived. Various methods and frameworks for segmentation have been proposed, and many are driven by the needs of medical image analysis. These provide valuable theoretical thoughts as the basis of knowledge-based segmentation, but only at a high level. Typically, such a method is shown to be generic as it works on a number of cases from various applications with reasonable successes. This is quite different from the requirement of medical image segmentation in the real world, which depend heavily on the specific application—the workflow of the medical procedure, the anatomy and pathology of interest, the performance and accuracy requirements and the user inputs. Given all the priors and conditions of a medical application, we need to design the algorithm that will be the best compromise between accuracy, speed, robustness and user inputs. The resulting system will be specific to the given application; not only the algorithm, but also the parameter settings. A medical image analysis algorithm will be put to tests on thousands of data sets before it can be made into a clinical product. Hence, even if it is application specific, such an algorithm is general in that it has to cover all possible variations of the application.

A developer in this field not only needs to master the various methods in computer vision, but also understand the situations each of them may be applied to, as well as their limitations. In the next sections, we will focus on real world issues of medical image segmentation. We will first

Figure 1. Lung nodule segmentation from multi-slice chest CT data

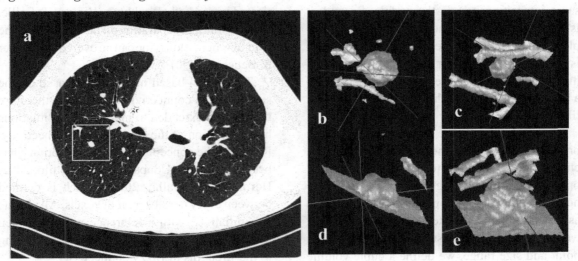

(a) An axial slice of the volume data. At the center of the marked box is the nodule to be segmented. Surface shaded display of the segmentation results are shown for nodules that are (b) solitary, (c) connected to vessels, (d) connected to chest wall, and (e) connected to both vessel and chest wall

give an overview of the relevant low-level methods with examples. We will then discuss the popular frameworks for incorporating global priors and their limitations. We will present the principles of a novel strategy that was developed recently (Shen, Shi, & Peng, 2005) for an sample application. Finally, we will conclude the chapter with an outlook on the future trends in this field.

APPLICATIONS USING LOW-LEVEL SEGMENTATION METHODS

In this section we will give 3D medical application examples that use low-level segmentation methods. We define low-level methods as those that do not incorporate global shape priors of the object to be segmented, but mostly rely on local image properties. Many surveys and textbooks (Sonka, Hlavac, & Boyle, 1998) give detailed descriptions of all the segmentation methods, and this short chapter will not serve as a duplication of these efforts. Instead, we will give examples to

show where each category of low-level method is adequate, and also review the recently developed methods.

Segmentation Using Regional and Morphological Methods

Region-based methods group together voxels that have some common properties. They are applicable when there is high contrast between object and background and intra-object variation is minimal. As shown in Figure 1, in a chest CT data, the lung area maps to dark regions, while the chest wall, the vessels, the airways and nodules map to bright regions of the same intensity range. A typical application is the segmentation of a lung nodule given a click point in the nodule. Since there is high contrast between object and background, a simple 3D region grow (Sonka et al., 1998; Adams & Bischof, 1984) is the best method to obtain the foreground voxels that are above a clear-cut threshold. The challenges are as follows: First, the nodule can be connected to a vessel and/or the chest wall, which has the same intensity range as the nodule. Second, it is required that the segmentation result be completely independent of the click point as long as it is within the nodule. Last, but not the least, is the high expectation from the user of success rate on a large number of cases due to the fact this looks like an easy problem.

These challenges are met by incorporating prior knowledge about the application. First, the click point is guaranteed to be in the nodule. Second, the nodule size range is known. Third, the nodule is known to be compact, while a vessel is assumed to be of elongated shape, and the chest wall is mostly a smooth surface. Given the click point and size range, we define a cubic volume of interest (VOI) centered at the click point, and hence isolate out the object and its immediate neighbors. In this VOI, methods such as mathematical morphology are applied to consistently find the nodule center and separate the nodule from the connected structures.

Mathematical morphology utilizes local shape information (Sonka et al., 1998; Haralick, Sternberg, & Zhuang, 1987). Although grayscale operations are also defined, this type of method is mostly used in binary images that are generated from an earlier process such as region grow. As illustrated in Figure 1(c), the foreground object contains a nodule connected to a vessel. The basic operators such as dilation, erosion, opening and closing can be used for boundary modifications and to separate two connected objects. However, the more effective separation techniques are based on the important concept of geodesic distance. A geodesic distance of a point inside the foreground object is the shortest travel distance to the background by any path that is completely inside the object.

Using a geodesic distance map, the vessel voxels can be removed from the nodule since their distance values are relatively small. Again, the knowledge about relative sizes between the nodule and the vessel are used to determine the distance thresholds. We could use more sophisticated watershed algorithms (Vincent & Soille, 1991) to find and separating distance basins, if the over-segmentation issue can be overcome (Meyer & Beucher, 1990).

The region-based methods are based on the similarity or connectivity of voxels, therefore they can be extended to more general situations by redefinition of the similarity or connectivity. Recently, the concept of fuzzy connectivity has been introduced (Udupa, Saha, & Lotufo, 2002; Herman & Carvalho, 2001), which is defined between every possible pair of voxels. All objects are initialized with a reference point and then grow by competition to acquire voxels according to the strengths of fuzzy connectivity.

Overall, region-based segmentation is robust, simple to implement and fast when the object is small. In some cases, region merging and splitting is necessary to the grown region according to other criterions (Sonka et al., 1998; Chang & Li, 1994). However, the more heuristics that have to be applied in order to get a decent result, the less reliable the algorithm will become. The bottom line is that region-based, low-level methods should be applied to regions with relatively homogenous intensities.

Segmentation Based on Primitive Detection

Image primitives are local properties such as edges, ridges and corners. Instead of looking for properties of all voxels inside the region, primitive-based methods look for the region boundaries. There are many recent developments in primitive detection, especially edge detection, which is the basis of most segmentation schemes. The detected primitives are usually fragmented, and the challenging problem of linking edges and lines into boundaries was the focus of many works in the early and middle 90s (Basak, Chanda, & Majumder, 1994; Wu & Leahy, 1992).

Basic edge detection is achieved by applying an edge operator (Sonka et al., 1998) followed by non-maxima suppression. A systematic treatment of edge detection was provided by Canny (1986), which is an optimal detector for step edges, and can be adapted to detect other features when different filters are selected. Recently, Brejl and Sonka (2000) invented a 3D edge detector that is particularly fit for anisotropic situations, which are typical in 3D medical data. Freeman and Edward (1991) proposed a method of systematically detecting all linear primitives, including step edges, ridges and valleys, as well as their orientations. They designed a basis of filters from which an arbitrarily-oriented filter can be generated to selectively detect the primitives of a specified orientation. This is particularly useful for high-level feature detection. For instance, if we know beforehand there should be a long ridge at a certain orientation and location, a ridge filter of that direction can be applied.

As a special type of primitive-based method, Hough Transform (Sonka et al., 1998; Shankar, Murthy, & Pal, 1998) utilizes a very powerful scheme for noisy medical images—voting. It is applicable when the object roughly fits a simple parametric model, such as a rectangle. Although in medical applications precisely regular shape is rare, some are roughly spherical or with a circular

cross-section. For instance, shown in Figure 2 are the segmentation results of the left ventricle from cardiac MR data. The outer and inner boundaries approximate a circle, which has three free parameters in its parametric equation. Edge detection followed by non-maxima suppression is performed within the region of interest, and each edge pixel casts one vote for every circle equation it satisfies. The circle with the highest vote is taken as the object boundary. To achieve good results, the parameter space needs to be carefully divided into cells. Sometimes the vote can be weighted by edge strengths.

The power of this algorithm comes from its strong assumption. It works in spite of noise, weak boundaries and even occlusions, as long as the good edges can form a majority over the outliers. Certainly, the parametric model has to be simple before the algorithm becomes too complex. However, in some cases even when the object shape is not regular, we may still use it to find at least the correct centroid of the object.

The Hough Transform is a type of robust estimation method. Its principle of utlizing the majority of pixels can be widely applied. In the presence of abnormality, noise and high complexity, the robustness of a segmentation algorithm is usually determined by the number of voxels the decision is made upon.

Figure 2. Segmentation of the left ventricle wall from cardiac MRI data. The white circles mark the inner and outer boundaries of the left ventricle.

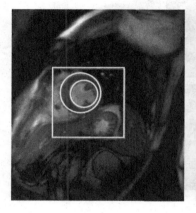 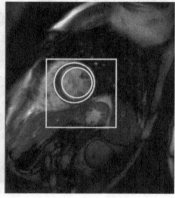 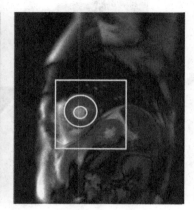

Statistical Segmentation Methods

Statistical methods treat the intensity of each voxel as an event, and model the local intensity variations by the estimation of probabilistic distributions. The goal is to use classification frameworks to determine whether a voxel belongs to a certain object. The set of voxels that are labeled as object points forms the segmented object. A simple scheme is to estimate the probability density functions (PDF) of different objects or background by computing the frequency of histograms from sample data. The estimated pdfs can then be applied to the test data. Each voxel can be classified using conventional classification methods, such as Bayesian classification or maximum likelihood decision. A more sophisticated algorithm would estimate the joint pdfs of the voxels in the neighborhood to capture the spatial local interaction properties between image labels. The most popular method is the Markov Random Field (MRF) framework, in which the pdfs are estimated with advanced algorithms such as EM algorithm. The segmentation is often obtained using a MAP estimator (Sun & Gu, 2004).

These type of methods can be applied when there is little knowledge about object shape and the intensities are nonhomogenous. A typical case, as shown in Figure 3, is the segmentation of ground glass nodules (GGN) from chest CT volume data, which has strong clinical significance due to the high malignance rate of GGNs (Zhang, Zhang, Novak, Naidich, & Moses, 2005). Due to large inter-nodule variations, an iterative approach is applied to gradually capture the local image properties. A rough intensity model is generated from training data and applied to the first round of classification. The resultant segmentation is then used to estimate a more specific distribution for the current nodule, which is in turn applied to the next round of classification. Several iterations combined with other heuristics give consistent segmentation results with respect to different user clickpoints. The same iterative strategy was used by Marroquin, Vemuri, Botello, and Calderon (2002) in the segmentation of brain MRIs. The establishment of pdfs is a learning process that requires large sample sets for each object, which may not be available for medical image segmentation. Further, large variations in

Figure 3. Segmentation of ground glass nodules (GGN) from chest CT data using Markov Random Field. Top row: Slices of volumes of interest (VOI). Bottom row: Slices of segmented GGN from the VOI above it. (Courtesy of Li Zhang from Siemens Corporate Research).

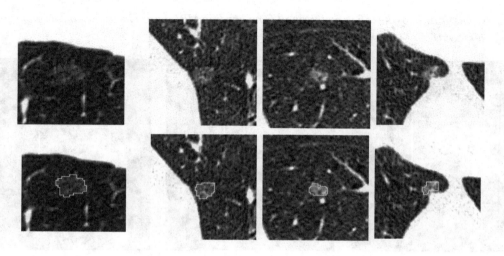

image properties often lead to overlapped pdfs. Usually, heuristics have to be combined to achieve a decent result.

SEGMENTATION INCORPORATING GLOBAL PRIORS

For more complex situations, low-level methods will not be successful. This is because the objects to be segmented in a medical application usually have high internal nonhomogeneity and strong internal edges. In these cases, a global prior is needed.

We first give as intuitive examples two special applications that utilize the global priors of object shapes—the tracing-based segmentation of tube-like structures. As shown in Figure 4, 3D tracing algorithms were developed for the segmentation of neurons from laser-scanning confocal image

stacks (Al-Kofahi et al., 2002), and of rib structures from chest CT data (Shen, Liang, Shao, & Qing, 2004). A tracing algorithm uses the global prior knowledge that the object has piecewise linear shapes with smooth surfaces. First, seed points are automatically detected for all objects by techniques such as sparse grid search or 2D cross-section analysis. From each seed, tracing proceeds iteratively along each object, using edge information to determine the tracing directions. Carefully designed stopping criteria are applied to terminate a trace.

This approach has the advantage of obtaining object centerlines and boundaries simultaneously, and all tube structures are naturally separated. Another significant advantage is the low computational cost. This type of algorithm is exploratory. Only the voxels on or near the objects are processed, which is a small portion of the image data.

Figure 4. 3D exploratory tracing-based segmentation

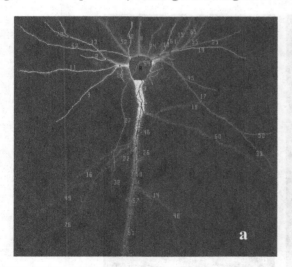 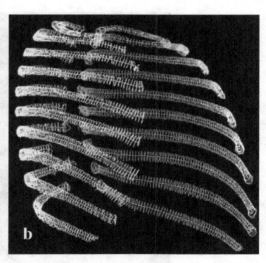

(a) Segmentation result of neuron from confocal image stacks, the centerlines are overlaid on original image (2D projection) (Courtesy of Khalid Al-kofahi from Thomson Legal & Regulatory, Eagan, MN); (b) Segmentation result of rib structures from chest CT image shown in Figure 1. Shown are the rib contours and centerlines. They are naturally separated. A graphical surface reconstruction algorithm can be applied to obtain the rib surfaces.

Deformable Models

The deformable models provide a framework that allows the incorporation of global priors. It is widely applied to medical data, and the potential is far from fully explored. Before global prior is introduced, a deformable model is a unified approach to the capture of local image properties through front evolution, without the need of local primitive grouping. Further, by the constraints that a smooth shape is to be maintained during evolution, the frontier points move with interaction rather than independently. Figure 5a and 5b show the two example segmentations using the level set method, which is one popular deformable model.

Kass, Witkin, and Terzopoulos (1988) proposed one of the first deformable models—snakes—in which they introduced the energy minimizing mechanism. By using gradient decent and variational approach, the 2D contour is attracted to the local energy minimum. Through contour or surface evolution, a deformable model integrates three factors to jointly determine the segmentation. First, the smoothness requirement of the shape constrains the relative motion of frontier points. These points are only allowed to move such that a smooth front is maintained. Second, the surface actively adapts to the local image primitives, such as edges, ridges, etc. Finally, it is possible to impose global geometrical constraints on the shape. In the initial treatment of snakes, these three factors are integrated as energy terms in the partial differential equation (PDE).

Accordingly, three issues are to be addressed when designing a deformable model. First of all, we need to decide how to represent a shape or surface. The other two major issues are the design of local image forces and the incorporation of global priors to constrain the front evolution.

The issue of shape representation becomes more challenging in a 3D situation. Pentland and Sclaroff (1991) used an approach based on finite element method (FEM) to establish a parametric

Figure 5. Surface evolving in the level set segmentation. The left column shows initialization, and the right column shows converged boundary.

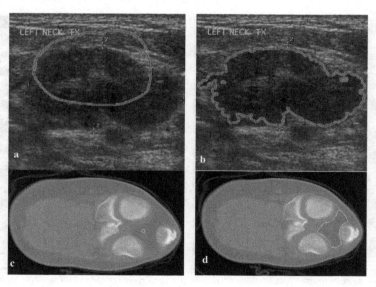

(a) and (b) Larynx tumor in ultrasound data (c) and (d) Hoffa pad in CT knee data. Courtesy of Gozde Unal and Greg Slabaugh from Siemens Corporate Research

model of shapes. Lorenz and Krahnstover (1999) used a 3D mesh to represent the vertebra shape. Recently, Slabaugh and Unal (2005) developed a more general deformable mesh for surface evolving.

The Level Set Method for Shape Representation and Evolution

In the past decades, the level set methods (Malladi, Sethian, & Vemuri, 1995; Adalsteinsson & Sethian, 1995) received much attention. The surface is represented implicitly. Typically, for a close surface, a signed distance function is defined in a volume that contains that surface. The value of each voxel is the geodesic distance of that voxel to the closest point on the surface. Since this value on the surface is zero, the set composed of all surface points is named the zero level set of the signed distance function. The distance values of voxels in and outside the surface are set to be negative and positive, respectively. This implicit representation of the surface by the zero level set of the signed distance function provides great simplicity at the cost of an increase in dimension. The implementation is relatively simple, and provides a flexible platform to design various algorithms. Further, level set is transparent to dimension, which makes it much more desirable than some other methods that are hard to adapt to 3D.

Until recently, most level set researchers focused their efforts on the problem of surface evolving under local image properties, such as defining local image force or speeds, either edge-based or region-based (Chan & Vese, 2001; Chakraborty, Staib, & Duncan, 1996). A recent survey by Suri, Liu, and Singh (2002) gave a systematic summary of all the important efforts that address in depth the local surface evolvement. Without a prior shape model, however, a deformable model such as level set only reacts to local properties. For edge-based force, the surface will converge at local edges. For region-based force, the surface will converge when the average intensity of voxels

in the object and background differs the most. A medical structure usually has complex local image properties, such as incomplete boundaries, noise, nonuniform internal intensities, etc. Therefore the most common problems for low-level segmentation methods also bother a deformable model—the leaking at weak boundaries or being caught by internal edges. The surface will truthfully conform to whatever local information it encounters. Even with the most advanced local constraining schemes, these problems persist.

Statistical Model as Global Prior Representation

Cootes, Taylor, Cooper, and Granham (1995) proposed the popular active shape models (ASM). Cootes, Edwards, and Taylor (2001) later proposed the active appearance models (AAM). Both of the two methods used statistical models to represent prior knowledge. The surface was represented by a point distribution model (PDM), which was a set of landmark points that were distributed on the object boundaries. For a given shape, the locations of all the landmarks were concatenated to form long vectors as the representation. The success of a PDM depends on correspondence of landmarks, which is challenging in 3D. Overall, the PDM models are difficult to implement in 3D. It is a very active field that attracts many contributions to solve these difficulties (Hill & Taylor, 1994; Walker, Cootes, & Taylor, 2002; Horkaew & Yang, 2003).

On the other hand, this was among the first systematic efforts to introduce statistical representation of global shape priors into a deformable model. Sample vectors were extracted from a set of registered training shapes and principal component analysis (PCA) is performed on the set of sample vectors. The dimension of the covariance matrix equals that of the sample vectors, but only the eigenvectors with the largest eigenvalues are taken to form the basis of the linear model space. The segmentation process first transforms the mean shape to the data, and then finds the correspondence of the mapped model landmarks by searching for strong edges in the contour's normal direction. Subsequently the shape vector computed from the correspondent points is projected onto the model basis to find the best matched model. This means a large number of residual components are discarded. The matched model is again matched onto the image data for next iteration. In a PDM, the representation of surface and the incorporation of global priors are combined and a shape is only allowed to vary within the model space. The local surface evolution is limited and for the only purpose of finding the matched model.

For the level set framework, recently Leventon, Grimson, and Faugeras (2000) introduced the similar PCA model. PCA analysis is performed on a set of registered training samples, each represented by a signed distance function defined in a volume. Compared to the PDM, the linear PCA model on signed distance function is only valid within the limited space centered at the mean shapes, which is clearly a disadvantage.

Limitations of the PCA Statistical Model

The PCA statistical models have limitations both in the representation and application of global priors. The representation is incomplete, especially when the structure is complex and with high variations due to age, gender, race and almost infinite types of pathological abnormalities. Coverage of these variations requires a large number of modes, in addition to the need for high-valued coefficients. Setting up such a large and high-dimension model space is impractical due to the limited size and coverage of the training set, in which every sample needs to be obtained by arduous manual segmentation. Further, searching in such a complex model space is also impractical if any reasonable performance is desired. Therefore, any practical PCA model space will be restricted to that of a relatively low dimensional, and the model shape can only vary in the neighborhood of the mean shape.

The established PCA model is applied to segmentation as follows. In an iteration of surface evolution, a model is identified from the PCA model space such that it has the minimum shape difference from the current surface. The difference is then used as a penalty term and added to the evolving force. In such a scheme, how to determine the relative strengths of model and local force is a critical issue. In a PDM, the local image force is only used to evolve the surface to its best model, and the shape residues not covered in the limited model space will be ignored. A level set scheme better understands the limitations of a model, and allows the surface to converge to a shape not covered by a model under local image force. The high-level model force and the local image force are added together, with a multiplier on one of the two terms to adjust the relative strength.

For a PDM, precise segmentation of a complex structure is obviously not possible, since the object is completely restricted to an inaccurate model space. In the literature, PDM showed its success mostly in 2D cases. Mitchell et al. (2002) extended it to 3D segmentation of a left ventricle from cardiac MR and Ultrasound images, in which the object of interest has a relatively simple shape and hence the issue of inaccurate model space is not severe. In some applications, such as ultrasound, the shape is not well defined. Even humans cannot consistently delineate the object boundaries. The goal is then to find a shape that best fits the visual clues of boundaries. This is where PDM is useful but, strictly speaking, it is geometric modeling rather than precise segmentation. On the other hand, geometric modeling sometimes is the best we can do since validation of results is not possible. Depending on application, geometric modeling may be a satisfactory solution even if it does not represent the actual object boundaries. When there is consistent ground truth from human, precise segmentation should be achieved.

In comparison, the level set scheme is fit for precise segmentation, since surface evolution is allowed to converge to local image primitives. However, the PCA model (Tsai et al., 2003; Yang, Staib, & Duncan, 2004) introduced the same-level competition scheme between global prior and local image forces. Because of the inaccurate model, the global prior term will often disagree with the local image term. In a situation where the shape is not well defined, the model term can be made very strong by adjusting the multiplier, and the resulting surface boundaries will be very close to that of a model shape. A example is shown in Figure 5c and 5d, in which a prior shape model was applied. In such a case, the user has only vague visual clues to identify the actual object boundary, therefore the boundaries suggested by a model shape are well accepted. Much work in the literature follows these types of strategies.

Figure 6. 3D level set segmentation of the vertebra

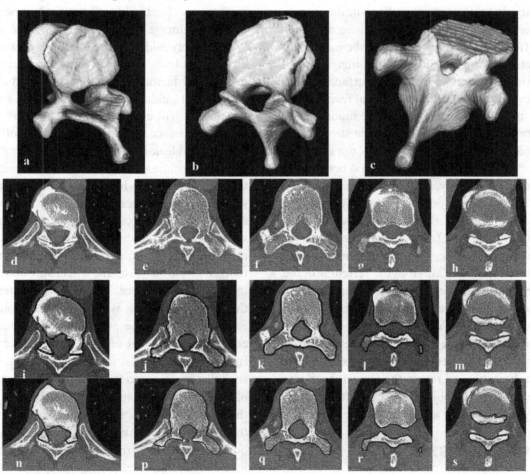

(a)-(c): 3D view of the complex structure of a vertebra shape. (d)-(h): Vertebra on selected axial slices, with its neighboring vertebra and rib structures. While the shape looks well defined for a human observer, local boundaries are far from clear. Also notice the pathology induced abnormal shape on the top-left of (d). (i)-(m): The 2D boundaries delineated by a human observer. Regions outside the contours belong to the neighboring vertebras and rib structures. (n)-(r): Converged 3D level set surface of segmented object projected onto selected axial slices.

In a situation where an object shape is well defined, the user would expect a precise segmentation. A good example is the human vertebra in high-contrast data, such as multi-slice CT images, as shown in Figure 6.

This 3D complex structure has a relatively well-defined shape, at least for a human observer, who can perform consistent delineation of the object boundaries on 2D slice images. However, there are many places where local boundaries are weak, diffused and have gaps. Further, such a structure is adjacent or even connected to a neighboring structure that has similar image properties. This is the typical case where we cannot afford an accurate model, and the inaccurate model will compete with the local image forces. If we make the model strong, the surface will not converge to some of the strong local features and abnormal shapes that are out of the model space. On the other hand, if we reduce the strengths of the model, then level set will leak out at places where local primitives are weak and hence need guidance. Obviously, this is a dilemma that cannot be completely addressed by adjusting the multiplier. In the work in which Leventon et al. (2000) defined this competition scheme, an attempt was made to segment the human vertebrae. The training shapes are from the vertebrae of the same data set, leaving the middle vertebrae out as the test data. The problem manifested itself. The not-well-fit model shape competes with local primitives to pull the evolving surface away from these strong features and the abnormal shapes. From the published result, the convergence was quite far from the object boundaries that can be easily delineated by a human observer.

A Better Strategy

The limitations of the PCA models for representing global prior knowledge can be understood from an alternative point of view. Mathematically, the PCA models are based on the moment average of the training samples, and hence high frequency

information will not be preserved. On the other hand, human observers to identify a complex structure most effectively use high frequency information, such as abrupt ridges, corners, etc. These are singular points, lines or planes where derivatives do not exist. A surface model represents smooth surfaces well, but does not incorporate these singular features. In other words, this important portion of the prior knowledge has to be represented more explicitly rather than implicitly embedded in the shape model.

Further, global prior knowledge, such as surface models, should not be put in competition with local image properties at the same level. When simply added to the local image force, a global prior loses it "global" status and degrades into a local factor. A global prior should act as a high level guidance to local evolution, so that the surface will converge to the "correct" local primitives, hence avoiding the problems of local minima and leak-out.

To determine what global priors are needed, we want to find out what causes the failure of the surface evolution when no global prior is applied. As shown in Figure 6, the internal intensity of the vertebra is very nonhomogenous, and there are many internal edges. A level set front when initialized inside the vertebrae will ensure converge to these internal edges. The only way to prevent this from happening is to keep these internal edges away from the evolution path. Since the convergence of level set depends on the initial front, a major effort is to design the initial front such that it is close to the boundaries but outside of the vertebrae. The surface will then converge to the outside boundaries before it even encounters the internal edges. Another problem is the weak boundary locations, from which the surface will leak out. We can carefully design the speed map according to the various local properties to avoid this problem. For instance, we can use region based speed at locations where edges are weak. Next, a more challenging issue is the adjacent, or even connected, ribs and vertebrae that have the same image properties. To separate them from the vertebrae of interest, we need to explicitly detect the high-level features formed between the vertebrae and its neighboring structures.

From the above, global priors should then include a surface model as a general description of shape, augmented by a set of known high-level features. The surface model is constructed as follows: First, a small number of vertebrae, roughly covering the spectrum of shape varia-

tions within the normal range, are selected and their surfaces are manually segmented. These surfaces are transformed into a common coordinate system using similarity transformation such that the spinal channel and inter-vertebrae planes are registered. We do not intend to match the surfaces themselves, since that is unnecessary and will require nonlinear warping of the surfaces. Afterwards, the registered surfaces are represented as a set of signed distance functions.

Figure 7. Representation and application of prior knowledge

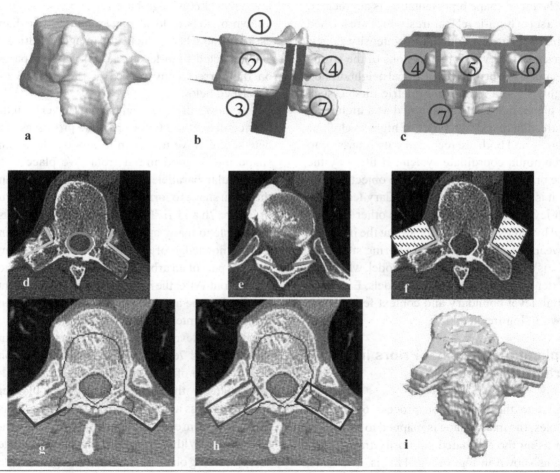

(a) The mean shape. (b)(c) The plane division of the volumes into regions. Each region has its specific speed design. (d)-(e) High-level boundary features and context features which are marked with black and gray, respectively. A context feature is not on object boundary, but is on the object interfaces. (f) Blocker speed regions. (g) Mean shape mapped to the image. Two high-level boundary features are detected. (h) The mean shape is augmented to make it close to the object boundaries. (i) 3D structure of the augmented mean shape to be used as the initial front for level set surface evolving.

We then compute the mean signed distance function, whose shape is shown in Figure 7a. It has the basic look and structure that belong to and characterize a vertebra. The mean shape model is used as a rough guide or template and hence does not need to cover the large variations. This low requirement allows a small sample size.

Using the mean shape as a reference system, we define planes that divide the volume into regions. For each region, the proper speed design is applied, which varies in the type of speed and the constants. The region division is shown in Figure 7b and 7c.

The mean shape representation is augmented with a set of high-level features, which are formed by linear primitives including intensity edges, ridges and valleys. If the locations of the strong and same-type primitives in a local neighborhood roughly fit to a simple parametric model, such as a plane, that plane is recorded as a high-level feature. There are two types of high-level plane features, and both are recorded with reference to the common coordinate system. If fitted by the ridge or edge primitives from the object boundary, it is named a high-level boundary feature. A high-level context feature, on the other hand, is fitted by valley primitives located at the interface between the object and a neighboring structure. Plane is the simplest parametric model, which can be extended to piecewise linear models. Examples of high level boundary and context features are shown in Figure 7d and 7e.

Application of Global Priors in Surface Evolution

Similar to the registration process of training samples, the mean shape is mapped to the image data using the estimated similarity transformation, as shown in Figure 7g. This is, of course, specific to this application. However, a transformation can be estimated with other more general methods to map the initial shape, and we have seen examples in the literature (Baillard, Hellier,

& Barillot, 2001). The boundaries of the mapped mean shape are usually close to the boundaries of the object, except that the surfaces at the two transverse processes are too far inside. Such an initial front will be captured by local minima and not converge to the outside true boundaries. It therefore needs to be modified, and we use the high level features to achieve this.

The high-level feature models are also mapped to the neighborhood of the features in the image data. The detection of high-level boundary and context features uses mainly parametric model-fitting techniques, such as Hough Transform. This is a typical knowledge-based strategy, which fits known models to local image data, rather than estimate models from detected image primitives. The detected high-level features have impacts on the correct convergence of the surface, as described below.

As shown in Figure 7g, the high-level boundary features at the two transverse processes are detected, and we use them to modify the mean shape into a good initial front. We place two rectangular parallelepipeds in connection with the mean shape to form the initial front, as shown in Figure 7h and 7i. This is a general idea that is applicable to many applications: If we are given a true knowledge of a partial boundary, we can use it as part of an arbitrary shape to augment the initial front. After the modification, the initial front is pulled to the actual boundary, which helps in avoiding the internal local minimums.

The high-level context features, as shown in Figure 7d and 7e, are used for the introduction of a new type of speed to affect level set evolution—namely the blocker speed. The blocker speed serves as an energy potential that prevents the surface from evolving beyond the detected context feature. With this we can prevent the leakage to neighboring objects. As shown in Figure 7f, the two plane context features divide the space into two regions. Using the center of the spinal channel as the reference, we can determine the region which the surface should not evolve into. For that region, the speed terms are made negative, which prevents the surface from evolving beyond the context features. Note that the high-level context features do not belong to object boundary; rather, they belong to background. The surface will not converge to the context feature, but will converge to the object boundary that is on the inner side of the context feature.

From the above, the leakage and local minimum issues that frequently bother a level set surface evolution are principally addressed. Finally, the separation planes associated with the mean shape are also mapped to the image data. Local primitive detection is performed to generate the speed terms specially designed for each region. Careful design of the speed is also an important part of this knowledge-based segmentation scheme.

As shown in Figure 6n-6s, after iterations of surface evolution, the level set surface converges to the correct object boundaries despite the internal inhomogeneity, the weak boundaries and the presence of neighboring structures. From this example we showed the power of prior knowledge when it is well represented, organized and applied to medical image segmentation. We only presented high level concepts in this example, and the reader is referred to the work of Shen et al. (2005) for a detailed treatment including mathematical deductions.

CONCLUSION, DISCUSSION, AND OUTLOOK

We have made an attempt in this chapter to give an intuitive introduction to the various methods and frameworks that are useful in 3D medical image segmentation. We also discussed the concepts of our approach of knowledge-based segmentation, in which the effective representation and application of prior knowledge is most important. From the discussion, the most prominent high-level features are of most value and need to be intensively explored before other image properties come into play.

The state-of-the-art medical image segmentation methods still leave much to be desired. Other than the difficulties of the segmentation problem itself, the relatively short time in which the 3D medical data become available is also one factor. The earlier scanners produced data in which the axial resolution is much lower than the other two directions. Therefore 3D correlation between two adjacent axial slices is weak, and a 3D segmentation method is not particularly more beneficial than 2D segmentation on each slice image. In the past two years, multi-slice CT scanners have achieved true isotropic voxels. With the development of medical instrument technology, 3D medical image segmentation will become increasingly popular. 3D methods are inherently better for the segmentation of complex structures, in that they implicitly involve the 3D structural information that is difficult to capture in 2D methods. On the other hand, it will still take time for people to have full awareness of the properties of these data and develop insights.

Medical imaging applications have now become an important driving force for the advance of computer vision. On the other hand, medical image analysis needs to address real-word issues that have been outside the realm of computer vision. These issues come largely from the fact that the end systems are mostly used by the physician. The human factor is essential, since any successful solution will have to be accepted by a physician and integrated into one's medical procedural workflow. This put strong constraints on the type of applicable methods. Because of this, there has been a discrepancy between the advanced frameworks presented in computer vision and the low-level and ad-hoc methods used by researchers working on real medical application solutions. Recently, we have seen the hope of practically applicable frameworks which are relatively simple in implementation, and reasonable in performance and robustness. In this respect, we foresee several trends. First, existing and coming frameworks from computer vision will improve themselves to be more practical and compete for their prevalence in medical image analysis. Second, more medical imaging researchers will make use of these frameworks, with their efforts focused on the incorporation of application-specific priors. Third, more efforts from the computer vision community will be attracted to solving real-world problems, and, hence, lead to the invention of more general methods for prior knowledge incorporation. As a byproduct, general frameworks will also be invented for the incorporation of user interaction into difficult segmentation problems.

ACKNOWLEDGMENT

I would like to thank my colleagues at Siemens Corporate Research: Dr. Gozde Unal, Dr. Greg Slabaugh, Dr. Leo Grady, Dr. Li Zhang, Dr. Zhizhou Wang, Zhigang Peng, Dr. Marie-Pierre Jolly, Ludek Hasa and Julien Nahed for their support in writing this chapter. Gratitude also goes to Dr. Khalid Al-Kofahi from Thomson Legal & Regulatory and Yonggang Shi from Boston University. They have provided useful images and references, and most importantly, insightful discussions, without which this chapter would not be possible.

REFERENCES

Adalsteinsson, D., & Sethian, J. (1995). A fast level set method for propagating interfaces. *Journal of Computational Physics, 118,* 269-277.

Adams, R., & Bischof, L. (1984). Seeded region growing. *IEEE Transactions on Pattern Analysis and Machine Intelligence, 16*(6), 641-647.

Al-Kofahi, K., Lasek, S., Szarowski, D., Pace, C., Nagy, G., Turner, J.N., et al. (2002). Rapid automated three-dimensional tracing of neurons from confocal image stacks. *IEEE Transactions on Information Technology in Biomedicine, 6*(2), 171-187.

Baillard, C., Hellier, P., & Barillot, C. (2001). Segmentation of brain images using level sets and dense registration. *Medical Image Analysis, 5,* 185-194.

Basak, J., Chanda, B., & Majumder, D. D. (1994). On edge and line linking with connectionist models. *IEEE Transactions on Systems, Man, and Cybernetics, 24*(3), 413-428.

Brejl, M., & Sonka, M. (2000). Directional 3D edge detection in anisotropic data: Detector design and performance assessment. *Computer Vision and Image Understanding, 77,* 84-110.

Canny, J. (1986). A computational approach to edge detection. *IEEE Transactions on Pattern Analysis and Machine Intelligence, 8*(6), 679-698.

Chakraborty, A., Staib, L. H., & Duncan, J. S. (1996). Deformable boundary finding in medical images by integrating gradient and region information. *IEEE Transactions on Medical Imaging, 15*(6), 859-870.

Chan, T., & Vese, L. (2001). An active contour model without edges. *IEEE Transactions on Image Processing, 10*(2), 266-277.

Chang, Y. L., & Li, X. (1994). Adaptive region growing. *IEEE Transactions on Image Processing, 3*(6), 868-72.

Cootes, T. F., Edwards, G. J., & Taylor, C. J. (2001). Active appearance models. *IEEE Transactions on Pattern Analysis and Machine Intelligence, 23*(6), 681-685.

Cootes, T. F., Taylor, C. J., Cooper, D. H., & Granham, J. (1995). Active shape models—their training and application. *Computer Vision and Image Understanding, 61*, 38-59.

Freeman, W. T., & Adelson, E. H. (1991). The design and use of steerable filters. *IEEE Transactions on Pattern Analysis and Machine Intelligence, 13*(9), 891-906.

Guy, G., & Medioni, G. (1996). Inferring global perceptual from local features. *International Journal of Computer Vision, 20*(1/2), 113-133.

Haralick, R. M., Sternberg, S. R., & Zhuang, X. (1987). Image analysis using mathematical morphology. *IEEE Transactions on Pattern Analysis and Machine Intelligence, 9*(4), 532-50.

Herman, G. T., & Carvalho, B. M., (2001). Multiseeded segmentation using fuzzy connectedness. *IEEE Transactions on Pattern Analysis and Machine Intelligence, 23*(5), 460-474.

Hill, A., & Taylor, C. J. (1994). Automatic landmark generation for point distribution models. *Proceedings of the 5th British Machine Vision Conference, 2*(2), 429-438.

Horkaew, P., & Yang, G. Z. (2003). Optimal deformable surface models for 3D medical image analysis. *IPMI*, 13-24.

Kass, M., Witkin, A., & Terzopoulos, D. (1988). Active contour models. *International Journal of Computer Vision, 1*(4), 321-331.

Leventon, M. E., Grimson, W. E., & Faugeras, O. (2000). Statistical shape influence in geodesic active contours. *Proceedings IEEE Conference on Computer Vision and Pattern Recognition, 1*(1), 316-323.

Lorenz, C., & Krahnstover, N. (1999). 3D statistical shape models for medical image segmentation. *International Conference on 3-D Digital Imaging and Modeling*, (pp. 414-423).

Malladi, R., Sethian, J. A., & Vemuri, B. C. (1995). Shape modeling with front propagation: A level set

approach. *IEEE Transactions on Pattern Analysis and Machine Intelligence, 17*(2), 158-75.

Marroquin, J. L., Vemuri, B. C., Botello, S., & Calderon, F. (2002). An accurate and efficient bayesian method for automatic segmentation of brain MRI. *Proceedings of ECCV* (pp. 560-574).

Meyer, F. & Beucher, S. (1990). Morphological segmentation. *Journal of Visual Communication and Image Representation, 1*(1), 21-46.

Mitchell, S. C., Bosch, J. G., Lelieveldt, B. P. F., van de Geest, R. J., Reiber, J. H. C., & Sonka, M. (2002). 3-D active appearance models: segmentation of cardiac MR and ultrasound images. *IEEE Transactions on Medical Imaging, 21*(9), 1167-1178.

Mohan, R., & Nevatia, R. (1989). Using perceptual organization to extract 3-D structures. *IEEE Transactions on Pattern Analysis and Machine Intelligence, 11*(11), 1121-1139.

Pentland, A. P., & Sclaroff, S. (1991). Closed-form solutions for physically based modeling and recognition. *IEEE Transactions on Pattern Analysis and Machine Intelligence, 13*(7), 715-729.

Sarkar, S., & Boyer, K. L. (1994). Computing perceptual organization in computer vision, *World Scientific Series on Machine Perception and Artificial Intelligence*. Singapore: World Scientific.

Shankar, B. U., Murthy, C. A., & Pal, S. K. (1998). A new gray level based Hough transform for region extraction, an application to IRS images, *Pattern Recognition Letters, 19*, 197-204.

Shen, H., Liang, L., Shao, M., & Qing, S. (2004). Tracing based segmentation for labeling of individual rib structures in chest CT volume data. *Proceedings of the 7th International Conference on Medical Image Computing and Computer Assisted Intervention* (pp. 967-974).

Shen, H., Shi, Y., & Peng, Z. (2005). Applying prior knowledge in the segmentation of 3D complex anatomic structures. *Computer Vision for Biomedical Image Applications: Current Techniques and Future Trends, An International Conference on Computer Vision Workshop, Lecture Notes of Computer Science, 3765* (pp.189-199). Beijing, China.

Slabaugh, G., & Unal, G. (2005). Active polyhedron: Surface evolution theory applied to deformable meshes. *Conference on Computer Vision and Pattern Recognition.*

Sonka, M., Hlavac, V., & Boyle, R. (1998). *Image processing, analysis, and machine vision* (2nd ed.). PWS Publishing.

Sun, J., & Gu, D. (2004). Bayesian image segmentation based on an inhomogeneous hidden Markov random field. *Proceedings of the 17th International Conference on Pattern Recognition* (pp. 596-599).

Suri, J. S., Liu, K., Singh, S., Laxminarayan, S.N., Zeng, X., & Reden, L. (2002). Shape recovery algorithm using level sets in 2-D/3-D medical imagery, a state-of-the-art review. *IEEE Transactions on Information Technology in Biomedicine, 6*(1), 8-28.

Tsai, A., Yezzi, A., Wells, W., Tempany, C., Tucker, D., Fan, A., et al. (2003). A shape-based approach to the segmentation of medical imagery using level sets. *IEEE Transactions on Medical Imaging, 22*(2), 137-154.

Udupa, J. K., Saha, P. K., & Lotufo, R. A. (2002). Relative fuzzy connectedness and object definition: Theory, algorithms, and applications in image segmentation. *IEEE Transactions on Pattern Analysis and Machine Intelligence, 24*(11), 1485-1500.

Vincent, L., & Soille, P. (1991). Watersheds in digital spaces: An efficient algorithm based on immersion simulations. *IEEE Transactions on Pattern Analysis and Machine Intelligence, 13*(6), 583-598.

Walker, K. N., Cootes, T. F., & Taylor, C. J. (2002). Automatically building appearance models from image sequences using salient features. *Image and Vision Computing, 20*(5-6), 435-440.

Wu, Z., & Leahy, R. (1992). Image segmentation via edge contour finding. *IEEE Computer Society Conference on Computer Vision and Pattern Recognition* (pp. 613-619).

Yang, J., Staib, H.S., & Duncan, J.S. (2004). Neighbor-constrained segmentation with level set based 3-D deformable models. *IEEE Transactions on Medical Imaging, 23*(8), 940-948.

Zhang, L., Zhang, T., Novak, C. L., Naidich, D. P., & Moses, D. A. (2005). A computer-based method of segmenting ground glass nodules in pulmonary CT images: Comparison to expert radiologists' interpretations. *Proceedings of SPIE Medical Imaging.*

This work was previously published in Advances in Image and Video Segmentation, edited by Y. Zhang, pp. 250-269, copyright 2006 by IRM Press (an imprint of IGI Global).

Chapter XVI
Parallel Segmentation of Multi–Channel Images Using Multi–Dimensional Mathematical Morphology

Antonio Plaza
University of Extremadura, Spain

Javier Plaza
University of Extremadura, Spain

David Valencia
University of Extremadura, Spain

Pablo Martinez
University of Extremadura, Spain

ABSTRACT

Multi-channel images are characteristic of certain applications, such as medical imaging or remotely sensed data analysis. Mathematical morphology-based segmentation of multi-channel imagery has not been fully accomplished yet, mainly due to the lack of vector-based strategies to extend classic morphological operations to multidimensional imagery. For instance, the most important morphological approach for image segmentation is the watershed transformation, a hybrid of seeded region growing and edge detection. In this chapter, we describe a vector-preserving framework to extend morphological operations to multi-channel images, and further propose a fully automatic multi-channel watershed segmentation algorithm that naturally combines spatial and spectral/temporal information. Due to the large data volumes often associated with multi-channel imaging, this chapter also develops a parallel implementation strategy to speed up performance. The proposed parallel algorithm is evaluated using magnetic resonance images and remotely sensed hyperspectral scenes collected by the NASA Jet Propulsion Laboratory Airborne Visible Infra-Red Imaging Spectrometer (AVIRIS).

INTRODUCTION

The segmentation of an image can be defined as its partition into different regions, each having certain properties (Zhang, 1996). In mathematical terms, a segmentation of an image f is a partition of its definition domain D_f into m disjoint, non-empty sets $s_1, s_2, ..., s_m$ called segments, so that $\bigcup_{i=1}^{m} S_i = D_f$ and $S_i \bigcap S_j = \varnothing$, $\forall i \neq j$. Segmentation of intensity images in the spatial domain usually involves four main approaches (Haralick & Shapiro, 1985). Thresholding techniques assume that all pixels whose value lies within a certain range belong to the same class. Boundary-based methods assume that the pixel values change rapidly at the boundary between two regions. Region-based segmentation algorithms postulate that neighboring pixels within the same region have similar intensity values, of which the split-and-merge technique is probably the most well known. Hybrid methods combine one or more of the above-mentioned criteria. This class includes variable-order surface fitting and active contour methods.

One of the most successful hybrid segmentation approaches is the morphological watershed transformation (Beucher, 1994), which consists of a combination of seeded region growing (Adams & Bischof, 1994; Mehnert & Jackway, 1997) and edge detection. It relies on a marker-controlled approach (Fan et al., 2001) that considers the image data as imaginary topographic relief; the brighter the intensity, the higher the corresponding elevation. Let us assume that a drop of water falls on such a topographic surface. The drop will flow down along the steepest slope path until it reaches a minimum. The set of points of the surface whose steepest slope path reaches a given minimum constitutes the *catchment basin* associated with that minimum, while the watersheds are the zones dividing adjacent catchment basins. Another way of visualizing the watershed concept is by analogy to immersion (Vincent & Soille, 1991). Starting from every minimum, the surface is progressively flooded until water coming from two different minima meet. At this point, a watershed line is erected. The watershed transformation can successfully partition the image into meaningful regions, provided that minima corresponding to relevant image objects, along with object boundaries, are available (Shafarenko et al., 1997). Despite its encouraging results in many applications, morphological techniques have not been fully exploited in applications that involve multi-channel imagery, where a vector of values rather than a single value is associated with each pixel location.

Many types of multi-channel images exist depending on the type of information collected for each pixel. For instance, color images are multi-channel images with three channels, one for each primary color in the RGB space. Images optically acquired in more than one spectral or wavelength interval are called multispectral. These images are characteristic in satellite imaging and aerial reconnaissance applications. The number of spectral channels can be extremely high, as in the case of hyperspectral images produced by imaging spectrometers (Chang, 2003). Finally, all image types above can be extended to the class of multitemporal images or image sequences, which consist of series of images defined over the same definition domain, but collected at more than a single time. Examples include magnetic resonance (MR) images in medical applications and video sequences.

Segmentation of multi-channel imagery has usually been accomplished in the spectral/temporal domain of the data only. Techniques include well known data clustering algorithms such as ISODATA (Richards & Jia, 1999). Other techniques, such as Soille's watershed-based multi-channel segmentation (Soille, 1996), are based on an initial spectral clustering followed by a post-classification using spatial information. This approach separates spatial information from spectral information, and thus the two types of information are not treated simultaneously.

In this chapter, we develop a novel watershed-based segmentation technique that naturally combines spatial and spectral/temporal information in simultaneous fashion. While such an integrated approach holds great promise in several applications, it also creates new processing challenges (Tilton, 1999). In particular, the price paid for the wealth of spatial and spectral/temporal information is an enormous amount of data to be processed. For that purpose, we develop a parallel implementation of the proposed segmentation algorithm that allows processing of high-dimensional images quickly enough for practical use. The chapter is structured as follows. The following section provides a mathematical formulation for multi-dimensional morphological operations, and relates the proposed framework to other existing approaches in the literature. A multi-dimensional watershed-based segmentation approach is described next, along with its parallel implementation. A quantitative segmentation evaluation comparison with regard to standard segmentation techniques is then provided, using both MR brain images and remotely sensed hyperspectral data collected by the 224-channel NASA Jet Propulsion Laboratory Airborne Visible Infra-Red Imaging Spectrometer (AVIRIS) system. The chapter concludes with some remarks.

MULTI-DIMENSIONAL MATHEMATICAL MORPHOLOGY

Our attention in this section focuses primarily on the development of a mechanism to extend basic morphological operations to multi-channel imagery. In the following, we provide a mathematical formulation for classic and extended morphological operations.

Classic Morphological Operations

Following a usual notation (Soille, 2003), let us consider a grayscale image f, defined on a space E. Typically, E is the 2-D continuous space R^2 or the 2-D discrete space Z^2. The classic erosion of f by $B \subset Z^2$ is given by the expression shown in Box 1.

Vector-Based Mathematical Morphology

Let us denote a multi-channel image with n channels as f, where the values of each pixel $f(x,y)$ of the definition domain D_f are given by an n-dimensional vector $f(x,y) = (f_1(x,y), f_1(x,y), ..., f_n(x,y))$. Extension of monochannel erosion and dilation above the images defined on the n-dimensional space is not straightforward. A simple approach consists in applying monochannel techniques to each image channel separately, an approach usually referred to as "marginal" morphology in the literature. This approach is unacceptable in

Box 1.

$$(f \ominus B)(x,y) = \min_{(s,t) \in Z^2(B)} \{f(x+s, y+t)\}, \qquad (x,y) \in Z^2 \qquad (1)$$

where $Z^2(B)$ denotes the set of discrete spatial coordinates associated to pixels lying within the neighborhood defined by a "flat" SE, designed by B. The term "flat" indicates that the SE is defined in the x-y plane. Similarly, the classic dilation of f by B is given by:

$$(f \oplus B)(x,y) = \max_{(s,t) \in Z^2(B)} \{f(x-s, y-t)\}, \qquad (x,y) \in Z^2 \qquad (2)$$

many applications because, when morphological techniques are applied independently to each image channel, there is a possibility for loss or corruption of information of the image due to the probable fact that new pixel vectors—not present in the original image—may be created as a result of processing the channels separately. In addition, no correlation between spectral/temporal components is taken into account. An alternative way to approach the problem of multi-dimensional morphology is to treat the data at each pixel as a vector. Unfortunately, there is no unambiguous means of defining the minimum and maximum values between two vectors of more than one dimension, and thus it is important to define an appropriate arrangement of vectors in the selected vector space.

Several vector-ordering schemes have been discussed in the literature (Plaza et al., 2004). Four classes of ordering will be shortly outlined here for illustrative purposes. Let us now consider an *n*-dimensional image f and let $f(x,y)$ and $f(x',y')$ denote two pixel vectors at spatial locations (x,y) and (x',y') respectively, with $f(x,y) = (f_1(x,y), ..., f_n(x,y))$ and $f(x',y') = f_1(x',y'), ..., f_n(x',y'))$. In marginal ordering (M-ordering), each pair of observations $f_i(x,y)$ and $f_i(x',y')$ would be ordered independently along each of the n channels. In reduced ordering (R-ordering), a scalar parameter function g would be computed for each pixel of the image, and the ordering would be performed according to the resulting scalar values. The ordered vectors would satisfy the relationship $f(x,y) \leq f(x',y') \Rightarrow g[f(x,y)] \leq g[f(x',y')]$. In partial ordering (P-ordering), the input multivariate samples would be partitioned into smaller groups, which would then be ordered. In conditional ordering (C-ordering), the pixel vectors would be initially ordered according to the ordered values of one of their components, for example, the first component, $f_1(x,y)$ and $f_1(x',y')$. As a second step, vectors with the same value for the first component would be ordered according to the ordered values of another component, e.g., the second component, $f_2(x,y)$ and $f_2(x',y')$, and so on.

In this chapter, we adopt a new distance-based vector ordering technique (D-ordering), where each pixel vector is ordered according to its distance from other neighboring pixel vectors in the data (Plaza et al., 2002). This type of ordering, which can be seen as a special class of R-ordering, has demonstrated success in the definition of multi-channel morphological operations in previous work. Specifically, we define a cumulative distance between one particular pixel $f(x,y)$ and all the pixel vectors in the spatial neighborhood given by B (*B*-neighborhood) as shown in Box 2.

It should be noted that the proposed basic multi-dimensional operators are vector-preserving in the sense that vectors which are not present in the input data cannot be generated as a result of the extension process (Plaza et al., 2002). Obviously, the choice of Dist is a key topic in the resulting multi-channel ordering relation. A common choice in remote sensing applications is the spectral angle (SAD), an illumination-insensitive metric defined between two vectors s_i and s_j as shown in Box 3.

In medical imaging, for instance, illumination effects not as relevant as noise or other types of interferers. In those cases, a most common choice is the Euclidean distance (ED). In the following, we respectively adopt SAD and ED as the baseline distances for remote sensing and medical imaging experiments discussed in this chapter.

MULTI-CHANNEL WATERSHED SEGMENTATION ALGORITHM

The segmentation paradigm of our multi-channel watershed segmentation algorithm consists of three stages. First, multi-dimensional morphological operations are used to collect a set of minima according to some measure of minima importance. Starting from the selected minima and using the multi-dimensional morphological gradient as a reference, a multi-channel watershed transformation by flooding is then applied.

Box 2.

$$C_B\left(f(x,y)\right) = \sum_{(s,t)} \mathrm{Dist}\left(f(x,y), f(s,t)\right), \qquad \forall (s,t) \in Z^2(B) \qquad (3)$$

where Dist is a linear point-wise distance measure between two N-dimensional vectors. As a result, $C_B(f(x,y))$ is given by the sum of Dist scores between $f(x,y)$ and every other pixel vector in the B-neighborhood. To be able to define the standard morphological operators in a complete lattice framework, we need to be able to define a *supremum* and an *infimum,* given an arbitrary set of vectors S=$\{v_1, v_2, ..., v_p\}$, where p is the number of vectors in the set. This can be achieved by computing $C_B(S) = C_B(v_1), C_B(v_2), ..., C_B(v_p)\}$ and selecting v_j, such that $C_B(v_j)$ is the minimum of $C_B(S)$, with $1 \leq j \leq p$. In similar fashion, we can select v_k, such that $C_B(v_k)$ is the maximum of $C_B(S)$, with $1 \leq k \leq p$. Based on the simple definitions above, the flat extended erosion of f by B consists of selecting of the B-neighborhood pixel vector that produces the minimum C_B value:

$$(f \ominus B)(x,y) = \left\{ f(x+s', y+t'), (s',t') = \arg\min_{(s,t) \in Z^2(B)} \left\{ C_B\left(f(x+s, y+t)\right) \right\} \right\} \qquad (x,y) \in Z^2$$

$$(4)$$

where the arg min operator selects the pixel vector that is most similar, according to the distance Dist, to all the other pixels in the in the B-neighborhood. On other hand, the flat extended dilation of f by B selects the B-neighborhood pixel vector that produces the maximum value for C_B:

$$(f \oplus B)(x,y) = \left\{ f(x-s', y-t'), (s',t') = \arg\max_{(s,t) \in Z^2(B)} \left\{ C_B\left(f(x-s, y-t)\right) \right\} \right\} \qquad (x,y) \in Z^2$$

$$1 \qquad (5)$$

where the arg max operator selects the pixel vector that is most different, according to Dist, from all the other pixels in the B-neighborhood. Using the above notation, the multi-channel morphological gradient at pixel $f(x,y)$ using B can be simply defined as follows:

$$G_B\left(f(x,y)\right) = Dist\left((f \oplus B)(x,y), (f \otimes B)(x,y)\right) \qquad (6)$$

Box 3.

$$SAD\left(s_i, s_j\right) = \cos^{-1}\left(s_i \cdot s_j / \|s_i\| \|s_j\|\right) = \cos^{-1}\left(\sum_{l=1}^{N} s_{il} s_{jl} \Big/ \left[\sum_{l=1}^{N} s_{il}^2\right]^{1/2} \left[\sum_{l=1}^{N} s_{jl}^2\right]^{1/2}\right) \qquad (7)$$

Finally, watershed regions are iteratively merged, according to a similarity criterion, to obtain the final segmentation.

Minima Selection

The key of an accurate segmentation resides in the first step, that is, the selection of "markers," or minima, from which the transform is started. Following a recent work (Malpica et al., 2003), we hierarchically order all minima according to their deepness, and then select only those above a threshold. This approach has the advantage that it provides an intuitive selection scheme controlled by a single parameter. The concept can be easily explained using the immersion simulation. The deepness of a basin would be the level the water would reach, coming in through the minimum of the basin, before the water would overflow into a neighboring basin, that is, the height from the minimum to the lowest point in the watershed line of the basin.

Deepness can be computed using morphological reconstruction applied to the multi-channel gradient in Equation 6. Reconstruction is a special class of morphological transformation that does not introduce discontinuities (Vincent, 1993). Given a "flat" SE of minimal size, designed by B, and the multi-channel gradient $G_B(f)$ of an n-dimensional image f, morphological reconstruction by erosion of $G_B(f)$ using B can be defined as shown in Box 4.

In the operation depicted in Box 4, $G_B(f) \otimes B$ is the standard erosion of the multi-channel gradient image, which acts as a "marker" image for the reconstruction, while $G_B(f)$ acts as a "mask" image. Reconstruction transformations always converge after a finite number of iterations t, that is, until the propagation of the marker image is totally impeded by the mask image. It can be proven that the morphological reconstruction $(G_B(f) \otimes B)^t$ of $G_B(f)$ from $G_B(f) \otimes B$ will have a watershed transform in which the regions with deepness lower than a certain value v have been joined to the neighboring region with closer spectral properties, that is, parameter v is a minima selection threshold.

Flooding

In this section, we formalize the flooding process following a standard notation (Soille, 2003). Let the set $P = \{p_1, p_2, \ldots, p_k\}$ denote the set of k minimum pixel vectors selected after multi-dimensional minima selection. Similarly, let the catchment basin associated with a minimum pixel p_i be denoted by $CB(p_i)$. The points of this catchment basin which have an altitude less than or equal to a certain deepness score d (Malpica et al., 2003) are denoted in Box 5.

Box 4.

$$\left(G_B(f) \otimes B \right)^t (x, y) = \bigvee_{k \geq 1} \left[\delta_B^t \left(G_B(f) \otimes B \mid G_B(f) \right) \right](x, y) \tag{8}$$

where

$$\left[\delta_B^t \left(G_B(f) \otimes B \mid G_B(f) \right) \right](x, y) = \left[\overbrace{\delta_B \delta_B \cdots \delta_B}^{t \; times} \left(G_B(f) \otimes B \mid G_B(f) \right) \right](x, y) \tag{9}$$

and

$$\left[\delta_B \left(G_B(f) \otimes B \mid G_B(f) \right) \right](x, y) = \vee \left\{ \left(G_B(f) \otimes B \right)(x, y), G_B(f(x, y)) \right\} \tag{10}$$

Box 5.

$$CB_d(\boldsymbol{p}_i) = \left\{ f(\mathrm{x,y}) \in CB(\boldsymbol{p}_i) \mid Dist\left(\boldsymbol{p}_i, f(\mathrm{x,y})\right) \le d \right\} \tag{11}$$

We also denote by $X_d = \bigcup_{i=1}^{k} CB_d(\boldsymbol{p}_i)$ the subset of all catchment basins which contain a pixel vector with a deepness value less than or equal to d. Finally, the set of points belonging to the regional minima of deepness d are denoted by $\mathrm{RMIN}_d(f(\mathrm{x,y}))$. The catchment basins are now progressively created by simulating the flooding process. The first pixel vectors reached by water are the points of highest deepness score. These points belong to $\mathrm{RMIN}_{pj}(f(\mathrm{x,y})) = X_{DB}(\boldsymbol{p}_j)$, where $\boldsymbol{p}_j$ is the deepest pixel in P, that is, $D_B(\boldsymbol{p}_j)$ is the minimum, with $1 \le j \le k$. From now on, the water either expands the region of the catchment basin already reached by water, or starts to flood the catchment basin whose minima have a deepness equal to $D_B(\boldsymbol{p}_l)$, where $\boldsymbol{p}_l$ is the deepest pixel in the set of P-$\{\boldsymbol{p}_j\}$. This operation is repeated until P=$\varnothing$. At each iteration, there are three possible relations of inclusion between a connected component $\boldsymbol{Y}$ and $\boldsymbol{Y} \cap X_{D_B(\boldsymbol{p}_j)}$:

1. If $\boldsymbol{Y} \cap X_{D_B(\boldsymbol{p}_j)} = \varnothing$ then it follows that a new minimum $\boldsymbol{Y}$ has been discovered at level $D_B(\boldsymbol{p}_j)$. In this case, the set of all minima at level $D_B(\boldsymbol{p}_j)$, that is, $\mathrm{RMIN}_{pj}(f(\mathrm{x,y}))$ will be used for defining $X_{D_B(\boldsymbol{p}_j)}$.

2. If $\boldsymbol{Y} \cap X_{D_B(\boldsymbol{p}_j)} \ne \varnothing$ and is connected, then the flooded region is expanding and $\boldsymbol{Y}$ corresponds to the pixels belonging to the catchment basin associated with the minimum and having a deepness score less than or equal to $D_B(\boldsymbol{p}_j)$, i.e. $\boldsymbol{Y} = CB_{D_B(\boldsymbol{p}_j)}(\boldsymbol{Y} \cap X_{D_B(\boldsymbol{p}_j)})$.

3. Finally, if $\boldsymbol{Y} \cap X_{D_B(\boldsymbol{p}_j)} \ne \varnothing$ and is not connected, then the flooded regions of the catchment basins of two distinct minima at level $D_B(\boldsymbol{p}_j)$ are expanding and merged together.

Once all levels have been flooded, the set of catchment basins of a multi-dimensional image f is equal to the set $X_{DB(\boldsymbol{p}_m)}$, where $\boldsymbol{p}_m$ is the least deep pixel in P, that is, $D_B(\boldsymbol{p}_m)$ is the maximum, with $1 \le m \le k$. The set of catchment basins after multi-dimensional watershed can be represented as a set $\left\{ CB(\boldsymbol{p}_i) \right\}_{i=1}^{k}$, where each element corresponds to the catchment basin of a regional minimum of the multi-channel input image f. This is the final segmentation output for the algorithm. A parallel algorithm for implementing the proposed flooding simulation is described in the following section.

Region Merging

To obtain the final segmentation, some of the regions $\left\{ CB(\boldsymbol{p}_i) \right\}_{i=1}^{k}$ resulting from the watershed can be merged to reduce the number of regions (Le Moigne & Tilton, 1995). This section briefly explains the region merging criteria and method employed. First, all regions are ordered into a region adjacency graph (RAG). The RAG is an undirected graph G=(V,E), where V = $\left\{ CB(\boldsymbol{p}_i) \right\}_{i=1}^{k}$ such that each region CB($\boldsymbol{p}_i$) is represented by a node, and e($\boldsymbol{p}_i$, $\boldsymbol{p}_j$)$\in$E if:

1. $\boldsymbol{p}_i, \boldsymbol{p}_j \in$V, and
2. CB($\boldsymbol{p}_i$), CB($\boldsymbol{p}_j$) are adjacent, or
3. Dist($\boldsymbol{p}_i, \boldsymbol{p}_j$) < S, where S is a pixel vector similarity threshold.

The merging process is based on graph G, where the weight of an edge e($\boldsymbol{p}_i$, $\boldsymbol{p}_j$) is the value of Dist($\boldsymbol{p}_i, \boldsymbol{p}_j$). Regions CB($\boldsymbol{p}_i$), CB($\boldsymbol{p}_j$) can be merged attending to spatial properties in the case of adjacent regions, and also according to pixel vector similarity criteria in the case of non-adjacent regions. Similar merging procedures have been successfully used before in the literature (Tilton, 1999). Finally, Kruskal's algorithm can be applied to generate the minimum spanning tree, denoted as T, by adding one edge at a time. Initially, the edges of G are sorted in a non-decreasing order of their weights. Then, the edges in the sorted list are examined one-by-one and checked to determine whether adding the edge that is currently being examined creates a cycle with the edges that were already added to T. If it does not, it is added to T; otherwise, it is discarded. It should be noted that adding $e(p_i, p_j)$ to T represents the merge of its two regions $CB(p_i)$ and $CB(p_j)$. On other hand, adding the edge with the minimum weight one-by-one in an increasing order to T using the sorted list is equivalent to the merge of the two most similar regions. Finally, when an edge is rejected because it creates a cycle in T, no merge is performed because its two regions have already been merged into one. The process is terminated when T contains k edges.

In order to summarize the different stages and parameters involved, Figure 1 shows a block diagram depicting our multi-dimensional morphological algorithm for segmentation of multi-channel images.

As noted, there are three input parameters: B, a "flat" SE of minimal size used in the morphological operations; v, a minima selection threshold used in the minima selection process and S, a pixel vector similarity threshold used in the region merging stage. First, a multi-channel gradient computation is performed by taking advantage of extended morphological operations. This step works as a multi-channel edge detector. Second, minima are selected from the resulting output by using the concept of deepness. Third, flooding from markers is accomplished by utilizing the spectral angle between pixel vectors. This operation makes use of the full spectral information (as opposed to traditional watershed-based segmentation algorithms), thus avoiding the problem of band selection from the input data. Finally, the resulting segmentation is refined by a region-merging procedure that integrates the spatial and spectral information. As can be deduced from the description above, one of the main contributions of the proposed algorithm is the fact that it naturally combines spatial/spectral information in all steps. The algorithm is fully automatic, and produces a segmentation output given by a set of watershed regions after region merging

Figure 1. Block diagram summarizing the multichannel watershed segmentation algorithm

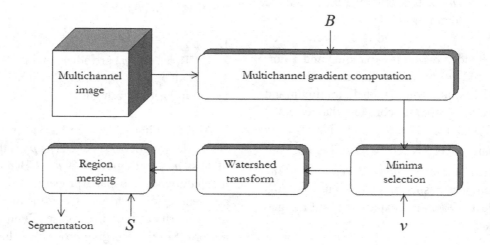

that we will denote from now on as $\{WS_i\}_{i=1}^{m}$, with $\bigcup_{i=1}^{m} WS_i = D_f$ and $WS_i \cap WS_j \neq \varnothing$, $\forall i \neq j$.

PARALLEL IMPLEMENTATION

Parallelization of watershed algorithms that simulate flooding is not a straightforward task. From a computational point of view, these algorithms are representative of the class of irregular and dynamic problems (Moga & Gabbouj, 1997). Moreover, the watershed process has an extremely volatile behavior, starting with a high degree of parallelism that very rapidly diminishes to a much lower degree. In this section, our goal is to develop an efficient and scalable parallel implementation of the algorithm proposed in the previous section.

Partitioning

Two types of partitioning strategies can be applied to image segmentation problems (Seinstra et al., 2002). One may decide whether the computation associated with the given problem should be split into pieces (functional decomposition), or the data on which the computation is applied (domain decomposition). Functional decomposition is inappropriate for segmentation with watersheds, where a sequence of operators are applied in a chain to the entire image. Our parallel algorithm uses domain decomposition, that is, the original multi-channel image f is decomposed into subimages. It is important to note that the subimages are made up of entire pixel vectors, that is, a single pixel vector is never split amongst several processing elements (PEs). If the computations for each pixel vector need to originate from several PEs, then they would require intensive inter-processor

message passing (Montoya et al., 2003). Thus, the global domain D_f is split among P processors in disjoint subdomains as shown in Box 6.

Task Replication

An important issue in SE-based morphological image processing operations is that accesses to pixels outside the domain D_f of the input image is possible. For instance, when the SE is centered on a pixel located in the border of the original image, a simple border-handling strategy can be applied (Seinstra et al., 2003). On the other hand, additional inter-processor communications may be required when the structuring element computation needs to be split amongst several different processing nodes, as shown by Figure 2. In the example, the computations for the pixel vector at spatial location (5,3) needs to originate from two processors. In order to avoid such an overhead, edge/corner pixels are replicated in the neighboring processors whose subdomains are thus enlarged with a so-called extension area. The extended subdomains are overlapping, and can be defined as follows:

$$D_{f_i}^e = \left\{ f(x,y) \in D_f \mid N_B\big(f(x,y)\big) \cap D_{f_i} \neq \varnothing \right\}$$

(13)

where $N_B(f(x,y))$ is the B-neighborhood of $f(x,y)$. Using the above notation, we can further denote the neighboring subimages of f_i as the set $N_B(f_i) = \left\{ f_j \mid D_{f_j} \cap D_{f_i}^e \neq \varnothing \right\}$. It should be noted that the task-replication strategy above enhances code reusability, which is highly recommended in order to build a robust parallel algorithm. As will be shown by experiments, the amount of redundant

Box 6.

$$D_f = D_{f_0} \cup D_{f_1} \cup \cdots \cup D_{f_{P-1}}, \text{ with } D_{f_i} \cap D_{f_j} = \varnothing, \forall \mathbf{i} \neq \mathbf{j}.$$

(12)

Figure 2. Morphological structuring element computation split between two processors

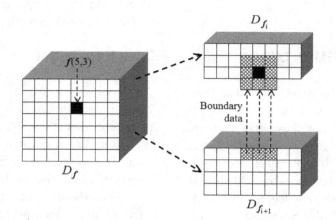

Figure 2. Morphological structuring element computation split between two processors

information introduced by the proposed framework can greatly reduce communication time.

Implementation

Our implementation of the parallel multi-channel watershed algorithm uses a simple master-slave model. The master processor divides the multi-channel image f into a set of subimages f_i which are sent to different processors, so that the domain of each subimage is an extended subdomain given by $D_{f_i}^e$. The slave processors run the segmentation algorithm on the respective subimages and also exchange data among themselves for uniform segmentation. After the segmented regions become stable, the slaves send the output to the master, which combines all of them in a proper way and provides the final segmentation. If we assume that the parallel system has p processors available, then one of the processors is reserved to act as the master, while each of the remaining p-1 processors create a local queue Q_i with $1 \leq i \leq p$-1. The minima selection algorithm is run locally at each processor to obtain a set of minima pixels surrounded by non-minima, which are then used to initialize each queue Q_i. Flooding is then performed locally in each processor as in the serial algorithm. However, due to the image

division, flooding is confined only to the local subdomain. Therefore, there may exist parts of the subimage that cannot be reached by flooding since they are contained in other subimages. Our approach to deal with this problem is to first flood locally at every deepness score in the subimage. Once the local flooding is finished, each processor exchanges segmentation labels of pixels in the boundary with appropriate neighboring processors. Subsequently, a processor can receive segmentation labels corresponding to pixels in the extended subdomain. The processor must now "reflood" the local subdomain from those pixels, a procedure that may introduce changes in segmentation labels of the local subdomain. Communication and reflooding are again repeated until stabilization (i.e., no more changes occur). When the flood-reflood process is finished, each slave processor sends the final segmentation labels to the master processor, which combines them together and performs region merging to produce final set of segmentation labels.

To conclude this section, we emphasize that although the flooding-reflooding scheme above seems complex, we have experimentally tested that this parallelization strategy is more effective than other approaches that exchange segmentation labels without first flooding locally at every deepness score. The proposed parallel framework guarantees that the processors are not tightly synchronized (Moga & Gabbouj, 1998). In addition, the processors execute a similar amount of work at approximately the same time, thus achieving load balance. Performance data for the parallel algorithm are given in the following subsection.

EXPERIMENTAL RESULTS

This section reports on the effectiveness of the proposed parallel segmentation algorithm in two specific applications. In the first one, phantom and real MR brain images are used to investigate the accuracy of multi-channel watershed segmentation in computer-aided medical diagnoses. In the second application, hyperspectral data collected by NASA's Airborne Visible Infra-Red Imaging Spectrometer (AVIRIS) are used to illustrate a remote sensing classification scenario.

MRI Brain Image Experiments

In medical applications, the detection and outlining of boundaries of organs and tumors in magnetic resonance imaging (MRI) are prerequisite. This is one of the most important steps in computer-aided surgery. In this section, we present two sets of experiments, one set of computer-generated phantom images and another set of real MRI

images, to show that the proposed algorithm has a good capability of segmentation.

Computer Simulations for Phantom Experiments

In this subsection, computer simulations are used to conduct a quantitative study and performance analysis of the proposed multi-channel watershed algorithm. The computer-generated phantom MRI images, shown in Figure 3, consist of four bands. The ellipses represent structural areas of three interesting cerebral tissues corresponding to gray matter (GM), white matter (WM) and cerebral spinal fluid (CSF). From the periphery to the center, the distribution of tissues is simulated as follows: background (BKG), GM, WM and CSF, given by the gray level values in Table 1. The gray level values of these areas in each band were simulated in such a fashion that these values reflect the average values of their respective tissues in real MRI images. A zero-mean Gaussian noise was added to the phantom images in Figure 3 to achieve different levels of signal-to-noise ratios (SNRs) ranging from 10 dB to 30 dB. Despite the fact that such MRI phantom images may be unrealistic, they only serve for the purpose of illustration of the proposed algorithm. This is done by using available absolute ground-truth information at a pixel level, known from the controlled simulation scenario in which the data were simulated.

Figure 3. Four band test phantoms for MRI simulation study

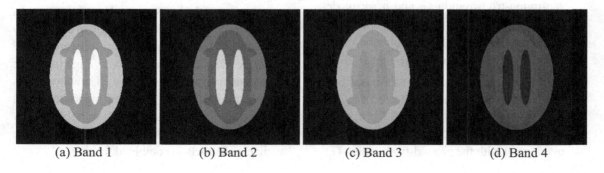

(a) Band 1   (b) Band 2   (c) Band 3   (d) Band 4

Table 1. Gray level values of the tissues of each band of the multichannel MRI phantom image

Band	GM	WM	CSF
1	209	180	253
2	150	124	232
3	207	188	182
4	95	94	42

In order to assess contour-fitting precision of the proposed multi-channel watershed algorithm, we use the following statistical measures (Hoover et al., 1996): correct detection, over-segmentation, under-segmentation and missed and noise region. Let D be the total number of regions detected by the algorithm, and let G be the number of ground-truth regions (four in the phantom example). Let the number of pixels in each detected region, D_i, be denoted as P_{D_i}. Similarly, let the number of pixels in each ground-truth region, G_i, be denoted as P_{G_i}. Let $0_{D_i G_i} = P_{D_i} \bigcap P_{G_i}$ be the number of overlapped pixels between P_{D_i} and P_{G_i}. Thus, if there is no overlap between P_{D_i} and P_{G_i}, then $0_{D_i G_i} = \varnothing$, while if there is complete overlap, then $0_{D_i G_i} = P_{D_i} = P_{G_i}$. Let a threshold value T be a measure of the strictness of the definition desired. With the above definitions in mind, the following segmentation accuracy metrics can be defined:

1. A pair made up of a detected region D_i and a ground-truth region G_i are classified as an instance of correct detection if $0_{D_i G_i} / P_{D_i} \geq T$, that is, at least T percent of the pixels in the detected region D_i are overlapped with the ground-truth region G_i;

2. A ground-truth region G_i and a set of detected regions D_j, j=1,...,n are classified as an instance of under-segmentation if: $\sum_{j=1}^{n} O_{D_j G_i} / P_{G_i} \geq T$, i.e. the ground-truth region G_i is at least T-percent overlapped with the compositin of the n detected regions, and, $\forall j \in [1, \cdots, n]$, $O_{D_j G_i} / P_{G_i} \geq T$, i.e. all of the detected regions D_j are at least T-percent overlapped with the ground-truth region G_i;

3. A set of ground-truth regions G_j, j=1,...,m and a detected region D_i are classified as an instance of over-segmentation if: $\sum_{j=1}^{m} O_{D_i G_j} / P_{D_i} \geq T$, i.e. the detected region D_i is at least T-percent overlapped with the composition f the m ground-truth regions, and, $\forall j \in [1, \cdots, m]$, $O_{D_i G_j} / P_{D_i} \geq T$, i.e. all of the ground truth regions G_j are at least T-percent overlapped with the detected region D_i;

4. A detected region D_i, not participating in any instance of correct detection, over-segmentation or under-segmentation, is classified as a missed region; and

5. A ground-truth region G_j not participating in any instance of correct detection, over-segmentation or under-segmentation is classified as noise region.

Using the five segmentation accuracy metrics above, Table 2 shows the number of correct detections, over-segmentations, under-segmentations, missed and noise regions obtained after applying the multi-channel watershed algorithm to the phantom image in Figure 3, corrupted by Gaussian noise in different proportions. The parameters used in experimental results were $B = B_5^{(\text{disk})}$, that is, a disk-shaped SE of radius equal to 5 pixels; v, a minima selection threshold automatically calculated from the data using the multi-level Otsu method (Plaza et al., 2002) and a pixel vector similarity threshold S that was set to 0.01 in experiments. The above values were selected empirically, although we experimentally observed that the algorithm behaved similarly with other parameter settings. In addition, several tolerance threshold values were considered in the computation of the five statistical metrics above. As shown by the table, most of the regions detected by the multi-channel watershed algorithm were labeled as correct detections, even for very high tolerance thresholds or signal-to-noise ratios. The above results demonstrated that the proposed algorithm could produce accurate results in the presence of noise by integrating the information available from all the available channels in combined fashion.

Table 2. Number of correct detections (C), over-segmentations (O), under-segmentations (U), missed (M) and noise (N) regions obtained after applying the multichannel watershed algorithm, using different tolerance (T) values, to the phantom image in Figure 3 corrupted by noise in different proportions

T	SNR = 30 dB					SNR = 20 dB					SNR = 10 dB				
	C	O	U	M	N	C	O	U	M	N	C	O	U	M	N
95%	4	0	0	0	0	2	1	1	0	2	2	0	2	0	4
90%	4	0	0	0	0	3	0	1	0	2	3	0	1	0	3
80%	4	0	0	0	0	4	0	0	0	1	3	0	1	0	1
70%	4	0	0	0	0	4	0	0	0	0	3	0	1	0	0
60%	4	0	0	0	0	4	0	0	0	0	4	0	0	0	0
50%	4	0	0	0	0	4	0	0	0	0	4	0	0	0	0

Real MRI Image Experiments

In the following experiments, a real MRI multi-channel image was used for performance evaluation. Figure 4 shows the four different slices of the considered case study. Since in many MRI applications the three cerebral tissues, GM, WM and CSF, are of major interest, Figure 5a shows five markers with higher *deepness* associated with these regions. They are shown as numbers superimposed on band 3 of the real image, where the order relates to their deepness score (the pixel labeled as "1" has the highest deepness). On other hand, Figure 5b shows the morphological gradient obtained for this case study. The result of the multi-channel flooding-based watershed algorithm (before region merging) from the markers in Figure 5a is given in Figure 5c, where

the considered parameter values were the same as those used for phantom experiments in the previous subsection. The final result after the region merging step is given in Figure 5d. For illustrative purposes, Figures 5e-g, respectively, show the segmentation result obtained by other standard algorithms. The first one is a standard single-channel watershed algorithm (Rajapakse et al., 1997) applied to the band with higher contrast, that is, band 2 in Figure 4b. The second one is a watershed clustering-based technique applied to the spectral feature space (Soille, 1996). This approach differs from our proposed combined method in that it separates the spectral and the spatial information. It first clusters the data in spectral space and then segments objects assuming that the pixels in a given class should have relatively homogeneous spectral intensities. The third

Figure 4. Four spectral bands of a real MRI brain image

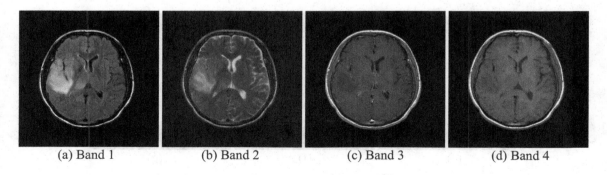

(a) Band 1   (b) Band 2   (c) Band 3   (d) Band 4

approach is the well known ISODATA segmentation procedure that is regarded as a benchmark for most unsupervised segmentation algorithms. The algorithm uses the Euclidean distance as a similarity measure to cluster data elements into different classes (Richards & Jia, 1999).

As observed in Figure 5, the multi-channel watershed algorithm in Figures 5c-d has several advantages over the other segmentation approaches tested. First, the proposed method was able to impose smoothness in the segmentation result. The segmentations produced by other methods often lack spatial consistency. For instance, the single-channel watershed algorithm in Figure 5e produced watershed lines which were rather noisy and jagged, even after region merging. This was because only one band was used, and the segmentation was dependent on intensity values at that particular band. In this work we selected the

band with higher contrast for the single-channel watershed run; this selection might not be optimal in other cases. On the other hand, the watershed-based clustering approach in Figure 5f produced a smoother segmentation as a consequence of the (separate) use of spatial and spectral information. However, this approach missed some important regions clearly visible in the results produced by all other algorithms. Finally, the ISODATA segmentation in Figure 5g was produced using the spectral information only, that is, a pixel was classified depending on its spectral values whatever those of its neighbors. This resulted in a rather noisy and disconnected output. As can be seen in Figures 5c and 5d, the region merging stage implemented in the proposed method improved the segmentation by associating together some disconnected regions resulting from the flooding. Overall, results in Figure 5 demonstrate the im-

Figure 5. (a) Five markers with highest deepness score, represented by numbers superimposed on band 3; (b) Multichannel morphological gradient; (c) Multichannel watershed segmentation (before merging); (d) Multichannel watershed segmentation (after merging); (e) Single-channel watershed segmentation; (f) Soille's watershed-based segmentation; (g) ISODATA segmentation

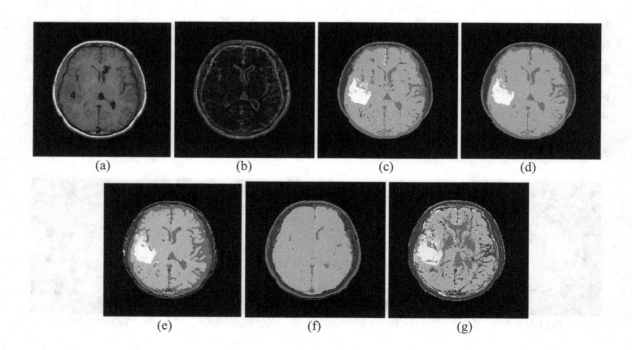

portance of using spatial and spectral information in simultaneous fashion.

Finally, it should be noted that no quantitative analysis was conducted for the real MRI experiments due to the lack of ground-truth information. However, a visual evaluation of the results in Figure 5 by an expert radiologist indicated a "better delineation of objects and superior spatial consistency of multi-channel watershed over the other tested approaches." As for computational complexity, we used a PC with an AMD Athlon 2.6 GHz processor and 512 Megabytes of RAM to run all the experiments in this section, and it was found that the multi-channel watershed algorithm produced segmentation results in less than 30 seconds in all cases. This was mainly due to the limited number of bands available. Subsequently, no parallelization strategies were deemed necessary for computer-aided diagnosis of MRI image experiments. However, multi-channel image data in other applications, such as hyperspectral images in remote sensing, are characterized by high-dimensional images with hundreds of spectral bands. As a result, further experimentation using real hyperspectral data sets with high dimensionality is pertinent.

Remotely Sensed Hyperspectral Data Experiments

The image data set used in experiments is a hyperspectral scene collected by the 224-band Airborne Visible Infra-Red Imaging Spectrometer (AVIRIS), a remote sensing instrument operated by NASA's Jet Propulsion Laboratory (Green et al., 1998). The data set was collected over an agricultural test site located in Salinas Valley, California, and represents a challenging segmentation problem. Fortunately, extensive ground-truth information is available for the area, allowing a quantitative assessment in terms of segmentation accuracy. Figure 6a shows the entire scene and a sub-scene of the dataset (called hereinafter Salinas A), dominated by directional regions. Figure 6b

shows the 15 available ground-truth regions. The available data volume (over 50 Mb) creates the need for parallel watershed-based analysis able to produce segmentation results quickly enough for practical use.

Table 3 displays the number of correct detections, over-segmentations, under-segmentations and missed regions obtained after applying the proposed multi-channel segmentation algorithm using disk-shaped SEs with different radiuses, measured using different tolerance thresholds. For illustrative purposes, results by two other standard algorithms, ISODATA and Soille's watershed-based clustering, are also displayed. It should be noted that the statistics for noise regions are not provided on purpose, due to the fact that available ground-truth information displayed in Figure 6b is not absolute. In all cases, parameter v was set automatically using the multi-level Otsu method, and parameter S was set to 0.01 empirically. As shown by Table 3, the use of appropriate structuring element sizes in the proposed method produced segmentation results which were superior to those found by ISODATA and Soille's watershed-based clustering algorithm. In particular, the best results were obtained when a disk-shaped SE $B = B_{15}^{(disk)}$ was used. This is mainly due to the relation between the SE and the spatial properties of regions of interest in the scene. Specifically, the usage of $B_{15}^{(disk)}$ resulted in a number of correct detections (11) which was the highest one in experiments, while the scores for all error metrics were minimized. Interestingly, no under-segmentation or missed instances were obtained in this case, while only one case of over-segmentation was observed. This case comprised the four lettuce romaine regions contained in the Salinas A subscene, which are at different weeks since planting (4, 5, 6 and 7 weeks, respectively), and covering the soil in different proportions. These four ground-truth regions were always detected as a single, over-segmented region, which is a reasonable segmentation result given the slight differences in the spectral characteristics of the

Figure 6. (a) Spectral band at 488 nm of an AVIRIS hyperspectral image comprising several agricultural fields in Salinas Valley, California, and a sub-scene of the dataset (Salinas A), outlined by a white rectangle; (b) land-cover ground truth regions

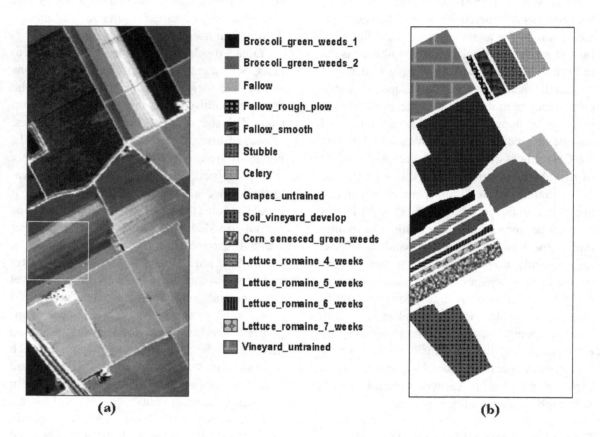

(a)

Broccoli_green_weeds_1
Broccoli_green_weeds_2
Fallow
Fallow_rough_plow
Fallow_smooth
Stubble
Celery
Grapes_untrained
Soil_vineyard_develop
Corn_senesced_green_weeds
Lettuce_romaine_4_weeks
Lettuce_romaine_5_weeks
Lettuce_romaine_6_weeks
Lettuce_romaine_7_weeks
Vineyard_untrained

(b)

Table 3. Number of correct detections (C), over-segmentations (O), under-segmentations (U) and missed (M) regions obtained after applying the proposed multichannel watershed algorithm, Soille's watershed-based clustering, and ISODATA to the AVIRIS Salinas scene in Fig. 6(a) using different tolerance (T) values

Method		T = 80%				T = 90%				T = 95%			
		C	O	U	M	C	O	U	M	C	O	U	M
Multichannel watershed Algorithm	$B_3^{(disk)}$	2	2	5	6	2	2	2	9	1	3	2	9
	$B_7^{(disk)}$	6	2	3	5	5	2	3	6	5	2	2	7
	$B_{11}^{(disk)}$	10	0	0	6	10	0	1	5	9	0	1	6
	$B_{15}^{(disk)}$	11	1	0	0	11	1	0	0	11	1	0	0
Watershed-based clustering		7	1	2	5	6	1	1	6	5	1	1	8
ISODATA		3	2	2	8	2	1	2	10	2	0	1	12

four lettuce fields. Overall, the results shown in Table 3 reveal that the proposed algorithm can achieve very accurate segmentation results in a complex analysis scenario given by agricultural classes with very similar spectral features.

It should be noted that the proposed algorithm required several hours of computation in the same computing environment described in MRI experiments, which created the need for a parallel implementation. In order to investigate the efficiency of our parallel multi-channel watershed implementation, we coded the algorithm using the C++ programming language with calls to a message passing interface (MPI). The parallel code was tested on a high-performance Beowulf cluster (Brightwell et al., 2000) available at NASA's Goddard Space Flight Center in Maryland. The system used in experiments, called Thunderhead, is composed of 256 dual 2.4 Ghz Intel Xeon nodes with 1 Gigabyte of local memory and 80 Gigabytes of main memory.

Table 4 shows execution times in seconds of the parallel algorithm with the AVIRIS scene for several combinations of SE sizes and number of processors. Processing times were considerably reduced as the number of processors was increased.

For instance, for the case of using $B_{15}^{(disk)}$, which resulted in the most accurate segmentation results as shown in Table 4, 36 processors were required to produce a segmentation result in less than ten minutes. If the application under study can tolerate less accurate segmentations, such as those obtained using $B_3^{(disk)}$, then the number of required processors to produce the output in about five minutes was only 16. In order to further analyze the scalability of the parallel code, Figure 7a plots the speed-up factors achieved by the parallel algorithm over a single-processor run of the algorithm as a function of the number of processors used in the parallel computation. The achieved speed-up factors were better for large SEs, a fact that reveals that the proposed parallel implementation is more effective as the volume of computations increases.

Finally, in order to investigate load balance, Figure 7b shows the execution times of the parallel algorithm for each of the processors on Thunderhead for a case study where 64 processors were used in the parallel computation; one processor (master or root processor) presents a slightly higher computational load as compared to the other processors. This comes as no surprise because the root processor is in charge of

Table 4. Execution time in seconds, T(K), and speed-up, S_K, achieved by the proposed multi-channel watershed algorithm with the AVIRIS Salinas scene in Figure 6a for several combinations of structuring element sizes and number of processors (K).

	$B_3^{(disk)}$		$B_7^{(disk)}$		$B_{11}^{(disk)}$		$B_{15}^{(disk)}$	
K	T(K)	S_K	T(K)	S_K	T(K)	S_K	T(K)	S_K
1	3145	1.00	7898	1.00	11756	1.00	16234	1.00
4	1195	2.63	2668	2.96	5090	2.31	5026	3.23
16	329	9.56	772	10.23	1112	10.58	1445	11.23
36	220	14.34	372	21.22	459	25.56	551	29.45
64	180	17.43	245	32.11	313	37.45	424	39.34
100	134	23.45	186	42.45	238	49.21	282	57.45
144	89	35.10	154	51.25	182	64.56	221	73.28
196	68	45.67	110	71.23	139	84.32	181	89.34
256	49	62.45	93	84.39	127	92.34	165	98.23

Figure 7. (a) Speed-up factors achieved by the parallel algorithm as a function of the number of processors; (b) execution times in seconds achieved for each of the processors using $B_{15}^{(disk)}$ as structuring element and 64 processors

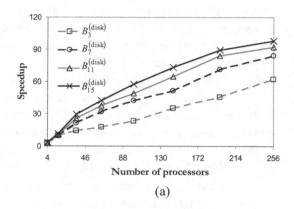

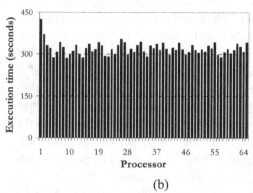

(a)

(b)

data partitioning, and also combines the partial results provided by every processor. It can be seen, however, that load balance is much better among the rest of the processors. Summarizing, we can conclude that the proposed multi-channel watershed segmentation algorithm, implemented on a commodity cluster of PCs, achieved good results in terms of segmentation accuracy, speed-up, scalability and load balance in the context of a high-dimensional image analysis application, dominated by large data volumes and complex patterns of communication and calculation.

CONCLUSION

This chapter has developed an approach to generalize the concepts of mathematical morphology to multi-channel image data. A new vector organization scheme was described, and fundamental morphological vector operations were defined by extension. Theoretical definitions of extended morphological operations were then used in the formal definition of a multi-channel watershed-based segmentation algorithm, which naturally combines the spatial and spectral/temporal in-

formation present in multi-channel images in simultaneous fashion. While such an integrated approach holds great promise in several applications, it also creates new processing challenges. For that purpose, this chapter also developed a parallel implementation which allows processing of large images quickly enough for practical use. A quantitative segmentation evaluation comparison with regard to standard techniques, using both MRI brain images and remotely sensed hyperspectral data collected by the NASA's Jet Propulsion Laboratory AVIRIS imaging spectrometer, revealed that the proposed parallel algorithm can produce highly accurate segmentation results in reasonable computation times, even when the computational requirements introduced by multi-channel imagery are extremely large.

ACKNOWLEDGMENT

The research in this chapter was supported by the European Commission through the project entitled "Performance analysis of endmember extraction and hyperspectral analysis algorithms" (contract no. HPRI–1999–00057). The authors would like to thank Professor Chein-I Chang for providing the MRI data and Dr. J. Anthony Gualtieri for providing the hyperspectral data. A. Plaza would also like to acknowledge support received from the Spanish Ministry of Education and Science (Fellowship PR2003-0360), which allowed him to conduct research as postdoctoral scientist at NASA's Goddard Space Flight Center and University of Maryland, Baltimore County.

REFERENCES

Adams, R., & Bischof, L. (1994). Seeded region growing. *IEEE Transactions on Pattern Analysis and Machine Intelligence, 16,* 641-647.

Beucher, S. (1994). Watershed, hierarchical segmentation and waterfall algorithm. In E. Dougherty (Ed.), *Mathematical morphology and its applications to image processing.* Boston: Kluwer.

Brightwell, R., Fisk, L. A., Greenberg, D. S., Hudson, T., Levenhagen, M., Maccabe, et al. (2000). Massively parallel computing using commodity components. *Parallel Computing, 26,* 243-266.

Chang, C.-I (2003). *Hyperspectral imaging: Techniques for spectral detection and classification.* New York: Kluwer.

Fan, J., Yau, D. K. Y., Elmargamid, A. K., & Aref, W. G. (2001). Automatic image segmentation by integrating color-edge extraction and seeded region growing. *IEEE Transactions on Image Processing, 10,* 1454-1466.

Green, R. O., et al. (1998). Imaging spectroscopy and the airborne visible/infrared imaging spectrometer (AVIRIS). *Remote Sensing of Environment, 65,* 227-248.

Haralick, R., & Shapiro, L. (1985). Image segmentation techniques. *Computer Vision, Graphics and Image Processing, 29,* 100-132.

Hoover, A., et al. (1996). An experimental comparison of range image segmentation algorithms. *IEEE Transactions on Pattern Analysis and Machine Intelligence, 18,* 673-689.

Le Moigne, J., & Tilton, J. C. (1995). Refining image segmentation by integration of edge and region data. *IEEE Transactions on Geoscience and Remote Sensing, 33,* 605-615.

Malpica, N., Ortuño, J. E., & Santos, A. (2003). A multi-channel watershed-based algorithm for supervised texture segmentation. *Pattern Recognition Letters, 24,* 1545-1554.

Mehnert, A., & Jackway, P. (1997). An improved seeded region growing algorithm. *Pattern Recognition Letters, 18,* 1065-1071.

Moga, A. N., & Gabbouj, M. (1997). Parallel image component labeling with watershed transformation. *IEEE Transactions on Pattern Analysis and Machine Intelligence, 19,* 441-450.

Moga, A. N., & Gabbouj, M. (1998). Parallel marker-based image segmentation with watershed transformation. *Journal of Parallel and Distributed Computing, 51,* 27-45.

Montoya, M. G., Gil, C., & García, I. (2003). The load unbalancing problem for region growing image segmentation algorithms. *Journal of Parallel and Distributed Computing, 63,* 387-395.

Plaza, A., Martinez, P., Perez, R., & Plaza, J. (2002). Spatial/spectral endmember extraction by multidimensional morphological operations. *IEEE Transactions on Geoscience and Remote Sensing, 40*(9), 2025-2041.

Plaza, A., Martinez, P., Perez, R., & Plaza, J. (2004). A new approach to mixed pixel classification of hyperspectral imagery based on extended morphological profiles. *Pattern Recognition, 37,* 1097-1116.

Rajapakse, J., Giedd, J., & Rapaport, J. (1997). Statistical approach to segmentation of single-channel cerebral MR images. *IEEE Transactions on Medical Imaging, 16,* 176-186.

Richards, J., & Jia, X. (1999). *Remote sensing digital image analysis* (3rd ed). Berlin: Springer.

Seinstra, F. J., Koelma, D., & Geusebroek, J. M. (2002). A software architecture for user transparent parallel image processing. *Parallel Computing, 28,* 967-993.

Shafarenko, L., Petrou, M., & Kittler, J. Automatic watershed segmentation of randomly textured color images. *IEEE Transactions on Image Processing, 6,* 1530-1544.

Soille, P. (1996). Morphological partitioning of multispectral images. *Journal of Electronic Imaging, 5,* 252-265.

Soille, P. (2003). *Morphological image analysis, principles and applications* (2nd ed.). Berlin: Springer.

Tilton, J. C. (1999). A recursive PVM implementation of an image segmentation algorithm with performance results comparing the HIVE and the Cray T3E. In *Proceedings of the 7th Symposium on the Frontiers of Massively Parallel Computation,* Annapolis, MD.

Vincent, L. (1993). Morphological grayscale reconstruction in image analysis: Applications and efficient algorithms. *IEEE Transactions on Image Processing, 2,* 176-201.

Vincent, L., & Soille, P. (1991). Watersheds in digital spaces: An efficient algorithm based on immersion simulations. *IEEE Transactions on Pattern Analysis and Machine Intelligence, 13,* 583-598.

Zhang, Y. J. (1996). A survey on evaluation methods for image segmentation. *Pattern Recognition, 29*(8), 1335-1346.

This work was previously published in Advances in Image and Video Segmentation, edited by Y. Zhang, pp. 270-291, copyright 2006 by IRM Press (an imprint of IGI Global).

Chapter XVII
Biomedical Image Registration for Diagnostic Decision Making and Treatment Monitoring

Xiu Ying Wang
The University of Sydney, Australia and Heilongjiang University, China

David Dagan Feng
The University of Sydney, Australia and Hong Kong Polytechnic University, Hong Kong, China

ABSTRACT

The chapter introduces biomedical image registration as a means of integrating and providing complementary and additional information from multiple medical images simultaneously to facilitate diagnostic decision-making and treatment monitoring. It focuses on the fundamental theories of biomedical image registration, major methodologies and contributions of this area, and the main applications of biomedical image registration in clinical contexts. Furthermore, discussions on the future challenges and possible research trends of this field are presented. The chapter aims to assist in a quick understanding of main methods and technologies, current issues, and major applications of biomedical image registration, to provide the connection between biomedical image registration and the related research areas, and finally to evoke novel and practical registration methods to improve the quality and safety of healthcare.

INTRODUCTION

Clinical knowledge management is a challenging and broad discipline related to the collection, processing, visualization, storage, preservation, and retrieval of health-related data and information to form useful knowledge for making critical clinical decisions. As an important part of clinical knowledge, medical images facilitate the understanding of anatomy and function, and are critical to research and healthcare. Medical imaging modalities can be divided into two major categories: anatomical modalities and functional modalities.

Anatomical modalities, mainly depicting morphology, include X-ray, computed tomography (CT), magnetic resonance imaging (MRI), ultrasound (US). Functional modalities, primarily describing information on the biochemistry of the underlying anatomy, include single photon emission computed tomography (SPECT) and positron emission tomography (PET). With the advances in medical imaging technologies, these imaging modalities are playing a more and more important role in improving the quality and efficiency of healthcare. For example, the functional imaging techniques can be used to image physiological and biochemical processes in different organs, such as brain, lung, liver, bone, thyroid, heart, and kidney (Figure 1). In such clinical settings, PET aids clinicians in choosing the most appropriate treatment and monitoring the patients' response to these therapies. Since information from multiple medical imaging modalities is usually of a complementary nature, proper extraction registration of the embedded information and knowledge is important in the healthcare decision making process and in clinical practice.

The combination of more advanced and user-friendly medical image databases is mak-

ing medical imaging results more accessible to clinical professionals. Starting in the early 1990s, the Visible Human Project and Human Brain Project at the US National Library of Medicine have produced a widely available reference of multimodal images of the human body. These projects provide users with labeled data and the connection of structural-anatomical knowledge with functional-physiological knowledge (Ackerman, 2001; Riva, 2003), and assist in making image data more usable for clinical training and surgery simulation and planning. A significant step in these virtual reality projects is the collection and registration of medical images from multiple imaging modalities.

Clinical practice often involves collecting and integrating considerable amounts of multimodality medical imaging data over time intervals to improve the optimization and precision of clinical decision making and to achieve better, faster, and more cost-effective healthcare. For example, in neurosurgical planning, the proper

Figure 1. Positron emission tomography (PET) (Courtesy of Hong Kong Sanatorium & Hospital)

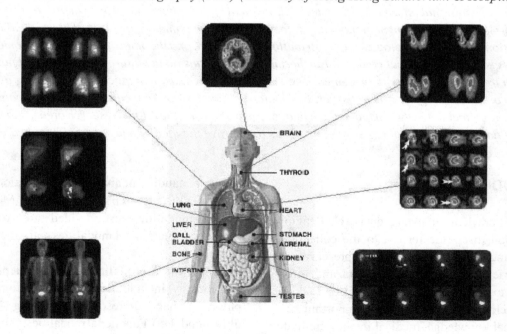

registration of the functional information with the detailed anatomical background enables the surgeon to optimize the operation with minimal damage to the healthy organs. The accurate and efficient registration of the complementary information available from different imaging modalities provides a basis for diagnostic and medical decision-making, treatment monitoring, and healthcare support.

A key issue in clinical knowledge management is biomedical image registration, which provides an effective mechanism to integrate the relevant information and knowledge in clinical and medical decision-making, operation planning, and image guided surgery. Registration algorithms also offer new possibilities to analyze and visualize multimodal image datasets simultaneously.

Using these algorithms, image data from multiple imaging modalities can be matched and presented in a common coordinate system, therefore,

anatomical and functional image information can be visualized simultaneously. Hence, biomedical image registration enables clinical professionals a complete insight into the patient data and can help to improve medical diagnosis and patient treatment (Handels, 2003).

Applications of biomedical image registration include radiation therapy, interventional radiology, diagnostic and clinical decision-making, image-guided surgery, procedure planning, and simulation, dynamic structural and functional change measurement, treatment, and disease progression monitoring, minimally invasive procedures, and the correlations between the function and morphology of human body. Furthermore, image registration is widely used in biomedical imaging, which includes methods developed for automated image labeling and pathology detection in individuals and groups. Moreover, registration algorithms can encode patterns of anatomic vari-

Figure 2. Registration of PET image scan with anatomic maps (Courtesy of Hong Kong Sanatorium & Hospital)

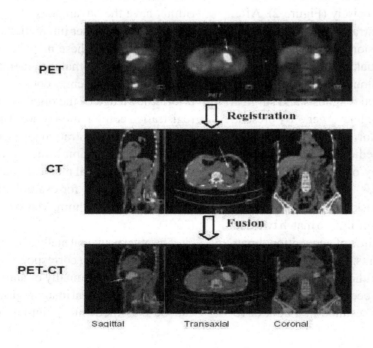

ability in large human populations, and can be used to create disease-specific, population-based atlases (Bankman, 2000).

Although biomedical image registration has been intensively investigated and enormous advances in imaging techniques have been achieved, the ever-increasing growth of imaging data and their applications in medical and clinical environments ensures the existence of future challenges in more precise and efficient biomedical image registration.

BACKGROUND

Accurate and efficient biomedical image registration can lead to additional clinical information not apparent in the isolated images and provide clinical professionals with sufficient information for diagnostic and medical decision-making. For example, functional imaging such as PET cannot provide very high-resolution image data, but by the registration of these functional images with anatomical images, for example, CT scanning, physiological and functional regions can be located more precisely (Figure 2). After automatic image registration to localize and identify anatomy and lesions, accurate diagnostic and clinical decision-making can be achieved. Such functional-to-anatomical data registration is very useful for clinical diagnosis and surgical operation, especially for telesurgery. By presenting relevant clinical information to clinicians at the point of care, biomedical image registration can improve the quality of care, patient safety, and healthcare benefits.

As a fundamental task in image processing, the process of registration aims to match two data sets that may differ in time of acquisition, imaging sensors, or viewpoints. Because of its crucial role in improving healthcare quality, medical image registration has been studied extensively for decades, which has resulted in a bulk of re-

views, surveys, and books, for example, Bankman (2000); Brown (1992); Fitzpatrick, Hill, and Maurer (2000); Lester and Arridge (1999); Maintz and Viergever (1998); Mäkelä (2002); Maurer and Fitzpatrick (1993); Rohr (2000); and van den Elsen, Pol, and Viergever (1993), . According to the registration feature space, principally, medical image registration can be distinguished into intensity-based registration and feature-based registration (Brown, 1992).

As one principal medical image registration methodology, intensity-based registration has attracted significant attention in the research community. As a result, numerous registration approaches have been proposed and used, for example, correlation based methods, Fourier-based approaches, the moment and principal axes methods [Alpert, Bradshaw, Kennedy, and Correia,(1990)], minimizing variance of intensity ratios (Woods, Mazziotta, and Cherry , 1993; Hill, Hawkes, Harrison, and Ruff, 1993), and mutual information methods (Collignon, Vandermeulen, Suetens, and Marchal 1995; Viola and Wells, 1995). Directly exploiting the image intensities, the intensity-based registration algorithms have the advantages of no segmentation required and few user interactions involved, and most importantly, these methods have potential to achieve fully automated registration. However, this category of schemes does not make use of a priori knowledge of the organ structure and the registration computation is not efficient. In order to improve the registration performance, speed, accuracy, and at same time to avoid the local minima, hierarchical medical image registration has been proposed, for example, Thevenaz and Unser (2000), and Pluim, Mainze, and Viergever (2001).

The other principal medical image registration category is based on corresponding features that can be extracted manually or automatically. The feature-based medical image registration methods can be classified into point-based approaches, for example, Besl and MaKey (1992); Bookstein (1992); and Fitzpatrick, West, and Maurer (1998); curve-based algorithms, for example, Maintz, van den Elsen, and Viergever (1996) and Subsol (1999); and surface-based methods, for example, Audette, Ferrie and Peters (2000) and Thompson and Toga (1996). One main advantage of feature-based registration is that the transformation can be stated in analytic form, which leads to efficient computational schemes. However, in the feature-based registration methodologies, a preprocessing step of detecting the features is needed and the registration results are highly dependent on the result of this preprocessing.

In medical image registration, a transformation which maps datasets obtained from different times, different viewpoints, and different sensors, must be determined. Depending on the characteristics of the differences between the medical images to be registered, generally, the registration transformations can be divided into rigid and non-rigid transformations. The rigid transformations can be used to cope with rotation and translation differences between the images. But usually, patient postures, tissue structures, and the shapes of the organs cannot always remain the same when they are imaged with different imaging devices or at different times, therefore, elastic or non-rigid registrations are required to cope with these differences between the images (Rohr, 2000). The elastic medical image registration was first introduced by Bajcsy (1989). As a challenging and active research topic, elastic medical image registration has attracted extensive attentions of researchers and a number of novel methods have been proposed; for example, a block matching strategy was used by Lin et al. (1994), and a flexible fluid model was proposed by Christensen, Kane, Marsh, and Vannier (1996). Elastic biomedical image registration is still an ongoing and challenging research topic and a lot of efforts are needed in this area.

TECHNOLOGICAL FUNDAMENTALS OF BIOMEDICAL IMAGE REGISTRATION

Biomedical Image Registration Definition

The problem of registration arises whenever images acquired from different sensors, at different times, or from different subjects need to be combined or compared for analysis or visualization. Biomedical image registration is the primary tool for comparing two or more medical images to discover the differences in the images or to combine information from multimodality medical images to reveal knowledge not accessible from individual images. Its main task is to determine a mapping to relate the pixels of one image to the corresponding pixels of a second image with respect to both space and intensity.

$$I_2 = g(I_1 (f(x,y,z))) \tag{1}$$

I_2 and I_1 are 3-D images, indexed by (x,y,z);
$f: (x,y,z) \rightarrow (x',y',z')$, spatial transformation;
g: One-dimensional intensity transformation.

Figure 3 illustrates the basic registration steps and the corresponding functions of each step.

Biomedical Registration Transformations

Biomedical image distortions must be taken into consideration when two sets of medical images are to be registered. There are many factors that can result in medical image distortions, for example, different underlying physics of imaging sensors, inter-subject differences, voluntary and involuntary movements of the subject during imaging. These distortions impose many challenges for biomedical image registration because image characteristics and distortions determine

Figure 3. Biomedical image registration procedure

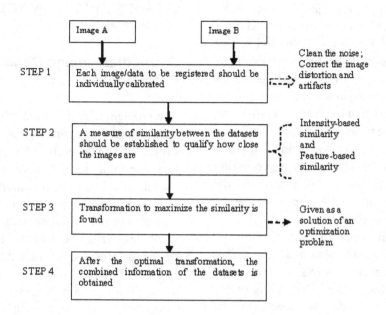

the registration transformations. For more details on medical imaging deformation characteristics and registration transformations, please refer to Bankman (2000); Fitzpatrick, Hill, and Maurer (2000); Turner and Ordidge (2000). According to its transformation type, biomedical image registration can be divided into rigid registration and non-rigid registration.

The rigid registration is used to correct the simplest distortions caused by rotation and translation. Because of the rigid structure of the skull, the distortions of the brain images are often assumed as rigid distortions. When the brain image registration is carried out, the rigid transformation, which preserves the lengths and angle measures, is often used to correct these translation and rotation displacements.

Affine transformation, which maps parallel lines into parallel lines, is used for the correction of translation, rotation, scaling, and skewing of the coordinate space. For example, affine transformation is useful for the correction of skewing distortion in CT caused by tilted gantry.

Non-rigid medical image deformations can be caused by the dramatic changes of the subject positions, tissue structures, and the shapes of the organs when the subject is imaged with different imaging devices or at different times. Usually, different imaging devices require the subject to pose differently to get optimal imaging results, therefore, rigid and affine transformations are not sufficient for correcting these non-rigid deformations. The involuntary motions of the lung and the heart lead to elastic deformations which cannot be registered using rigid and affine transformations as well. Even brain structure cannot always be considered as the same over time because of the differences between pre-operation and post-operation. Non-rigid image registration is an active research area, which is important for correcting the soft tissue deformations, temporal displacements due to disease progression and surgical intervention, and individual variations. In elastic transformations, the straightness of lines cannot be preserved and the transformations can be arbitrarily complex.

Implementation Issues

Interpolation is required when an image needs to undergo transformations. Usually, the intra-slice resolution is higher than the inter-slice resolution, hence, the interpolation operation should be carried out to compensate for this difference. Images from different imaging modalities have different resolution, therefore in a multimodal image registration, lower resolution images are often interpolated to the sample space of the higher resolution images. Lehmann, Gönner, and Spitzer (1999) presented a survey of interpolation methods in medical image processing.

In biomedical image registration, the most frequently used interpolation methods include nearest neighbor, linear, bilinear, trilinear, cubic, bicubic, tricubic, quadrilinear, and cubic convolution interpolation. The more complex the interpolation methods, the more surrounding points concerned, and the slower the registration speed. In order to speed up the registration procedure, low cost interpolation techniques are often preferred. Because of its good trade-off between accuracy and computational complexity, the bilinear interpolation is the most commonly used method (Zitová and Flusser, 2003). According to the research of Thévenaz, Blu, and Unser (2000), in cardiac and thorax image registration, trilinear interpolation can help to achieve good registration performance.

The optimization algorithm is required by almost every registration procedure, which serves as a searching strategy. There are several optimization algorithms often used in the biomedical image registration. The exhaustive searching method has been selected as optimization strategy by researchers. However, because of its high computational complexity, the exhaustive method for searching for the global optimization is not an efficient choice. The Powell algorithm by Powell (1964) and Simplex method by Nelder and Mead (1965) are more efficient than the exhaustive searching strategy in finding an optimum solution.

The Powell algorithm has been used frequently as an optimization strategy for biomedical image registration, for example, Collignon et al. (1995), Maes, Collignon, Vandermeulen, Marchal, and Suetens (1997), Wang and Feng (2005). The Powell algorithm performs a succession of one-dimensional optimizations, finding in turn the best solution along each freedom degree, and then returning to the first degree of freedom. The algorithm stops when it is unable to find a new solution with a significant improvement to the current solution.

The Downhill-Simplex algorithm has been used by, for example, Hill et al. (1993) and van Herk and Kooy (1994). Rohlfing and Maurer (2003) adopted a variant of the Downhill-Simplex algorithm restricted to the direction of the steepest ascent.

In order to search a vast number of parameters, which represent the complex deformation fields, multi-resolution optimization algorithms have been adopted by researchers in the biomedical image registration community, for example, Penny (1998). Initially, the registration is performed at coarse spatial scales, then to the finer ones. These multi-resolution or coarse-to-fine optimization algorithms can accelerate computation and help to escape from the local minima.

Performance Validation of Biomedical Image Registration

For all types of registration, assessment of the registration accuracy is very important. A medical image registration method cannot be accepted as a clinical tool to make decisions about patient management until it has been proved to be accurate enough. Important criteria for assessing the performance of registration schemes are accuracy, robustness, usability, and computational complexity. The often used validation methods include Fiducial landmarks, Phantom studies, and Visual inspection.

Fiducial landmarks, which can predict the expected error distribution, have been devised to assess the registration accuracy. To a certain extent, assessment using fiducial landmarks provides a "gold standard" for medical image registration. However, the fiducial landmarks can either suffer from the movement of skin mobility or are highly invasive. Also, these validation measures cannot be applied retrospectively.

Phantom studies are important for the estimation of the registration accuracy because the data and displacement information is fully known beforehand. Phantom-based validations provide measures for mean transformation errors and computational complexity for different methods, and they are especially useful for estimating the accuracy of intra-modality registration methods.

Visual inspection, which provides a qualitative assessment, is the most intuitive method for evaluation of the registration accuracy. This assessment method may involve the inspection of subtraction images, contour overlays, or viewing anatomical landmarks. It has been used widely in both rigid and non-rigid registration assessment, but it may be considered as an informal and insufficient approach.

Researchers have been developing novel and practical validation techniques, for example, Hellier, Barillot, Memin and Perez (2001) proposed a hierarchical estimation method for 3-D registration. The measurement of the consistency of transformations has been proposed to serve as accuracy qualification method by, for example, Holden et al. (2000). Wang, Feng, Yeh, and Huang (2001) proposed a novel automatic method to estimate confidence intervals of the resulting registration parameters and allow the precision of registration results to be objectively assessed for 2-D and 3-D medical images. Fitzpatrick, Hill, and Maurer (2000); Mäkelä, Clarysse, Sipilä, Pauna, Pham, Katila, and Magnin (2002), and Zitová and Flusser (2003) presented good discussions and summaries about performance validation methods for medical image registration.

However, validation of registration accuracy is a difficult task because of the lack of the ground truth. Objective performance validation still remains a challenge in the field of biomedical image registration.

MAJOR BIOMEDICAL IMAGE REGISTRATION METHODOLOGIES

As described previously, the biomedical image registration methods can be divided into intensity-based category and feature-based category.

Intensity-Based Medical Image Registration

Intensity-based medical image registration fully and directly exploits the image raw intensities, and an explicit segmentation of the images is not required. Therefore, this category of registration provides high registration accuracy. Because of little or no user interaction involved in this kind of registration, fully automated registration and quantitative assessment become possible. However, this category of schemes does not make use of knowledge of the organ structure and also the registration computation is not very efficient. The well-established intensity-based similarity measures used in the biomedical image registration area include minimizing the intensity differences, correlation-based techniques, and entropy-based techniques.

Similarity measures by minimizing the intensity differences include the Sum of Squared Differences (SSD) and the Sum of Absolute Differences (SAD), which exhibit a minimum in the case of perfect matching. Although they are efficient to calculate, these methods are sensitive to intesity changes.

$$SSD = \sum_{i}^{N} \left| R(i) - T(S(i) \right|^{2} \qquad (2)$$

$$SAD = \frac{1}{N} \sum_{i}^{N} |R(i) - T(S(i)|$$ (3)

Where $R(i)$ is the intensity value at position i of reference image R and $S(i)$ is the corresponding intensity value in study image S; T is geometric transformation.

Correlation techniques were proposed to aim at multimodal biomedical image registration, for example, Maintz, van den Elsen, and Viergeve (1996). The cross-correlation technique has also been used for rigid motion correction of SPECT cardiac images, for example, Mäkelä et al. (2002). However, because usually the geometric deformations of the image modalities are not likely to be linear, these correlation methods, which require a linear dependence between the intensity of the images, cannot always achieve reliable registration results. The normalized cross correlation is defined as:

$$R = \frac{\sum_{i}(I_R(i)) - \overline{I}_R)(I_S(i) - \overline{I}_S)}{\sqrt{\sum_{i}(I_R(i) - \overline{I}_R)^2}\sqrt{\sum_{i}(I_S(i) - \overline{I}_S)^2}}$$ (4)

Where $I_R(i)$ is the intensity value at position i of reference image R and $I_S(i)$ is the corresponding intensity value in study image S; $\overline{I}_R$ and $\overline{I}_S$ are the mean intensity value of reference and study image respectively.

Information theoretic techniques play an essential role in multimodality medical image registration.

The Shannon entropy is widely used as a measure of information in many branches of engineering. It was originally developed as a part of information theory in the 1940s and describes the average information supplied by a set of symbols $\{x\}$ whose probabilities are given by $\{p(x)\}$.

$$H = -\sum_{x} p(x) \log p(x)$$ (5)

In image registration area, when the images are correctly aligned, the joint histograms have

tight clusters and the joint entropy is minimized. These clusters disperse as the images become less well registered, and correspondingly, the joint entropy is increased. Because minimizing the entropy does not require that the histograms are unimodal, the joint entropy is generally applicable to multimodality registration and obviates the need of segmentation of images.

Mutual information (MI) was first proposed by Collignon et al. (1995) and Viola et al. (1995), and it is a promising and powerful criterion for multimodality medical image registration, for example, Maes, et al. (1997); Roche, Malandain, and Ayache (2000); Thevenaz and Unser (2000); and Likar and Pernus (2001).

Let R be the reference data presented by m samples $\{r_0, r_1, ..., r_{m-1}\}$ with a marginal probability distribution $P_R(r)$. Analogously, the study data S consists of n samples $\{s_0, s_1, ..., s_{n-1}\}$ with a marginal probability distribution $P_S(s)$. The mutual information I of the reference image R and study image S measures the degree of dependence of R and S by measuring distance between the joint distribution $P_{RS}(r,s)$ and the distribution associated to $P_R(r)$ and $P_S(s)$. MI can be defined as:

$$I_{R,S} = \sum_{(r,s)} P_{RS}(r,s) \log(\frac{P_{RS}(r,s)}{P_R(r)P_S(s)})$$ (6)

With $H(R)$ and $H(s)$ being the entropy of R and S, respectively, $H(R,S)$ is their joint entropy.

$$H(R) = -\sum_{r} P_R(r) \log P_R(r)$$ (7)

$$H(S) = -\sum_{s} P_S(s) \log P_S(s)$$ (8)

$$H(R,S) = -\sum_{r,s} P_{RS}(r,s) \log P_{RS}(r,s)$$ (9)

MI is related to entropy by the equation:

$$I_{R,s} = H(R) + H(S) - H(R,S)$$ (10)

Under the assumption that the mutual information of the two images is maximum when the images are in registration, registration can be performed by maximizing the mutual information as a function of a geometric transformation T of the study image S:

$$S_T = T(S) \qquad (11)$$

$$I_{R,S_T} = \sum_{(r,T(s))} P_{R,S_T}(r,T(s)) \ \log(\frac{P_{R_T}(r,T(s))}{P_R(r)P_{S_T}(T(s))}) \qquad (12)$$

$$T_{reg} = \arg\max_T(I_{R,S_T}) \qquad (13)$$

T_{reg} is the transformation that will bring the images into registration.

Mutual information registration does not assume a linear relationship among intensity values of the images to be registered and is one of the few intensity-based measures that are well suited to the multimodality image registration.

Feature-Based Medical Image Registration

In feature-based registration approaches, transformations often can be stated in analytic form, hence efficient computational schemes can be achieved. However, in most of these methods, the preprocess step is needed and the registration results are highly dependent on the result of this preprocess. Because registration algorithms using landmarks often require users to specify corresponding landmarks from the two images manually or semi-automatically, such methods cannot always provide very accurate registration.

The feature-based medical image registration methods can be classified into point-based approaches, for example, Fitzpatrick, West, and Maurer (1998), curve-based algorithms, for example, Maintz et al. (1996), and Subsol (1999), and surface-based methods, for example, Chen, Pellizari, Chen, Cooper, and Levin (1987); Borgefors (1988), and Pellizari, Chen, Spelbring, Weichselbaum, and Chen (1989). Figure 4 illustrates the feature-based registration procedure. Point-based registration involves identifying the corresponding points, matching the points, and inferring the image transformation.

The corresponding points are also called homologous landmarks to emphasize that they should present the same feature in the different images. These points can either be anatomical features or markers attached to the patient, which can be identified in both images modalities. Anatomical landmark based registration methods have the

Figure 4. Feature-based registration procedure

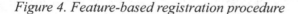
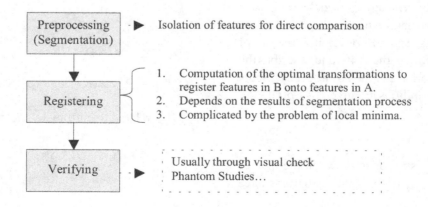

drawback of user interaction being required. Registration algorithms based on extrinsic landmarks which maybe invasive or non-invasive, are comparatively easy to implement, fast, and can be automated, but they may have drawbacks of invasiveness and less accurate results. As a successful example, iterative closest points (ICP) method proposed by Besl and McKay (1992), maybe the most widely used medical image registration approach in medical imaging applications, for example, Fitzpatrick, West, and Maurer (1998).

When points are available, Thin-Plate Splines (TPS) which produce a smoothly interpolated spatial mapping, are often used to determine the transformation for 2-D medical image registration, for example, Bookstein (1989).

Boundaries or surfaces are distinct features in medical image registration due to various segmentation algorithms which can successfully locate such features. Surface-based registration methods can be rigid or deformable.

In rigid surface-based registration methods, the same anatomical structure surfaces are extracted from the images and used as input for the registration procedure. The Head-and-Hat algorithm, proposed by Chen et al. (1987) and Pellizari, Chen, Spelbring, Weichselbaum, and Chen (1989), is one successful surface fitting technique for multimodal image registration. In this method, two equivalent surfaces are identified in the images. The first surface extracted from the higher-resolution images, is represented as a stack of discs, and is referred to as "head". The second surface, referred to as "hat", is represented as a list of unconnected 3D points. The registration is determined by iteratively transforming the hat surface with respect to the head surface, until the closest fit of the hat onto the head is found. Because the segmentation task is comparatively easy, and the computational cost is relatively low, this method remains popular. However, this method is prone to error for convoluted surfaces.

In deformable surface-based registration methods, the extracted surfaces or curves from

one image is elastically deformed to fit the second image. The deformable curves are known as snakes or active contours which help to fit contours or surfaces to image data. Snakes operate by simulating a controllable elastic material, much like a thin, flexible sheet. We can initially position the model by using information from anatomical atlases; then, the model is allowed to relax to a stationary position. This minimum energy position seeks to find the best position to trade off internal and external forces. The internal forces are due to the elastic nature of the material and the external forces stem from sharp boundaries in image intensity. Important deformable surface-based registration approaches include, for example, the elastic matching approach proposed by Bajcsy and Kovacic (1989), and the finite-element model technique proposed by Terzopoulos and Metaxas (1991), and so on. Deformable surface-based registration is suited for intersubject and atlas registration. A drawback of these methods is that a good initial pre-registration is required to achieve a proper convergence.

APPLICATIONS OF BIOMEDICAL IMAGE REGISTRATION

Clinical and Surgical Applications

Biomedical image registration algorithms can combine information from multiple imaging modalities, allowing the evaluation of the progress of disease or treatment from time series of data, and the measurement of dynamic patterns of structural changes, tumor growth, or degenerative disease processes. Biomedical image registration can be used in medical and surgical areas, including diagnostic planning and simulation, treatment monitoring, image-guided surgery, pathology detection, and radiotherapy treatment.

Multimodal image registration methods play a central role in therapeutic systems, for example, Hill et al. (2000), and Lee, Nagano, Duerk, Sodee, and Wilson (2003). By registering the information from different imaging modalities, better and more accurate information can be obtained to aid the therapy planning. For example, the registration of functional images with anatomical images helps early diagnosis and better localization of pathological areas. Also, by quantitative comparison of images taken at different times, the information about evolution over time can be referred, for example, the monitoring of tumor growth in image sequences.

Many surgical procedures require highly precise 3D localization to extract deeply buried targeted tissue while minimizing collateral damage to adjacent structures (Grimson, 1995). Image-guided surgery (Figure 5) emerged to meet this end. In surgical practice, surgeons usually examine 2-D anatomical images (MRI or CT) and then mentally transfer the information to the patient. Thus, there is a clear need for registered visualization technique which allows the surgeons

to directly visualize important structures to guide the surgical procedure.

Biomedical image registration is important for telemedicine, which is the integration of telecommunication technologies, information technologies, human-machine interface technologies, and medical care technologies, when distance separates the participants. In the case of healthcare, a telemedicine system should be able to register multiple sources of patient data, diagnostic images, and integrate other information to enhance healthcare delivery across space and time. For example, biomedical image registration is an important component in teleradiology, which is a primary image-related application.

Biomedical Image Registration for Different Organs

Medical image registration has been applied to the diagnosis of breast cancer, cardiac studies,

Figure 5. Image-guided surgical system

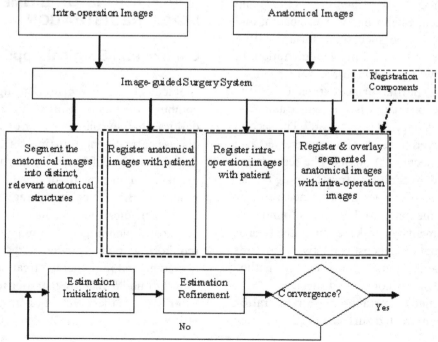

wrist and other injuries, and different neurological disorders including brain tumors, and so on.

Brain image registration is the most intensively studied subject in the biomedical image registration field. Numerous rigid and non-rigid registration algorithms for monomodal and multimodal images have been proposed. Feature-based biomedical image registration includes, for examples, crest-line-based registration (Guéziec and Ayache 1992, etc.), chamfer-matching-based registration (van Herk and Kooy 1994; Xiao and Jackson 1995), head-hat surface matching technique (Pelizzari et al. 1989), and ICP algorithm (Besl and McKay 1992). Intensity-based head image registration algorithms include: minimization of variation ratios (Woods 1993; Hill 1993), correlation-based registration (Collins, Neelin, Peters, and Evans 1994), and mutual information registration (Collignon et al. 1995), and so on. Figure 6 illustrates the main methodologies of brain medical image registration.

The registration of cardiac images from multiple imaging modalities is a preliminary step to combine anatomic and functional information. The integration of the complementary data provides a more comprehensive analysis of the cardiac functions and pathologies, and additional and useful information for physiologic understanding and diagnosis.

Because of the lack of anatomical landmarks and the low image resolution, the cardiac image registration is more complex than brain image registration. The non-rigid and mixed motion of the heart and the thorax structures makes the task even more difficult. Researchers have proposed numerous registration approaches for cardiac images, for example, Mäkelä et al. (2002); McLeish, Hill, Atkinson, Blackall, and Razavi; Pallotta et

Figure 6. Brain image registration

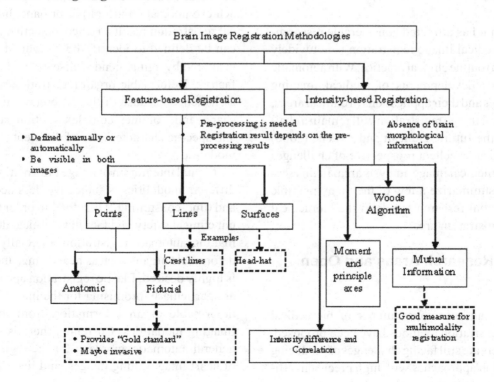

al. (1995); Thirion (1998) published a good review of cardiac image registration methods. However, cardiac image registration remains a challenge because of a number of problems related to the existing registration methods. For example, point-based registration approaches for the heart are not always accurate because of the lack of accurate anatomical landmark points in the cardiac; using heart surfaces can result in better registration of the region of interest, but the registration result is highly dependent on the surfaces selected and the imaging modalities. In intensity-based cardiac image registration, the use of image intensity difference and correlation methods relies on the assumption that intensity values in the registered images are strongly correlated. However, this assumption, especially in multimodal registration, is frequently violated, which would lead to unsatisfactory results.

CHALLENGES AND FUTURE TRENDS

Although it has attracted considerable researchers, biomedical image registration is not widely applied in routine clinical practice. With automatic continuous developments of medical imaging techniques and their applications in clinical areas, biomedical image registration will remain a challenge in the future. Duncan and Ayache (2000) presented an excellent prospective of challenges ahead in medical image analysis area. In this section, we summarize a few of the many possible and potential research trends in the biomedical image registration area.

Active Research Areas and Open Issues

Although an enormous number of biomedical image registration methods have been proposed, researchers are still facing challenges of producing registration approaches with high precision, effi-ciency, and validity, which can be used in clinical practice. Hierarchical biomedical image registration and hybrid biomedical image registration are two registration schemes that have advantages of both increased computation efficiency and the ability to find better solutions.

In the hierarchical registration methods, the images are first registered at coarse, lower-resolution scales, and then the transformation solution obtained at this resolution scale is used as the initial estimation for the registration at a higher-resolution scale. The advantages of the hierarchical biomedical image registration approaches include accelerating computation efficiency and avoiding local minima, and therefore, improving the registration performance (Lester & Addridge, 1999).

The challenges created by inter-subject variations in the organ structures promote researchers to explore the hybrid approaches for biomedical image registration. Hybrid registration approaches, combining the intensity-based algorithms with landmark-based methods and making use of the merits of both these methods, have potential to achieve automatic and high performance biomedical registration results. Hence, objective criteria can be defined to identify how organ structure is altered by aging, gender, disease, and genetic factors. Deformable organ registration remains a challenge because of the differences in organ shape and volume, complex motion sources, and specific characteristics of different imaging modalities.

Mental integration of image information from different modalities is subjective, less accurate, and time-consuming. Therefore, in order to benefit clinical safety and facilitate clinical decision making, automatic registration, especially for the deformable organs such as heart, lung, and liver, is highly desired. Elastic registration approaches are particularly promising for the integration of deformable organ information from multiple imaging modalities. Currently, there is still no general automatic approach for the registration of heart images, lung images, and liver images.

Hybrid methods, combining similarity measures with morphological information may provide possibilities for elastic registration.

The validation of the registration performance is particularly important. Although a wide variety of registration approaches have been proposed, objective validation of these methods is not well established. Image databases may in the future provide a source for the objective comparison of different registration methods.

Future Trends

Precise and efficient biomedical image registration is not only a big challenge, but also provides exciting opportunities to improve the quality and safety of diagnostic and medical decision making, treatment monitoring, and healthcare support. Although the more advanced imaging system, the PET scanner containing a CT scanner, has been developed, there is still a need for multi-dimensional, multimodality image registration techniques to assist the analysis of temporal changes and the integration of necessary information from different imaging modalities. With ever-increasing growth of medical datasets with higher resolution, higher dimensionality, and wider range of scanned areas, the demand for more efficient biomedical image registration will increase.

The applications of multimedia techniques, for example, electronic patient records and medical images, greatly push the advance of telemedicine and e-health. As an important component and technique of telemedicine and e-health, accurate and efficient biomedical image registration will play a more and more important role in remote diagnosis, patient monitoring, teleradiology, and overcoming the barriers of distance in healthcare service.

Although the existing image-based virtual human can provide the healthcare professionals with a quality of anatomical information and knowledge, there is a need to produce virtual humans with both anatomical and functional information and knowledge. Hence, whole-body multimodality image registration needs further efforts to support the virtual human projects which are essential in surgery simulation and virtual and augmented reality in medicine.

As an active research area, biomedical image registration will continue attracting researchers to develop automatic, non-rigid registration methods, which will facilitate clinical decision making, treatment monitoring, and surgical planning. The research of biomedical image registration will greatly promote the development and advance of medical imaging techniques, patient care service, and medical education. The multimodality biomedical image registration will be more and more important in medical diagnosis, surgery planning as well as intraoperative navigation, and in the future, biomedical image registration will play a more essential role in helping people to discover the mysteries of the human body and its complicated functions.

CONCLUSION

Biomedical image registration of different medical images, which aims to extract and combine the complementary and useful information and knowledge provided by the individual images, is an important step to a more comprehensive and accurate analysis of the organ functions and pathologies. Biomedical image registration has been extensively investigated and numerous methodologies have been proposed in this area.

Monomodality image registration is essential for follow-up treatment and disease monitoring, while multimodality image registration provides complementary and additional information for diagnosis, surgical planning, and treatment assessment. Rigid registration is often used to correct translation and rotation displacement, but it is not sufficient for correcting the complex, non-linear distortions, which may result from factors such as differences between the imaging modalities, the temporal displacements due to disease progression and surgical intervention, and individual variations. Non-rigid biomedical image registration remains an active and challenging area for both brain and other deformable organs.

As an important issue of clinical knowledge management, biomedical image registration is helpful in preparing medical data to be more useful for diagnostic and clinical decision making, treatment monitoring, and healthcare supporting, and it provides critical solutions in some cases for achieving better and more efficient healthcare.

ACKNOWLEDGMENT

This work is supported by the ARC, UGC, HLJNSF and HLJE grants.

REFERENCES

Ackerman, M.J., Yoo, T., & Jenkins, D. (2001). From data to knowledge: The visible human project continues. *Medinfo, 10*(2), 887-890.

Alpert, N.M., Bradshaw, J.F., Kennedy, D. & Correia, J.A. (1990). The principal axes transformation: A method for image registration. *Journal of Nuclear Medicine, 31*, 1717-1722.

Audette, M., Ferrie, F. & Peters, T. (2000). An algorithm overview of surface registration techniques for medical imaging. *Medical Image Analysis, 4*(4), 201-217.

Bajcsy, R. & Kovacic, S. (1989). Multiresolution elastic matching. *Computer Vision, Graphics, and Image Processing, 46*, 1-21.

Bankman, I. (2000). *Handbook of medical imaging: Processing and analysis*. Academic Press.

Besl, P.J. & MaKey, N.D. (1992). A method for registration of 3-D shapes. *IEEE Transactions on Pattern Analysis and Machine Intelligence, 14*(2), 239-256.

Bookstein, F. L. (1989). Principal warps: Thin-plate splines and the decomposition of deformations. *IEEE Transactions on Pattern Analysis and Machine Intelligence, 11*(6), 567-585.

Borgefors, G. (1988). Hierarchical chamfer matching: A parametric edge matching algorithm. *IEEE Transactions on Pattern Analysis and Machine Intelligence, 10*, 849-865.

Brown, L.G. (1992). A survey of image registration techniques. *ACM Computing Surveys 24*(4), 325-376.

Chen, C., Pellizari, C.A., Chen, G.T.Y., Cooper, M.D. & Levin, D.N. (1987). Image analysis of PET data with the aid of CT and MR images. *Information Processing in Medical Imaging*, 601-611.

Christensen, G.E., Kane, A.A., Marsh, J.L. & Vannier, M.W. (1996). Synthesis of an individual cranial atlas with dysmorphic shape. *Mathematical methods in biomedical image analysis* (pp. 309-318). Los Alamitos, CA: IEEE Computer Society Press.

Collignon, A., Vandermeulen, D., Suetens, P. & Marchal, G. (1995). 3D multi-modality image registration using feature space clustering. In N. Ayche (Ed.), *Computer Vision, Virtual Reality, and Robotic Mechine, 905, of Lecture Notes in Computer Science* (pp. 195-204). Berlin: Springer-Verlag.

Collins, D.L., Neelin, P., Peters, T.M. & Evans, A.C. (1994). Automatic 3D intersubject registration of MR volumetric data in standardized Talairach space. *Journal of Computer Assisted Tomography, 18*(2), 192-205.

Davatzikos, C.A., Prince, J.L. & Bryan, R.N. (1996). Image registration based on boundary mapping. *IEEE Transactions on Medical Imaging, 15*, 112-115.

Dey, D., Slomka, P.J., Hahn, L.J., & Kloiber, R. (1999). Automatic three-dimensional multimodality registration using radionuclide transmission

CT attenuation maps: A phantom study. *Journal of Nuclear Medicine, 40*(3), 448-455.

Duncan, J.S. & Ayache, N. (2000). Medical image analysis: Progress over two decades and the challenges ahead. *IEEE Transactions on Pattern and Machine Intelligence, 22*(1), 58-106.

Fitzpatrick, J.M. (2001). Detecting failure, assessing success. In J.V. Hajnal, D.L.G. Hill & D.J.E. Hawkes (Eds.), *Medical image registration* (pp. 117-139). CRC Press.

Fitzpatrick, J.M., Hill, D.L.G. & Maurer, C.R. (2000). *Handbook of medical imaging.* Bellingham, WA: SPIE Press.

Fitzpatrick, J.M., West, J. B. & Maurer, C. R. (1998). Predicting error in rigid-body point-based registration. *IEEE Transactions on Medical Imaging, 17*, 694-702.

Grimson, W.E.L. (1995). Medical applications of image understanding. *IEEE Expert, 10*(5), 18-28.

Guéziec, A. & Ayache, N. (1992). Smoothing and matching of 3-D space curves. In R.A. Robb (Ed.), *Visualization in biomedical computing,* 1808, Proc. SPIE (pp. 259-273). Bellingham, WA: SPIE PRESS.

Hajnal, J., Saeed, N., Soar, E., Oatridge, A., Young, I. & Bydder, G. (1995). Detection of subtle brain changes using subvoxel registration and subtraction of serial MR images. *Journal of Computer Assisted Tomography, 19*(5) , 677-691.

Handels, H. (2003). Medical image processing: New perspectives in computer supported diagnostics, computer aided surgery and medical education and training. *Year Book of Medical Informatics*, 503-505.

Hellier, P., Barillot, C., Memin, E. & Perez, P. (2001). Hierarchical estimation of a dense deformation field for 3-D robust registration. *IEEE Transactions on Medical Imaging, 20,* 388-402.

Hill, D. L. G., Batchelor, P. G., Holden, M. H. & Hawkes, D. J. (2001). Medical image registration. *Physics in Medicine and Biology, 46*(1), 1-45.

Hill, D. L. G., Hawkes, D. J., Harrison, N. A. & Ruff, C.F. (1993). A strategy for automated multimodality image registration incorporating anatomical knowledge and imager characteristics. In H.H. Barrett & A.F. Gmitro (Eds.), *Lecture Notes in Computer Science. Proceedings of the 13th International Conference on Information Processing in Medical Imaging* (pp. 182-196). New York: Springer-Verlag.

Hill, D. L. G., Smith, A.D., Mauerer, C.R., Cox, T.C.S., Elwes, R., Brammer, M.J., Hawkes, D.J. & Polkey, C.E. (2000). Sources of error in comparing functional magnetic resonance imaging and invasive electrophysiology recordings. *Journal of Neurosurgery, 93*, 214-223.

Holden, M., Hill, D.L.G., Denton, E.R.E., Jarosz, J.M., Cox, T.C.S., Rohlfing, T., Goodey, J. & Hawkes, D.J. (2000). Voxel similarity measures for 3D serial MR image registration. *IEEE Transactions on Medical Imaging, 19*, 94-102.

Lee, Z., Nagano, K.K., Duerk, J.L., Sodee, D.B. & Wilson, D.L. (2003). Automatic registration of MR and SPECT images for treatment planning in prostate cancer. *Academic Radiology, 10*, 673-684.

Lehmann, T.M., Gönner, C. & Spitzer, K. (1999). Survey: Interpolation methods in medical image processing. *IEEE Transactions on Medical Imaging, 18*(11), 1049-1075.

Lester, H. & Arridge, S.R. (1999). A survey of hierarchical non-linear medical image registration. *Patter Recognition, 32*, 129-149.

Likar, B. & Pernus, F. (2001). A hierarchical approach to elastic registration based on mutual information. *Image and Vision Computing, 19*, 33-44.

Lin, K. P., Huang, S. C., Baxter, L. & Phelp, M.E. (1994). A general technique for interstudy registration of multifunction and multimodality images. *IEEE Transactions on Nuclear Science, 41*, 2850-2855.

Maes, F., Collignon, A., Vandermeulen, D., Marchal, G. & Suetens, P. (1997). Multimodality image registration by maximisation of mutual information. *IEEE Transaction on Medical Imaging, 6*(2), 187-198.

Maes, F., Vandermeulen, D. & Suetens, P. (1999). Comparative evaluation of multiresolution optimisation strategies for multimodality image registration by maximisation of mutual information. *Medical Image Analysis, 3*(4), 373-386.

Mäkelä, T., Clarysse, P., Sipilä, O., Pauna, N., Pham, Q.C., Katila, T. & Magnin, I.E. (2002). A review of cardiac image registration methods. *IEEE Transaction on Medical Imaging, 21*(9), 1011-1021.

Maintz, J.B.A. & Viergever, M.A. (1998). A survey of medical image registration. *Medical Image Analysis, 2*(1), 1-36.

Maintz, J.B.A., van den Elsen, P.A. & Viergever, M.A. (1996). Evaluation of ridge seeking operators for multimodality medical image registration. *IEEE Transactions on Pattern Analysis and Machine Intelligence, 18*(4), 353-365.

Maurer, C. R. & Fitzpatrick, J. M. (1993). A review of medical image registration. In R.J. Maciunas (Ed.), *Interactive image guided neurosurgery* (pp. 17-44). Parkridge, IL: American Association of Neurological Surgeons.

McLeish, K., Hill, D.J.G., Atkinson, D., Blackall, J.M. & Razavi, Reza. (2002). A study of motion and deformation of the heart due to respiration. *IEEE Transactions on Medical Imaging, 21*(9), 1142-1150.

Nelder, J. & Mead, R.A. (1965). A simplex method for function minimization. *Computer Journal, 17*, 308-313.

Pallotta, S., Gilardi, M.C., Bettinardi, V., Rizzo, G., Landoni, C., Striano, G., Masi, R., & Fazio, F. (1995). Application of a surface matching image registration technique to the correlation of cardiac studies in positron emission tomography by transmission images. *Physics in Medicine and Biology, 40*, 1695-1708.

Pellizari, C.A., Chen, G.T.Y., Spelbring, D.R., Weichselbaum, R.R. & Chen, C.T. (1989). Accurate three-dimensional registration of CT, PET, and/or MR images of the brain. *Computer Assisted Tomography, 13*(1), 20-26.

Penny, G.P., Weese, J., Little, J.A., Desmedt, P., Hill, D.L.G. & Hawkes, D.J. (1998). A comparison of similarity measures for use in 2D-3D medical image registration. *IEEE Transactions on Medical Imaging, 17*, 586-595.

Pluim, J.P.W., Maintz, J.B.A. & Viergever, M.A. (2001). Mutual information matching in multiresolution contexts. *Image and Vision Computing, 19*(1-2), 45-52.

Powell, M.J.D. (1964). An efficient method for finding the minimum of a function of several variables without calculating derivatives. *Computuer Journal, 7*, 155-163.

Riva, G. (2003). Review paper: Medical applications of virtual environments. *Year Book of Medical Informatics*, 159-169.

Roche, A., Malandain, G. & Ayache, N. (2000). Unifying maximum likelihood approaches in medical image registration. *International Journal of Imaging Systems and Technology, 11*, 71-80.

Rohlfing, T. & Maurer, C.C. (2003). Nonrigid image registration in shared-memory multiprocessor environments with application to brains, breasts, and bees. *IEEE Transactions on Information Technology in Biomedicine, 7*(1), 16-25.

Rohr, K. (2000). Elastic registration of multimodal medical images: A survey. *Auszug aus: Kunstliche Intelligenz, Heft.*

Subsol, G. (1999). Crest lines for curve-based warping. *Brain Warping* (pp. 241-262). San Diego: Academic.

Subsol, G., Thirion, J.-P. & Ayache, N. (1998). A scheme for automatically building three-dimensional morphometric anatomical atlases: application to a skull atlas. *Medical Image Analysis, 2*(1), 37-60.

Terzopoulos, D. & Metaxas, D. (1991). Dynamic 3D models with local and global deformations: Deformable superquadrics. *IEEE Trans. PAMI, 13*(7), 703-714.

Thévenaz P., Blu, T. & Unser, M. (2000). Image interpolation and resampling. In I. Bankman (Ed.), *Handbook of medical imaging: Processing and analysis* (pp. 393-418). Academic Press.

Thévenaz, P. & Unser, M. (2000). Optimization of mutual information for multiresolution registration. *IEEE Transaction on Image Processing, 9*(12), 2083-2099.

Thirion, J.P. (1998). Image matching as a diffusion process: An analogy with Maxwell's demons. *Med. Image Anal., 2*, 243-260.

Thompson, P. & Toga, A.W. (1996). A surface-based technique for warping three-dimensional images of the brain. *IEEE Transaction on Medical Imaging, 15*(4), 402-417.

Turner, R. & Ordidge, R.J. (2000). Technical challenges of functional magnetic resonance imaging: The biophysics and technology behind a reliable neuroscientific tool for mapping the human brain. *IEEE Engineering in Medicine and Biology*, 42-54.

van den Elsen, P.A., Pol, E.J.D. & Viergever, M.A. (1993). Medical image matching—A review with classification. *IEEE Engineering in Medicine and Biology, 12*, 26-39.

van Herk, M. & Kooy, H.M. (1994). Automatic three-dimensional correlation of CT-CT, CT-MRI, and CT-SPECT using chamfer matching. *Medical Physics, 21*(7), 1163-1177.

Viola, P. & Wells, W.M. (1995). Alignment by maximization of mutual information. *The Fifth International Conference on Computer Vision* (pp. 16-23).

Wang, H.S., Feng, D., Yeh, E. & Huang, S. C. (2001). Objective assessment of image registration results using statistical confidence intervals. *IEEE Transactions on Nuclear Science, 48*, 106-110.

Wang, X. & Feng, D. (to be published in Vol.3, 2005). Automatic elastic medical image registration based on image intensity. *International Journal of Image and Graphic (IJIG)*, World Scientific.

Xiao, H. & Jackson, I.T. (1995). Surface matching: Application in poat-surgical/post-treatment evaluation. In H.U. Lemke, K. Inamura, C.C. Jaffe & M.W. Vannier (Eds.), *Computer assisted radiology* (pp. 804-811). Berlin: Springer-Verlag.

Zitová, B. & Flusser, J. (2003). Image registration methods: A survey. *Image and Vision Computing, 21*, 977-1000.

This work was previously published in Clinical Knowledge Management: Opportunities and Challenges, edited by B. Bali, pp. 159-181, copyright 2005 by IGI Publishing, formerly known as Idea Group Publishing (an imprint of IGI Global).

Chapter XVIII
A Software Tool for Reading DICOM Directory Files

Ricardo Villegas
Universidad de Carabobo, Venezuela

Guillermo Montilla
Universidad de Carabobo, Venezuela

Hyxia Villegas
Universidad de Carabobo, Venezuela

ABSTRACT

DICOMDIR directory files are useful in medical software applications because they allow organized access to images and information sets that come from radiological studies that are stored in conformance with the digital imaging and communication in medicine (DICOM) standard. During the medical application software development, specialized programming libraries are commonly used in order to solve the requirements of computation and scientific visualization. However, these libraries do not provide suitable tools for reading DICOMDIR files, making necessary the implementation of a flexible tool for reading these files, which can be also easily integrated into applications under development. To solve this problem, this work introduces an object-oriented design and an open-source implementation for such reading tool. It produces an output data tree containing the information of the DICOM images and their related radiological studies, which can be browsed easily in a structured way through navigation interfaces coupled to it.

INTRODUCTION

The digital imaging and communications in medicine (DICOM) standard (National Electrical Manufacturers Association (NEMA0, 2004a; Revet, 1997) was published in 1993. Its main goal was to establish norms for handling, storing, and interchanging medical images and associated digi-

tal information within open systems. Also it was to facilitate the interoperability among acquisition equipments and other medical devices, as well as their integration within specialized information systems in the medical and health care area.

Since then, the appearance and use of computer-assisted medical applications have increased, as a result of the accelerated technological development and the standardization process of medical information representation and handling, which generated a greater demand of development tools for those applications.

These applications range from health care information systems and picture archiving and communication systems (PACS) () solutions, to technological support systems for medical procedures, such as image-based diagnosis and surgical planning, which previously depended on the knowledge and expertise of the physicians.

In such applications, the handling of images coming from different acquisition modalities is essential. These images generated from radiological studies and stored according to the specifications of parts 10, 11 and 12 of the DICOM standard (NEMA, 2004e, f,& g) must be retrieved from storage media as a bidimensional display or in tridimensional reconstructions and other special processes, such as fusion and segmentation of images. The use of DICOMDIR directory files is almost mandatory for searching, accessing, and browsing medical images because they index the files belonging to the patient on whom the studies were performed, thus making it easier to access to those images and their associated medical information.

During the medical application software development, the use of programming interfaces (APIs) or class libraries is frequent in order to solve the computation and visualization needs, as well as for providing DICOM support to the applications. In that sense, there exist numerous public domain applications that can be used by radiologists and other specialists for reading and displaying DICOM images files and even for reading DICOMDIR index files, which cannot be integrated into applications under development because of their proprietary code.

Companies, such as Lead Technologies, ETIAM, Merge, Laurel Bridge, and DeJarnette, have commercial software development kits (SDKs) that provide complete implementations of the DICOM standard, but the acquisition costs for these SDKs are high. Open-source libraries are an alternative choice for integrating DICOM support into applications. Regarding this matter, libraries, such as visualization tool kit (VTK) (), insight segmentation and registration tool kit (ITK), DICOM tool kit (DCMTK), and virtual vision machine (VVM), allow the reading of DICOM images, but they do not provide mechanisms for reading DICOMDIR files. Like in the DCMTK case, there are other libraries that provide tools for a basic and low-level access to the information contained in the files. However, they have disadvantages, such as troublesome information retrieving process and reading tools, which are difficult to integrate into the applications.

Due to the lack of an adequate tool for reading and handling DICOMDIR files in a structured and simple way, which could be also easily coupled to browsing interfaces and attached to medical application under development, we introduce in this article the design and implementation of a DICOMDIR files reader. This tool has been successfully integrated into an application for neurosurgery preoperative planning (Montilla, Bosnjak, Jara, & Villegas, 2005), but it also can be attached to any other software under development that requires the handling of DICOM images and DICOMDIR directory files.

The next sections include the revision of related works, the essential theoretical background that frames this work within the DICOM standard context; the description of the methodology used for the implementation of the tool; and, finally, the discussion and conclusions obtained from the integration and test of the implemented reader into a medical application.

ANTECEDENTS AND RELATED WORKS

The creation of the American College of Radiology (ACR)-NEMA committee in 1983 was the product of earlier attempts by the American College of Radiology (ACR) and the National Electrical Manufacturers Association (NEMA) to establish a normative for exchanging, transmitting, and storing medical images and their associated information. The version 1.0 of the standard was published by this joint committee in 1985, under the document ACR-NEMA No. 300-1985, followed in 1988 by the document ACR-NEMA No. 300-1988 of version 2.0. Previous to these normatives, medical images were stored in files by the acquisition devices under their own proprietary formats and transferred through point-to-point communication or by removable storage media. Versions 1.0 and 2.0 established a standardized terminology and information structure, as well as hardware interfaces, software commands sets, and consistent data formats.

The most recent version, known as DICOM 3.0 (NEMA, 2004a) was published in 1993, and it was structured in parts, or documents, to facilitate its support and extension. In the last version, objects for the representation of patients, studies, reports, and other data sets were added, as well as unique identifiers for these objects, enabling the transmission of information through communication networks using the TCP/IP protocol. The DICOM 3.0 standard facilitates the transfer of images and related information within open systems containing different medical equipments and the integration with medical information systems and applications.

DICOM parts 3, 6, 10, and 12 (NEMA, 2004b, d, 4e, & g) were of particular interest for our tool design. They define and describe the DICOMDIR directory object and other information objects; attributes and representation values of DICOM information model entities; and specifications for files formats and information storage in physical media.

We have not found formal research papers related to the design and implementation of open-source tools for reading DICOMDIR files and their integration within medical applications. Nevertheless, there exist documented development libraries that include support for this kind of file. On the other hand, regarding the complexity of searching and decoding information contained in DICOM files and the fact that the tool had to be integrated into a medical application developed with C++ language, we decided to search for open-source development libraries, based upon C++ and with DICOM support in order to use them as a base for the tool development.

Just a few development libraries, besides the expensive commercial ones, enable the reading and analysis of DICOMDIR files. Due to their structures or features only three open-source libraries, based upon C++ language, were deemed appropriate to be used as reference for the tool design and implementation; the remaining APIs were found either to have a complicated structure or were based upon Java language.

GDCM (GDCM, 2005) is an API supported by Centre de Recherche et d'Applications en Traitement de l'Image et du Signal (CREATIS), which provides a fairly complete support for reading DICOMDIR files and a simple access to the information extracted from them. However, it implements only part 5 of the DICOM standard; therefore, it would be of little use as a base library for medical applications that require the implementation of other features defined by the standard.

Dicomlib library (DicomLib, 2005) provides a fuller implementation of the DICOM standard, and it also features the reading of DICOMDIR files. Although this library tries to ease the huge intrinsic complexity in the use of the DICOM standard, its access and presentation of the DICOMDIR compiled information is not the best one to be integrated into the applications.

Finally, DICOM tool kit (DCMTK) (DC-MTK, 2005) from Oldenburger Forschungs und Entwicklungsinstitut für Informatik-Werkzeuge und Systeme (OFFIS) is another complete library, having several years of evolution and continous use in medical applications development. Although DCMTK provides support for the creation, modification, and opening of DICOMDIR files, it does not offer structured and simple access to the information gathered from the files. However, we selected DCMTK as the base library for the reader development due to its robustness, flexibility, and ability to handle of DICOM images.

Thus, starting from the basic functions for information searches and decoding that provides DCMTK, it was possible to develop the tool for reading the information contained in DICOMDIR files and attach this tool to medical applications that require organized access to DICOM image sets from medical studies.

THEORETICAL BACKGROUND.

A lot has been written about the DICOM standard ever since it was published, including revisions and extensions. The scope of DICOM is so wide that the researcher certainly gets overwhelmed by the amount and complexity of the information contained in the standard documents. In our case, as in any other case of software development that involves the handling of information within the

DICOM scope, the revision of basic fundamentals for real-world information representation according to the DICOM standard was necessary.

Within DICOM's structure, the term "information" refers to medical images coming from different acquisition modalities, signals, curves, look-up tables, and structured reports, as well as to other information gathered during patient visits to the healthcare specialist and the studies derived from them. This information and its generating agents are represented by the standard through models.

DICOM Application and Information Models

DICOM structures and organizes medical data and information through models that emulate the real-world hypothetical situation, where a patient visits a health care specialist, who later orders a set of radiological studies as shown in Figure 1.

An application model is defined as an entity/relationship diagram (see Figure 2) that relates real-world objects inside the standard scope. Its diagram derives from the way hospitals' radiol-

Figure 1. Correspondence between the radiological exam environment and the DICOM Information Model

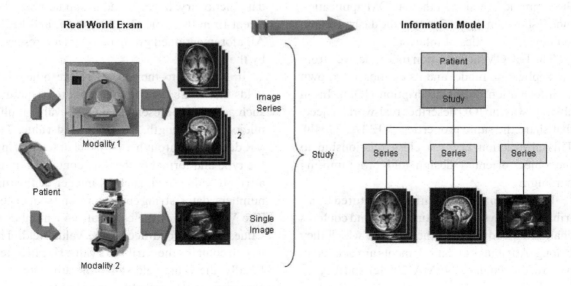

Figure 2. Simplified DICOM application model showing information entities and relationships among them

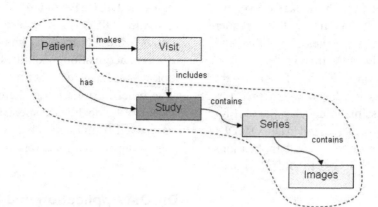

ogy departments handle images from one or more acquisition modalities. Those images are ordered in a series, according to some spatial or temporal relationship, and then stored in a folder for each patient.

Although the application model contains entities for representing several DICOM objects, such as exams results, medical reports, and study procedures, in this work only the patient, study, series, and image entities were considered because they are directly associated to data contained within the images. This consideration produces the simplified version of the DICOM application model shown in Figure 2, where the dashed region contains the entities of interest.

The DICOM information model derives from the application model and its entities are known as information object description (IOD). In an abstract way, an IOD describes real-world objects that share the same properties (NEMA, 2004b). This abstraction keeps a close relationship to the object-oriented design and programming paradigm.

Information model entities are featured by attributes whose types, multiplicities, and contents change depending upon the entity to which they belong. Attributes or data elements are defined in part 5 of the standard (NEMA, 2004c), and they are

cataloged in part 6 of the data dictionary (NEMA, 2004d). An attribute is classified according to its presence in obligatory (types 1 and 2), conditional (types 1C and 2C), and optional (type 3).

Attributes are identified in the data dictionary through a tag composed from an ordered 16-bit number duple (*gggg,eeee*) expressed in hexadecimal form. These numbers represent the group and the element number within that group. The standard attributes have an even group number, different from 0000, 0002, 0004, and 0006, whereas private attributes, not contained in the data dictionary, have an odd group number, different from 0001, 0003, 0005, 0007, and FFFF. All aforementioned group numbers are reserved by the standard.

In addition to the tag, there are other data fields that also belong to the attributes structure, such as value representation (VR), value multiplicity (VM), length, and contained value. The VR describes, through a 2-byte character string, the type and format of the data contained in the attribute value field, such as integer or floating numbers, dates, string characters, and sequences. The VM specifies the cardinality or number of values that are codified in the value field. The length contains the attribute's value size in bytes. Finally, the value field stores the attribute data, according to its respective presence type.

For each IOD there are defined operation sets and named services that are executed on the information objects. When an entity needs to perform an operation over an IOD, it must request the proper service to another entity, which behaves as a server. Each object-defined service establishes a service-object pair (SOP), and the whole service set that is applicable to a particular IOD is a named SOP class.

The *media storage service class* and the *queryrRetrieve service class* are examples of SOP classes. The first one comprises the M-READ, M-WRITE, and M-DELETE services set, applied to the reading, writing, and deleting of files with image IODs coming from acquisition modalities. The second class groups the C-FIND, C-MOVE, and C-GET services that can be requested for querying and transferring information from IODs associated with different entities.

An SOP instance is the occurrence of an IOD that is operated within a communication context, through a specific service set. For example, DICOMDIR directory files are SOP products from requesting the information writing service from a directory IOD to a physical storage media.

The simplified model from our research considers only four entities and their corresponding IODs. The patient entity contains data of the patient for whom radiological studies were performed as described by the study entity. The series entity models information resulting from radiological studies, such as images or signals, and keeps some kind of spatial or temporal relationship among them. The image entity represents the images coming from some of the existing acquisition modalities, for example, computed tomography (CT), magnetic image resonance (MRI), or ultra sound (US).

DICOM File Format

The DICOM file format, described in part 10 of the standard (NEMA, 2004e), defines the way data representing a SOP instance is stored in a physical storage media. The data is encapsulated as a stream of bytes, preceded by a header with metainformation required for identifying the SOP instance and class.

The header has an organized sequence of components, named file ID, which organizes files hierarchically. An ID has up to eight components, where each one is a string of one to eight characters separated by backslashes. The file ID generally corresponds to a directory path and to a filename, for example, SUBDIR1\SUBDIR2\SUBDIR3\ABCDEFGH.

Located after the header is the data set associated with the information model entity that is stored in the file. Depending upon the entity nature, this stream of bytes could represent some of the following objects: images, curves, signals, overlay annotations, lookup tables for transforming images pixel values according to acquisition modalities or values of interest, presentation images descriptions, structure reports, or raw data.

Within the context and scope of our research, we considered only DICOM files containing images associated with studies performed on patients. Therefore, the stored data describes the image plane and the pixels features, as well as values for mapping the image to color or gray scales, overlay planes, and other specific features.

DICOM files are gathered in collections sharing a common name space, such as storage volumes or directory trees, and having unique file identifiers within it. The file collection is an abstraction of a container where files can be created or read. Each collection must be accompanied by an index file with a DICOMDIR identifier, corresponding to a DICOM directory object instance. Part 12 of the standard (NEMA, 2004g) describes the way the DICOM file information is encoded inside the physical storage media. It depends upon the file system used by the computer system for the files creation and interchange, as well as the physical media used for it.

DICOMDIR File Format

The DICOM standard defines a special object class as a named basic directory object, whose purpose is to serve as an organizing index for DICOM files stored in a physical media. The instance of a DICOM directory class object is a file with a unique filename and ID named DICOMDIR. The formal definition of the DICOMDIR object and its content are in part 3 annex F of the DICOM standard (NEMA, 2004b), whereas its structure complies with the DICOM files format specified in section 7 of part 10 (NEMA, 2004e).

There are registers in the DICOMDIR file with the information associated to objects stored in a DICOM files set, and it does not make reference to files that do not belong to the set. Each register contains a field identifying the represented

information type, such as patient, study, series, and image, besides a group of specific fields with attributes extracted from the stored SOP instance. The registers are hierarchically sorted, and they are linked among themselves in the same hierarchy level and to the next lower level in the hierarchy (Figure 3).

The preceding information is generally present in the file, such as indicated in the standard, but some data fields can be optional, such as those related to the complementary information of the patient (birth date, sex, and age) and the studies (referring physician, institution, protocols, and diagnoses), as well as image descriptive information, for example, dimensions, samples by pixel, photometric interpretation, and gray-level window.

Figure 3. Structure of a DICOMDIR file and its representation in a physical storage media

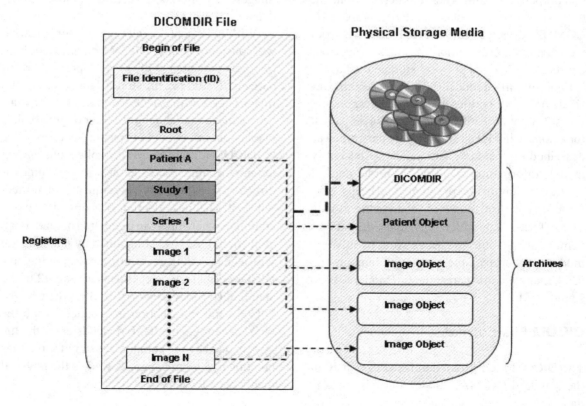

There should be a unique DICOMDIR file for each DICOM files set contained in a storage media. The DICOMDIR file location is related to the storage media directory organization, and it is commonly found at the root directory. DICOM-DIR files help to make fast queries and searches throughout media contained images, without the need for reading whole file sets. Otherwise, searching and browsing images and information within file sets becomes an intensive, tedious, and difficult task.

DICOMDIR FILE READER IMPLEMENTATION

Description

The implemented tool enables DICOMDIR files to be opened in order to obtain the most relevant information from the DICOM-file collection they index. This information is organized in a hierarchical data structure, which can be easily

consulted, and when coupled to a suitable graphic interface, permits the interactive browsing of the information related to the collection. The implementation was made using C++ language, based upon an object-oriented design that allows new DICOM data fields to be added to the reader. Some DCMTK library classes and methods (DCMTK, 2005) were used to facilitate the searching and decoding of the data contained within DICOM-DIR files, thus avoiding the inherent complexity in the handling of the information stored under DICOM standard specifications.

Data Structures

The references to SOP instances contained in DICOMDIR files are linked according to the entities' hierarchy of PATIENT-STUDY-SERIES-IMAGE, which is implicitly established in the DICOM information model, thus establishing a natural correspondence between the hierarchy and a tree data structure. This tree has heterogeneous content nodes that correspond to the DICOM

Figure 4. Structure of the data tree structure built by the reading tool

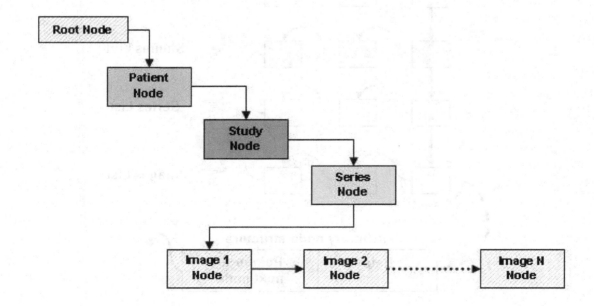

simplified application model (Figure 2), so there are five node types: root, patient, study, series, and image. The entities' relationship cardinality sets the offspring multiplicity, that is, a patient could be object from several studies, whereas each one of them could have several image series.

During the reading of a directory file, all of the file's hierarchical links are traveled, and the related collection file information is gathered for filling the nodes' specific fields, thus building the data tree structure. At the end of the reading process, the tree has the relevant collection information, having a structure similar to that shown in Figure 4. This data structure could be browsed in order to consult the information without the need of accessing the whole file set again.An approach was considered for the tree structure implementation where the nodes behave simultaneously as structural elements and data containers. In this way, the nodes establish the tree hierarchical structure and each one of them also stores the information associated to the corresponding entity. Hierarchy levels are made up of linked node lists, and each one of these lists have a children's list, corresponding to elements from the next lower hierarchy level (Figure 5). This approach facilitates the travelling of the tree and its coupling to browsing interfaces.

A class hierarchy was defined for enabling the nodes polymorphic handling through virtual methods. In this hierarchy, the base class, DICOMDIRNode, defines the basic structure for the other nodes, as well as the virtual methods for accessing and travelling the tree. All subclasses deriving from it, that is, DICOMDIRRootNode, DICOMDIRPatientNode, DICOMDIRStudyN-

Figure 5. Data tree implementation using linked node lists as data containers

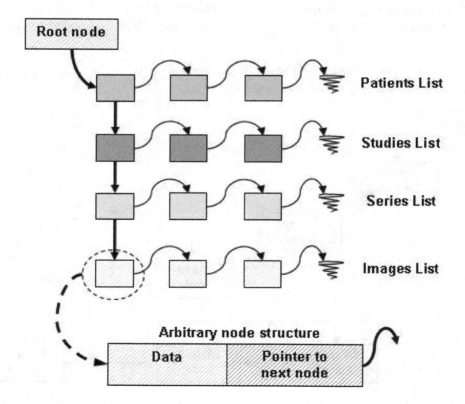

ode, DICOMDIRSeriesNode, and DICOMDIR-ImageNode, redefine their contents and behavior according to the corresponding DICOM application model entity to which they belong.

Collected DICOM Data Fields

DICOM files contain rather large data-element groups that are cataloged in the DICOM data dictionary (NEMA, 2004d). However, not all of these elements are useful in the scope of software applications that handle medical images, and for that reason, a selection of relevant elements was made in order to limit the number of data fields gathered during the DICOMDIR files reading process. Table 1 shows the collected data fields with their tags, value representations, multiplicities, presence attributes, and corresponding DCMTK classes and C++ standard types.

Algorithm 1.

```
Open DICOMDIR file for reading
Assign DICOMDIR file root register to NODE variable
With NODE, do recursively    /* Begin of recursive block */
{
        Assign NODE first child to Next_Register variable
        While (Next_Register <> NULL)
        {
                Select according to Next_Register type
                {
                Case PATIENT:
                        Get patient node related information
                        Create a new DICOMDIR_PatientNode node object
                        Fill node members with gathered information
                        Insert node in the data tree
                        Assign Next_Register to NODE
                        Call recursive block with new NODE value
                        Complete missing patient information extracted from related image file
                Case STUDY:
                        Get study node related information
                        Create a new DICOMDIR_StudyNode node object
                        Fill node members with gathered information
                        Insert node in the data tree
                        Assign Next_Register to NODE
                        Call recursive block with new NODE value
                        Complete missing study information extracted from related image file
                Case SERIES:
                        Get series node related information
                        Create a new DICOMDIR_SerieNode node object
                        Fill node members with gathered information
                        Insert node in the data tree
                        Assign Next_Register to NODE
                        Call recursive block with new NODE value
                        Complete missing series information extracted from related image file
                Case IMAGE:
                        Get image node related information
                        Create a new DICOMDIR_ImageNode node object
                        Fill node members with gathered information
                        Insert node in the data tree
                        Assign Next_Register to NODE
                        Call recursive block with new NODE value
                }
                Assign NODE next child to Next_Register
        }
}           /* End of recursive block */
```

Table 1. DICOM attributes compiled during DICOMDIR file reading process. Attributes are grouped by node type, showing main DICOM data fields and corresponding DCMTK/ C++ data types for each one of them (source: NEMA, 2004d)

Node type	Tag	Field name	VR	VM	Presence	DCMTK data type	C++ data type
PATIENT	(0010,0010)	Patient name	PN	1	Obligatory	DcmPersonName	char[ ]
	(0010,0020)	Patient ID	LO	1	Obligatory	DcmLongString	char[ ]
	(0010,0030)	Birth date	DA	1	Optional	DcmDate	char[ ]
	(0010,0040)	Sex	CS	1	Optional	DcmCodeString	char[ ]
	(0010,1010)	Age	AS	1	Optional	DcmAgeString	char[ ]
STUDY	(0020,0010)	Study ID	SH	1	Obligatory	DcmShortString	char[ ]
	(0008,0020)	Study date	DA	1	Obligatory	DcmDate	char[ ]
	(0008,0030)	Study time	TM	1	Obligatory	DcmTime	char[ ]
	(0008,1030)	Description	LO	1	Obligatory	DcmLongString	char[ ]
	(0018,1030)	Protocol name	LO	1	Optional	DcmLongString	char[ ]
	(0008,0090)	Referring physician	PN	1	Optional	DcmPersonName	char[ ]
	(0008,0080)	Institution	LO	1	Optional	DcmLongString	char[ ]
	(0008,1080)	Diagnoses	LO	1..N	Optional	DcmLongString	char[ ]
SERIE	(0020,0011)	Serie number	IS	1	Obligatory	DcmIntegerString	signed long
	(0008,0060)	Modality	CS	1	Obligatory	DcmCodeString	char[ ]
	(0018,0015)	Body part	CS	1	Optional	DcmCodeString	char[ ]
	(0008,0021)	Serie date	DA	1	Optional	DcmDate	char[ ]
	(0008,0031)	Serie time	TM	1	Optional	DcmTime	char[ ]
	(0008,103E)	Description	LO	1	Optional	DcmLongString	char[ ]
	(0008,1050)	Performing physician	PN	1..N	Optional	DcmPersonName	char[ ]
IMAGE	(0020,0013)	Image number	IS	1	Obligatory	DcmIntegerString	signed long
	(0008,0008)	Image type	CS	1..N	Optional	DcmCodeString	char[ ]
	(0008,0023)	Image date	DA	1	Optional	DcmDate	char[ ]
	(0008,0033)	Image time	TM	1	Optional	DcmTime	char[ ]
	(0028,0010)	Rows number	US	1	Optional	Uint16	unsigned short
	(0028,0011)	Columns number	US	1	Optional	Uint16	unsigned short
	(0028,0100)	Bits allocated	US	1	Optional	Uint16	unsigned short
	(0028,0101)	Bits stored	US	1	Optional	Uint16	unsigned short
	(0028,0102)	High bit	US	1	Optional	Uint16	unsigned short
	(0028,0002)	Samples per pixel	US	1	Optional	Uint16	unsigned short
	(0028,0103)	Pixel representation	US	1	Optional	Uint16	unsigned short
	(0028,0004)	Photometric interpretation	CS	1	Optional	DcmCodeString	char[ ]
	(0018,0050)	Slice thickness	DS	1	Optional	DcmDecimalString	float
	(0028,0030)	Pixel spacing	DS	2	Optional	DcmDecimalString	float
	(0028,1050)	Window center	DS	1..N	Optional	DcmDecimalString	signed long
	(0028,1051)	Window width	DS	1..N	Optional	DcmDecimalString	unsigned long
	(0028,1053)	Rescale slope	DS	1	Optional	DcmDecimalString	float
	(0028,1052)	Rescale Intersection	DS	1	Optional	DcmDecimalString	float
	(0004,1500)	Referenced file ID	CS	1..8	Optional	DcmCodeString	char[ ]

One selection criteria for the data fields is based upon the information provided by the image processing. Among the selected fields are the image dimensions, the samples per pixel number, and the gray-level window. Another criterion is the general information that guides the user during the search and selection of images, for example, patient's data, description, and modality of the study. Complementary fields that do not provide significant information for the image processing or to the user applications were not used for the gathering process, for example, address, occupation, and medical antecedents of the patient, and the technical information from the image acquisition devices.

Reading Process

The reader uses Algorithm 1 for the DICOMDIR information retrieving process.

It can be observed that in this algorithm starting from the parent nodes, each tree node and its children's nodes are recursively travelled, level by level, until reaching the deepest tree level. Only nodes from PATIENT, STUDY, SERIES, and IMAGE types are taken into account, though it is possible to extend the consideration to other types of nodes. For each visited node, the selected fields are compiled according to the node type (see Table 1). However, as explained in the DICOMDIR File Format section, not all the fields have an obligatory presence inside the DICOMDIR file, therefore the missing information must be completed from the corresponding DICOM image file, once its file identifier is known.

Some methods from the DCMTK library are used to travel through the DICOMDIR structure and retrieve its data. These methods can handle data elements encoded either in *big Endian* or *little Endian* byte ordering, or with any kind of representation values and cardinalities. The retrieving methods are invoked by the data element tag each time a node is visited, whereas the travelling methods are used during recursive calls to the tool's main reading method.

Figure 6. Results achieved from the integration of the DICOMDIR reading tool into a medical application for neurosurgery planning. The tool is coupled with a graphical interface for browsing throughout studies, series and images.

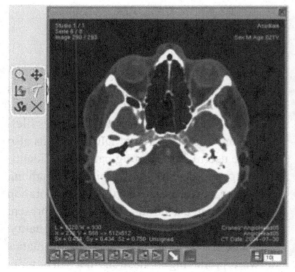 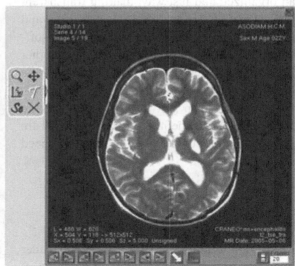

RESULTS AND DISSCUSSION

The DICOMDIR reader was integrated for its test and validation into software for neurosurgery and brachytherapy planning, developed with the VVM library (Montilla, Bosnjak, & Villegas, 2003). A graphical interface was coupled to the reader in order to enable the navigation of the information in a simple way. By just opening the associated DICOMDIR file, users will be able to have the interface display the patients' study images and their related medical information. Control widgets provided by the interface were used for interactively browsing and selecting the images.

The reading process was verified with DICOMDIR files associated to several image sets, coming from studies of CT and MRI performed on different patients. It could be proved that the reader recollected the information specified by the class definitions for each type of node, enabling display of its structure through the interface. Two examples from the tests are shown in Figure 6. In both examples, the studies were made on the patient's head but with two different modalities. The CT study has an eight-image series, whereas the MRI study contains 14 images.

It was observed that access to the information collected from the studies can be made in an organized and fast way, making transparent the navigation process of data structures and improving the efficiency in the use of the software. The tool is able to be integrated with other applications under development that require the handling of DICOM images and DICOMDIR files.As is usual in software projects implying code reusability, benefits from using our tool are going to be directly reflected in ease and speed of development.

CONCLUSION

The design used for the DICOMDIR file reader allows the medical application programmer to ef-

fortlessly incorporate the feature for the handling of this kind of file in software under development. Also, it avoids exhaustively understanding the DICOM standard and DCMTK classes and methods, which can be really hard and bothersome, enabling the programmer to focus on the integration of the tool into the application, as well as on the development of a navigation interface, according to the application's needs. Because the reading tool has open-source code, it can be reused and modified at will by the programmers. In addition, the design used for the tool development enables inclusion of new data fields to the presently used entities, as well as to add other information model entities to the data tree structure.

By integrating the tool into a medical application that handles DICOM image sets, it was proved it facilitates the browsing and searching of the information contained in the image sets, accelerating the fulfillment of these tasks and improving the efficiency and performance of the application. Open-source programming tools of this type also facilitate the development of medical applications and help to reduce software costs, thus making it more accessible to health institutions, physicians, and patients, particularly in regions where investment in health care solutions is either limited or not a priority issue.

FUTURE WORKS

We are considering the future implementation of tools for converting images from other formats to the DICOM format and for the creation of DICOMDIR files from nonindexed studies files. A tool for anonymization of DICOM fields also could be useful in protecting patient confidentiality during the sharing of clinical data among research teams. We hope that the implementation and subsequent use of this tool set will represent an incremental increase in the efficiency, quality, and speed of development of medical informatics software, producing applications that will be more complete and flexible at same time.

ACKNOWLEDGMENT

The authors want to express their gratitude to Dr. Luis Iván Jara, a neurosurgeon appointed to the Hospital Metropolitano del Norte (Valencia-Venezuela), for providing us the DICOM image sets used for the functional verification and evaluation of the reading tool. Financial support for this research was granted by Scientific and Humanistic Development Council of the University of Carabobo, Venezuela, under project CDCH-UC No. 0461-06.

REFERENCES

Digital imaging and communications in medicine took kit (DCMTK). (2005). *DICOM toolkit software documentation*. Oldenburger Forschungs und Entwicklungsinstitut für Informatik-Werkzeuge und Systeme (OFFIS). Retrieved on September 29, 2005, from http://dicom.offis.de/dcmtk.php.en

DicomLib. (2005). *DICOM software documentation*. Sunnybrook and Women's College Health Sciences Center Imaging Research Group. Retrieved on September 29, 2005, from http://dicomlib.swri.ca/dicomlib/html/index.htm

GDCM. (2005). *Grass roots DICOM software documentation*. Centre de Recherche et d'Applications en Traitement de l'Image et du Signal (CREATIS). Retrieved on September 29, 2005, from http://www.creatis.insa-lyon.fr/Public/Gdcm

Montilla, G., Bosnjak, A., Jara, L. I., & Villegas, H. (2005). Computer assisted planning using dependent texture mapping and multiple rendering projections in medical applications. *Proceedings from 3rd European Medical & Biological Engineering Conference and Ifmbe European Conference on Biomedical Engineering. Ifmbe* (pp. 4420-4425). Praga, Czech Republic: .

Montilla, G., Bosnjak, A., & Villegas, H. (2003). Visualización de mundos virtuales en la medicina. bioingeniería en Iberoamérica: Avances y desarrollos. In C. Müller-Karger & M. Cerrolaza (Eds.), *Centro internacional de métodos numéricos en ingeniería CIMNE* (pp. 519-545). Barcelona: .

National Electrical Manufacturers Association (NEMA). (2004a). *Digital imaging and communications in medicine. Part 1: Introduction and overview* (NEMA Standards Pub., PS3.1).

National Electrical Manufacturers Association (NEMA). (2004b). *Digital imaging and communications in medicine. Part 3: Information object definitions* (NEMA Standards Pub., PS3.3).

National Electrical Manufacturers Association (NEMA). (2004c). *Digital imaging and communications in medicine. Part 5: Data structures and encoding* (NEMA Standards Pub., PS3.5).

National Electrical Manufacturers Association (NEMA). (2004d). *Digital imaging and communications in medicine. Part 6: Data dictionary* (NEMA Standards Pub., PS3.6).

National Electrical Manufacturers Association (NEMA). (2004e). *Digital imaging and communications in medicine. Part 10: Media storage and file format for media interchange* (NEMA Standards Pub., PS3.10).

National Electrical Manufacturers Association (NEMA). (2004f). *Digital imaging and communications in medicine. Part 11: Media storage application profiles* (NEMA Standards Pub., PS3.11).

National Electrical Manufacturers Association (NEMA). (2004g). *Digital imaging and communications in medicine. Part 12: Media formats and physical media for media interchange* (NEMA Standards Pub., PS3.12).

Revet, B. (1997). *DICOM cookbook for implementations in modalities* (Tech. Rep.). Philips Medical Systems.

APPENDIX: GLOSSARY OF TERMS

American College of Radiology(ACR)/ National Electrical Manufacturers Association (NEMA)(ACR): This joint committee is responsible for the development and maintenance of the DICOM standard.

Acquisition modalities: These imaging techniques and devices provide radiological images from patients' anatomy. Most commonly used modalities are CT (computed tomography), MRI (magnetic resonance imaging) and US (ultra sound).

Application programming interfaces (APIs): A set of specialized functions, class libraries, and tools used by software programmers to facilitate the application development process.

Attribute: A property of an information object represented as a data element.

Big Endian: An encoding scheme where multiple byte values are encoded with the most significant byte first, followed by the remaining bytes in decreasing order of significance.

Browsing interfaces: These mechanisms and widgets provide a way to navigate information within software applications.

Data element: This is a single atomic information unit that is related to a real-world object attribute and is defined by an entry in the DICOM data dictionary.

Digital imaging and communications in medicine (DICOM): This standard establishes norms for handling, storing, and interchanging medical images and associated digital information.

DICOM application model: An entity/relationship diagram used to model the relationships existing between real-world objects within the DICOM standard's scope.

DICOM data dictionary: This is a catalog of DICOM data elements that describes the semantics and contents of each one of them.

DICOM information model: An entity/relationship diagram used to model the relationships between the information-object definitions representing classes of real-world objects defined by the DICOM application model.

DICOMDIR file: This is a unique and mandatory file that accompanies a file set and indexes these files.

Entity/relationship diagram: This is a graphical representation of a set of objects and the relationships existing among them.

Image-based diagnosis: Techniques used by health care specialists to diagnose patients' diseases through analysis of radiological imaging studies.

Information object description (IOD): This is an abstract definition for real-world objects that share the same properties.

Little Endian: An encoding scheme where multiple byte values are encoded with the least significant byte first, followed by the remaining bytes in increasing order of significance.

Open source: Programming paradigm based upon software engineering principles that pursues software code reutilization to facilitate the development of applications.

Proprietary code: Programming paradigm that establishes that the software applications code is protected and is not available either for modification or reutilization.

Software development kits (SDKs): See APIs.

Service: This is an operation that can be requested for acting over an information object.

Service-object pair (SOP): This is a relationship that is established between an information object and an operation or the service applicable over it.

SOP class: This is the whole set of services applicable over an information object.

Surgical planning: This describes the preoperative procedure where the surgeon determines surgical protocols and approaching trajectories to be followed during the intraoperative stage of the surgery.

Value multiplicity (VM): This is the DICOM data field that specifies the cardinality or number of values existing for a data element.

Value representation (VR): This is the DICOM data field that specifies the data type and format of values existing for a data element.

This work was previously published in International Journal of Healthcare Information Systems and Informatics, Vol. 2, Issue 1, edited by J. Tan, pp. 54-70, copyright 2007 by IGI Publishing, formerly known as Idea Group Publishing (an imprint of IGI Global).

Compilation of References

Ackerman, M.J., Yoo, T., & Jenkins, D. (2001). From data to knowledge: The visible human project continues. *Medinfo, 10*(2), 887-890.

Adalsteinsson, D., & Sethian, J. (1995). A fast level set method for propagating interfaces. *Journal of Computational Physics, 118,* 269-277.

Adams, R., & Bischof, L. (1994). Seeded region growing. *IEEE Transactions on Pattern Analysis and Machine Intelligence, 16,* 641-647.

Aeschlimann, M., Dinda, P., Kallivokas, L., López, J., Lowekamp, B., & O'Hallaron, D. (1999). Preliminary report on the design of a framework for distributed isualization. *Proceedings of the International Conference on Parallel and Distributed Processing Techniques and Applications* (PDPTA'99). Las Vegas, NV.

Alan, R., & Tria, A. (2006). Quadriceps-sparing total knee arthroplasty using the posterior stabilized TKA design. *The journal of knee surgery, 19*(1), 71-76.

Al-Kofahi, K., Lasek, S., Szarowski, D., Pace, C., Nagy, G., Turner, J.N., et al. (2002). Rapid automated three-dimensional tracing of neurons from confocal image stacks. *IEEE Transactions on Information Technology in Biomedicine, 6*(2), 171-187.

Alpert, N.M., Bradshaw, J.F., Kennedy, D. & Correia, J.A. (1990). The principal axes transformation: A method for image registration. *Journal of Nuclear Medicine, 31,* 1717-1722.

Anbar, N., Milescu, L., Naumov, A., Brown, C., Button, T., Carly, C., & AlDulaimi, K. (2001). Detection of cancerous breasts by dynamic area telethermometry. *IEEE Engineering in Medicine and Biology Magazine, 20*(5), 80-91.

Anderson, K., Buehler, K., & Markel, D. (2005). Computer-assisted navigation in total knee arthroplasty. *The Journal of Arthroplasty, 20*(7), 132-138.

Antani, S., Lee, D. J., Long, L. R., & Thoma, G. R. (2004). Evaluation of shape similarity measurement methods for spine X-ray images. *Journal of Visual Communication and Image Representation, 15*(3), 285-302.

Antani, S., Long, L. R., Thoma, G. R., & Lee, D. J. (2003). Evaluation of shape indexing methods for content-based retrieval of X-ray images. In *Proceedings of IS&T/SPIE 15th Annual Symposium on Electronic Imaging, Storage, and Retrieval for Media Databases* (pp. 405-416). Santa Clara, CA: SPIE.

Antani, S., Xu, X., Long, L. R., & Thoma, G. R. (2004). Partial shape matching for CBIR of spine X-ray images. In *Proceedings of IS&T/SPIE Electronic Imaging — Storage and Retrieval Methods and Applications for Multimedia 2004* (pp. 1-8). San Jose, CA: SPIE.

Arthur, K., Booth, K., & Ware, C. (1993). Evaluating 3D task performance for fish tank virtual worlds. *ACM Trans. Inf. Syst, 11*(3), 239-265.

Arya, S., & Mount, D. (1993). Approximate nearest neighbor searching. *Proceedings of ACM-SIAM Symposium on Discrete Algorithms (SODA'93),* (pp. 271-280).

Audette, M., Ferrie, F. & Peters, T. (2000). An algorithm overview of surface registration techniques for medical imaging. *Medical Image Analysis, 4*(4), 201-217.

Austern, M. (1999). *Generic programming and the STL: Professional computing series.* Addison-Wesley.

Aziz, O., Panesar, S., Netuveli, G., Paraskeva, P., Sheikh, A., & Darzi, A. (2005). Handheld computers and the 21st century team: A pilot study. *BMS Medical Informatics and Decision Making, 5*(28).

Baeza-Yates, R., & Ribeiro-Neto, B. (Eds.). (1999). *Modern information retrieval.* Boston: Addison-Wesley.

Bailey, M., & Clark, D. (1998). Using chromadepth to obtain inexpensive single-image stereovision for scientific visualization. *Journal of Graphics Tools, 3*(3), 1-9.

Baillard, C., Hellier, P., & Barillot, C. (2001). Segmentation of brain images using level sets and dense registration. *Medical Image Analysis, 5*, 185-194.

Bajaj, C., Pascucci, V., & Schikore, D. (1997). The contour spectrum. *Proceedings of IEEE Visualization 1997,* (pp. 167-173).

Bajcsy, R. & Kovacic, S. (1989). Multiresolution elastic matching. *Computer Vision, Graphics, and Image Processing, 46*, 1-21.

Ballard, D. H., Hayhoe, M. M., Pook, P. K., and Rao, R. P. N. (1997). Deictic codes for the embodiment of cognition. *Behavioral and Brain Sciences, 20*, 723-742.

Bankman, I. (2000). *Handbook of medical imaging: Processing and analysis.* Academic Press.

Barger, A., Block, W., Toropov, Y., Grist, T., & Mistretta, C. (2002). Time-resolved contrast-enhanced imaging with isotropic resolution and broad coverage using an undersampled 3D projection trajectory. *Magnetic Resonance in Medicine, 48*(2), 297-305.

Barratt, D., Penney, G., Chan, C., Slomczykowski, M., Carter, T., Edwards, P., & Hawkes, D. (2006). Self-calibrating 3D-ultrasound-based bone registration for minimally invasive orthopedic surgery. *IEEE transactions on medical imaging, 25*(3), 312-323.

Barton, G., & Lees, A. (1997). An application of neural networks for distinguishing gait patterns on the basis of hip-knee joint angle diagrams. *Gait and Posture, 5*,

28-35. Gage, J. (1991). *Gait analysis in cerebral palsy.* London: Mac Keith Press.

Basak, J., Chanda, B., & Majumder, D. D. (1994). On edge and line linking with connectionist models. *IEEE Transactions on Systems, Man, and Cybernetics, 24*(3), 413-428.

Beckmann, N., Kriegel, H.-P., Schneider, R., & Seeger, B. (1990). The R*-tree: An efficient and robust access method for points and rectangles. In *Proceedings of ACM SIGMOD International Conference on Management of Data* (pp. 322-331). Atlantic City, NJ: ACM Press.

Belloum, A., Groep, D., Hendrikse, Z., Hertzberger, B., Korkhov, V., et al. (2003). VLAM-G: A grid-based virtual laboratory. *Future Generation Computer Systems, 19*(2), 209-217.

Bennis, C., Vezien, J., & Iglesias, G. (1991). Piecewise surface flattening for non-distorted texture mapping. *Computer Graphics, 25*, 237-246.

Berman, F., Fox, G., & Hey, T. (2002). Grid computing—making the global infrastructure a reality. John Wiley & Sons, Ltd.

Besl, P.J. & MaKey, N.D. (1992). A method for registration of 3-D shapes. *IEEE Transactions on Pattern Analysis and Machine Intelligence, 14*(2), 239-256.

Bethel, E., & Shalf, J. (2003). Cactus and visapult: An ultra-high performance grid-distributed visualization architecture using connectionless protocols. *IEEE Computer Graphics and Applications, 23*(2), 51-59.

Betrancourt, M. (2005). The animation and interactivity principles in multimedia learning. In R. E. Mayer (Ed.), *The Cambridge Handbook of Multimedia Learning* (pp. 287-296). New York, NY: Cambridge University Press.

Beucher, S. (1994). Watershed, hierarchical segmentation and waterfall algorithm. In E. Dougherty (Ed.), *Mathematical morphology and its applications to image processing.* Boston: Kluwer.

Beyer, H., and Holtzblatt, K. (1997). *Contextual Design: A Customer-Centered Approach to Systems Designs*: Morgan Kaufman.

Bird, S., & Lane, D. (2006). House officer procedure documentation using a personal digital assistant: A longitudinal study. *BMC Medical Informatics and Decision Making, 6*(5).

Black, C., Murray, K., Howell, K., Harper, J., Atherton, D., Woo, P., et al. (2002). Juvenile-onset localized scleroderma activity detection by infrared thermography. *Rheumatology, 41*(10), 1178-1182.

Boad, I., Navazo, I., & Scopigno, R. (2001). Multi-resolution volume visualization with a texture-based octree. *The Visual Computer, 17,* 185-197.

Bookstein, F. L. (1989). Principal warps: Thin-plate splines and the decomposition of deformations. *IEEE Transactions on Pattern Analysis and Machine Intelligence, 11*(6), 567-585.

Borgefors, G. (1988). Hierarchical chamfer matching: A parametric edge matching algorithm. *IEEE Transactions on Pattern Analysis and Machine Intelligence, 10,* 849-865.

Botha C., & Post, F. (2002). New technique for transfer function specification in direct volume rendering using real-time visual feedback. *Proceedings of SPIE Symposium on Medical Imaging, 4681,* 349-356.

Bowman, D., Datey, A., Ryu, Y., Farooq, U., & Vasnaik, O. (2002). Empirical comparison of human behavior and performance with different display devices for virtual environments. *Proceedings of the Human Factors and Ergonomics Society Annual Meeting,* (pp. 2134-2138).

Bowman, D., Kruijff, E., LaViola, J., Jr., & Poupyrev, I. (2001). An introduction to 3D user interface design. *Presence, 10*(1), 96-108.

Brederson, J., Ikits, M., Johnson, C., & Hansen, C. (2000). The visual haptic workbench. *Proceedings of PHANToM Users Group Workshop,* (pp. 46-49).

Brejl, M., & Sonka, M. (2000). Directional 3D edge detection in anisotropic data: Detector design and performance assessment. *Computer Vision and Image Understanding, 77,* 84-110.

Brightwell, R., Fisk, L. A., Greenberg, D. S., Hudson, T., Levenhagen, M., Maccabe, et al. (2000). Massively parallel computing using commodity components. *Parallel Computing, 26,* 243-266.

Brodley, C. E., Kak, A, Dy, J., Shyu, C. R., Aisen, A., & Broderick, L. (1999). Content-based retrieval from medical image database: A synergy of human interaction, machine learning, and computer vision. In *Proceedings of the Sixteenth National Conference on Artificial Intelligence* (pp. 760-767). Orlando, FL: AAAI Press / MIT Press.

Brodsky, E., & Block, W. (2003). Interactive visualization of time-resolved contrast-enhanced magnetic resonance angiography (CE-MRA). *Proceedings of the 14ᵗʰ IEEE Visualization 2003,* (pp. 108). Seattle, WA: IEEE Computer Society.

Brodsky, E., Isaacs, D., Grist, T., & Block, W. (2006). 3D fluoroscopy with real-time 3D non-cartesian phased-array contrast-enhanced MRA. *Magnetic Resonance in Medicine, 56*(2), 247-254.

Brooks, F. (1999). What's real about virtual reality?. *IEEE Computer Graphics and Applications, 9,* 16-27.

Brooks, F., Ouh-Young, M., Batter, J., & Kilpatrick, P. (1990). Project GROPE- haptic displays for scientific visualization. *Computer Graphics, 24*(4), 177-185.

Brown, L.G. (1992). A survey of image registration techniques. *ACM Computing Surveys 24*(4), 325-376.

Bruno, N., & Cutting, J. (1988). Minimodality and the perception of layout. *Journal of Experimental Psychology, 117,* 161-170.

Buhler, P., Just, U., Will, E., Kotzerke, J., & van den Hoff, J. (2004). An accurate method for correction of head movement in PET. *IEEE Transactions on Medical Imaging, 23*(9), 1176-1185.

Cabral, B., Cam, N., & Foran, J. (1994). Accelerated volume rendering and tomographic reconstruction using texture mapping hardware. *Proceedings of the 1994 Symposium on Volume Visualization,* (pp. 91-98). New York, NY: ACM Press.

Cactus. http://www.cactuscode.org.

Canny, J. (1986). A computational approach to edge detection. *IEEE Transactions on Pattern Analysis and Machine Intelligence, 8*(6), 679-698.

Card, S. K., MacKinlay, J. D., & Shneiderman, B. (1999). *Readings in information visualization: Using vision to think.* San Francisco: Morgan Kaufmann.

Carroll, J. (1993). *Human cognitive abilities: A survey of factor-analytic studies.* New York: Cambridge University Press.

Center for Computational Visualization of University of Texas at Austin. (2003). *Grid- enabled visualization.* Poster of NPACI All-hands Meeting. San Diego, CA.

Chadwick, J., Haumann, D., & Parent, R. (1989). Layered construction for deformable animated characters. *Computer Graphics, 23,* 243-252.

Chakraborty, A., Staib, L. H., & Duncan, J. S. (1996). Deformable boundary finding in medical images by integrating gradient and region information. *IEEE Transactions on Medical Imaging, 15*(6), 859-870.

Chan, T., & Vese, L. (2001). An active contour model without edges. *IEEE Transactions on Image Processing, 10*(2), 266-277.

Chang, C.-I (2003). *Hyperspectral imaging: Techniques for spectral detection and classification.* New York: Kluwer.

Chang, C.-L., Cheng, B.-W., & Su, J.-L. (2004). Using case-based reasoning to establish a continuing care information system of discharge planning. *Expert Systems with Applications, 26*(4), 601-613.

Chang, Y. L., & Li, X. (1994). Adaptive region growing. *IEEE Transactions on Image Processing, 3*(6), 868-72.

Chau, T. (2001). A review of analytical techniques for gait data. Part 1, Fuzzy, statistical and fractal methods. *Gait and Posture, 13,* 49-66.

Chau, T. (2001). A review of analytical techniques for gait data. Part 2, Neural networks and wavelet methods. *Gait and Posture, 13,* 102-120.

Chen, C., Pellizari, C.A., Chen, G.T.Y., Cooper, M.D. & Levin, D.N. (1987). Image analysis of PET data with the aid of CT and MR images. *Information Processing in Medical Imaging,* 601-611.

Chen, D., & Zeltzer, D. (1992). Pump it up: Computer animation of a biomechanically- based model of muscle using the finite element method. *Computer Graphics, 26*(2), 89-98.\

Chen, K., Lin, J., & Moa, C. (1996). The applications of competitive Hopfield neural network to medical image segmentation. *IEEE Transactions on Medical Imaging, 15*(4), 560-567.

Chen, M., Mountford, S., & Sellen, A. (1988). A study in interactive 3D rotation using 2D control devices. *Computer Graphics, 22*(4), 121-129.

Cheng, H. D., & Cui, M. (2004). Mass lesion detection with a fuzzy neural network. *Pattern Recognition, 37*(6), 1189-1200.

Chiueh, T., & Ma, K. (1997). A parallel pipelined renderer for time-varying volume data. *International Symposium on Parallel Architectures, Algorithms and Networks 1997 (I-SPAN '97),* (pp. 9-15). Taipei, Taiwan: IEEE.

Christensen, G.E., Kane, A.A., Marsh, J.L. & Vannier, M.W. (1996). Synthesis of an individual cranial atlas with dysmorphic shape. *Mathematical methods in biomedical image analysis* (pp. 309-318). Los Alamitos, CA: IEEE Computer Society Press.

Christou, C. G., & Bülthoff, H. H. (1999). View dependence in scene recognition after active learning. *Memory & Cognition, 27,* 996-1007.

Cmake software introduction. (2007). http://www.cmake.org/HTML/Index.html.

Cohen, M. (1992). Interactive spacetime control for animation. *Computer Graphics Proceedings, 26*(2), 293-302.

Coleman, J., Goettsch, A., Savchenko, A., Kollmann, H., Wang, K., Klement, E., & Bono, P. (1996). TeleInViVoTM: Towards collaborative volume visualization environments. *Computers & Graphics, 20*(6), 801-811.

Collen, M. F. (1995). *A history of medical informatics in the United States, 1950 to 1990*. Indianapolis, IN: American Medical Informatics Association.

Collignon, A., Vandermeulen, D., Suetens, P. & Marchal, G. (1995). 3D multi-modality image registration using feature space clustering. In N. Ayche (Ed.), *Computer Vision, Virtual Reality, and Robotic Mechine, 905, of Lecture Notes in Computer Science* (pp. 195-204). Berlin: Springer-Verlag.

Collins, D.L., Neelin, P., Peters, T.M. & Evans, A.C. (1994). Automatic 3D intersubject registration of MR volumetric data in standardized Talairach space. *Journal of Computer Assisted Tomography, 18*(2), 192-205.

Condor. http://www.cs.wisc.edu/condor/.

Confalonieri, N., Manzotti, A., Pullen, C., & Ragone, V. (2005). Computer-assisted technique versus intramedullary and extramedullary alignment system in total knee replacement: A radiological comparison. *Acta orthopaedica Belgica, 71,* 703-709.

Connecting for Health. Retrieved April 1, 2007, from http://www.connectingforhealth.nhs.uk/.

Cootes, T. F., Edwards, G. J., & Taylor, C. J. (2001). Active appearance models. *IEEE Transactions on Pattern Analysis and Machine Intelligence, 23*(6), 681-685.

Cootes, T. F., Taylor, C. J., Cooper, D. H., & Granham, J. (1995). Active shape models—their training and application. *Computer Vision and Image Understanding, 61,* 38-59.

Cruz-Neira, C., Sandin, D., & DeFanti, T. (1993). Surround-screen projection-based virtual reality: The design and implementation of the CAVE. *ACM Computer Graphics, 27*(2), 135-142.

Cullip, T., & Neumann, U. (1993). *Accelerating volume reconstruction with 3D texture mapping hardware*. Chapel Hill, NC: University of North Carolina.

Czajkowski, K., Foster, I., & Kesselman, C. (1999). Resource co-allocation in computational grids. *Proceedings of the 8ᵗʰ IEEE International Symposium on High Performance Distributed Computing* (HPDC-8), (pp. 219-228).

Daubresse, F., Vajeu, C., & Loquet, J. (2005). Total knee arthroplasty with conventional or navigated technique: comparison of the learning curves in a community hospital. *Acta orthopaedica Belgica, 71*(6), 710-713.

Davatzikos, C., Vaillant, M., Resnick, S., Prince, J., Letovsky, S., & Bryan, R. (1996). A computerized method for morphological analysis of the corpus callosum. *Journal of Computer-Assisted Tomography, 20,* 88-97.

Davatzikos, C.A., Prince, J.L. & Bryan, R.N. (1996). Image registration based on boundary mapping. *IEEE Transactions on Medical Imaging, 15,* 112-115.

Davis, R., Ounpuu, S., Tyburski, D., & Gage, J. (1991). A gait analysis data collection and reduction technique. *Human Movement Science, 10,* 575-587.

DCE. http://www.opengroup.org/dce/.

De Dombal, F. T. (1996). *Medical informatics: The essentials*. Oxford, Boston: Butterworth-Heinemann.

De Guzman, E., Ho-Ching, F., Matthews, T., Rattenbury, T., Back, M., & Harrison, S. (2003). Eewww!: Tangible instruments for navigating into the human body. *Extended Abstracts of CHI 2003,* 806-807.

De Momi, E., Cerveri, P., Audrito, M., Facchini, A., & Ferrigno G. (2006). 3D shape iterative reconstruction method based on statistical models. In: F. Langlotz, B. Davies, & R. Ellis (Eds.), 6ᵗʰ Annual Meeting of CAOS-International. *Computer Assisted Orthopaedic Surgery* (pp. 123-126).

De Momi, E., Cerveri, P., Audrito, M., Facchini, A., Ferrigno G. (2006). A new Algorithm for hip joint center computation in TKR. In: F. Langlotz, B. Davies, & R. Ellis (Eds.), 6ᵗʰ Annual Meeting of CAOS-International. *Computer-Assisted Orthopaedic Surgery* (pp. 119-122).

Delp, S., Stulberg, S., Davies, B., Picard, F., & Leitner, F. (1998). Computer-assisted knee replacement. *Clinical Orthopaedics, 354,* 49-56.

Demiralp, C., Laidlaw, D., Jackson, C., Keefe, D., & Zhang, S. (2003). Subjective usefulness of CAVE and fish tank VR display systems for a scientific visualization application. *Proceedings of IEEE Visualization.* Seattle, WA.

Department of Health. (2000). *The NHS plan: A plan for investment, a plan for reform.* London: HMSO.

Department of Health. *The creation of the National Health Service.* Retrieved April 13, 2006, from http://www.dh.gov.uk/AboutUs/HowDHWorks/HistoryOfDH/HistoryOfDHArticle/fs/en?CONTENT_ID=4106108&chk=ujPIOa.

Desbrun, M., & Gascuel, M-P. (1995). Animating soft substances with implicit surfaces. *Proceedings of SIGGRAPH'95,* (pp. 287-290).

Dey, D., Slomka, P.J., Hahn, L.J., & Kloiber, R. (1999). Automatic three-dimensional multimodality registration using radionuclide transmission CT attenuation maps: A phantom study. *Journal of Nuclear Medicine, 40*(3), 448-455.

DicomLib. (2005). *DICOM software documentation.* Sunnybrook and Women's College Health Sciences Center Imaging Research Group. Retrieved on September 29, 2005, from http://dicomlib.swri.ca/dicomlib/html/index.htm

DiGioia, A., Jaramaz, B., Blackwell, M., Simon, D., Morgan, F., Moody, J., et al. (1998). Image-guided navigation system to measure intraoperatively acetabular implant alignment. *Clinical orthopaedics and related research, 355,* 8-22.

Digital imaging and communications in medicine took kit (DCMTK). (2005). *DICOM toolkit software documentation.* Oldenburger Forschungs und Entwicklungsinstitut für Informatik-Werkzeuge und Systeme (OFFIS). Retrieved on September 29, 2005, from http://dicom.offis.de/dcmtk.php.en

DoE Department of Energy Science Grid. http://www.doesciencegird.org.

Domini, F., Caudek, C., & Skirko, P. (2003). Temporal integration of motion and stereo cues to depth. *Perception & Psychophysics, 65,* 48-57.

Dong, F., Krokos, M., & Clapworthy, G. (2000). Fast volume rendering and data classification using multi-resolution min-max octrees. *Computer Graphics Forum, 19*(3), 359-368.

Dosher, B., Sperling, G., & Wurst, S. (1986). Tradeoffs between stereopsis and proximity luminance covariance as determinants of perceived 3D structure. *Journal of Vision Research, 26*(6), 973-990.

Drebin, R., Carpenter, L., & Hanrahan, P. (1988). Volume rendering. *Computer Graphics, 22*(4), 65-73.

Duncan, J.S. & Ayache, N. (2000). Medical image analysis: Progress over two decades and the challenges ahead. *IEEE Transactions on Pattern and Machine Intelligence, 22*(1), 58-106.

DVR. http://www.aus-vo.org/soft_dvr.html.

Eakins, J. P. (2002). Towards in intelligent image retrieval. *Pattern Recognition, 35*(1), 3-14.

Egecioglu, O., Ferhatosmanoglu, H., & Ogras, U. (2004). Dimensionality reduction and similarity computation by inner-product approximations. *IEEE Transactions on Knowledge and Data Engineering, 16*(6), 714-726.

Eliot, J., & Smith, I. M. (1983). *An international directory of spatial tests.* Windsor, Berks: Nfer-Nelson.

El-Naqa, I., Yang, Y., Galatsanos, N. P., & Wernick, M. N. (2003). Relevance feedback based on incremental learning for mammogram retrieval. In *Proceedings of the International Conference of Image Processing 2003* (pp. 729-732). Barcelona, Spain: IEEE Press.

El-Naqa, I., Yang, Y., Galatsanos, N. P., Nishikawa, R. M., & Wernick, M. N. (2004). A similarity learning approach to content-based image retrieval: Application to digital mammography. *IEEE Transactions on Medical Imaging, 23*(10), 1233-1244.

Ernst, M., & Banks, M. (2002). Humans integrate visual and haptic information in a statistically optimal fashion. *Nature, 415*(6870), 429-433.

e-Science. http://www.e-science.clrc.ac.uk and http://www.escience-grid.org.uk/.

FAFNER. http://www.npac.syr.edu/factoring.html.

Fan, J., Yau, D. K. Y., Elmargamid, A. K., & Aref, W. G. (2001). Automatic image segmentation by integrating color-edge extraction and seeded region growing. *IEEE Transactions on Image Processing, 10,* 1454-1466.

Feldman, A., & Acredolo, L. P. (1979). The effect of active versus passive exploration on memory for spatial location in children. *Child Development, 50*, 698-704.

Feng, D., Siu, W. C., & Zhang, H. J. (Eds.). (2003). *Multimedia information retrieval and management: Technological fundamentals and applications.* Berlin: Springer.

Ferecatu, M., Crucianu, M., & Boujemaa, N. (2004). Retrieval of difficult image classes using SVM-based relevance feedback. In *Proceedings of the 6th ACM SIGMM International Workshop on Multimedia Information Retrieval* (pp. 23-30). New York: ACM Press.

Ferecatu, M., Crucianu, M., & Boujemaa, N. (2004). Sample selection strategies for relevance feedback in region-based image retrieval. In *Pacific-Rim Conference on Multimedia 2004* (pp. 497-504). Tokyo, Japan: IEEE Press.

Ferrigno, G., & Pedotti, A. (1985). ELITE: A digital dedicated hardware system for movement analysis via real-time TV-signal processing. *IEEE Transaction on Biomedical Engineering, 32*, 943-950.

Fitzpatrick, J.M. (2001). Detecting failure, assessing success. In J.V. Hajnal, D.L.G. Hill & D.J.E. Hawkes (Eds.), *Medical image registration* (pp. 117-139). CRC Press.

Fitzpatrick, J.M., Hill, D.L.G. & Maurer, C.R. (2000). *Handbook of medical imaging.* Bellingham, WA: SPIE Press.

Fitzpatrick, J.M., West, J. B. & Maurer, C. R. (1998). Predicting error in rigid-body point-based registration. *IEEE Transactions on Medical Imaging, 17*, 694-702.

Flavell, J. H., Green, F. L., Flavell, E. R., Harris, P. L., & Astington, J. W. (1995). Young children's knowledge about thinking. *Monographs of the Society for Research in Child Development, 60*(1), 1-113.

Fleck, M., Forsyth, D., & Bregler, C. (1996). Finding naked people. *4th European Conference on Computer Vision, 2*, 593-602.

Fleute, M., Lavallee, S., & Julliard, R. (1999). Incorporating a statistically-based shape model into a system for computer-assisted anterior cruciate ligament surgery. *Medical Image Analysis, 3*(3), 209-222.

Florance, V. & Masys, D. (2002). *Next generation IAIMS: Binding knowledge to effective action.* Report Number N01-LM-9-3523. Washington, DC: Association of American Medical Colleges.

Florance, V. & Moller, M. T. (2002). *Better Health 2010: A report by the AAMC's better_health 2010 Advisory Board.* Washington, DC: Association of American Medical Colleges.

Fonseca, M. J., & Jorge, J. A. (2003). Indexing high-dimensional data for content-based retrieval in large database. In *Proceedings of the Eighth International Conference on Database Systems for Advanced Applications* (pp. 267-274). Kyoto, Japan: IEEE Press.

Foreman, N., Sandamas, G., and Newson, D. (2004). Distance underestimation in virtual space is sensitive to gender but not activity-passivity or mode of interaction. *CyberPsychology & Behavior, 7*(4), 451-457.

Foster, I., & Kesselman, C. (1999). *The grid: Blueprint for a new computing infrastructure.* San Francisco, CA: Morgan Kaufmann.

Foster, I., & Kesselman, C. (2003). *The grid 2: Blueprint for a new computing infrastructure.* San Francisco, CA: Morgan Kaufmann Publishers.

Foster, I., Geisler, J., Nickless, W., Smith, W., & Tuecke, S. (1997). Software infrastructure for the I-WAY high performance distributed computing experiment. *Proceedings of the 5th IEEE Symposium on High Performance Distributed Computing,* (pp. 562-571).

Foster, I., Kesselman, C., & Tuecke, S. (2001). The anatomy of the grid: Enabling scalable virtual organizations. *International J. Supercomputer Applications, 15*(3).

Foster, I., Kesselman, C., Nick, J., & Tuecke, S. (2002). The physiology of the grid: An open grid services architecture for distributed systems integration. *Open Grid Service Infrastructure WG, Global Grid Forum.*

Freeman, W. T., & Adelson, E. H. (1991). The design and use of steerable filters. *IEEE Transactions on Pattern Analysis and Machine Intelligence, 13*(9), 891-906.

Froehlich, B., & Plate, J. (2000). The cubic mouse: A new device for three-dimensional input. *Proceedings of the SIGCHI conference on Human factors in computing systems,* (pp. 526-531).

Fuchs, H., Levoy, M., & Pizer, S. (1989). Interactive visualization of 3D medical data. *IEEE Computer,* 46-50.

Funge, J., Tu, X., & Terzopoulos, D. (1999). Cognitive modeling: Knowledge, reasoning and planning for intelligent characters. *Proceedings of SIGGRAPH'99,* (pp. 29-38).

Garg, A. X., Norman, G. R., Spero, L., & Maheshwari, P. (1999). Do virtual computer models hinder anatomy learning? *Academic Medicine, 74*(10), S87-S89.

Garg, A. X., Norman, G., & Sperotable, L. (2001). How medical students learn spatial anatomy. *The Lancet, 357,* 363-364.

GDCM. (2005). *Grass roots DICOM software documentation.* Centre de Recherche et d'Applications en Traitement de l'Image et du Signal (CREATIS). Retrieved on September 29, 2005, from http://www.creatis.insa-lyon.fr/Public/Gdcm

Gelder, A., & Kim, K. (1996). Direct volume rendering with shading via three-dimensional textures. *Volume Visualization Symposium 96,* (pp. 23-30).

Gerig, G., Koller, T., Szekely, G., Brechbühler, C., & Kübler, O. (1993). Symbolic description of 3-D structures applied to cerebral vessel tree obtained from MR angiography volume data. IPMI '93: *Proceedings of the 13th International Conference on Information Processing in Medical Imaging* (pp. 94-111). Springer-Verlag.

Gevers, T., & Stokman, H. (2003). Classifying color edges in video into shadow-geometry, highlight, or material transitions. *IEEE Transactions on Multimedia, 5*(2), 237-243.

Gevers, T., (2001). Color-based retrieval. In M. S. Lew (Ed.), *Principles of visual information retrieval* (pp. 11-49). London: Springer.

Gibbs, S. (2000). *Guide to the interpretation of gait deviations.* Scotland: The Dundee Royal Infirmary.

Gilder, G. (2002). *Gilder's law on network performance. Telecosm: The world after bandwidth abundance.* Touchstone Books.

Glatard, T., Montagnat, J., & Magnin, I. E. (2004). Texture based medical image indexing and retrieval: Application to cardiac imaging. In *Proceedings of the ACM SIGMM International Workshop on Multimedia Information Retrieval* (pp. 135-142). New York: ACM Press.

Gleicher, M. (1998). Retargeting motion to new characters. *Proceedings of SIGGRAPH'98,* (pp. 33-42).

Global Grid Forum. http://www.ggf.org.

Goldfinger, E. (1991). *Human anatomy for artists.* New York, NY, Oxford: Oxford University Press.

Gonzalez, R. C., & Woods, R. E. (2002). *Digital image processing.* Upper Saddle River, NJ: Prentice Hall.

Gordin, D. N., & Pea, R. D. (1995). Prospects for scientific visualization as an educational technology. *The Journal of the Learning Sciences, 4,* 249-279.

Gorte, B., & Stein, A. (1998). Bayesian classification and class area estimation of satellite images using stratification. *Trans.GeoRS, 36*(3), 803-812.

Gourret, J., Magnenat Thalmann, N., & Thalmann, D. (1989). Simulation of object and human skin deformations in a grasping task. *Computer Graphics, 23,* 21-30.

Gray, W. D., & Fu, W.-T. (2004). Soft constraints in interactive behavior: The case of ignoring perfect knowledge in-the-world for imperfect knowledge in-the-head. *Cognitive Science, 28*(3), 359-382.

Gray, W. D., Sims, C. R., Fu, W.-T., & Schoelles, M. J. (2006). The soft constraints hypothesis: A rational analysis approach to resource allocation for interactive behavior. *Psychological Review, 113*(3) 461-482.

Green, R. O., et al. (1998). Imaging spectroscopy and the airborne visible/infrared imaging spectrometer (AVIRIS). *Remote Sensing of Environment, 65,* 227-248.

Gridport. http://gridport.net/main.

GriKSL. http://www.aei.mpg.de/~tradke/GriKSL/.

Grimshaw, A., Wulf, W., et al. (1997). The legion visio of a worldwide virtual computer. *Communications of the ACM, 40*(1).

Grimson, W.E.L. (1995). Medical applications of image understanding. *IEEE Expert, 10*(5), 18-28.

Grimstead, I., Avis, N., & Walker D. (2003). Automatic distribution of rendering workloads in a grid-enabled collaborative visualization environment. *Proceedings of the 2004 ACM/IEEE conference on Supercomputing.*

Guan, H. & Wada, S. (2002). Flexible color texture retrieval method using multi-resolution mosaic for image classification. In *Proceedings of the 6th International Conference on Signal Processing: Vol. 1* (pp. 612-615). Beijing, China: IEEE Press.

Guéziec, A. & Ayache, N. (1992). Smoothing and matching of 3-D space curves. In R.A. Robb (Ed.), *Visualization in biomedical computing*, 1808, Proc. SPIE (pp. 259-273). Bellingham, WA: SPIE PRESS.

Guthe, S., Wand, M., Gosner, J., & Straßer, W. (2002). Interactive rendering of large volume data sets. *Proceedings of IEEE Visualization 2002,* (pp. 53-60).

Guttman, A. (1984). R-trees: A dynamic index structure for spatial searching. In *Proceedings of ACM SIGMOD International Conference on Management of Data* (pp. 47-54). New York: ACM Press.

Guy, G., & Medioni, G. (1996). Inferring global perceptual from local features. *International Journal of Computer Vision, 20*(1/2), 113-133.

gViz. http://www.visualization.leeds.ac.uk/gViz/.

Haaker, R., Stockheim, M., Kamp, M., Proff, G., Breitenfelder, J., & Ottersbach, A. (2005). Computer-assisted navigation increases precision of component placement in total knee arthroplasty. *Clinical Orthopaedics and Related Research, 433,* 152-159.

Haber, R., & McNabb, D. (1990). Visualization idioms: A conceptual model for scientific visualization systems. In: G. Nielson, B. Shriver, & L. Rosenblum (Eds.), *Visualization in scientific computing,* (pp.74-93). Los Alamitos, NM: IEEE Computer Society Press.

Hadwiger, M., Berger, C., & Hauser, H. (2003). High-quality two-level volume rendering of segment data sets on consumer graphics hardware. *Proceedings of the IEEE Visualization 2003 Conference,* (pp. 301-308).

Haeghen, Y. V., Naeyaert, J. M. A. D., Lemahieu, I., & Philips, W. (2000). An imaging system with calibrated color image acquisition for use in dermatology. *IEEE Transaction on Medical Imaging, 19*(7), 722-730.

Hahn, H., Preim, B., Selle, D., & Peitgen, H. (2001). Visualization and interaction techniques for the exploration of vascular structures. *VIS '01: Proceedings of the conference on Visualization* (pp. 395-402). IEEE Computer Society.

Hajnal, J., Saeed, N., Soar, E., Oatridge, A., Young, I. & Bydder, G. (1995). Detection of subtle brain changes using subvoxel registration and subtraction of serial MR images. *Journal of Computer Assisted Tomography, 19*(5) , 677-691.

Ham, C. (2004). *Health policy in Britain: The politics and organisation of the National Health Service* (5th ed.). Hampshire: Palgrave Macmillan.

Handels, H. (2003). Medical image processing: New perspectives in computer supported diagnostics, computer aided surgery and medical education and training. *Year Book of Medical Informatics*, 503-505.

Hansen, C., & Johnson, C. (2004). *The visualization handbook*. MA: Elsevier Butterworth Heinemann.

Haralick, R. M. (1979). Statistical and structural approaches to texture. In *Proceedings of the IEEE, 67*(5), 786-804.

Haralick, R. M., Shanmugan, K., & Dinstein, I. (1973). Textural features for image classification. *IEEE Transactions on Systems, Man and Cybernetics, 3*(6), 610-621.

Haralick, R. M., Sternberg, S. R., & Zhuang, X. (1987). Image analysis using mathematical morphology. *IEEE Transactions on Pattern Analysis and Machine Intelligence, 9*(4), 532-50.

Haralick, R., & Shapiro, L. (1985). Image segmentation techniques. *Computer Vision, Graphics and Image Processing, 29*, 100-132.

Harman, K. L., Humphrey, G. K., & Goodale, M. A. (1999). Active manual control of object views facilitates visual recognition. *Current Biology, 9,* 1315-1318.

Head, J., Wang, F., Lipari, C., & Elliott, R. (2000). The important role of infrared imaging in breast cancer. *IEEE Engineering in Medicine and Biology Magazine, 19,* 52-57.

Healthcare Commission. (2004). Retrieved April 13, 2006, from http://ratings2004.healthcarecommission. org.uk/.

Heer, J., & Khooshabeh, P. (2004, May 25-28). *Seeing the Invisible.* Paper presented at the Association for Computing Machinery Conference on Advanced Visual Interfaces Conference, Lecce, Italy.

Hegarty, M. & Waller, D. (2005). Individual differences in spatial abilities. In P. Shah & A. Miyake (Eds.). *The Cambridge Handbook of Visuospatial Thinking* (pp. 121 – 169). New York: Cambridge University Press.

Hegarty, M. (2004). Commentary: Dynamic visualizations and learning: Getting to the difficult questions. *Learning and Instruction, 14,* 343-351.

Hegarty, M., Keehner, M., Cohen, C., Montello, D. R. & Lippa, Y. (2007). The role of spatial cognition in medicine: Applications for selecting and training professionals. In G. Allen (Ed.) *Applied Spatial Cognition* (pp. 285-315). Mahwah, NJ: Lawrence Erlbaum.

Heger, S., Portheine, F., Ohnsorge, J., Schkommodau, E., & Radermacher, K. (2005). *IEEE engineering in medicine and biology magazine, 24*(2), 85-95.

Hellier, P., Barillot, C., Memin, E. & Perez, P. (2001). Hierarchical estimation of a dense deformation field for 3-D robust registration. *IEEE Transactions on Medical Imaging, 20,* 388-402.

Herman, G. T., & Carvalho, B. M., (2001). Multi-seeded segmentation using fuzzy connectedness. *IEEE Transactions on Pattern Analysis and Machine Intelligence, 23*(5), 460-474.

Herman, G., & Liu, H. (1979). Three-dimensional display of human organs from computer tomograms. *Computer Graphics and Image Processing, 9*(1), 1-21.

Herzog, W., Nigg, B., Read, L., & Olsson, E. (1989). Asymmetries in ground reaction force patterns in normal human gait. *Medicine and Science in Sports and Exercise, 21,* 110-114.

Hill, A., & Taylor, C. J. (1994). Automatic landmark generation for point distribution models. *Proceedings of the 5th British Machine Vision Conference, 2*(2), 429-438.

Hill, D. L. G., Batchelor, P. G., Holden, M. H. & Hawkes, D. J. (2001). Medical image registration. *Physics in Medicine and Biology, 46*(1), 1-45.

Hill, D. L. G., Hawkes, D. J., Harrison, N. A. & Ruff, C.F. (1993). A strategy for automated multimodality image registration incorporating anatomical knowledge and imager characteristics. In H.H. Barrett & A.F. Gmitro (Eds.), *Lecture Notes in Computer Science. Proceedings of the 13th International Conference on Information Processing in Medical Imaging* (pp. 182-196). New York: Springer-Verlag.

Hill, D. L. G., Smith, A.D., Mauerer, C.R., Cox, T.C.S., Elwes, R., Brammer, M.J., Hawkes, D.J. & Polkey, C.E. (2000). Sources of error in comparing functional magnetic resonance imaging and invasive electrophysiology recordings. *Journal of Neurosurgery, 93,* 214-223.

Hinckley, K., Pausch, R., Kassell, N., & Goble, J. (1994). A three-dimensional user interface for neurosurgical visualization. *The SPIE Conf. on Medical Imaging,* (pp. 126-136).

Hinckley, K., Tullio, J., Pausch, R., Profftt, D., & Kassell, N. (1997). Usability analysis of 3D rotation techniques. *Proceedings of the 10th Annual ACM Symposium on User Interface Software and Technology,* (pp. 1-10).

Hodgins, J., & Pollard, N. (1997). Adapting simulated behaviors for new characters. *Proceeding of SIGGRAPH'97,* (pp. 153-162).

Hoi, C.-H., Chan, C.-H., Huang, K., Lyu, M. R., & King, I. (2004). Biased support vector machine for relevance feedback in image retrieval. In *Proceedings of International Joint Conference on Neural Networks* (pp. 3189-3194). Budapest, Hungary: IEEE Press.

Holden, M., Hill, D.L.G., Denton, E.R.E., Jarosz, J.M., Cox, T.C.S., Rohlfing, T., Goodey, J. & Hawkes, D.J. (2000). Voxel similarity measures for 3D serial MR image registration. *IEEE Transactions on Medical Imaging, 19,* 94-102.

Hollan, J., Hutchins, E., & Kirsh, D. (2000). Distributed cognition: Toward a new foundation for human-computer interaction research. *ACM Transactions on Computer-Human Interaction, 7*(2), 174-196.

Hollnagel, E., & Woods, D. (2005). *Joint Cognitive Systems: Foundations of Cognitive Systems Engineering.* Boca Rotan: CRC Press - Taylor and Francis.

Hoover, A., et al. (1996). An experimental comparison of range image segmentation algorithms. *IEEE Transactions on Pattern Analysis and Machine Intelligence, 18,* 673-689.

Hoppe, H., DeRose, T., Duchamp, T., Halstead, M., Jin, H., McDonald, J., et al. (1994). Piecewise smooth surface reconstruction. *Proceedings of SIGGRAPH '94,* (pp. 295-302).

Horkaew, P., & Yang, G. Z. (2003). Optimal deformable surface models for 3D medical image analysis. *IPMI,* 13-24.

Hsi, S., Linn, M. C., & Bell, J. E. (1997). The role of spatial reasoning in engineering and the design of spatial instruction. *Journal of Engineering Education, April,* 151-158.

Hsu, C.-C., & Ho, C.-S. (2004). A new hybrid case-based architecture for medical diagnosis. *Information Sciences, 166*(1-4), 231-247.

Huang, H. K. (2003). PACS, image management, and imaging informatics. In D. Feng, W. C. Siu, & H. J. Zhang (Eds.), *Multimedia information retrieval and management: Technological fundamentals and applications* (pp. 347-365). New York: Springer.

Huang, J., Mueller, K., Shareef, N., et al. (2000). Fast-Splats: Optimized splatting on rectilinear grids. *Proceedings of IEEE Visualization 2000,* (pp. 219-226).

Huk, T. (2006). Who benefits from learning with 3D models? The case of spatial ability. *Journal of Computer Assisted Learning, 22,* 392-404.

Humphreys, G., Houston, M., Ng, R., Frank, R., Ahern, S., Kirchner, P., & Klosowki, J. (2002). Chromium: A stream-processing framework for interactive rendering on clusters. *SIGGRAPH 2002, Proceedings of the 29th annual conference on computer graphics and interactive techniques, 21*(3), 693-702. San Antonio, TX: ACM Press.

Hutchins, E. L., Hollan, J. D., & Norman, D. A. (1985). Direct manipulation interfaces. *Human-Computer Interaction, 1,* 311-338.

Huttenlocher, J. (1962). Effects of manipulation of attributes on efficiency of concept formation. *Psychological Reports, 10,* 503-509.

Iles, V., & Sutherland, K. (2001). *Organisational change.* NCC SDO.

Ilsar, I., Joskowicz, L., Kandel, L., Matan, Y., & Liebergall, M. (2006). Navigated total knee replacement—a comprehensive clinical state of the art study. In: F. Langlotz, B. Davies, & R. Ellis (Eds.), 6th Annual Meeting of CAOS-International. *Computer-Assisted Orthopaedic Surgery* (pp. 229-231).

Ishii, H., Ben-Joseph, E., Underkoer, J., Yeung, L., Chak, D., Kanji, Z., & Piper, B. (2002). Augmented urban planning workbench: Overlaying drawings, physical models and digital simulation. *ISMAR '02: Proceedings of the International Symposium on Mixed and Augmented Reality (ISMAR'02),* (pp. 203). Washington, D.C.: IEEE Computer Society.

ITK insight segmentation and registration toolkit. (2007). http://www.itk.org.

Jain A., et al. (1992). Text segmentation using Gabor filters for automatic document processing. *Machine Vision and Applications, 5,* 169-184.

James, D., & Pai, D. (1999). ArtDefo: Accurate real-time deformable objects. *Proceedings of SIGGRAPH '99,* (pp. 65-72).

James, K. H., Humphrey, G. K., & Goodale, M. A. (2001). Manipulating and recognizing virtual objects: Where the action is. *Canadian Journal of Experimental Psychology, 55*, 111-120.

James, K. H., Humphrey, G. K., Vilis, T., Corrie, B., Baddour, R., & Goodale, M. A. (2002). "Active" and "passive" learning of three-dimensional object structure within an immersive virtual reality environment. *Behavior Research Methods, Instruments, & Computers, 34*, 383-390.

Janes, D., Schulte, M., Brodsky, E., & Block, W. (2006). Rapid vascular rendering using 4D cluster visualization. *ISMRM workshop on real-time MRI, (p. 6)*. Santa Monica, CA.

Jaramaz, B., DiGioia, A., Blackwell, M., & Nikou, C. (1998). Computer-assisted measurement of cup placement in total hip replacement. *Clinical orthopaedics and related research, 354*, 70-81.

JavaTM 2 SDK. Standard edition documentation version 1.4.2 http://java.sun.com/j2se/1.4.2/docs.

Jeffery, R., Morris, R., & Denham, R. (1991). Coronal alignment after total knee replacement. *The Journal of bone and joint surgery. British volume, 73*(5), 709-714.

JOGL. Java-openGL binding. https://jogl.dev.java.net/.

Jones, A. (2003). *Grand Research Challenges in Information Systems Final Report*. Warrenton, Virginia: Computing Research Associates (CRA).

Jones, B. (1998). A reappraisal of infrared thermal image analysis for medicine. *IEEE Trans. Medical Imaging, 17*(6), 1019-1027.

Kadaba, M., Ramakrishnan, H., Wootten, M., Gainey, J., Gorton, G., & Cochran, G. (1989). Repeatability of kinematic, kinetic, and electromyographic data in normal adult gait. *Journal of Orthopaedic Research, 7*, 849-860.

Kajiya, J., & Herzen, B. (1984). Ray tracing volume densities. *Computer Graphics, 18*(3), 165-174.

Kali, Y., & Orion, N. (1996). Spatial abilities of high school students in the perception of geologic structures. *Journal of Research in Science Teaching, 33*, 369-391.

Kalitzin, S., Staal, J., Romeny, B., & Viergever, M. (2000). Image segmentation and object recognition by Bayesian grouping. *IEEE Image Processing, Proceedings 2000 International Conference, 3*, 580-583.

Kalra, P., Magnenat Thalmann, N., Moccozet, L., Sannier, G., Aubel, A., & Thalmann, D. (1998). Real-time animation of realistic virtual humans. *IEEE Computer Graphics and Applications, 18*(5), 42-55.

Kanitsar, A., Fleischmann, D., Wegenkittl, R., Felkel, P., & Gröller, E. (2002). Cpr: Curved planar reformation. *VIS '02: Proceedings of the conference on Visualization* (pp. 37-44). IEEE Computer Society.

Kass, M., Witkin, A., & Terzopoulos, D. (1988). Active contour models. *International Journal of Computer Vision, 1*(4), 321-331.

Kaufman, A. (1991). *Volume visualization*. IEEE Computer Society Press.

Kaufman, A. (1997). Volume visualization: Principles and advances. *Proceedings of SIGGRAPH*. Los Angeles, CA.

Keehner, M., Hegarty, M., Cohen, C., Khooshabeh, P., and Montello, D. R. (in press). Spatial reasoning with interactive computer visualizations: The role of individual differences in distributed cognition. *Cognitive Science*.

Kennedy, I. (2001). *Learning from Bristol: Public inquiry into children's heart surgery at the Bristol Royal Infirmary 1984-1995*. London: The Stationery Office.

Khooshabeh, P. (2004). *Learning Spatial Relationships: Ethnography and Experiment of an Echographic Training Simulation*. Unpublished Undergraduate Honors Thesis, Primary Reader: Professor Richard Ivry. Secondary Reader: Professor Frank Tendick, University of California, Berkeley.

Khooshabeh, P. (2006). *Quality of Information: Mental Representations and Small Scale Space*. Unpublished

Masters Thesis, University of California, Santa Barbara.

Kimmel, R., Amir, A., & Bruckstein, A. (1994). Finding shortest paths on surfaces. In: P-J. Laurent (Ed.), *Curves and surfaces in geometric design,* (pp. 259-268). Wellesley, MA: A.K. Peters.

Kindlmann, G. (2002). Transfer functions in direct volume rendering: Design, interface, interaction. *Proceedings of SIGGRAPH '02 Course Notes.*

Kindlmann, G., & Durkin, J. (1998). Semi-automatic generation of transfer functions for direct volume rendering. *Proceedings of IEEE Symp. Volume Visualization,* (pp. 79-86).

Kirsh, D. & Maglio, P. (1994). On distinguishing epistemic from pragmatic action. *Cognitive Science, 18*(4), 513-549.

Kirsh, D. (1997). Interactivity and multimedia interfaces. *Instructional Science, 25,* 79-96.

Kirsh, D. (2005). Metacognition, distributed cognition and visual design. In P. Gardinfors & P. Johansson (Eds). *Cognition, Education, and Communication Technology* (pp. 147-180). Mahwah, NJ: Lawrence Erlbaum.

Knill, D. (2005). Reaching for visual cues to depth: The brain combines depth cues differently for motor control and perception. *Journal of Vision, 5*(2), 103-115.

Kniss, J., Kindlmann, G., & Hansen, C. (2001). Interactive volume rendering using multi-dimensional transfer functions and direct manipulation widgets. *Proceedings of IEEE Visualization'01 Conference,* (pp. 255-262).

Kniss, J., Kindlmann, G., & Hansen, C. (2002). Multi-dimensional transfer functions for interactive volume rendering. *IEEE Transactions on Visualization and Computer Graphics, 8*(3), 270-285

Knosp, B., Wang, S., & Ni, J. (2002). Grid-based volume rendering. *Proceedings of the International Conference of Supercomputing.* Baltimore, MD.

Kosara, R., Healey, C., Interrante, V., Laidlaw, D., & Ware, C. (2003). User studies: Why, how, and when?. *IEEE Computer Graphics and Applications,* (pp. 20-25).

Kranzlmüller, D., Heinzlreiter, P., & Volkert, J. (2003). Grid-enabled visualization with GVK. *Proceedings of 1st European Across Grids Conference 2003.* Santiago, Spain.

Kreuger, W., Bohn, C., Froehlich, B., Schueth, Strauss, H., & Wesche, G. (1995). The responsive workbench: A virtual work environment. *IEEE Computer, 28*(7), 42-48.

Krokos, M., Savenko, A., Clapworthy G.., et al. (2004). Real-time visualisation within the multimod application framework. *Proceedings of Information Visualization 04,* (pp. 21-26). IEEE Computer Society Press.

Krygier, J., Reeves, C., Cupp, J., & DiBiase, D. (1997). *Multimedia in geographic education: Design, implementation, and evaluation.* Retrieved March 16, 2006, http://horizon.unc.edu/projects/monograph/CD/Science_Mathematics/Krygier.asp

Kuhn, D., & Ho, V. (1980). Self-directed activity and cognitive development. *Journal of Applied Developmental Psychology, 1,* 119-133.

Lacroute, P., & Levoy, M. (1994). Fast volume rendering using a shear-warp factorization of the viewing transformation. *Computer Graphics, 28*(4), 451-458.

LaMar, E., Hamann, B., & Joy, K. (1999). Multi-resolution techniques for interactive texture-based volume visualization. *Proceedings of IEEE Visualization'99,* (pp. 355-361).

Lapinsky, S., Weshler, J., Mehta, S., Varkul, M., Hallett, D., & Stewart, T. (2001). Handheld computers in critical care. *Critical Care, 5*(4), 227-231.

Laszlo, J. (1996). Limit cycle control and its application to the animation of balancing and walking. *Proceeding of SIGGRAPH'96,* (pp. 155-162).

Laur, D., & Hanrahan, P. (1991). Hierarchical splating: A progressive refinement algorithm for volume rendering, *Proceedings of ACM SIGGRAPH 1991,* (pp. 285-287).

Lazarus, F., Coquillart, S., & Jancene, P. (1994). Axial deformations: An intuitive deformation technique. *Computer-Aided Design, 26*(8), 607-613.

Le Moigne, J., & Tilton, J. C. (1995). Refining image segmentation by integration of edge and region data. *IEEE Transactions on Geoscience and Remote Sensing, 33,* 605-615.

Lee, Z., Nagano, K.K., Duerk, J.L., Sodee, D.B. & Wilson, D.L. (2003). Automatic registration of MR and SPECT images for treatment planning in prostate cancer. *Academic Radiology, 10,* 673-684.

Legion. http://www.cs.virginia.edu/~legion/.

Lehmann, T. M., Guld, M. O., Keysers, D, Deselaers, T., Schubert, H., Wein B. B., & Spitzer, K. (2004). Similarity of medical images computed from global feature vectors for content-based retrieval. (LNAI, pp. 989-995).

Lehmann, T. M., Guld, M. O., Thies, C., Plodowski, B., Keysers, D., Ott, B., & Schubert, H. (2004). IRMA—Content-based image retrieval in medical applications. In *Proceedings of the 14th World Congress on Medical Informatics* (pp. 842-848).

Lehmann, T. M., Wein, B. B., & Greenspan, H. (2003). Integration of content-based image retrieval to picture archiving and communication systems. In *Proceedings of Medical Informatics Europe.* Amsterdam, The Netherlands: IOS Press.

Lehmann, T.M., Gönner, C. & Spitzer, K. (1999). Survey: Interpolation methods in medical image processing. *IEEE Transactions on Medical Imaging, 18*(11), 1049-1075.

Lester, H. & Arridge, S.R. (1999). A survey of hierarchical non-linear medical image registration. *Patter Recognition, 32,* 129-149.

Leventon, M. E., Grimson, W. E., & Faugeras, O. (2000). Statistical shape influence in geodesic active contours. *Proceedings IEEE Conference on Computer Vision and Pattern Recognition, 1*(1), 316-323.

Levitt, R., Wall, A., & Appleby, J. (1999). *The reorganized National Health Service* (6th ed.). United Kingdom: Stanley Thornes Ltd.

Levoy, M. (1998). Display of surfaces from volume data. *IEEE Computer Graphics and Applications, 8*(5), 29-37.

Lewinnek, G., Lewis, J., Tarr, R., Compere, C., & Zimmerman, J. (1978). Dislocations after total hip-replacement arthroplasties. *The Journal of bone and joint surgery. American volume, 60,* 217-220.

Li, C. H., & Yuen, P. C. (2000). Regularized color clustering in medical image database. *IEEE Transaction on Medical Imaging, 19*(11), 1150-1155.

Li, C.-T. (1998). *Unsupervised texture segmentation using multi-resolution Markov random fields.* Doctoral dissertation, University of Warwick, Coventry, UK.

Likar, B. & Pernus, F. (2001). A hierarchical approach to elastic registration based on mutual information. *Image and Vision Computing, 19,* 33-44.

Lin, K. P., Huang, S. C., Baxter, L. & Phelp, M.E. (1994). A general technique for interstudy registration of multi-function and multimodality images. *IEEE Transactions on Nuclear Science, 41,* 2850-2855.

Lipton, L. (1997). *Stereographics developers handbook.* StereoGraphics Corporation.

Liu, A., Tharp, G., French, L., Lai, S., & Stark, L. (1993). Some of what one needs to know about using head-mounted displays to improve teleoperator performance. *Robotics and Automation, IEEE Transactions on, 9*(5), 638-648.

Liu, J., Redmond, M., Brodsky, E., Alexander, A., Lu, A., Thornton, F., et al. (2006). Generation and visualization of four-dimensional MR angiography data using an undersampled 3-D projection trajectory. *IEEE Transactions on Medical Imaging, 25*(2), 148-157.

Lohman, D. F. (1988). Spatial abilities as traits, processes and knowledge. In R. J. Sternberg (Ed.), *Advances in the psychology of human intelligence* (Vol. 4, pp. 181-248). Hillsdale, NJ: Erlbaum.

Lorensen, W., & Cline, H. (1985). Marching cubes: A high resolution 3D surface construction algorithm. *Computer Graphics, 21*(4),163-169.

Lorenz, C., & Krahnstover, N. (1999). 3D statistical shape models for medical image segmentation. *International Conference on 3-D Digital Imaging and Modeling,* (pp. 414-423).

Lowe, R. K. (1999). Extracting information from an animation during complex visual learning. *European Journal of Psychology of Education. 14*, 225-244.

Lowe, R. K. (2004). Interrogation of a dynamic visualization during learning. *Learning and Instruction, 14*, 257-274.

Luft, T., Colditz, C., & Deussen, O. (2006). Image enhancement by Unsharp masking the depth buffer. *SIGGRAPH '06: Proceedings of the 33rd annual conference on Computer graphics and interactive techniques* (pp. 1206-1213). ACM Press.

Lum, E., & Ma, K. (2002). Hardware-accelerated parallel non-photorealistic volume rendering. *Proceeding of NPAR 2002 Symposium on Non-Photorealistic Animation and Rendering,* (pp. 67-75).

Maes, F., Collignon, A., Vandermeulen, D., Marchal, G., & Suetens, P. (1997). Multimodality image registration by maximisation of mutual information. *IEEE Transaction on Medical Imaging, 6*(2), 187-198.

Maes, F., Vandermeulen, D. & Suetens, P. (1999). Comparative evaluation of multiresolution optimisation strategies for multimodality image registration by maximisation of mutual information. *Medical Image Analysis, 3*(4), 373-386.

MAF—Multimod Project introduction. (2007). http://www.tecno.ior.it/multimod/.

Maillot, J., Yahia, H., & Verroust, A. (1993). Interactive texture mapping. *Computer Graphics, 27,* 27-34.

Maintz, J.B.A. & Viergever, M.A. (1998). A survey of medical image registration. *Medical Image Analysis, 2*(1), 1-36.

Maintz, J.B.A., van den Elsen, P.A. & Viergever, M.A. (1996). Evaluation of ridge seeking operators for multimodality medical image registration. *IEEE Transactions on Pattern Analysis and Machine Intelligence, 18*(4), 353-365.

Majumdar, S., Kothari, M., Augat, P., Newitt, D. C., Link, T. M., Lin, J. C., & Lang, T. (1998). High-resolution magnetic resonance imaging: Three-dimensional trabecular bone architecture and biomechanical properties. *Bone, 22,* 445-454.

Mäkelä, T., Clarysse, P., Sipilä, O., Pauna, N., Pham, Q.C., Katila, T. & Magnin, I.E. (2002). A review of cardiac image registration methods. *IEEE Transaction on Medical Imaging, 21*(9), 1011-1021.

Malladi, R., Sethian, J. A., & Vemuri, B. C. (1995). Shape modeling with front propagation: A level set approach. *IEEE Transactions on Pattern Analysis and Machine Intelligence, 17*(2), 158-75.

Malpica, N., Ortuño, J. E., & Santos, A. (2003). A multi-channel watershed-based algorithm for supervised texture segmentation. *Pattern Recognition Letters, 24,* 1545-1554.

Manal, K., & Stanhope, S. (2004). A novel method for displaying gait and clinical movement analysis data. *Gait and Posture, 20,* 222-226.

Marchak, F. M., & Marchak, L. C. (1991). Interactive versus passive dynamics and the exploratory analysis of multivariate data. *Behavior Research Methods, Instruments, & Computers, 23,* 296-300.

Marchak, F. M., & Zulager, D. D. (1992). The effectiveness of dynamic graphics in revealing structure in multivariate data. *Behavior Research Methods, Instruments, & Computers, 24,* 253-257.

Marks, J., Andalman, B., Beardsley, P., et al. (1997). Design galleries: A general approach to setting parameters for computer graphics and animation. *ACM Comp. Graphics (SIGGRAPH '94),* (pp. 389-400).

Marroquin, J. L., Vemuri, B. C., Botello, S., & Calderon, F. (2002). An accurate and efficient bayesian method for automatic segmentation of brain MRI. *Proceedings of ECCV* (pp. 560-574).

Martelli, S., Nofrini, L., Vendruscolo, P., & Visani, A. (2003). Criteria of interface evaluation for computer-assisted surgery systems. *International Journal of Medical Informatics, 72,* 35-45.

Martens, J., van Liere, R., & Kok, A. (2007). Widget manipulation revisited: A case study in modeling interactions between experimental conditions. *IPT-EGVE 2007*. The Eurographics Association.

Maurel, W., & Thalmann, D. (1999). A case study analysis on human upper limb modeling for dynamic simulation. *Journal of Computer Methods in Biomechanics and Biomechanical Engineering, 2*(1), 65-82.

Maurer, C. R. & Fitzpatrick, J. M. (1993). A review of medical image registration. In R.J. Maciunas (Ed.), *Interactive image guided neurosurgery* (pp. 17-44). Parkridge, IL: American Association of Neurological Surgeons.

Mayr, E., Moctezuma de la Barrera, J., Krismer, M., & Nogler, M. (2005). The impact of fixation type and location on tracker stability in navigated THA—a cadaver study. In: F. Langlotz, B. Davies, & R. Ellis (Eds.), 5th Annual Meeting of CAOS-International. *Computer-Assisted Orthopaedic Surgery* (pp. 314-315).

Mccloy, R., & Stone, R. (2001). Virtual reality in surgery. *British Medical Journal, 323,* 912-915.

McLeish, K., Hill, D.J.G., Atkinson, D., Blackall, J.M. & Razavi, Reza. (2002). A study of motion and deformation of the heart due to respiration. *IEEE Transactions on Medical Imaging, 21*(9), 1142-1150.

McNulty, T., & Ferlie, E. (2002*). Re-engineering healthcare: The complexities of organisational transformation.* Oxford: Oxford University Press.

Meehan, M., Whitton, M., & Brooks, F., Jr. (2002). Physiological measures of presence in stressful virtual environments. *Proceedings of ACM SIGGRAPH2002, 21,* (pp. 645-652).

Mehnert, A., & Jackway, P. (1997). An improved seeded region growing algorithm. *Pattern Recognition Letters, 18,* 1065-1071.

Melanson, B., Kelso, J., & Bowman, D. (2002). *Effects of active exploration and passive observation on spatial learning in a CAVE.* Retrieved October 2005, from http://eprints.cs.vt.edu/archive/00000602/

Merla, A., Di Donato, L., Di Luzio, S., Farina, G., Pisarri, S., Proietti, M., et al. (2002). Infrared functional imaging applied to Raynaud's phenomenon. *IEEE Engineering in Medicine and Biology Magazine, 21*(6), 73-79.

Merloz, P., Tonetti, J., Pittet, L., Coulomb, M., Lavallee, S., Troccaz, J., et al. (1998). Computer-assisted spine surgery. *Comput-Aided Surgery, 3*(6), 297-305.

Message Passing Interface. http://www.mpi-forum.org/.

Meyer, F. & Beucher, S. (1990). Morphological segmentation. *Journal of Visual Communication and Image Representation, 1*(1), 21-46.

Mitchell, S. C., Bosch, J. G., Lelieveldt, B. P. F., van de Geest, R. J., Reiber, J. H. C., & Sonka, M. (2002). 3-D active appearance models: segmentation of cardiac MR and ultrasound images. *IEEE Transactions on Medical Imaging, 21*(9), 1167-1178.

MITK—The Medical Imaging ToolKit. (2007). http://www.mitk.net.

Moga, A. N., & Gabbouj, M. (1997). Parallel image component labeling with watershed transformation. *IEEE Transactions on Pattern Analysis and Machine Intelligence, 19,* 441-450.

Moga, A. N., & Gabbouj, M. (1998). Parallel marker-based image segmentation with watershed transformation. *Journal of Parallel and Distributed Computing, 51,* 27-45.

Moghaddam, H. A., Khajoie, T. T., & Rouhi, A. H. (2003). A new algorithm for image indexing and retrieval using wavelet correlogram. In *Proceedings of the International Conference on Image Processing 2003: Vol. 3* (pp. 497-500). Barcelona, Catalonia, Spain: IEEE Press.

Mohan, R., & Nevatia, R. (1989). Using perceptual organization to extract 3-D structures. *IEEE Transactions on Pattern Analysis and Machine Intelligence, 11*(11), 1121-1139.

Molnar, S., Cox, M., Ellsworth, D., & Fuchs, H. (1994). A sorting classification of parallel rendering . *IEEE Computer Graphics and Applications, 14*(4), 23-32.

Montilla, G., Bosnjak, A., & Villegas, H. (2003). Visualización de mundos virtuales en la medicina. bioingeniería en Iberoamérica: Avances y desarrollos. In C. Müller-Karger & M. Cerrolaza (Eds.), *Centro internacional de métodos numéricos en ingeniería CIMNE* (pp. 519-545). Barcelona: .

Montilla, G., Bosnjak, A., Jara, L. I., & Villegas, H. (2005). Computer assisted planning using dependent texture mapping and multiple rendering projections in medical applications. *Proceedings from 3rd European Medical & Biological Engineering Conference and Ifmbe European Conference on Biomedical Engineering. Ifmbe* (pp. 4420-4425). Praga, Czech Republic: .

Montoya, M. G., Gil, C., & García, I. (2003). The load unbalancing problem for region growing image segmentation algorithms. *Journal of Parallel and Distributed Computing, 63,* 387-395.

Moore's Law as Explained by Intel. http://www.intel.com/research/silicon/mooreslaw.htm.

Mulder, J., & van Liere, R. (2002). The personal space station: Bringing interaction within reach. *Proceedings of VRIC 2002 Conference* (pp. 73-81).

Muller, H., Michous, N., Bandon, D., & Geissbuhler, A. (2004). A review of content-based image retrieval systems in medical applications — Clinical benefits and future directions. *International Journal of Medical Informatics, 73*(1), 1-23.

Muller, H., Rosset, A. Vallee, J.-P., & Geissbuhler, A. (2004). Comparing features sets for content-based image retrieval in a medical-case database. In *Proceedings of IS&T/SPIE Medical Imaging 2004: PACS and Imaging Informatics* (pp. 99-109).

Najarian, K. (2006). *Biomedical signal and image processing.* CRC.

National Electrical Manufacturers Association (NEMA). (2004). *Digital imaging and communications in medicine. Part 1: Introduction and overview* (NEMA Standards Pub., PS3.1).

National Electrical Manufacturers Association (NEMA). (2004). *Digital imaging and communications in medicine. Part 3: Information object definitions* (NEMA Standards Pub., PS3.3).

National Electrical Manufacturers Association (NEMA). (2004). *Digital imaging and communications in medicine. Part 5: Data structures and encoding* (NEMA Standards Pub., PS3.5).

National Electrical Manufacturers Association (NEMA). (2004). *Digital imaging and communications in medicine. Part 6: Data dictionary* (NEMA Standards Pub., PS3.6).

National Electrical Manufacturers Association (NEMA). (2004). *Digital imaging and communications in medicine. Part 10: Media storage and file format for media interchange* (NEMA Standards Pub., PS3.10).

National Electrical Manufacturers Association (NEMA). (2004). *Digital imaging and communications in medicine. Part 11: Media storage application profiles* (NEMA Standards Pub., PS3.11).

National Electrical Manufacturers Association (NEMA). (2004). *Digital imaging and communications in medicine. Part 12: Media formats and physical media for media interchange* (NEMA Standards Pub., PS3.12).

Nelder, J. & Mead, R.A. (1965). A simplex method for function minimization. *Computer Journal, 17,* 308-313.

Newlan, S., van Dam, T., Klootwijk, P., & Meij, S. (2002). Ubiquitous mobile access to real-time patient monitoring data. *Computers in Cardiology, 22-25,* 557-560.

Ng-Thow-Hing, V. (1998). Reconstruction of multiple regions of muscle fiber architecture using B-Spline solid models. *Proceedings of NACOB'98,* the Third North American Congress on Biomechanics, (pp. 219-220).

NHS Modernisation Agency. (2005). *Improvement leaders' guide: Process mapping, analysis and redesign.* London: HMSO.

NHS.UK. (2006). *About the NHS.* Retrieved April 12, 2006, from http://www.nhs.uk/england/aboutTheNHS/history/default.cmsx.

Nielson, G., & Hamann, B. (1999). Techniques for the interactive visualization of volumetric data. *Proceeding of IEEE Visualization 1999 Conference,* (pp. 45-50).

Nishibori, M. (2000). Problems and solutions in medical color imaging. In *Proceedings of the Second International Symposium on Multi-Spectral Imaging and High Accurate Color Reproduction* (pp. 9-17). Chiba, Japan: SPIE.

Nishibori, M., Tsumura, N., & Miyake, Y. (2004). Why multi-spectral imaging in medicine? *Journal of Imaging Science and Technology, 48*(2), 125-129.

Nixon, M. (2002). Feature extraction and image processing. Newnes.

Noble, R., & Clapworthy, G. (1998). Sculpting & animating in a desktop VR environment. *Proceedings of Computer Graphics International '98,* (pp. 187-195). Hanover (Germany), IEEE Computer Society Press.

Noble, R., & White, R. (2005). Visualisation of gait analysis data. *Paper presented at the International Conference on Information Visualisation.* London.

Norman, D. A. (1990). *Cognitive artifacts.* La Jolla, CA: Dept. of Cognitive Science, University of California, San Diego.

Oeltze, S., & Preim, B. (2005). Visualization of vascular structures: method, validation and rvaluation. *IEEE Transactions on Medical Imaging, 24*(4), 540-548.

Open Grid Services Infrastructure (OGSI) Version 1.0. S. Tuecke, Czajkowski K., Foster, I., Frey, J., Graham, S., Kesselman, C., Maguire, T., Sandholm, T., Vanderbilt, P., Snelling, D.; Global Grid Forum Draft Recommendation, 6/27/2003.

OpenLDAP. http://www.openldap.org.

Orion, N., Ben-Chaim, D., & Kali, Y. (1997). Relationship between earth-science education and spatial visualization. *Journal of Geoscience Education, 45,* 129-132.

Otsu, N. (1979). A threshold selection method from gray-level histograms. *IEEE Trans. Systems, Man, and Cybernetics, 9*(1), 62-66.

Ouyang, A., & Tan, Y. P (2002). A novel multi-scale spatial-color descriptor for content-based image retrieval. In *Proceedings of the 7th International Conference on Control, Automation, Robotics and Vision: Vol. 3* (pp. 1204-1209).

Oyama, L., Tannas, H., & Moulton, S. (2002). Desktop and mobile software development for surgical practice. *Journal of Pediatric Surgery, 37*(3), 477-481.

Pallotta, S., Gilardi, M.C., Bettinardi, V., Rizzo, G., Landoni, C., Striano, G., Masi, R., & Fazio, F. (1995). Application of a surface matching image registration technique to the correlation of cardiac studies in positron emission tomography by transmission images. *Physics in Medicine and Biology, 40,* 1695-1708.

Partridge, M., & Calvo, R. A. (1998). Fast dimensionality reduction and simple PCA. *Intelligent Data Analysis, 2*(1-4), 203-214.

Pattichis, C., Kyriacou, E., Voskarides, S., Pattichis, M., Istepanian, R., & Schizas, C. (2002). Wireless telemedicine systems: An overview. *IEEE Antenna's and Propogation Magazine, 44*(2), 143-153.

Pedersen, H. (1995). Decorating implicit surface. *Proceedings of the SIGGRAPH'95,* (pp. 291-300).

Pekar, V., Wiemker, R., & Hempel, D. (2001). Fast detection of meaningful isosurfaces for volume data visualization. In: T. Ertl, K. Joy, & A. Varshney (Eds.), *Proceedings of IEEE Visualization 2001,* (pp. 223-230).

Pellizari, C.A., Chen, G.T.Y., Spelbring, D.R., Weichselbaum, R.R. & Chen, C.T. (1989). Accurate three-dimensional registration of CT, PET, and/or MR images of the brain. *Computer Assisted Tomography, 13*(1), 20-26.

Penny, G.P., Weese, J., Little, J.A., Desmedt, P., Hill, D.L.G. & Hawkes, D.J. (1998). A comparison of similarity measures for use in 2D-3D medical image registration. *IEEE Transactions on Medical Imaging, 17,* 586-595.

Pentland, A. P., & Sclaroff, S. (1991). Closed-form solutions for physically based modeling and recognition. *IEEE Transactions on Pattern Analysis and Machine Intelligence, 13*(7), 715-729.

Peruch, P., Vercher, J.L., & Gauthier, G. M. (1995). Acquisition of spatial knowledge through visual exploration of simulated environments. *Ecological Psychology, 7*(1), 1-20.

Petrou, M. (2006). *Image processing: Dealing with texture.* John Wiley and sons Ltd.

Pfautz, J. (2000). *Depth perception in computer graphics.* Doctoral dissertation, University of Cambridge, UK.

Pfister, H., Lorensen, B., Bajaj, C., Kindlmann, G., Schroeder, W., Sobeierajski A., et al. (2001). The transfer function bake-off. *IEEE Computer Graphics and Applications,* 16-22.

Pham, D., Xu, C., & Prince, J. (1999). *A survey of current methods in medical image segmentation.* Technical Report JHU/ECE 99-01, Department of Electrical and Computer Engineering, John Hopkins University, Baltimore, MD. Retrieved May 16, 2007, from http://www.rfai.li.univtours.fr/webrfai/chercheurs/rousselle/Docu-m/pdf /p124r.pdf.

Philbeck, J. W., Klatzky, R. L., Behrmann, M., Loomis, J. M., & Goodridge, J. (2001). Active control of locomotion facilitates nonvisual navigation. *Journal of Experimental Psychology: Human Perception and Performance, 27,* 141-153.

Picard, F., DiGioia, A., Moody, J., Martinek, V., Fu, F., Rytel, M., et al. (2001). Accuracy in tunnel placement for ACL reconstruction. Comparison of traditional arthroscopic and computer-assisted navigation techniques. *Comput-Aided Surgery, 6*(5), 279-89

Pierrynowski, M. (1995). Analytic representation of muscle line of action and geometry. In: P. Allard, I. Stokes, J. Blanchi, (Eds.), *Three-dimensional analysis of human movement.* Human Kineticss, (chap. 11, pp. 215-256).

Plassmann, P., & Ring, E. (1997). An open system for the acquisition and evaluation of medical thermological images. *European Journal of Thermology, 7,* 216-220.

Platt, S., & Badler, N. (1981). Animating facial expressions. *Computer Graphics, 15*(3), 245-252.

Plaza, A., Martinez, P., Perez, R., & Plaza, J. (2002). Spatial/spectral endmember extraction by multidimensional morphological operations. *IEEE Transactions on Geoscience and Remote Sensing, 40*(9), 2025-2041.

Plaza, A., Martinez, P., Perez, R., & Plaza, J. (2004). A new approach to mixed pixel classification of hyperspectral imagery based on extended morphological profiles. *Pattern Recognition, 37,* 1097-1116.

Pluim, J., Maintz, J., & Viergever, M. (2003). Mutual information-based registration of medical images: A survey. *IEEE Transactions on Medical Imaging, 22,* 986-1004.

Pluim, J.P.W., Maintz, J.B.A. & Viergever, M.A. (2001). Mutual information matching in multiresolution contexts. *Image and Vision Computing, 19*(1-2), 45-52.

Poon, C., & Braun, M. (1997). Image segmentation by a deformable contour model incorporating region analysis. *Physics in Medicine and Biology, 42,* 1833-1841.

Powell, M.J.D. (1964). An efficient method for finding the minimum of a function of several variables without calculating derivatives. *Computuer Journal, 7,* 155-163.

Qi, W., Taylor, R., Healey, C., & Martens, J. (2006). A comparison of immersive HMD, fish tank VR and fish tank with haptics displays for volume visualization. *Proceedings of the 3rd symposium on Applied perception in graphics and visualization 2006,* (pp. 51-58).

Qian, G.., Sural, S., Gu, Y., & Pramanik, S. (2004). Similarity between Euclidean and cosine angle distance for nearest neighbor queries. In *Proceedings of 2004 ACM Symposium on Applied Computing* (pp. 1232-1237). Nicosia, Cyprus: ACM Press.

Qiu, Y., Shi, J., Zhao, Y., & Chen, W. (2005). GVis: An architecture for grid-enabled interactive parallel visualization. *Proceedings of the 5th Conference on Virtual Reality and Visualization 2005* (CCVRV'05). Bejing, China (in Chinese). *Journal of Computer Research and Development, 42,* Supplement A, 612-617.

Rajapakse, J., Giedd, J., & Rapaport, J. (1997). Statistical approach to segmentation of single-channel cerebral

MR images. *IEEE Transactions on Medical Imaging, 16*, 176-186.

Razzaque, S., & Whitton, M. (2001). Redirected walking. *Proceedings of Eurographics 2001*, (pp. 289-294).

Redmond, M., Brodsky, E., Hu, Y., Grist, T., Schulte, M., & Block, W. (2004). The 4D cluster visualization project. *Proceedings of the SPIE medical imaging 2004: Visualization, image-guided procedures, and display, 5367*, 28-38. San Diego, CA: *SPIE*.

Rencher, A. C. (1998). *Multi-variate statistical inference and applications*. New York: John Wiley & Sons.

Revet, B. (1997). *DICOM cookbook for implementations in modalities* (Tech. Rep.). Philips Medical Systems.

Richards, J., & Jia, X. (1999). *Remote sensing digital image analysis* (3rd ed). Berlin: Springer.

Richardson, B. L., Wuillemin, D. B., & MacKintosh, G. J. (1981). Can passive touch be better than active touch? A comparison of active and passive tactile maze learning. *British Journal of Psychology, 72*, 353-362.

Rieber, L. P., Tzeng, S-C., & Tribble, K. (2004). Discovery learning, representation, and explanation within a computer-based simulation: Finding the right mix. *Learning and Instruction, 14*, 307-323.

Riva, G. (2003). Review paper: Medical applications of virtual environments. *Year Book of Medical Informatics*, 159-169.

Robb, R., Greenleaf, J., Ritman, E., et al. (1974). Three-dimensional visualization of the intact thorax and contents: A technique for cross-sectional reconstruction from multi-planar x-ray views. *Comput. Biomedl Res, 7*, 395-419.

Rocchio, J. J. (1971). Relevance feedback in information retrieval. In G. Salton (Ed.), *The SMART retrieval system-experiments in automatic document processing* (pp.313-323). Englewood Cliffs, NJ: Prentice Hall.

Roche, A., Malandain, G. & Ayache, N. (2000). Unifying maximum likelihood approaches in medical image registration. *International Journal of Imaging Systems and Technology, 11*, 71-80.

Rochford, K. (1985). Spatial learning disabilities and underachievement among university anatomy students. *Medical Education, 19*, 13-26.

Roettger, S., Bauer, M., & Stamminger, M. (2005). Spatialized transfer functions. *Proceedings IEEE/Euro-Graphics Symposium on Visualization*, (pp. 271-278).

Rohlfing, T. & Maurer, C.C. (2003). Nonrigid image registration in shared-memory multiprocessor environments with application to brains, breasts, and bees. *IEEE Transactions on Information Technology in Biomedicine, 7*(1), 16-25.

Rohr, K. (2000). Elastic registration of multimodal medical images: A survey. *Auszug aus: Kunstliche Intelligenz, Heft*.

Ropinski, T., Steinicke, F., Hinrichs, K. (2006). Visually supporting depth perception in angiography imaging. *Proceedings of the 6th International Symposium on Smart Graphics* (pp. 93-104). Springer.

Rosenthal, M., & Wolford, R. (2000). Resident procedure and resuscitation tracking using a palm computer. *Academic Emergency Medicine, 7*(10), 1171.

Rosset, A., Ratib, O., Geissbuhler, A., & Vallee, J. P. (2002). Integration of a multimedia teaching and reference database in a PACS environment. *Radiographics, 22*(6), 1567-1577.

Rui, Y., & Huang, T. (2002). Learning based relevance feedback in image retrieval. In A. C. Bovik, C. W. Chen, & D. Goldfof (Eds.), *Advances in image processing and understanding: A festschrift for Thomas S. Huang* (pp. 163-182). New York: World Scientific Publishing.

Rusinkiewicz S., Burns, M., & DeCarlo, D. (2006). Exaggerated shading for depicting shape and detail. *SIGGRAPH '06: Proceedings of the 33rd annual conference on Computer graphics and interactive techniques* (pp. 1199-1205). ACM Press.

Russell, G., & Miles, R. (1987). Display and perception of 3D space filling data. *Applied Optics, 26*(6), 973-982.

Russell-Gebbett, J. (1985). Skills and strategies: Pupils' approaches to three-dimensional problems in biology. *Journal of Biological Education, 19*, 293-298.

Saito, T., & Takahashi, T. (1990). Comprehensible rendering of 3-D shapes. *SIGGRAPH '90: Proceedings of the 17th annual conference on Computer graphics and interactive techniques* (pp. 197-206). ACM Press.

Sarkar, S., & Boyer, K. L. (1994). Computing perceptual organization in computer vision, *World Scientific Series on Machine Perception and Artificial Intelligence.* Singapore: World Scientific.

Savenko, A., Van Sint Jan, S., & Clapworthy, G. (1999). A biomechanics-based model for the animation of human locomotion. *Proceedings of GraphiCon '99*, (pp. 82-87). Moscow: Dialog-MGU Press.

Schaefer, G., Tait, R., & Zhu, S. (2006). Overlay of thermal and visual medical images using skin detection and image registration. *28th IEEE Int. Conference Engineering in Medicine and Biology,* (pp. 965-967).

Scheepers, F., Parent, R., Carlson, W., & May, S. (1997). Anatomy-based modeling of the human musculature. *Proceedings of SIGGRAPH'97,* (pp. 163-172).

Schmidt, R., Montani, S., Bellazzi, R., Portinale, L., & Gierl, L. (2001). Cased-based reasoning for medical knowledge-based systems. *International Journal of Medical Informatics, 64*(2-3), 355-367.

Schroeder, W., Avila, L., & Hoffman, W. (2000). Visualizing with VTK: A tutorial. *IEEE Comput. Graph. App., 20*(5), 20-27.

Schroeder, W., Martin, K., & Lorensen, B. (Ed.). (2002). *The visualization toolkit an object-oriented approach to 3D graphics* (3rd ed.). Kitware.

Schulze, J., Kraus, M., Lang, U., et al. (2003). Integrating pre-integration into the Shear-Warp Algorithm. *Proceedings of the 3rd International Workshop on Volume Graphics,* (pp. 109-118).

Schulze, J., Zeleznik, J., Forsberg, A., & Laidlaw, D. (2005). Characterizing the effect of level of immersion on a 3D marking task. *Proceedings of HCI International,* (pp. 447-452). HCI International.

Schutte, L., Narayanan, U., Stout, J., Selber, P., & Gage, J. (2000). An index for quantifying deviations from normal gait. *Gait and Posture, 11,* 25-31.

Schwan, S. & Riempp, R. (2004). The cognitive benefits of interactive videos: learning to tie nautical knots. *Learning and Instruction, 14,* 293-305.

Schwartz, D. L. & Holton, D. L. (2000). Tool use and the effect of action on the imagination. *Journal of Experimental Psychology: Learning Memory and Cognition, 26,* 1655-1665.

Sebe, N., & Lew, M. S. (2002). Texture features for content-based retrieval. In M. S. Lew (Ed.), *Principles of visual information retrieval* (pp.51-85), London: Springer.

Sederberg, T., & Parry, S. (1986). Free-form deformation of solid geometric models. *Computer Graphics, 20,* 151-160.

Seinstra, F. J., Koelma, D., & Geusebroek, J. M. (2002). A software architecture for user transparent parallel image processing. *Parallel Computing, 28,* 967-993.

Semwal, S., & Hallauer, J. (1994). Biomechanical modeling: Implementation line-of-action algorithm for human muscles and bones using generalized cylinders. *Computers & Graphics, 18*(1), 105-112.

Serdobolskii, V. (2000). *Multivariate statistical analysis: A high-dimensional approach.* London: Kluwer Academic Publishers.

Serif, T., Ghinea, G., & Frank, A. (2005). A ubiquitous approach for visualizing back pain data. *Proceedings of the International Conference on Computational Science and its Applications* (ICCSA 2005), (pp. 1018-1027).

Shafarenko, L., Petrou, M., & Kittler, J. Automatic watershed segmentation of randomly textured color images. *IEEE Transactions on Image Processing, 6,* 1530-1544.

Shah, B., Raghavan, V., & Dhatric, P. (2004). Efficient and effective content-based image retrieval using space transformation. *Proceedings of the 10th International Multimedia Modelling Conferenc* (p. 279). Brisbane, Australia. IEEE Press.

Shankar, B. U., Murthy, C. A., & Pal, S. K. (1998). A new gray level based Hough transform for region extraction, an application to IRS images, *Pattern Recognition Letters*, 19, 197-204.

Shen, H., Liang, L., Shao, M., & Qing, S. (2004). Tracing based segmentation for labeling of individual rib structures in chest CT volume data. *Proceedings of the 7th International Conference on Medical Image Computing and Computer Assisted Intervention* (pp. 967-974).

Shen, H., Shi, Y., & Peng, Z. (2005). Applying prior knowledge in the segmentation of 3D complex anatomic structures. *Computer Vision for Biomedical Image Applications: Current Techniques and Future Trends, An International Conference on Computer Vision Workshop, Lecture Notes of Computer Science, 3765* (pp.189-199). Beijing, China.

Shi, J., & Cai, W. (1995). *Algorithms and systems of scientific visualization.* Science Press (in Chinese).

Shi, J., Zhao, Y., Qiu, Y., & Chen, W. (2004). A case study on grid-enabled visualization. *Journal of Computer Research and Development, 41*(2), 2231-2236 (in Chinese).

Shneiderman, B. (1983). Direct manipulation: A step beyond programming languages. *Computer, 16*(8), 57-69.

Shreiner, D., Woo, M., Neider, J., & Davis, T. (Ed.). (2005). *OpenGL programming guide: The official guide to learning OpenGL, version 2.* Addison-Wesley.

Shyu, C., Brodley, C., Kak, A., Kosaka, A., Aisen, A., & Broderick, L. (1999). ASSERT: A physician-in-the-loop content-based image retrieval system for HRCT image databases. *Computer Vision and Image Understanding, 75*(1/2), 111-132.

Shyu, C.-R., Pavlopoulou, C., Kak, A. C., Brodly, C. E., & Broderick, L. (2002). Using human perceptual categories for content-based retrieval from a medical image database. *Computer Vision and Image Understanding, 88*(3), 119-151.

Simple Object Access Protocol (SOAP). http://www.w3.org/TR/soap/.

Sinha, U., & Kangarloo, H. (2002). Principal component analysis for content-based image retrieval. *RadioGraphics, 22*, 1271-1289.

Siston, R., & Delp, S. (2006). Evaluation of a new algorithm to determine the hip joint center. *Journal of Biomechanics, 39,* 125-130.

Slabaugh, G., & Unal, G. (2005). Active polyhedron: Surface evolution theory applied to deformable meshes. *Conference on Computer Vision and Pattern Recognition.*

Smeaton, A. F., & Over, P. (2003). TRECVID: Benchmarking the effectiveness of information retrieval tasks on digital video. In *International Conference on Image and Video Retrieval*, 18-27.

Smeulders, A. W. M., Worring, M., Santini, S., Gupta, A., & Jain, R. (2000). Content-based image retrieval at the end of the early years. *IEEE Transactions on Pattern Analysis and Machine Intelligence, 22*(12), 1349-1380.

Soille, P. (1996). Morphological partitioning of multispectral images. *Journal of Electronic Imaging, 5*, 252-265.

Soille, P. (2003). *Morphological image analysis, principles and applications* (2nd ed.). Berlin: Springer.

Sommers, K., Hesler, J., & Bostick, J. (2001). Little guys make a big splash: PDA projects at Virginia Commonwealth University. *Proceedings of the 29th annual ACM SIGUCCS conference on User services,* (pp. 190-193).

Sonka, M., Hlavac, V., & Boyle, R. (1998). *Image processing, analysis, and machine vision* (2nd ed.). PWS Publishing.

Spence, R. (2001). *Information visualization.* Essex: ACM Press.

Squire, D. M., Muller, H., Muller, W., Marchand-Maillet, S., & Pun, T. (2001). Design and evaluation of a content-based image retrieval system. In S. M. Rahman (Ed.), *Design and management of multimedia information systems: Opportunities and challenges* (pp. 125-151). Hershey, PA: Idea Group Publishing.

Squire, D. M., Muller, W., Muller, H., & Pun, T. (2000). Content-based query of image databases: inspirations from text retrieval, *Pattern Recognition Letters, 21*(13-14), 1193-1198.

Steenblik, R. (1987). The chromostereoscopic process: A novel single image stereoscopic process. *Proceedings of SPIE - True 3D Imaging Techniques and Display Technologies.*

Stindel, E., Gil, D., Briard, J., Merloz, P., Dubrana, F., & Lefevre, C. (2005). Detection of the center of the hip joint in computer-assisted surgery: An evaluation study of the Surgetics algorithm. *Computer-Aided Surgery, 10*(3), 133-139.

Stoeckl, B., Nogler, M., Rosiek, R., Fischer, M., Krismer, M., & Kessler, O. (2004). Navigation improves accuracy of rotational alignment in total knee arthroplasty. *Clinical Orthopaedics and Related Research, 426,* 180-186.

Straka, M., Cervenansky, M., Cruz, A., Kochl, A., Sramek, M., Gröller, E., & Fleischmann, D. (2004). The vesselglyph: Focus & context visualization in ct-angiography. *VIS '04: Proceedings of the conference on Visualization* (pp. 385-392). IEEE Computer Society.

Subsol, G. (1999). Crest lines for curve-based warping. *Brain Warping* (pp. 241-262). San Diego: Academic.

Subsol, G., Thirion, J.-P. & Ayache, N. (1998). A scheme for automatically building three-dimensional morphometric anatomical atlases: application to a skull atlas. *Medical Image Analysis, 2*(1), 37-60.

Suckling, J., Parker, J., Dance, D. R., Astley, S., Hutt, I., Boggis, C. R. M., Ricketts, I., Stamatakis, E., Cerneaz, N., Kok, S.-L., Taylor, P., Betal, D., & Savage, J. (1994). The mammographic image analysis society digital mammogram database. In *Proceedings of the 2nd International Workshop on Digital Mammography*, 375-378.

Sun, J., & Gu, D. (2004). Bayesian image segmentation based on an inhomogeneous hidden Markov random field. *Proceedings of the 17th International Conference on Pattern Recognition* (pp. 596-599).

Suri, J. S., Liu, K., Singh, S., Laxminarayan, S.N., Zeng, X., & Reden, L. (2002). Shape recovery algorithm using level sets in 2-D/3-D medical imagery, a state-of-the-art review. *IEEE Transactions on Information Technology in Biomedicine, 6*(1), 8-28.

Sutherland, I. (1968). A head-mounted three-dimensional display. *Proceeding of the Fall Joint Computer Conference,* (pp. 757-764).

Swain, M. J., & Ballard, D. H. (1991). Color Indexing. *International Journal of Computer Vision, 7*(1), 11-32.

Tait, R., Schaefer, G., Hopgood, A., & Nolle, L. (2006). Automated visual inspection using a distributed blackboard architecture. *Int. Journal of Simulation: Systems, Science & Technology, 7*(3), 12-20.

Tait, R., Schaefer, G., Hopgood, A., & Zhu, S. (2006). Efficient 3-D medical image registration using a distributed blackboard system. *28th IEEE Int. Conference Engineering in Medicine and Biology,* (pp. 3045-3048).

Tamai, S. (1999). The color of digital imaging in pathology and cytology. *Proceedings of the First Symposium of the "Color" of Digital Imaging in Medicine.* Tokyo, Japan: SPIE.

Tao, D., & Tang, X. (2004). Random sampling based SVM for relevance feedback image retrieval. In *The IEEE Computer Society Conference on Computer Vision and Pattern Recognition 2004,* 647-652. Washington, DC: IEEE Press.

Tarini, M., Cignoni, P., & Montani, C. (2006). Ambient occlusion and edge cueing to enhance real-time molecular visualization. *IEEE Transactions on Visualization and Computer Graphics, 12*(6).

Taylor, R., Chen, J., Okimoto, S., Llopis-Artime, N., Chi, V., Brooks, F., et al. (1997). Pearls found on the way to the ideal interface for scanned-probe microscopes. *Proceedings of Proceedings of IEEE Visualization,* (pp. 467-470).

Taylor, R., Hudson, T., Seeger, A., Weber, H., Juliano, J., & Helser, A. (2001). VRPN: A device-independent, network-transparent VR peripheral system. *VRST'01: Proceedings of the ACM symposium on Virtual reality software and technology,* (pp. 55-61).

Tenginakai, S., Lee, J., & Machiraju, R. (2001). Salient iso-surface detection with model-independent statistical signatures. In: T. Ertl, K. Joy, & A. Varshney (Eds.), *Proceedings of IEEE Visualization 2001,* (pp. 231-238).

Terzopoulos, D. & Metaxas, D. (1991). Dynamic 3D models with local and global deformations: Deformable superquadrics. *IEEE Trans. PAMI, 13*(7), 703-714.

Terzopoulos, D., & Waters, K. (1990). Physically-based facial modeling, analysis and animation. *Journal of Visualization and Computer Animation, 1*(2), 73-80.

The Globus Projects. http://www.globus.org.

The Open Grid Services Architecture. http://www.globus.org/ogsa/.

Thévenaz P., Blu, T. & Unser, M. (2000). Image interpolation and resampling. In I. Bankman (Ed.), *Handbook of medical imaging: Processing and analysis* (pp. 393-418). Academic Press.

Thévenaz, P. & Unser, M. (2000). Optimization of mutual information for multiresolution registration. *IEEE Transaction on Image Processing, 9*(12), 2083-2099.

Thirion, J.P. (1998). Image matching as a diffusion process: An analogy with Maxwell's demons. *Med. Image Anal., 2*, 243-260.

Thompson, P. & Toga, A.W. (1996). A surface-based technique for warping three-dimensional images of the brain. *IEEE Transaction on Medical Imaging, 15*(4), 402-417.

Tilton, J. C. (1999). A recursive PVM implementation of an image segmentation algorithm with performance results comparing the HIVE and the Cray T3E. In *Proceedings of the 7th Symposium on the Frontiers of Massively Parallel Computation*, Annapolis, MD.

Tomov, S., Bennett, R., McGuigan, M., Peskin, A., Smith, G., & Spiletic, J. (2004). Application of interactive parallel visualization for commodity-based clusters using visualization APIs. *Computers & Graphics, 28*(2), 273-278.

Tourassi, G. D. (1999). Journey toward computer-aided diagnosis: Role of image texture analysis. *Radiology*, 317-320.

Tria, A. (2006). The evolving role of navigation in minimally invasive total knee arthroplasty. *The American journal of orthopedics, 35*(7), 18-22.

Tsai, A., Yezzi, A., Wells, W., Tempany, C., Tucker, D., Fan, A., et al. (2003). A shape-based approach to the segmentation of medical imagery using level sets. *IEEE Transactions on Medical Imaging, 22*(2), 137-154.

Turner, P., Milne, G., Kubitscheck, M., Penman, I., & Turner, S. (2005). Implementing a wireless network of PDAs in a hospital setting. *Personal and Ubiquitous Computing, 9*(4), 209-217.

Turner, R. & Ordidge, R.J. (2000). Technical challenges of functional magnetic resonance imaging: The biophysics and technology behind a reliable neuroscientific tool for mapping the human brain. *IEEE Engineering in Medicine and Biology*, 42-54.

Turner, R., & Thalmann, D. (1993). The Elastic Surface Layer Model for animated character construction. In: N. Magnenat-Thalmann & D. Thalmann, (Eds.), *Communicating with virtual worlds*, (pp. 399-412). Springer Verlag.

UDDI.org. http://www.uddi.org/.

Udupa, J. K., Saha, P. K., & Lotufo, R. A. (2002). Relative fuzzy connectedness and object definition: Theory, algorithms, and applications in image segmentation. *IEEE Transactions on Pattern Analysis and Machine Intelligence, 24*(11), 1485-1500.

Udupa, J., & Herman G. (1989). Volume rendering vs. surface rendering. *Communication of ACM, 32*, 1344-1366.

Uematsu, S. (1985). Symmetry of skin temperature comparing one side of the body to the other. *Thermology, 1*, 4-7.

Ullmer, B., & Ishii, H. (2001). Emerging frameworks for tangible user interfaces. In: J. Carroll (Ed.), *Human-computer interaction in the new millennium*, (pp. 579-601). Addison-Wesley.

Ullmer, B., Ishii, H., & Glas, D. (1998). Mediablocks: Physical containers, transports, and controls for online media. *Proceedings of SIGGRAPH '98*, (pp. 379-386).

van 'Bemmel, J. H., & Musen, M. A. (Eds.) (1997). *Handbook of medical informatics*. Heidelberg, Germany: Springer-Verlag.

van den Elsen, P.A., Pol, E.J.D. & Viergever, M.A. (1993). Medical image matching—A review with classification. *IEEE Engineering in Medicine and Biology, 12,* 26-39.

van Herk, M. & Kooy, H.M. (1994). Automatic three-dimensional correlation of CT-CT, CT-MRI, and CT-SPECT using chamfer matching. *Medical Physics, 21*(7), 1163-1177.

van Liere, R., & Mulder, J. (2003). Optical tracking using projective invariant marker pattern properties. *Proceedings of the IEEE Virtual Reality Conference 2003,* (pp. 191-198).

Van Sint Jan, S., Clapworthy, G., & Rooze, M. (1998). Visualization of combined motions in human joints. *IEEE Computer Graphics & Applications, 18*(6), 10-14.

Van Sint Jan, S., Salvia, P., Clapworthy, G., & Rooze, M. (1999). Joint-motion visualization using both medical imaging and 3D-electrogoniometry. *Proceedings of the 17ᵗʰ Congress International Society of Biomechanics.* Calgary (Canada).

Van Sint Jan, S., Viceconti, M., & Clapworthy, G. (2004). Modern visualisation tools for research and education in biomechanics. *Proceedings of Information Visualization 04,* (pp. 9-14). IEEE Computer Society Press.

Veenland, J. F., Grashuis, J. L., Weinans, H., Ding, M., & Vrooman, H. A. (2002). Suitability of texture features to assess changes in trabecular bone architecture. *Pattern Recognition Letters, 23*(4), 395-403.

Veltkamp, R. C., & Hagedoorn, M. (2002). State of the art in shape matching. In M. S. Lew (Ed.), *Principles of visual information retrieval* (pp.87-119), London: Springer.

Viceconti, M., Leardini, A., Zannoni, C., et al. (2004). The multi-mod application framework. *Proceedings of Information Visualization 04,* (pp. 15-20). IEEE Computer Society Press.

Viceconti, M., Zannoni, C., Testi, D., & Cappello, A. (1999). CT data sets surface extraction for biomechanical modeling of long bones. *Computer Methods and Programs in Biomedicine, 59,* 159-166.

Vincent, L. (1993). Morphological grayscale reconstruction in image analysis: Applications and efficient algorithms. *IEEE Transactions on Image Processing, 2,* 176-201.

Vincent, L., & Soille, P. (1991). Watersheds in digital spaces: An efficient algorithm based on immersion simulations. *IEEE Transactions on Pattern Analysis and Machine Intelligence, 13*(6), 583-598.

Viola, P. & Wells, W.M. (1995). Alignment by maximization of mutual information. *The Fifth International Conference on Computer Vision* (pp. 16-23).

Viola, P., & Wells, W. (1997). Alignment by maximization of mutual information, *International Journal of Computer Vision, 24,* 137-154.

VolumePro. (2007). http://www.terarecon.com.

VTK—the visualization toolkit. (2007). http://public.kitware.com/VTK/index.php.

Walker, K. N., Cootes, T. F., & Taylor, C. J. (2002). Automatically building appearance models from image sequences using salient features. *Image and Vision Computing, 20*(5-6), 435-440.

Wang, H.-C., Li, T.-Y., & Chang, C.-Y. (2006). A web-based tutoring system with styles-matching strategy for spatial geometric transformation. *Interacting with Computers, 18*(3), 331-355.

Wang, H.S., Feng, D., Yeh, E. & Huang, S. C. (2001). Objective assessment of image registration results using statistical confidence intervals. *IEEE Transactions on Nuclear Science, 48,* 106-110.

Wang, R. X.-F., & Simons, D. J. (1999). Active and passive scene recognition across views. *Cognition, 70,* 191-210.

Wang, X. & Feng, D. (to be published in Vol.3, 2005). Automatic elastic medical image registration based on image intensity. *International Journal of Image and Graphic (IJIG),* World Scientific.

Wanger, L., Ferwerda, J., & Greenberg, D. (1992). Perceiving spatial relationships in computer-generated images. *IEEE Computer Graphics and Applications, 12*(3), 44-51, 54-58.

Ware, C. (2004). *Information visualization.* San Francisco, CA: Morgan Kaufmann.

Ware, C., & Franck, G. (1996). Evaluating stereo and motion cues for visualizing information nets in three dimensions. *ACM Trans. Graph., 15*(2), 121-140.

Ware, C., Arthur, K., & Booth, K. (1993). Fish tank virtual reality. *Proceedings of CHI 93,* (pp. 37-42).

Waters, K. (1987). A muscle model for animating three-dimensional facial expression. *Computer Graphics, 21*(4), 17-24.

Web Service Resource Framework. http://www.globus.org/wsrf/.

Web Service. http://www.w3.org/2002/ws/.

Web Services Description Language. http://www.w3.org/TR/wsdl/.

Web Services Flow Language (WSFL 1.0). (2001). Frank Leymann, IBM Software Group. http://www-306.ibm.com/software/solutions/webservices/pdf/WSFL.pdf.

Wei, C.-H, & Li, C.-T. (2005). Design of content-based multimedia retrieval. In M. Pagani (Ed.), *Encyclopedia of multimedia technology and networking* (pp. 116-122). Hershey, PA: Idea Group Reference.

Welch, W., & Witkin, A. (1992). Variational surface modeling. *Computer Graphics, 26,* 157-166

Wernecke, J. (1994). *The inventor mentor: Programming object-oriented 3D graphics with open inventor, release 2.* Addison-Wesley.

West, J., & Maurer, C. (2004). Designing optically tracked instruments for image-guided surgery. *IEEE Transactions on Medical Imaging, 23*(5), 533-545.

Westermann, R., & Ertl, T. (1998). Efficiently using graphics hardware in volume rendering applications. *Proceedings of SIGGRAPH 98,* (pp. 169-177).

Westermann, R., & Sevenich, B. (2001). Accelerated volume ray-casting using texture mapping. *Proceedings of IEEE Visualization 2001,* (pp. 271- 278).

Westover, L. (1990). Footprint evaluation for volume rendering. *Proceedings of SIGGRAPH'90. ACM SIGGRAPH Computer Graphics, 24*(4), 367-376.

Wexler, M., Kosslyn, S. M. & Berthoz, A. (1998). Motor processes in mental rotation. *Cognition, 68,* 77-94.

Wiecek, B., Zwolenik, S., Jung, A., & Zuber, J. (1999). Advanced thermal, visual and radiological image processing for clinical diagnostics. *21ˢᵗ IEEE Int. Conference on Engineering in Medicine and Biology,* (p. 1108).

Wilhelms, J., & Gelder, A. (1997). Anatomically-based modeling. *Proceedings of SIGGRAPH'97,* (pp. 173-180).

Wilson, M. (2002). Six views of embodied cognition. *Psychonomic Bulletin and Review, 9,* 625-636.

Wilson, P. N. (1999). Active exploration of a virtual environment does not promote orientation or memory for objects. *Environment and Behavior, 31,* 752-763.

Wilson, P. N., Foreman, N., Gillett, R., & Stanton, D. (1997). Active versus passive processing of spatial information in a computer simulated environment. *Ecological Psychology, 9,* 207-222.

Winnemöller, H., Olsen, S., & Gooch B. (2006). Real-time video abstraction. *SIGGRAPH '06: Proceedings of the 33ʳᵈ annual conference on Computer graphics and interactive techniques* (pp. 1221-1226). ACM Press.

Wohlschlager, A., & Wohlschlager, A. (1998). Mental and manual rotation. *Journal of Experimental Psychology: Human Perception and Performance, 24,* 397-412.

Wong, S. T. C. (1998). CBIR in medicine: Still a long way to go. In *Proceedings of the IEEE Workshop on Content-Based Access of Image and Video Libraries,* 114. Santa Barbara, CA: IEEE Press.

Wong, S., & Hoo, K. S. (2002). Medical imagery. In V. Castelli, & L. D. Bergman (Eds.), *Image databases:*

Search and retrieval of digital imagery (pp. 83-105). New York: John Wiley & Sons.

Woods, R., Mazziotta, J., & Cherry, S. (1993). MRI-PET registration with an automated algorithm. *Journal of Computer Assisted Tomography, 17,* 536-546.

Wu, Z., & Leahy, R. (1992). Image segmentation via edge contour finding. *IEEE Computer Society Conference on Computer Vision and Pattern Recognition* (pp. 613-619).

Xiao, H. & Jackson, I.T. (1995). Surface matching: Application in poat-surgical/post-treatment evaluation. In H.U. Lemke, K. Inamura, C.C. Jaffe & M.W. Vannier (Eds.), *Computer assisted radiology* (pp. 804-811). Berlin: Springer-Verlag.

Yang, J., Staib, H.S., & Duncan, J.S. (2004). Neighbor-constrained segmentation with level set based 3-D deformable models. *IEEE Transactions on Medical Imaging, 23*(8), 940-948.

Young, M., Landy, M., & Maloney, L. (1993). A perturbation analysis of depth perception from combinations of texture and motion cues. *Journal of Vision Research, 33*(18), 2685-2696.

Yu, H., Li, M., Zhang, H.-J., & Feng, J. (2002). Color texture moments for content-based image retrieval. In *Proceedings of the International Conference on Image Processing 2002: Vol. 3* (pp. 929-932).

Zelkowitz, M. V., Wallace, D.R. (1998). Experimental models for validating technology. *IEEE Computer, 31*(5), 23-31.

Zhai, S. (1995). *Human performance in six degrees of freedom input control.* Doctoral Thesis, University of Toronto, Toronto.

Zhang, J. & Norman, D.A. (1994). Representations in distributed cognitive tasks. *Cognitive Science, 18,* 87-122.

Zhang, L., Zhang, T., Novak, C. L., Naidich, D. P., & Moses, D. A. (2005). A computer-based method of segmenting ground glass nodules in pulmonary CT images: Comparison to expert radiologists' interpretations. *Proceedings of SPIE Medical Imaging.*

Zhang, Y. J. (1996). A survey on evaluation methods for image segmentation. *Pattern Recognition, 29*(8), 1335-1346.

Zhao, Y., Chen, W., Qiu, Y., & Shi, J. (2004). GVis: A Java-based architecture for grid- enabled interactive visualization. *Proceedings of the 3rd international conference on grid and cooperative computing-* GCC. *Lecture Notes in Computer Science, 3252,* 704-711. Wuhan, China: Springer-Verlag.

Zheng, G., Marx, A., Langlotz, U., Widmer, K., Buttaro, M., & Nolte, L. (2002). A hybrid CT-free navigation system for total hip arthroplasty. *Computer-Aided Surgery, 7*(3), 129-145.

Zitova, B., & Flusser, J. (2003). Image registration methods: A survey. *Image and Vision Computing, 21,* 977-1000.

Zumbach, J., Reimann, P., & Koch, S. (2001). Influence of passive versus active information access to hypertextual information resources on cognitive and emotional parameters. *Journal of Educational Computing Research, 25*(3), 301-318.

About the Contributors

Feng Dong is a lecturer in computer graphics in the Department of Information Systems and Computing, Brunel University, Uxbridge, UK. His research interests include fundamental computer graphics algorithms, texture synthesis, image-based rendering, medical visualization, volume rendering, human modeling and rendering, and VR. Dong has a PhD in computer science from Zhejiang University, China.

* * *

Walter F. Block is an associate professor in the Biomedical Engineering, Medical Physics, and Radiology Departments at the University of Wisconsin-Madison. He received his BS in electrical engineering at the University of Illinois- Champaign and a master's in electrical engineering at Stanford University. After serving as a systems engineer with General Electric Healthcare for five years, he returned to Stanford where he developed rapid abdominal methods during his PhD training. At the University of Wisconsin, Dr. Block runs an interdisciplinary team that develops rapid MRI techniques for musculoskeletal, vascular, and interventional imaging.

Ethan K. Brodsky is an assistant scientist in the Medical Physics and Radiology Departments at the University of Wisconsin-Madison. He received his BS in electrical engineering at the University of Wisconsin-Madison. After a short time in industry working on embedded systems and device drivers, he returned to Madison to develop techniques for rapid and real-time imaging during his MS and PhD studies. He currently works at the University of Wisconsin as part of teams investigating interventional imaging techniques, water/fat imaging, and gradient system characterization.

Pietro Cerveri received his master's in electronic engineering from Politecnico di Milano, Milano Italy, in 1994 and his doctorate in bioengineering in 2001. He is a research scientist and contract professor of cognitive system engineering at Bioengineering Department–Politecnico di Milano, Milan, Italy. He spent research periods at U.S.-NIH (Bethesda, MD-USA), Electronic Arts (Vancouver, CA), and University of Campinas (Campinas, BR). His scientific interests cover human emotion analysis and biomechanical simulation, vision science, computer-assisted surgery, neural networks, knowledge representation database and bioinformatics.

Dongbin Chen received his doctorate from the School of Computing and Technology, University of East London, London, UK, in 2003. He received his master's of engineering degree and was a senior engineer with the Second Academy of Aero-Space from 1988 to 1998. He is currently a research assistant with the School of Information System and Computing, Brunel University, Middlesex, UK. His research interests include image processing, image inspection, computer vision, machine vision, photogrammetry, integration of vision application systems and 3D graphic applications.

Lorraine De Souza is professor in rehabilitation and head of school in the School of Health Sciences and Social Care at Brunel University. She is also a physiotherapist, and a fellow of the Chartered Society of Physiotherapy. Her research interests are in the management of multiple sclerosis, together with disability caused by spinal pain, and the quality of life of very severely disabled people. Professor De Souza has recently been the chairperson of the Multiple Sclerosis Professional Network, and is currently a member of the Professional Advisory Committee for Care, a committee of the Motor Neurone Disease Association.

Giancarlo Ferrigno received his MS in electronic engineering in 1983 and his PhD in bioengineering in 1990 from the Politecnico di Milano where he teaches foundations of bioengineering (electronics) and biosensors and microtechnologies for the bachelor's degree and the master's degree in biomedical engineering, respectively. He is full professor at the Politecnico di Milano and he is author of about 70 full papers on international scientific journals and 16 patents in the biomedical field. He is currently director of the Bioengineering Department. He is responsible for the laboratories of neuroscience & IT and computer-aided surgery. He is responsible for several projects funded by Italian Space Agency, Italian Institute of Technology and industrial partners in the biomedical field.

Justin Gore is health services researcher and evaluation lead at North West London Hospitals NHS Trust. After several years working as a research associate and lecturer in Social Research and Policy at Hull University, in 2001 he transferred his activities into a healthcare environment. His main interests and publications are in the areas of quality of life, patient experience, chronic obstructive pulmonary disease, change management, process redesign and 'multi-method' evaluations. He is involved in teaching healthcare professionals how to conduct research and provide evidence-based practice, and is 'industrial supervisor' for two PhD students.

John Harper is professor and academic head of paediatric dermatology at Great Ormond Street Hospital for Children and the Institute of Child Health, London. He trained at St. Mary's Hospital, University in London and was promoted to professor in 2001. He was the president of the European Society of Paediatric Dermatology from 1993 to 1996, and is the senior editor of the *Textbook of Pediatric Dermatology*, (2nd edition) published in 2006. His research interests include atopic dermatitis, in particular genetics and new treatments, and localized scleroderma/morphoea.

Christopher G. Healey is an associate professor in the Department of Computer Science at North Carolina State University. Healey received a bachelor's in Computer Science at the University of Waterloo in Waterloo, Canada, and an MS and PhD in Computer Science at the University of British Columbia in Vancouver, Canada. He completed a postdoctoral fellowship at the University of California at Berkeley. Healey received a National Science Foundation CARRER award for research in perception and visualization in 2001. Healey's research interests include scientific and information visualization, computer graphics, human perception, artificial intelligence techniques for mixed-initiative interaction, data compression, navigation in virtual worlds, and the role of aesthetics in information representation.

Mary Hegarty received her BA and MA from University College Dublin, Ireland. She worked as a research assistant for three years at the Irish National Educational Research Centre before attending Carnegie Mellon, where she received her PhD in Psychology in 1988. She has been on the faculty of the Department of Psychology, UCSB since then. The author of over 60 articles and chapters on spatial cognition, diagrammatic reasoning, and individual differences, she is co-editor of a book on diagrammatic reasoning and inference. She is a fellow of the American Psychological Society. A former Spencer Postdoctoral Fellow, Mary Hegarty is on the editorial board of *Journal of Experimental Psychology: Learning, Memory and Cognition*, and is a member of the governing board of the Cognitive Science Society. Her current research is funded by the Office of Naval Research and the National Science Foundation.

Klaus Hinrichs received his diploma degree in mathematics with a minor in computer science from the University of Hannover, Germany, in 1979, and the PhD degree in computer science from the Swiss Federal Institute of Technology (ETH) in Zurich, Switzerland, in 1985. Since 1991, he is a full professor at the Department of Computer Science at the Westfälische Wilhelms-Universität in Münster, Germany. He is also the head of the Visualization and Computer Graphics Research group (VisCG). His research interests include medical visualization, medical visualization, city visualization, computational geometry and data structures and databases for spatial data.

Adrian Hopgood is professor and dean of the Faculty of Computing Sciences and Engineering at De Montford University, UK. He is also a visiting professor at the Open University. His main research interests are in intelligent systems and their practical applications. He graduated with a BSc (Hons) in physics from the University of Bristol in 1981 and obtained a PhD from the University of Oxford in 1984. He is a fellow of the British Computer Society and a committee member for its specialist group on artificial intelligence.

Kevin Howell is a clinical scientist at the Rheumatology Department of the Royal Free Hospital, London, UK. He gained a BSc in physics from the University of Birmingham in 1991. In 1995 he completed the MSc in medical electronics and physics at St. Bartholomew's Medical School in London. The Royal Free scleroderma unit is now the UK's busiest center for thermal imaging in scleroderma, and interests include the application of thermography for the assessment of both Raynaud's phenomenon and inflammation in childhood localized scleroderma. Kevin also has experience in the assessment of the microcirculation by use of the laser Doppler technique.

Douglas R. Janes is a PhD student in the Electrical Engineering department at the University of Wisconsin–Madison. He received his BS in electrical engineering at Arizona State University and MS in electrical engineering at the University of Wisconsin–Madison. His research interests include computer architecture, high-performance embedded processors, programming languages, and compilers. His industry experience includes four years on the Motorola PowerPC team and a Co-op at Intel on the Micro Signal Architecture team. His current research is focused on visualization and MRI reconstruction of high resolution images in real time.

Madeleine Keehner received her PhD in experimental psychology from the University of Bristol, UK. She spent two years as a research fellow in a joint position at the University of California, San

Francisco (Department of Surgery) and Berkeley (Department of Bioengineering), studying spatial cognitive abilities and performance in minimally invasive surgery (NSF-funded). After this, she held a three-year postdoctoral position in the Department of Psychology, UC Santa Barbara (NSF-funded), continuing her work on individual differences in spatial abilities, and expanding this to explore factors involved in learning and reasoning with interactive 3D computer visualizations analogous to those used in medical education. Following her postdoctoral research, she spent a year as a lecturer at Curtin University in Western Australia, and is now based in the School of Psychology at the University of Dundee, Scotland.

Peter Khooshabeh received his bachelor's degree in cognitive science from UC Berkeley, and is currently a PhD student at the University of California, Santa Barbara in the Department of Psychology, working closely with Professor Mary Hegarty. His emphasis is cognition, perception, and cognitive neuroscience and he is affiliated with the Interactive Digital Multimedia Research group. In particular, Peter studies spatial thinking and human-computer interaction in several different domains and with different user populations, including a specific interest in individual differences. Some of these domains range from social network visualization to supporting intelligence analysts to biomedical visualizations in dentistry, diagnostics, and surgery.

Ronghua Liang obtained his PhD in computer science and technology from the College of Computer Science at Zhejiang University in China in June 2003. He is now an associate professor at the College of Information Engineering in Zhejiang University of Technology, and he is the acting director of Computer Network and Multimedia Lab. He worked as a research fellow from April of 2004 to July of 2005 at the University of Luton in the UK. His current activities include teaching and research in the areas of medical visualization and graphics in Zhejiang University of Technology. He has written more than 30 publications in the fields of computer graphics, computer vision, and medical visualization.

Hai Lin is a professor in State Key Laboratory of CAD&CG, Zhejiang University since 2004. He was a research fellow in computer graphics in the Department of Computer and Information Sciences, De Montfort University, UK from 2000 to 2003. His research interests include medical visualization, volume rendering and virtual reality. Lin received his PhD in computer science from Zhejiang University, China.

Jean-Bernard Martens is a full-time professor in the area of Visual Interaction in the Department of Industrial Design of the Eindhoven University of Technology. His chosen research area addresses aspects such as tangible user interfaces, augmented and virtual environment for activities such as design, medical image diagnosis, gaming, co-located collaborative work, and so forth. In the past, he has performed research in other related areas, such as image processing and analysis (visual pattern recognition), visual perception in humans, quantitative research methods and statistical models. Some of these topics are covered in this book "Image Technology Design—A Perceptual Approach" (published by Kluwer Academic Publishers in 2003). In the more recent past, he has also started research that aims at acquiring a better understanding of end-user technology acceptance and user complaints (so-called soft product failures).

Elena De Momi has a master's degree in biomedical engineering from the Politecnico di Milano (2002) and a PhD in bioengineering in 2006 in computer-assisted surgery. She stayed several months at MEM Research Center Institute for Surgical Technology and Biomechanics, University of Bern, Switzerland, and at ICAOS Lab, Western Pennsylvania Hospital, Carnegie Mellon University, Pittsburgh, Pennsylvania, U.S. Since April 2006, she has had a research grant at the Department of Bioengineering of Politecnico di Milano. Her teaching activities are in the field of navigation systems and computer-assisted orthopaedic surgery. She is author of four peer-reviewed international papers in the field of biomedical technologies.

Robert Noble was born in Manchester, England, in 1951. He obtained a BA in mathematics from Oxford University in 1972 and an MSc in electronics from Southampton University in 1973. After five years as an electronic development engineer, he joined the research division of the Central Electricity Generating Board, working on the control and visualization of reactor robots. This interest in computer graphics led to his moving to De Montfort University earn a PhD, in virtual sculpting, which he obtained in 1999. Since 1997, he has been a lecturer in graphics and visualization at the Robert Gordon University, Aberdeen. His research interests are virtual sculpting and visualization.

Sarah Pajak graduated from the University of Leicester in 2000 with an honors degree in psychology with sociology. She completed her MSc in occupational psychology at the University of Nottingham in 2001. Sarah went on to work as a researcher for the Royal College of Psychiatrists' Research Unit, London, focusing on workforce-related issues in psychiatry. Her research interests include organizational culture, change and patient and staff experience. Sarah is currently working as a researcher at an acute NHS hospital trust while completing her PhD in health services research at Brunel University, West London.

Wen Qi is a PhD candidate in the Department of Industrial Design at the University of Technology Eindhoven. He is working on the IOP-MMI project "*3D Interaction with Scientific Data*" that is sponsored by the SenterNovem under Dutch Minister of Economic Affairs. His primary research interests include virtual reality, 3D interaction techniques, and scientific visualization. He is a student member of ACM and the UK ergonomic society.

Yingjun Qiu is an assistant researcher in the UI group of Microsoft Research Asia in Beijing. He received his master's degree from the Computer Science and Technology college of Zhejiang University in Hangzhou, the capital city of Zhejiang province, China, in 2006. Before that he studied at the State key Lab of Computer-Aided Design and Computer Graphics at Zhejiang University for three years. The topics he studied at college included distributed computing, grid computing and scientific visualization. He has published three papers on these topics. The subject of the dissertation for his master's degree is *Research On and Implementation of Interactive Grid Visualization System GVIS*. He joined Microsoft Research Asia at 2006 after graduation and worked on user interface field.

Timo Ropinski received his PhD in computer science in 2004, and his diploma in computer science in 2002, and passed his exam in biology/computer science in 2001. He is a research assistant at the Department of Computer Science at the Westfälische Wilhelms-Universität in Münster, Germany since 2001, working in the group of Klaus Hinrichs. His research interests are medical visualization and real-time rendering.

Gerald Schaefer received his BSc in computing from the University of Derby and his PhD in computer vision from the University of East Anglia. He worked at the Colour & Imaging Institute, University of Derby as a research associate (1997-1999), as senior research fellow at the School of Information Systems, University of East Anglia (2000-2001), and as senior lecturer in computing at the School of Computing and Informatics at Nottingham Trent University (2001-2006). In September 2006, he joined the School of Engineering and Applied Science at Aston University. His research interests include medical imaging, color image analysis, physics-based vision, and image retrieval.

Michael Schulte received his BS degree in electrical engineering from the University of Wisconsin-Madison, and his MS and PhD degrees in electrical engineering from the University of Texas at Austin. He is currently an associate professor at the University of Wisconsin-Madison, where he leads the Madison Embedded Systems and Architectures Group. His research interests include high-performance embedded processors, computer architecture, domain-specific systems, computer arithmetic, and reconfigurable computing. He is a senior member of the IEEE and the IEEE Computer Society, and an associate editor for the IEEE Transactions on Computers and the Journal of VLSI Signal Processing.

Jiaoying Shi is a professor in the Department of Computer Science and Engineering of Zhejiang University, which is located in Hangzhou, the capital city of Zhejiang Province of China. He graduated in the Department of Physics at formal Leningrad of USSR in 1960. Since the early 1970s, he has worked in the field of computer science and engineering. He is one of the founders of the State key Lab of Computer-Aided Design and Computer Graphics at Zhejiang University and served as the director of the lab for 10 years. His research interests include computer graphics, visualization in scientific computing and virtual reality. He has published more than 200 papers and four books.

Jennis Meyer-Spradow received his diploma in mathematics in 2005. He has been a PhD student since 2005 in the Department of Computer Science at the Westfälische Wilhelms-Universität in Münster, Germany, working in the group of Klaus Hinrichs. His research interests are medical visualization and real-time rendering.

Frank Steinicke received his PhD in computer science in 2006, and his diploma in mathematics in 2002. He is a research assistant at the Department of Computer Science at the Westfälische Wilhelms-Universität in Münster (Germany) in the Visualization and Computer Graphics (VisCG) research group headed by Klaus Hinrichs, since 2002. Since 2006, he works as the CEO of university spin-off iVisTec GbR (supplier for interactive visualization technologies). His research interests are computer graphics, human-computer interaction and 3D user interfaces and virtual reality.

Roger Tait received a BSc and a PhD in computer science, both from Nottingham Trent University. During his PhD, he was carrying out research into image processing and artificial intelligence for use in non-destructive evaluation and in medical imaging. He is currently working as a research fellow in the School of Computing and Information at Nottingham Trent University.

Russell Taylor is a research professor of computer science, physics and astronomy, and applied and materials sciences at the University of North Carolina at Chapel Hill. He is the co-director of the UNC NIH National Research Resource for Computer Integrated Systems for Microscopy and Manipulation.

His research interests include scientific visualization, distributed virtual worlds, haptic display, and interactive 3D computer graphics. All of these come together in his role as the director of the computer science team in the UNC Nano-scale Science Research Group, a multidisciplinary team working together to develop improved interfaces for scanned probe and other microscopes.

Raymond White originally qualified as an engineer with Rolls Royce and completed a degree in mechanical engineering in 1974. A lectureship in prosthetic and orthotic mechanics was followed by a lectureship in bioengineering at the University of Aberdeen. During this post, he had both academic and clinical responsibilities. He completed his PhD in 1993 and he has supervised numerous medical and paramedical staff undertaking postgraduate research. As manager and scientific director of the gait laboratory in Aberdeen, many gait assessments have been carried out on children with cerebral palsy and with other loco-motor disorders. His research interests include gait and human movement studies.

Christopher Williams is an IT graduate specializing in many areas of computer science and systems development. Having worked for over seven years as the head of IT systems at a medium-sized law firm based in South Wales, UK, he currently works as a software engineer for General Dynamics UK Ltd. He received his BSc degree in computer science and MSc in enterprise systems development from Brunel University, West London in 2005 and 2006 respectively. He is a professional member of the British Computer Society and an active member of its young professionals group.

Patricia Woo is professor of paediatric rheumatology at University College London (UCL), and director of the Centre for Paediatric and Adolescent Rheumatology at UCL. The centre comprises clinical service and research at great Ormond Street hospital/institute of child health and at the University college hospital/UCL.

Xujiong Ye is a senior research scientist at Medicsight, London. Her research interests include medical image analysis, computer graphics, texture analysis, computer vision and visualization. Ye has a PhD in electronic engineering from Zhejiang University, China.

Youbing Zhao is an innovator in Simense Technology, Shanghai, China. He received his PhD from the Computer and Science and Technology college of Zhejiang University in Hangzhou, the capital city of Zhejiang province, China in 2005. Before that, he studied at the State key Lab of Computer-Aided Design and Computer Graphics at Zhejiang University for five years. His interests are mainly on scientific visualization, parallel rendering, and distributed/grid computing. He has published nine papers on these topics. After graduating from Zhejinag University in 2005, he joined Simense Technology, Shanghai and has been working on several computer graphics-related research projects.

Index